I0044679

Clinical Frontiers in Medical Genetics

Clinical Frontiers in Medical Genetics

Edited by Ellie Peyton

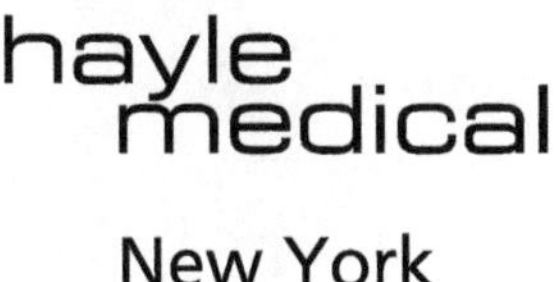

New York

Hayle Medical,
750 Third Avenue, 9th Floor,
New York, NY 10017, USA

Visit us on the World Wide Web at:
www.haylemedical.com

ISBN: 978-1-63241-653-7

Cataloging-in-Publication Data

Clinical frontiers in medical genetics / edited by Ellie Peyton.
p. cm.
Includes bibliographical references and index.
ISBN 978-1-63241-653-7
1. Medical genetics. 2. Human genetics. 3. Genetic disorders. I. Peyton, Ellie.
RB155 .C55 2019
616.042--dc23

Table of Contents

Preface ... IX

Chapter 1 **Association between H19 SNP rs217727 and lung cancer risk in a Chinese population** ... 1
Lingling Li, Genyan Guo, Haibo Zhang, Baosen Zhou, Lu Bai, He Chen, Yuxia Zhao and Ying Yan

Chapter 2 **Fc receptor-like 3 (*−169T>C*) polymorphism increases the risk of tendinopathy in volleyball athletes** ... 7
José Inácio Salles, Lucas Rafael Lopes, Maria Eugenia Leite Duarte, Dylan Morrissey, Marilena Bezerra Martins, Daniel Escorsim Machado, João Antonio Matheus Guimarães and Jamila Alessandra Perini

Chapter 3 **Novel digenic inheritance of *PCDH15* and *USH1G* underlies profound non-syndromic hearing impairment** ... 17
Isabelle Schrauwen, Imen Chakchouk, Anushree Acharya, Khurram Liaqat, Irfanullah, Deborah A. Nickerson, Michael J. Bamshad, Khadim Shah, Wasim Ahmad and Suzanne M. Leal

Chapter 4 **The altered activity of P53 signaling pathway by *STK11* gene mutations and its cancer phenotype in Peutz-Jeghers syndrome** ... 23
Yu-Liang Jiang, Zi-Ye Zhao, Bai-Rong Li, Fu Yang, Jing Li, Xiao-Wei Jin, Hao Wang, En-Da Yu, Shu-Han Sun and Shou-Bin Ning

Chapter 5 **Functional study on new *FOXL2* mutations found in Chinese patients with blepharophimosis, ptosis, epicanthus inversus syndrome** ... 33
Lu Zhou, Jiaqi Wang and Tailing Wang

Chapter 6 **Role of DFNB1 mutations in hereditary hearing loss among assortative mating hearing impaired families from South India** ... 39
Pavithra Amritkumar, Justin Margret Jeffrey, Jayasankaran Chandru, Paridhy Vanniya S, M. Kalaimathi, Rajagopalan Ramakrishnan, N. P. Karthikeyen and C. R. Srikumari Srisailapathy

Chapter 7 **Novel mutations in *HSF4* cause congenital cataracts in Chinese families** ... 63
Zongfu Cao, Yihua Zhu, Lijuan Liu, Shuangqing Wu, Bing Liu, Jianfu Zhuang, Yi Tong, Xiaole Chen, Yongqing Xie, Kaimei Nie, Cailing Lu, Xu Ma and Juhua Yang

Chapter 8 **Clinical and molecular characterization of *POU3F4* mutations in multiple DFNX2 Chinese families** ... 71
Yu Su, Xue Gao, Sha-Sha Huang, Jing-Ning Mao, Bang-Qing Huang, Jian-Dong Zhao, Dong-Yang Kang, Xin Zhang and Pu Dai

Chapter 9 **Association of Catechol-Omethyltransferase (COMT Val^{158}Met) with future risk of cardiovascular disease in depressed individuals** 81
Aysha Almas, Yvonne Forsell, Vincent Millischer, Jette Möller and Catharina Lavebratt

Chapter 10 **Identification of *ANKDD1B* variants in an ankylosing spondylitis pedigree and a sporadic patient** 88
Zhiping Tan, Hui Zeng, Zhaofa Xu, Qi Tian, Xiaoyang Gao, Chuanman Zhou, Yu Zheng, Jian Wang, Guanghui Ling, Bing Wang, Yifeng Yang and Long Ma

Chapter 11 **Common variant of *BCAS3* is associated with gout risk in Japanese population: the first replication study after gout GWAS in Han Chinese** 96
Masayuki Sakiyama, Hirotaka Matsuo, Hirofumi Nakaoka, Yusuke Kawamura, Makoto Kawaguchi, Toshihide Higashino, Akiyoshi Nakayama, Airi Akashi, Jun Ueyama, Takaaki Kondo, Kenji Wakai, Yutaka Sakurai, Ken Yamamoto, Hiroshi Ooyama and Nariyoshi Shinomiya

Chapter 12 **A variant in *KCNQ1* gene predicts metabolic syndrome among Northern urban Han Chinese women** 102
Yafei Liu, Chunxia Wang, Yafei Chen, Zhongshang Yuan, Tao Yu, Wenchao Zhang, Fang Tang, Jianhua Gu, Qinqin Xu, Xiaotong Chi, Lijie Ding, Fuzhong Xue and Chengqi Zhang

Chapter 13 **Genome-wide association study of nocturnal blood pressure dipping in hypertensive patients** 109
Jenni M. Rimpelä, Ilkka H. Pörsti, Antti Jula, Terho Lehtimäki, Teemu J. Niiranen, Lasse Oikarinen, Kimmo Porthan, Antti Tikkakoski, Juha Virolainen, Kimmo K. Kontula and Timo P. Hiltunen

Chapter 14 **Exome sequencing identifies novel dysferlin mutation in a family with paucisymptomatic heterozygous carriers** 120
Mahjoubeh Jalali-Sefid-Dashti, Melissa Nel, Jeannine M. Heckmann and Junaid Gamieldien

Chapter 15 **Identification of deletion-duplication in *HEXA* gene in five children with Tay-Sachs disease from India** 126
Jayesh Sheth, Mehul Mistri, Lakshmi Mahadevan, Sanjeev Mehta, Dhaval Solanki, Mahesh Kamate and Frenny Sheth

Chapter 16 **Clinical characteristics and spectrum of *NF1* mutations in 12 unrelated Chinese families with neurofibromatosis type 1** 131
Bin Mao, Siyu Chen, Xin Chen, Xiumei Yu, Xiaojia Zhai, Tao Yang, Lulu Li, Zheng Wang, Xiuli Zhao and Xue Zhang

Chapter 17 **Heterozygous versus homozygous phenotype caused by the same *MC4R* mutation: novel mutation affecting a large consanguineous kindred** 140
Max Drabkin, Ohad S. Birk and Ruth Birk

Chapter 18 **An African perspective on the genetic risk of chronic kidney disease** 147
Cindy George, Yandiswa Y Yako, Ikechi G Okpechi, Tandi E Matsha, Francois J. Kaze Folefack and Andre P Kengne

Chapter 19 **Factor XIII polymorphism and risk of aneurysmal subarachnoid haemorrhage in a South Indian population** **161**
Arati Suvatha, M. K. Sibin, Dhananjaya I. Bhat, K. V. L. Narasingarao, Vikas Vazhayil and G. K. Chetan

Chapter 20 **Novel mutations in *ALDH1A3* associated with autosomal recessive anophthalmia/microphthalmia** **169**
Siying Lin, Gaurav V. Harlalka, Abdul Hameed, Hadia Moattar Reham, Muhammad Yasin, Noor Muhammad, Saadullah Khan, Emma L. Baple, Andrew H. Crosby and Shamim Saleha

Chapter 21 **Novel mutations of PKD genes in Chinese patients suffering from autosomal dominant polycystic kidney disease and seeking assisted reproduction** **177**
Wen-Bin He, Wen-Juan Xiao, Yue-Qiu Tan, Xiao-Meng Zhao, Wen Li, Qian-Jun Zhang, Chang-Gao Zhong, Xiu-Rong Li, Liang Hu, Guang-Xiu Lu, Ge Lin and Juan Du

Chapter 22 **Common *FTO* rs9939609 variant and risk of type 2 diabetes in Palestine** **190**
Anas Sabarneh, Suheir Ereqat, Stéphane Cauchi, Omar AbuShamma, Mohammad Abdelhafez, Murad Ibrahim and Abdelmajeed Nasereddin

Chapter 23 **Expanding the clinical phenotype of *IARS2*-related mitochondrial disease** **196**
Barbara Vona, Reza Maroofian, Emanuele Bellacchio, Maryam Najafi, Kyle Thompson, Ahmad Alahmad, Langping He, Najmeh Ahangari, Abolfazl Rad, Sima Shahrokhzadeh, Paulina Bahena, Falk Mittag, Frank Traub, Jebrail Movaffagh, Nafise Amiri, Mohammad Doosti, Reza Boostani, Ebrahim Shirzadeh, Thomas Haaf, Daria Diodato, Miriam Schmidts, Robert W. Taylor and Ehsan Ghayoor Karimiani

Chapter 24 **The estrogen receptor 1 gene affects bone mineral density and osteoporosis treatment efficiency in Slovak postmenopausal women** **212**
Vladimira Mondockova, Maria Adamkovicova, Martina Lukacova, Birgit Grosskopf, Ramona Babosova, Drahomir Galbavy, Monika Martiniakova and Radoslav Omelka

Chapter 25 **Multimodal imaging in a pedigree of X-linked Retinoschisis with a novel *RS1* variant** **225**
Kirk Stephenson, Adrian Dockery, Niamh Wynne, Matthew Carrigan, Paul Kenna, G. Jane Farrar and David Keegan

Chapter 26 **First molecular study in Lebanese patients with Cockayne syndrome and report of a novel mutation in *ERCC8* gene** **235**
Alain Chebly, Sandra Corbani, Joelle Abou Ghoch, Cybel Mehawej, André Megarbane and Eliane Chouery

Chapter 27 **Preliminary study showing no association between G238A (rs361525) tumor necrosis factor-α (TNF-α) gene polymorphism and its serum level, hormonal and biochemical aspects of polycystic ovary syndrome** **242**
Fahimeh Kordestani, Sahar Mazloomi, Yousef Mortazavi, Saeideh Mazloomzadeh, Mojtaba Fathi, Haleh Rahmanpour and Abolfazl Nazarian

Chapter 28 **Targeted gene panel for genetic testing of South Indian children with steroid resistant nephrotic syndrome 250**
Annes Siji, K. N. Karthik, Varsha Chhotusing Pardeshi, P. S. Hari and Anil Vasudevan

Permissions

List of Contributors

Index

Preface

Every book is a source of knowledge and this one is no exception. The idea that led to the conceptualization of this book was the fact that the world is advancing rapidly; which makes it crucial to document the progress in every field. I am aware that a lot of data is already available, yet, there is a lot more to learn. Hence, I accepted the responsibility of editing this book and contributing my knowledge to the community.

Medical genetics is a branch of medicine concerned with the application of genetics to medical care, particularly to hereditary disorders. It encompasses the areas of personalized medicine, gene therapy and predictive medicine. Certain genetic syndromes are Down syndrome, chromosomal rearrangements, fragile X syndrome, neurofibromatosis, Turner syndrome, etc. Chromosome studies are used to determine the cause of birth defects, developmental delay, autism, or dysmorphic features. For cases with a suspicion of metabolic condition, quantitative amino acid analysis, urine organic acid analysis, enzyme testing, etc. are performed. Diet, medication and enzyme replacement therapy may be used to reduce or manage long-term complications. This book elucidates the concepts and innovative models around prospective developments with respect to medical genetics. It explores all the important aspects of medical genetics in the present day scenario. It is appropriate for students seeking detailed information in this area as well as for experts.

While editing this book, I had multiple visions for it. Then I finally narrowed down to make every chapter a sole standing text explaining a particular topic, so that they can be used independently. However, the umbrella subject sinews them into a common theme. This makes the book a unique platform of knowledge.

I would like to give the major credit of this book to the experts from every corner of the world, who took the time to share their expertise with us. Also, I owe the completion of this book to the never-ending support of my family, who supported me throughout the project.

Editor

1

Association between H19 SNP rs217727 and lung cancer risk in a Chinese population: a case control study

Lingling Li[1†], Genyan Guo[1†], Haibo Zhang[2], Baosen Zhou[3], Lu Bai[4], He Chen[1], Yuxia Zhao[1*] and Ying Yan[2*]

Abstract

Background: H19 was the first long non-coding RNA (lncRNA) to be confirmed. Recently, studies have suggested that H19 may participate in lung cancer (LC) development and progression. This study assessed whether single nucleotide polymorphisms (SNPs) in H19 are associated with the risk of LC in a Chinese population.

Methods: A case-control study was performed, and H19 SNP rs217727 was analyzed in 555 lung cancer patients from two hospitals and 618 healthy controls to test the association between this SNP and the susceptibility to LC.

Results: The A/A homozygous genotype of rs217727 was significantly associated with an increased LC risk (odds ratio (OR) = 1.661, 95% confidence interval (CI) = 1.155 to 2.388, $P = 0.006$). Significant associations remained after stratification by smoking status ($P < 0.001$). Furthermore, the A/A genotype had a higher risk of LC than those of G/G in the squamous cell carcinoma (OR = 2.022, $P = 0.004$) and adenocarcinoma (OR = 1.606, $P = 0.045$) subgroups.

Conclusions: The rs217727 SNP in lncRNA H19 was significantly associated with susceptibility to LC, particularly in squamous cell carcinoma and adenocarcinoma, and identified the homozygous A/A genotype as a risk factor for LC.

Keywords: Lung cancer, H19, Susceptibility, SNP

Background

Lung cancer (LC) has a high incidence and will continue to be the most common cause of cancer-related death around the world [1]. In China, this malignancy has the highest mortality and accounts for an estimated 25% of cancer-related deaths [2]. LC is a complex pathological process. The major risk factors by far are cigarette smoking and air pollution. Because a proportion of individuals exposed to carcinogens may have genetic factors associated with the development of cancer, predisposing genic elements should be weighed as risk factors for LC.

Long non-coding RNAs (lncRNAs) are longer than 200 nucleotides and are defined as non-protein-coding transcripts that are universally transcribed in the genome [3]. LncRNAs are transcribed as sense, antisense, bidirectional, intronic, or intergenic [4]. They can work by binding to chromatin-modifying complexes to specifically silence genomic loci both in cis and trans [5]. Increasingly, more studies have revealed that lncRNAs play a major role in many aspects of tumorigenesis at the epigenetic, transcriptional, and posttranscriptional levels, including cell growth, apoptosis, invasion, and metastasis. Based on the latest studies, there is evidence that lncRNAs can control gene expression through multiple mechanisms, such as transcription, translation, imprinting, genome rearrangement, and chromatin modification [6]. H19 is a maternally expressed imprinted gene on chromosome 11p15.5 that encodes for a capped and spliced RNA and has been implicated in cancer [7]. It was the first lncRNA discovered in the human genome and plays a crucial role in mammalian development [8, 9].

Single nucleotide polymorphisms (SNPs) have been widely used in plant, livestock, and animal genetic analyses. SNPs may affect gene expression and function. In addition, SNPs can be associated with the susceptibility to cancer. To date, there have been rare reports of

* Correspondence: zyx_yd@163.com; yanyingdoctor@sina.com
†Lingling Li and Genyan Guo contributed equally to this work.
[1]Department of Radiotherapy Oncology, The Fourth Affiliated Hospital of China Medical University, No.4 Chongshan East Road, Huanggu District, Shenyang, Liaoning 110032, People's Republic of China
[2]Department of Radiation Oncology, The General Hospital of Shenyang Military Command, No.83 Wenhua Road, Shenhe District, Shenyang, Liaoning 110016, People's Republic of China
Full list of author information is available at the end of the article

genetic mutations in lncRNAs and their possible correlations to LC susceptibility. Thus far, the association between H19_rs217727 polymorphisms and LC has not been studied in the Chinese population.

In this hospital-based case-control study, we hypothesized a possible association between variant genotypes of the human H19 gene (rs217727) and LC. To test our hypothesis, SNPs within the H19 gene were genotyped from blood DNA samples of 555 LC patients and 618 age- and gender-matched general population controls.

Methods

Study population

The study population consisted of 555 LC patients and 618 healthy controls. The LC patients were consecutively recruited between September 2010 and November 2015 from the First Affiliated Hospital of China Medical University and the Fourth Affiliated Hospital of China Medical University. Each patient was histopathologically diagnosed including squamous cell carcinoma (SCC), adenocarcinoma (AD) and small cell lung cancer (SCLC). These control subjects were picked out throughout the same period in the Fourth Affiliated Hospital of China Medical University from the health examination center. Allowing for a better condition, the following exclusion criteria were used: history of LC; history of significant concomitant tumors; any cancer-related metastasis; chemotherapy or radiotherapy; non autologous transfusion. All subjects (LC patients and healthy controls) participated had no family history of LC in this study. Then, we randomly took sample of 618 healthy controls, which were frequency matched to the LC cases on age and gender. All participants who were unrelated ethnic Chinese resided in or near Liaoning province. All individual participants voluntarily joined this study with informed consents. Information was collected by a structured questionnaire. Smoking was defined as ≥10 cigarettes per day for at least 2 years.

SNPs selection and genotyping

The location of the 2.7 kb human H19 gene (Gene ID: 283120) including the DMR (differentially methylated regions) and the promoter region was pinpointed to chromosome 11, position (1972982–1981641). The HapMap project has established a common pattern in the human genome for most of the population on the basis of DNA sequence variation. Based on the HapMap data and the criteria of minor allele frequency (MAF) > 0.05 in CB population, we found two SNPs rs217727 and rs2107425 in H19, and they are in high linkage disequilibrium (LD). Some researchers had found that H19_rs2107425 and H19_rs217727 play roles in carcinoma susceptibility. The role of rs2107425 polymorphism had been identified in lung cancer. So, we chose the other one SNP, rs217727.

Genomic DNA was extracted from venous blood. Usually, about 5 ml venous blood samples were collected from each participant. The blood samples are registered and stored at – 80 °C. Genomic DNA was extracted from leukocytes, and separated from the whole blood using a standard phenol-chloroform protocol. Genotyping was performed by pre-designed TaqMan probes (Applied Biosystems, Foster City, CA, USA). The assay ID is C___2603707_10 (part number: 4351379), and the specific amplicon context sequence is TGTGGTGGCTGGTGGTCAACCGTCC[A/G]CCGCAGGGGGTGGCCATGAAGATGG (Table 1) The H19_rs217727 polymorphism was amplified and genotyped through the TaqMan SNP Genotyping Assay by using the ABI 7500 Real-time PCR system (Applied Biosystems, Foster City, CA, USA) in 96-well plates. The reaction mixture (5 μl) contained 2.5 μl TaqMan® Genotyping Master Mix (Applied Biosystems, Foster City, CA, USA), 0.125 μl hydrolysis probe, 1.375 μl ddH2O and 30 ng genomic DNA for each SNP, according to the following PCR protocol: 95 °C for 10 min for 1 cycle; 95 °C for 15 s and 60 °C for 1 min for 40 cycles; followed by a cycle of 60 °C for 1 min which is a stage of analysis for genotypes. Controls (known genotype and water) were included in each reaction plate to ensure that the genotyping were accuracy. The deionized water was used as a negative control and the rs3219073/GG SNP of PARP-1 was used as a positive control, which was previously detected in many lung cancer samples [10]. Two researchers analyses the genotype individually in a blind method. Approximately 10% samples were randomly selected to repeat detection, the results for random sampling were 100% concordant as quality control samples.

Statistical analysis

The data obtained were computed and analyzed via SPSS, version 16.0 (SPSS Inc., Chicago, IL, USA). Continuous variables without skewness were estimated via means ± standard derivation (SD) and compared with the Student's t tests. Categorical variables were used through frequency counts and compared by the Chi-

Table 1 Genotyped SNP ordered according to the position in the H19 gene

dbSNP	NCBI assembly location (Build 37)	TaqMan assay ID	Base change	Tag SNP (CHB population; HapMap)	Cinfirmed functional effect of SNP
rs217727	Chr.11:2016908	C___2603707_10	A/G	Yes	No
Context Sequence: TGTGGTGGCTGGTGGTCAACCGTCC[A/G]CCGCAGGGGGTGGCCATGAAGATGG					

square (χ^2) test [11]. The Hardy–Weinberg equilibrium (HWE) was estimated by the goodness-of-χ^2 test. When the HWE was respected, the allele comparison and the additive model were asymptotically equivalent [12]. Correlations between the genotype and the susceptibility of LC were assessed via odds ratio (OR) with 95% confidence interval (CI) by logistic regression analyses with adjustment for age and smoking status [13]. OR was also evaluated subgroup, viz. tumors of different pathological types. A value of $P < 0.05$ was considered statistically significant.

Results

Characteristics of the study population

The demographics of the 555 LC patients and 618 healthy controls are summarized in Table 2. The majority of the LC patients were diagnosed with adenocarcinoma (44.6%) followed by squamous cell carcinoma (38.7%) and small cell carcinoma (16.7%). The mean ages of the LC patients and healthy controls were 60.15 ± 9.896 and 60.05 ± 10.170 years, respectively. There was no significant difference in the frequency distributions of age or gender ($P = 0.517$ and 0.798) between the LC patients and the controls. However, the data was significantly higher (61.8%) in cases with the smoking status than that in controls ($P < 0.001$), which is consistent with the epidemiological distribution of LC.

H19 polymorphisms and the susceptibility of LC

The genotype of H19_rs217727 and its association with the risk of LC are presented in Table 3. The genotype distribution of the rs217727 in the controls did not deviate from those expected under HWE ($P = 0.167$). A statistically significant increase in the risk of LC was found for carriers of the A/A genotype compared to the homozygous carriers of the wild-type G/G genotype (OR = 1.661, 95%CI = 1.155–2.388, $P = 0.006$). After adjustment for the smoking status, the A/A genotype was also significant ($P = 0.002$). However, when the combined A/G + A/A genotypes were compared to the wild-type G/G genotype, there was no significant difference.

Stratified analysis of H19 polymorphisms and the risk of LC

We carried out stratified analysis to assess the relationship between the H19 lncRNA SNPs and the risk of LC according to the pathological subtypes (Table 4). We found that the rs217727 A/A genotype was associated with an increased cancer risk for squamous cell carcinoma ($P = 0.004$, adjusted OR = 1.996, 95% CI = 1.142 to 3.489, $P = 0.015$) and adenocarcinoma ($P = 0.045$, adjusted OR = 1.767, 95% CI = 1.096 to 2.850, $P = 0.019$), but not for small cell carcinoma ($P = 0.123$, adjusted OR = 1.799, 95% CI = 0.846 to 3.827, $P = 0.127$). There was no significant association between this polymorphism and the susceptibility of LC with other genotypes.

Discussion

LncRNAs, which characterize a functionally varied class of transcripts, have been found in many different species, such as humans, animals, plants, yeast, and viruses [14–17]. Many researchers suggest that lncRNAs play a key role in tumorigenesis and during cellular development, differentiation, and many other biological processes. Furthermore, several studies have reported that lncRNAs are misregulated in various types of cancers [18–20]. Significant overexpression of lncRNAs-CCAT2 was found in lung adenocarcinoma [21]. Nie et al. [22] reported that the lncRNA ANRIL was overexpressed in NSCLC patient tissues and associated with advanced "tumor node metastasis (TNM)" subsets, tumor size, and prognosis. Therefore, abnormalities of the expression of lncRNAs may be involved in the tumorigenesis of LC. Genetic variants in lncRNAs could be a biomarker for the prediction of cancer susceptibility in humans. Liu et al. [23] found that lncRNAs-MALAT1_rs619586

Table 2 Baseline characteristics of study subjects

Characteristics	Case ($n = 555$)	Controls ($n = 618$)	P value
Age (year)	60.15 ± 9.896	60.05 ± 10.170	0.517
Sex			0.798
Male (%)	394 (70.1)	434 (70.2)	
Female (%)	161 (29.9)	184 (29.8)	
Smoking status			< 0.001
Ever (%)	343 (61.8)	143 (23.1)	
Never (%)	212 (38.2)	475 (76.9)	
Pathological types			–
Squamous Cells Carcinoma (%)	215 (38.7)	–	
Adenocarcinoma (%)	248 (44.6)	–	
Small Cell Carcinoma (%)	92 (16.7)	–	

Table 3 H19 polymorphisms (rs217727) among the cases and controls and the associations with risk of LC

Genotype	Case, *n* (%)	Control, *n* (%)	Crude OR, (95%CI)	*P* value	Adjusted OR, (95%CI)[a]	P^a value
G/G	210 (37.9)	246 (39.8)	1.0(ref.)		1.0(ref.)	
A/G	250 (45.0)	305 (49.4)	0.960 (0.749~ 1.231)	0.749	0.957 (0.730~ 1.255)	0.751
A/A	95 (17.1)	67 (10.8)	**1.661 (1.155~ 2.388)**	**0.006**	**1.849 (1.248~ 2.740)**	**0.002**
A/G + A/A	345 (62.1)	372 (60.2)	1.086 (0.859~ 1.375)	0.490	1.111 (0.860~ 1.435)	0.420

The bold values mean statistically significance with $P < 0.05$
LC lung cancer, *OR* odds ratio, *CI* confidence interval
[a]Adjusted for smoking status

was associated with decreased hepatocellular carcinoma risk. LncRNAs-HOTAIR_rs12826786 in strong linkage disequilibrium with rs1899663 ($r^2 = 1$) was associated with the risk of gastric cardia adenocarcinoma [24]. However, their definitive roles in cancer development and progression remain largely unclear.

The H19 lncRNA gene does not encode a protein, but an oncofetal RNA [25, 26]. Deregulation of oncofetal RNA plays a critical role in tumorigenesis [26]. Accumulating evidence suggests that loss of imprinting and deregulation of the H19 gene are associated with human cancer, and its overexpression is a frequent event in lung cancer development [27, 28]. H19 is abnormally expressed in many types of cancers, including gastric [29], liver [30], colorectal [31], bladder [32], and pancreatic cancer [33], and increases the tumorigenic properties of tumor cells [34–37]. In addition, studies have shown that H19 enhances invasion and migration of pancreatic ductal adenocarcinoma cells by decreasing let-7 and subsequently increasing the HMGA2-mediated epithelial-mesenchymal transition (EMT) [33]. Barsyte-Lovejoy et al. [34] found that the knockdown of H19 inhibited colony formation and anchorage-independent growth in lung cancer cells. Other studies have reported that H19 could be induced under hypoxic stress through the p53/HIF1-α pathway. Moreover, the knockdown of H19 could significantly suppress hypoxia-induced cancer cell proliferation in vivo [36]. Furthermore, high expression of H19 was positively associated with advanced TNM stage and was a predictor of overall survival (OS) in gastric cancer patients [38, 39]. Studies have shown that the H19_rs2107425 SNP was related to the susceptibility of bladder cancer, and showed a significant correlation with LC susceptibility ($P = 0.02$, age under 50 years) [40, 41]. However, Riaz et al. [42] found that H19_rs2107425 did not alter H19 mRNA expression in breast cancer. Yang et al. [43] reported that the variant H19 genotypes (CT + TT rs217727, CT + TT rs2839698) were correlated with an increased risk of gastric cancer ($P = 0.040$, $P = 0.033$), and the CT and TT genotypes in rs2839698 were also related to higher H19 mRNA levels in serum. In contrast, the rs217727 polymorphism did

Table 4 Stratification analyses of H19 polymorphisms (rs217727) and risk of LC

Pathological types	Case, *n* (%)	Control, *n* (%)	Crude OR, (95%CI)	*P* value	Adjusted OR, (95%CI)[a]	P^a value
Squamous Cells Carcinoma						
G/G	81 (37.7)	217 (41.6)	1.0 (ref.)		1.0 (ref.)	
A/G	94 (43.7)	252 (48.3)	0.999 (0.705~ 1.416)	0.997	0.790 (0.532~ 1.174)	0.244
A/A	**40 (18.6)**	**53 (10.1)**	**2.022 (1.247~ 3.279)**	**0.004**	**1.996 (1.142~ 3.489)**	**0.015**
A/G + A/A	134 (62.3)	305 (58.4)	1.177 (0.849~ 1.631)	0.327	0.977 (0.675~ 1.414)	0.903
Adenocarcinoma						
G/G	97 (39.1)	228 (40.1)	1.0 (ref.)		1.0 (ref.)	
A/G	110 (44.4)	281 (49.4)	0.920 (0.665~ 1.272)	0.615	0.904 (0.647~ 1.262)	0.552
A/A	**41 (16.5)**	**60 (10.5)**	**1.606 (1.011~ 2.551)**	**0.045**	**1.767 (1.096~ 2.850)**	**0.019**
A/G + A/A	151 (60.9)	341 (59.9)	1.041 (0.767~ 1.412)	0.797	1.047 (0.765~ 1.433)	0.776
Small Cell Carcinoma						
G/G	32 (34.8)	187 (41.6)	1.0 (ref.)		1.0 (ref.)	
A/G	46 (50.0)	216 (48)	1.245 (0.761~ 2.035)	0.383	1.114 (0.680~ 1.926)	0.612
A/A	14 (15.2)	47 (10.4)	1.741 (0.860~ 3.522)	0.123	1.799 (0.846~ 3.827)	0.127
A/G + A/A	60 (65.2)	263 (58.4)	1.333 (0.835~ 2.129)	0.229	1.253 (0.764~ 2.056)	0.372

The bold values indicate statistical significance ($P < 0.05$)
LC lung cancer, *OR* odds ratio, *CI* confidence interval
[a] Adjusted for smoking status

not affect the H19 mRNA level. To the best of our knowledge, the role of the H19_rs217727 polymorphism in LC susceptibility is still unknown in the Chinese population. Accordingly, we investigated whether this polymorphism was associated with the risk of LC in the Chinese population.

In this study, the A/A genotype of H19_rs217727 was significantly higher in the LC patients than in the controls ($P = 0.006$). In particular, there was a significantly increased risk of squamous cells carcinoma ($P = 0.004$) and adenocarcinoma ($P = 0.045$). However, when the combined A/G + A/A genotypes were compared with the wild-type G/G genotype, there was no significant difference. Therefore, the G allele may be a protective factor and people who carry this allele may be less likely to develop lung cancer. However, the present research was limited with respect to geographical variation, nation, and sample size. These factors may greatly affect the accuracy of this experiment. Additional studies that encompass more geographical regions, additional ethnic groups, and larger sample size should be performed. Although all subjects were enrolled from only two hospitals and selection bias could not be avoided, the genotype distribution of the controls in our study did accord with the HWE. Additional studies are also necessary to understand the mechanism by which the rs217727 SNP affects H19 mRNA expression, alters the translational efficiency, or leads to alterations in the H19 structure in LC.

Conclusions

In the current study, we found that the H19_rs217727 polymorphism plays a crucial role in the risk of LC in a Chinese population. Larger population-based studies are required to confirm the relationship between H19 expression levels and the susceptibility to LC. H19_rs217727 SNPs may be potential clinical markers for predicting the risk of LC.

Abbreviations

AD: Adenocarcinoma; CI: Confidence interval; DMR: Differentially methylated regions; HWE: Hardy–Weinberg equilibrium; LC: Lung cancer; LD: Linkage disequilibrium; lncRNA: Long non-coding RNA; MAF: Minor allele frequency; OR: Odds ratio; SCC: Squamous cell carcinoma; SCLC: Small cell lung cancer; SD: Standard derivation; SNPs: Single nucleotide polymorphisms

Acknowledgments

The authors thank all patients and control subjects for their participation and all personnel participating in our study for help in preparing blood samples, interviewing subjects, analyzing data and supporting experiments.

Funding

This work was supported by the Clinical Capability Construction Project for Liaoning Provincial Hospitals (grant number LNCCC-B08–2014).

Authors' contributions

LL analyzed and interpreted the patient data regarding the lung cancer and was a major contributor in writing the manuscript. GG screened out the gene loci and took part in writing the manuscript. LB, HC and HZ participated in sample collection. BZ provided experimental conditions. BZ, YY and YZ guided the experiment. All authors read and approved the final manuscript.

Competing interests

The authors declare that they have no competing interests.

Author details

[1]Department of Radiotherapy Oncology, The Fourth Affiliated Hospital of China Medical University, No.4 Chongshan East Road, Huanggu District, Shenyang, Liaoning 110032, People's Republic of China. [2]Department of Radiation Oncology, The General Hospital of Shenyang Military Command, No.83 Wenhua Road, Shenhe District, Shenyang, Liaoning 110016, People's Republic of China. [3]Department of Epidemiology, China Medical University, Shenyang, Liaoning, China. [4]Department of Radiotherapy Oncology, The First Affiliated Hospital of China Medical University, Shenyang, Liaoning, China.

References

1. Siegel R, Ma J, Zou Z, et al. Cancer statistics. CA Cancer J Clin. 2014;64:9–29.
2. Chen W, Zheng R, Zeng H, et al. Annual report on status of cancer in China, 2011. Chin J Cancer Res. 2015;27:2.
3. Ponting CP, Oliver PL, Reik W. Evolution and functions of long noncoding RNAs. Cell. 2009;136:629–41.
4. Nakaqawa S, Kageyama Y. Nuclear lncRNAs as epigenetic regulators-beyond skepticism. Biochim Biophys Acta. 2014;1839(3):215–22.
5. Koziol MJ, Rinn JL. RNA traffic control of chromatin complexes. Curr Opin Genet Dev. 2010;20:142–8.
6. Fatica A, Bozzoni I. Long non-coding RNAs: new players in cell differentiation and development. Nat Rev Genet. 2014;15:7–21.
7. Kallen AN, Zhou XB, Xu J, et al. The imprinted H19 lncRNA antagonizes let-7 microRNAs. Mol Cell. 2013;52:101–12.
8. Brannan CI, Dees EC, Ingram RS, et al. The product of the H19 gene may function as an RNA. Mol Cell Biol. 1990;10(1):28–36.
9. Keniry A, Oxley D, Monnier P, et al. The H19 lincRNA is a developmental reservoir of miR-675 that suppresses growth and Igf1r. Nat Cell Biol. 2012;14:659–65.
10. Wang HT, Gao Y, Zhao YX, et al. PARP-1 rs3219073 polymorphism may contribute to susceptibility to lung cancer. Genet Test Mol Biomarkers. 2014;18(11):736–40.
11. Adamec C. Example of the use of the nonparametric test. Test χ^2 for comparison of 2 independent examples. Cesk Zdrav. 1964;12:613–9.
12. Guedj M, Nuel G, Prum B. A note on allelic tests in case-control association studies. Ann Hum Genet. 2008;72:407–9.
13. Woolf B. On estimating the relation between blood group and disease. Ann Hum Genet. 1955;19:251–3.
14. Pauli A, Valen E, Lin MF, et al. Systematic identification of long noncoding RNAs expressed during zebrafish embryogenesis. Genome Res. 2012;22(3):577–91.
15. Swiezewski S, Liu F, Magusin A, et al. Cold-induced silencing by long antisense transcripts of an Arabidopsis Polycomb target. Nature. 2009; 462(7274):799–802.
16. Houseley J, Rubbi L, Grunstein M, et al. A ncRNA modulates histone modification and mRNA induction in the yeast GAL gene cluster. Mol Cell. 2008;32(5):685–95.
17. Reeves MB, Davies AA, McSharry BP, et al. Complex I binding by a virally encoded RNA regulates mitochondria-induced cell death. Science. 2007;316(5829):1345–8.
18. Cesana M, Cacchiarelli D, Legnini I, et al. A long noncoding RNA controls muscle differentiation by functioning as a competing endogenous RNA. Cell. 2011;147:358–69.
19. Guffanti A, Iacono M, Pelucchi P, et al. A transcriptional sketch of a primary human breast cancer by 454 deep sequencing. BMC. Genomics. 2009;10:163.
20. Khaitan D, Dinger ME, Mazar J, et al. Themelanoma-upregulated long noncoding RNASPRY4-IT1 modulates apoptosis and invasion. Cancer Res. 2011;71:3852–62.
21. Qiu M, Xu Y, Yang X, et al. Ccat2 is a lung adenocarcinoma-specific long non-coding RNA and promotes invasion of non-small cell lung cancer. Tumor Biol. 2014;35:5375–80.

22. Nie FQ, Sun M, Yang JS, et al. Long noncoding RNA ANRIL promotes non–small cell lung cancer cell proliferation and inhibits apoptosis by silencing KLF2 and P21 expression. Mol Cancer Ther. 2015;14:268–77.
23. Liu Y, Pan S, Liu L, et al. A genetic variant in long non-coding RNA HULC contributes to risk of HBV-related hepatocellular carcinoma in a Chinese population. PLoS One. 2012;7:e35145.
24. Guo W, Dong Z, Bai Y, et al. Associations between polymorphisms of hotair and risk of gastric cardia adenocarcinoma in a population of North China. Tumor Biol. 2015;36:2845–54.
25. Poirier F, Chan C, Timmons P, et al. The murine H19 gene is activated during embryonic stem cell differentiation in vitro and at the time of implantation in the developing embryo. Development. 1991;113:1105–14.
26. Ariel L, Ayesh S, Periman EJ, et al. The product of the imprinted H19 gene is an oncofetal RNA. Mol Pathol. 1997;50(1):33–4.
27. Hibi K, Nakamura H, Hirai A, et al. Loss of H19 imprinting in esophageal cancer. Cancer Res. 1996;56:480–2.
28. Kondo M, Suzuki H, Ueda R, et al. Frequent loss of imprinting of the h19 gene is often associated with its overexpression in human lung cancers. Oncogene. 1995;10:1193–8.
29. Wang J, Song YX, Wang ZN. Non-coding RNAs in gastric cancer. Gene. 2015;560:1–8.
30. Zhang L, Yang F, Yuan JH, et al. Epigenetic activation of the MiR-200 family contributes to H19-mediated metastasis suppression in hepatocellular carcinoma. Carcinogenesis. 2013;34:577–86.
31. Tsang WP, Ng EK, Ng SS, et al. Oncofetal H19-derived miR-675 regulates tumor suppressor RB in human colorectal cancer. Carcinogenesis. 2010;31:350–8.
32. Luo M, Li Z, Wang W, Zeng Y, et al. Upregulated H19 contributes to bladder cancer cell proliferation by regulating ID2 expression. FEBS J. 2013;280:1709–16.
33. Ma C, Nong K, Zhu H, et al. H19 promotes pancreatic cancer metastasis by derepressing let-7's suppression on its target HMGA2-mediated EMT. Tumor Biol. 2014;35:9163–9.
34. Barsyte-Lovejoy D, Lau SK, Boutros PC, et al. The c-Myc oncogene directly induces the H19 noncoding RNA by allele-specific binding to potentiate tumorigenesis. Cancer Res. 2006;66:5330–7.
35. Lottin S, Adriaenssens E, Dupressoir T, et al. Overexpression of an ectopic H19 gene enhances the tumorigenic properties of breast cancer cells. Carcinogenesis. 2002;23:1885–95.
36. Ayesh S, Matouk I, Schneider T, et al. Possible physiological role of H19 RNA. Mol Carcinog. 2002;35:63–74.
37. Matouk IJ, Mezan S, Mizrahi A, et al. The oncofetal H19 RNA connection: hypoxia, p53 and cancer. Biochim biophys Acta. 2010;1803:443–51.
38. Yang F, Bi J, Xue X, et al. Up-regulated long non-coding RNA H19 contributes to proliferation of gastric cancer cells. FEBS J. 2012;279:3159–65.
39. Zhang EB, Han L, Yin DD, et al. C-Myc-induced, long, non-coding H19 affects cell proliferation and predicts a poor prognosis in patients with gastric cancer. Med Oncol. 2014;31:914.
40. Verhaegh GW, Verkleij L, Vermeulen SH, et al. Polymorphisms in the h19 gene and the risk of bladder cancer. Eur Urol. 2008;54:1118–26.
41. Gong W-J, Yin J-Y, Li X-P, et al. Association of well-characterized lung cancer lncRNA polymorphisms with lung cancer susceptibility and platinum-based chemotherapy response. Tumor Biol. 2016;37:8349–58.
42. Riaz M, Berns EM, Sieuwerts AM, et al. Correlation of breast cancer susceptibility loci with patient characteristics, metastasis-free survival, and mRNA expression of the nearest genes. Breast Cancer Res Treat. 2012;133(3):843–51.
43. Yang C, Tang R, Ma X, et al. Tag SNPs in long non-coding RNA H19 contribute to susceptibility to gastric cancer in the Chinese Han population. Oncotarget. 2015;6(17):15311–20.

2

Fc receptor-like 3 (*−169T>C*) polymorphism increases the risk of tendinopathy in volleyball athletes: a case control study

José Inácio Salles[1,2,4], Lucas Rafael Lopes[1,3,5], Maria Eugenia Leite Duarte[1], Dylan Morrissey[4], Marilena Bezerra Martins[1], Daniel Escorsim Machado[3], João Antonio Matheus Guimarães[1] and Jamila Alessandra Perini[1,3,5*]

Abstract

Background: Tendinopathy pathogenesis is associated with inflammation. Regulatory T (Treg) cells contribute to early tissue repair through an anti-inflammatory action, with the forkhead box P3 (FOXP3) transcription factor being essential for Treg function, and the FC-receptor-like 3 (FCRL3) possibly negatively regulating Treg function. *FCRL3 −169T>C* and *FOXP3 −2383C>T* polymorphisms are located near elements that regulate respective genes expression, thus it was deemed relevant to evaluate these polymorphisms as risk factors for tendinopathy development in athletes.

Methods: This case-control study included 271 volleyball athletes (146 tendinopathy cases and 125 controls) recruited from the Brazilian Volleyball Federation. Genotyping analyses were performed using TaqMan assays, and the association of the polymorphisms with tendinopathy evaluated by multivariate logistic regression.

Results: Tendinopathy frequency was 63% patellar, 22% rotator cuff and 15% Achilles tendons respectively. Tendinopathy was more common in men (OR = 2.87; 95% CI = 1.67–4.93). Higher age (OR = 8.75; 95% CI = 4.33–17.69) and more years of volleyball practice (OR = 8.38; 95% CI = 3.56–19.73) were risk factors for tendinopathy. The *FCRL3 −169T>C* frequency was significantly different between cases and controls. After adjustment for potential confounding factors, the *FCRL3 −169C* polymorphism was associated with increased tendinopathy risk (OR = 1.44; 95% CI = 1.02–2.04), either considering athletes playing with tendon pain (OR = 1.98; 95% CI = 1.30–3.01) or unable to train due to pain (OR = 1.89; 95% CI = 1.01–3.53). The combined variant genotypes, *FCRL3 −169TC* or *−169CC* and *FOXP3 −2383CT* or *−2383TT*, were associated with an increased risk of tendinopathy among athletes with tendon pain (OR = 2.24; 95% CI: 1.14–4.40 and OR = 2.60; 95% CI: 1.11–6.10). The combined analysis of *FCRL3 −169T>C* and *FOXP3 −2383C>T* suggests a gene-gene interaction in the susceptibility to tendinopathy.

Conclusions: *FCRL3 −169C* allele may increase the risk of developing tendinopathy, and together with knowledge of potential risk factors (age, gender and years playing) could be used to personalize elite athletes' training or treatment in combination with other approaches, with the aim of minimizing pathology development risk.

Keywords: Fc receptor-like 3, Forkhead box P3 gene, Single nucleotide polymorphism, Tendinopathy, Volleyball athletes

* Correspondence: jamilaperini@yahoo.com.br; japerini@into.saude.gov.br
[1]Research Division, National Institute of Traumatology and Orthopaedics, Avenida Brasil, 500, Rio de Janeiro, RJ 20940-070, Brazil
[3]Research Laboratory of Pharmaceutical Sciences, West Zone State University, Rio de Janeiro, Brazil
Full list of author information is available at the end of the article

Background

The viscoelastic properties of tendons are fundamental for transmitting the force generated by muscle for sport performance. However, the tissue deformation during repetitive and continuous stress makes the tendons susceptible to injury [1]. High-level volleyball players have an inherently high training load and the constant repetition of technical movements may increases the risk for tendinopathy [2].

Historically, tendinopathy has been considered an inflammatory disease, nevertheless a failed healing response of the tendon is regarded as being the main disruption [3, 4]. Previous analysis of tissue samples with tendon pathologies has shown collagen fiber degeneration and disorientation, hypercellularity, angiogenesis and decrease in inflammatory cells [5–7]. In addition, further evidence has suggested that tendons submitted to repetitive mechanical stress and its damage to stromal tissues plays a critical role in the immune system response to regeneration [8]. Thus, the influx of immune cells and their subsequent cytokine production and the critical interactions with resident tenocytes were determinants of the inflammatory effect on the tendon repair or degeneration [9]. Recently, several studies with animal models and tissue samples of tendinopathy patients have reinforce that the immune cells play a key role in the pathophysiology of this disease. [4, 10, 11]. Moreover, other studies have exposed the presence of T lymphocytes in tendinopathic tissue samples and indicated that this cell population may be more immunologically active than was previously thought [11–13].

CD4 + Foxp3+ regulatory T cells (Treg) are a subset of T lymphocytes that mediate an inhibitory effect on immune activity by suppressing the proliferation and function of effector T cells [14, 15]. The forkhead box P3 (FOXP3) is a transcription factor that plays an essential role in the function of Treg cells, in regulating the immune response and maintaining immune tolerance [16]. The FOXP3, encoded by the gene with the same name, is located in chromosome Xp11.23, and consists of 11 exons and encode a 431 amino-acid protein [17]. Polymorphisms in *FOXP3* gene may interfere in the suppressive function of Treg cells, lead to immune system instability, and hence, to the development of disease [18, 19]. The *FOXP3 –2383C>T* (rs3761549) polymorphism is located in the first intron, close to the *FOXP3* promoter region, and has been associated with susceptibility to autoimmune diseases [20–22]. These results have suggest a discussion about the Treg cell functions in relation to the pathogenic mechanisms of tendinopathy.

Since the Treg cells maintain immunological tolerance and prevent autoimmune and inflammatory diseases [14, 23], understanding of the genes involved in these pathways is essential for a better understanding of the pathological mechanisms. In this context, Fc receptor-like 3 (FCRL3) is a glycoprotein of the immunoglobulin receptor superfamily, expressed in Treg cells that may play a role as a negative regulator of Treg function [24–26]. The FCRL3, encoded by the gene with the same name, is located in chromosome 1q21–23, and has a functional polymorphism in the promoter region (*FCRL3 -169T>C*, rs7528684) that changes promoter activity and consequently alters nuclear factor-κB (NFκB) binding [27]. Moreover, *FCRL3 –169C* polymorphism has been associated with higher expression of FCRL3 in Treg cells [24, 27]. Due to the importance of their signaling domains in various immune cell types, the *FCRL3* gene probably modulates immune cell functions, and affects signaling pathways.

We hypothesized that polymorphisms in *FCRL3* and *FOXP3* genes may influence the onset and/or the progression of tendinopathy. The main aim of this study was to investigate the contribution of *FCRL3 –169T>C* and *FOXP3 –2383C>T* polymorphisms as risk factors for tendinopathy development in volleyball athletes, as well as their association with tendinopathy symptoms and sports activities.

Methods

Study design

The study protocol was approved by the Human Ethics Committee of the Brazilian National Institute of Traumatology and Orthopedics (Protocol number 0037.0.305.000/2011 and 17373613.8.0000.5273/2013). Two hundred and seventy one athletes recruited via the Brazilian Volleyball Federation in Rio de Janeiro, Brazil. A study flowchart (Fig. 1) describes the athlete recruitment period (tendinopathy cases and controls), and the number of samples successfully genotyped for each polymorphism.

Inclusion criteria were volleyball players from the Brazilian Volleyball Federation. All participating athletes or their parents/legal guardians provided written informed consent and answered a questionnaire detailing demographics, sports activities, medical history, personal tendon injury and painful symptoms. The questionnaires were personally administered in two periods, December 2011–March 2012 and January 2014–July 2014, during training and the competition. The questionnaires included questions about ethnicity, self-identified according to the classification scheme adopted by the Brazilian Census (http://www.ibge.gov.br), which relies on self-perception of skin color. Accordingly, individuals were distributed in three "race/color" groups: *branco* (white, $n = 103$), *pardo* (meaning brown, here denoted as intermediate, $n = 7$), and *preto* (black, $n = 22$). One hundred thirty-nine athletes (51.3%) declined to give information about ethnicity.

The athletes were separated into cases ($n = 146$) and controls ($n = 125$) group (Fig. 1), according the presence

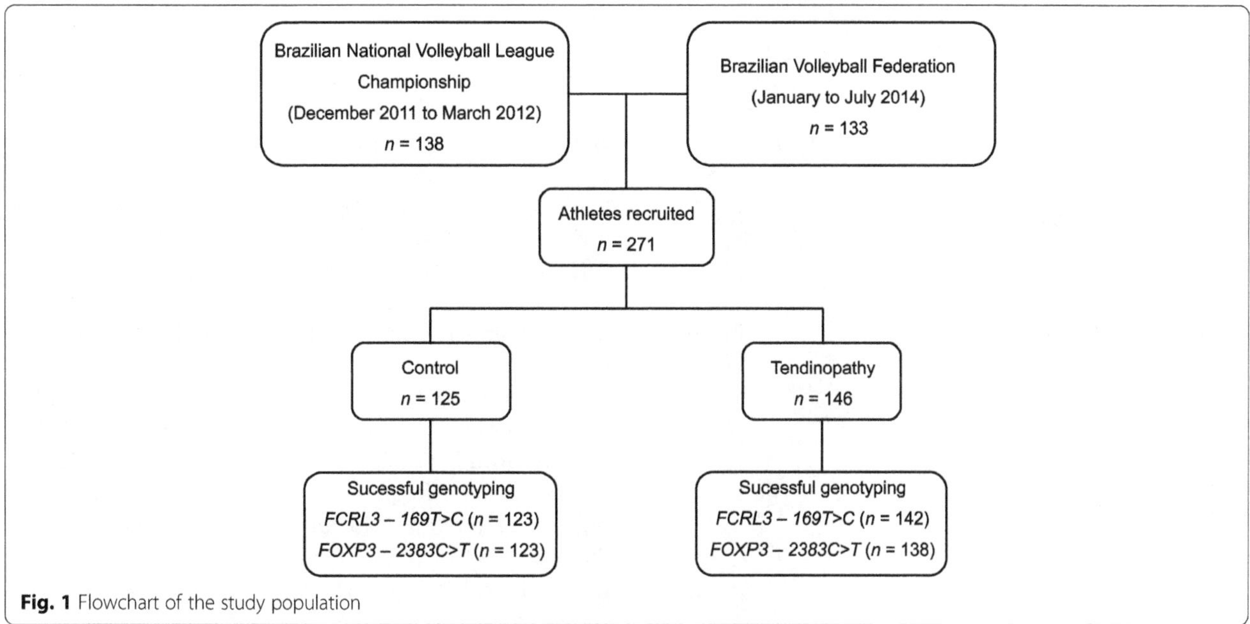

Fig. 1 Flowchart of the study population

or absence of tendinopathy clinically diagnosed by medical practitioners and confirmed with magnetic resonance image examination (MRI). The confirmatory MRI was performed during the Volleyball National Championship (December 2011 to March 2012) and the training of Brazilian Volleyball Federation carried out from January through July 2014. All diagnoses were confirmed by two blinded radiologists. As described in our previous studies [28, 29], the chronic tendinopathy diagnostic were (i) progressive pain related to training in the last 6 months and during clinical examination; and at least one of the following criteria: (ii) palpable nodular thickening over the tendon; (iii) tenderness on tendon palpation; (iv) history of swelling over the tendon area. The control group consisted of athletes with absence of tendinopathy history in any joint and who present no previous diagnosis of tendinopathy.

Genotyping of polymorphisms

Genomic DNA was obtained from saliva samples as previously described [28]. The genotyping analyses of *FCRL3 –169T>C* (rs7528684) and *FOXP3 –2383C>T* (rs3761549) polymorphisms were performed using a TaqMan allelic discrimination assay obtained from Applied Biosystems (C_1741825_10 and C_27058744_10, respectively). For all polymorphisms real-time polymerase chain reaction (PCR) reactions were performed on a 7500 Real-Time System (Applied Biosystems, Foster City, CA, USA), and the genotypes were then determined directly.

Statistical analysis

The sample size was calculated using Epi Info 7, version 7.1.3. (http://wwwn.cdc.gov/epiinfo/ html/downloads.htm) to detect a difference between case and control groups, assuming an odds ratio of 2.0 with a power of 0.8 and 5% type I error.

The Student's *t*-test was conducted to compare continuous variables between tendinopathy cases and controls and were expressed as the mean ± standard deviation (SD). Chi-square ($\chi 2$) test or Fisher's exact test, when applicable, was applied to compare differences in nominal data, as well as for the statistical analysis of the distribution frequencies of genotypes and alleles between the two groups. Additionally, Hardy-Weinberg equilibrium (HWE) was calculated by the $\chi 2$ test for goodness-of-fit. *FCRL3 –169T>C* and *FOXP3 –2383C>T* allele frequency and genotype distribution were derived by gene counting.

Multivariate logistic regression analyses were performed to identify possible confounding factors in the associations between polymorphisms and tendinopathy or between polymorphisms and tendinopathy features, which was estimated by the odds ratio (OR) with a 95% confidence interval (95% CI). The difference was statistically significant when $p < 0.05$. All analyses were performed using the Statistical Package for Social Sciences (SPSS Inc., Chicago, IL, USA), version 20.0.

Results

Table 1 presents the demographic, clinical and sport characteristics of the volleyball athletes. There were significant differences between the tendinopathy cases and controls with regard to mean age (26.86 ± 6.03 and 21.62 ± 5.39, respectively, $p = 0.0001$), average time of years of practice in volleyball (12.27 ± 5.35 and 8.27 ± 4.92, respectively, $p = 0.0001$), gender and tendinopathy clinical symptoms (tendon pain and away from training due pain).

Table 1 Characteristics of the volleyball athletes ($n = 271$)

Variables	Controls ($n = 125$)	Tendinopathy ($n = 146$)	p-value[a]	OR (95% CI)
Age group	n (%)			
Sub - 18	47 (37.6)	14 (9.6)	< 0.001	1[b]
Sub - 23	40 (32.0)	33 (22.6)		2.77 (1.30–5.89)
Adult	38 (30.4)	99 (67.8)		8.75 (4.33–17.69)
Gender				
Female	52 (41.6)	29 (19.9)	< 0.001	1[b]
Male	73 (58.4)	117 (80.1)		2.87 (1.67–4.93)
Ethnicity[c]				
White	67 (74.4)	36 (85.7)	0.41	1[b]
Intermediate	5 (5.6)	2 (4.8)		0.74 (0.14–4.03)
Black	18 (20.0)	4 (9.5)		0.41 (0.13–1.31)
Years of practice in volleyball				
0–5	45 (36.0)	17 (11.6)	< 0.001	1[b]
6–10	46 (36.8)	40 (27.4)		2.30 (1.14–4.64)
11–15	22 (17.6)	51 (34.9)		6.14 (2.90–12.98)
> 15	12 (9.6)	38 (26.1)		8.38 (3.56–19.73)
Declared preference				
Right	120 (96.0)	141 (96.6)	0.53	1[b]
Left	5 (4.0)	5 (3.4)		0.85 (0.24–3.01)
Function				
Spiker	90 (72.0)	115 (78.8)	0.34	1[b]
Setter	22 (17.6)	22 (15.1)		0.78 (0.41–1.50)
Libero	13 (10.4)	9 (6.1)		0.54 (0.22–1.32)
Traumatic lesion				
No	85 (68.0)	88 (60.3)	0.23	1[b]
Yes	40 (32.0)	58 (39.7)		1.40 (0.85–2.31)
Tendon pain				
No	47 (37.6)	14 (9.6)	< 0.001	1[b]
Yes	78 (62.4)	132 (90.4)		5.68 (2.94–10.98)
Away from training due pain				
No	91 (72.8)	80 (54.8)	0.003	1[b]
Yes	34 (27.2)	66 (45.2)		2.21 (1.32–3.68)

Notes: *OR* odds ratio; *CI* confidence interval
[a]Chi-Square Test or Fisher's exact test
[b]Reference group
[c]There are ethnicity information of 132 athletes

The evaluation of demographic and clinical characteristics revealed the athlete male gender (moderate risk), older age and higher years of practice in volleyball (very large risk) were risk factors for tendinopathy (Table 1). However, there were no significant differences between the two groups concerning the average time of practice in volleyball by age group (Student T test, Fig. 2a). The frequency of tendinopathy by tendon among elite volleyball athletes is shown in Fig. 2b. There was a significant gender difference among to the affected tendon type ($p = 0.003$, $\chi 2$ test).

The *FCRL3 −169T>C* and *FOXP3 −2383C>T* polymorphisms were in Hardy–Weinberg equilibrium. The allelic and genotypic frequencies and association's analyses of both polymorphisms are summarized in Table 2. Athletes with tendinopathy showed a significant higher frequency of the variant allele *FCRL3 −169C* compared with the controls. After adjusting for confounding factors (age, years of practice in volleyball, gender and pain), evaluated in multivariate logistic regression models, *FCRL3 −169C* polymorphism was associated with a higher risk of tendinopathy. By contrast, no significant differences were detected in the *FOXP3 −2383C>T* polymorphism frequency between the two groups (Table 2). In addition, *FCRL3 −169T>C* polymorphism frequency was significantly different regards to tendon pain and were away from training due pain between cases and controls who presented these clinical symptoms complaints (Table 3). After adjusting for confounding factors, the *FCRL3 −169C* allele increases the risk (approximate 2-fold) of developing tendinopathy among athletes who present pain or were away from training due pain. Moreover, a combined analysis of the *FCRL3 −169T>C* and *FOXP3 −2383C>T* polymorphisms was performed to investigate if their interaction would increase the risk of developing of tendinopathy among athletes who present tendon pain or were away from training due pain (Fig. 3). It has been observed that relative to the combined wild-type genotype (*FCRL3 −169TT* and *FOXP3 −2383CC*), the combined variant genotype (*FCRL3 −169TC* or *−169CC* and *FOXP3 −2383CT* or *−2383TT*) were associated with an increased risk of developing tendinopathy among athletes who present tendon pain (WT/VAR: OR = 2.24; 95% CI: 1.14–4.40 and *VAR/VAR*: OR = 2.60; 95% CI: 1.11–6.10) or were away from training due pain (*VAR/VAR*: OR = 5.00; 95% CI: 1.12–22.30).

Based on the results of this study and the previous ones, we propose a hypothesis for the role of *FCRL3 −169T>C* polymorphism in the tendinopathy development (Fig. 4).

Discussion

High incidence of tendon overuse injuries prevails in elite volleyball athletes mainly because they have to go through many hours of practice [2]. Moreover, the biomechanical characteristics of the skills required in volleyball associated with the joint anatomy of the players are accepted as being the risk factors for overuse injuries [30]. Among the ball-related sports, volleyball is one of the types that cause a high rate of overuse injury by demanding repetition of similar movement patterns [31] with an professional volleyball attacker performing approximately 40,000 spikes a year [32]. This volume of spikes may be represented by the fact that from 8 to

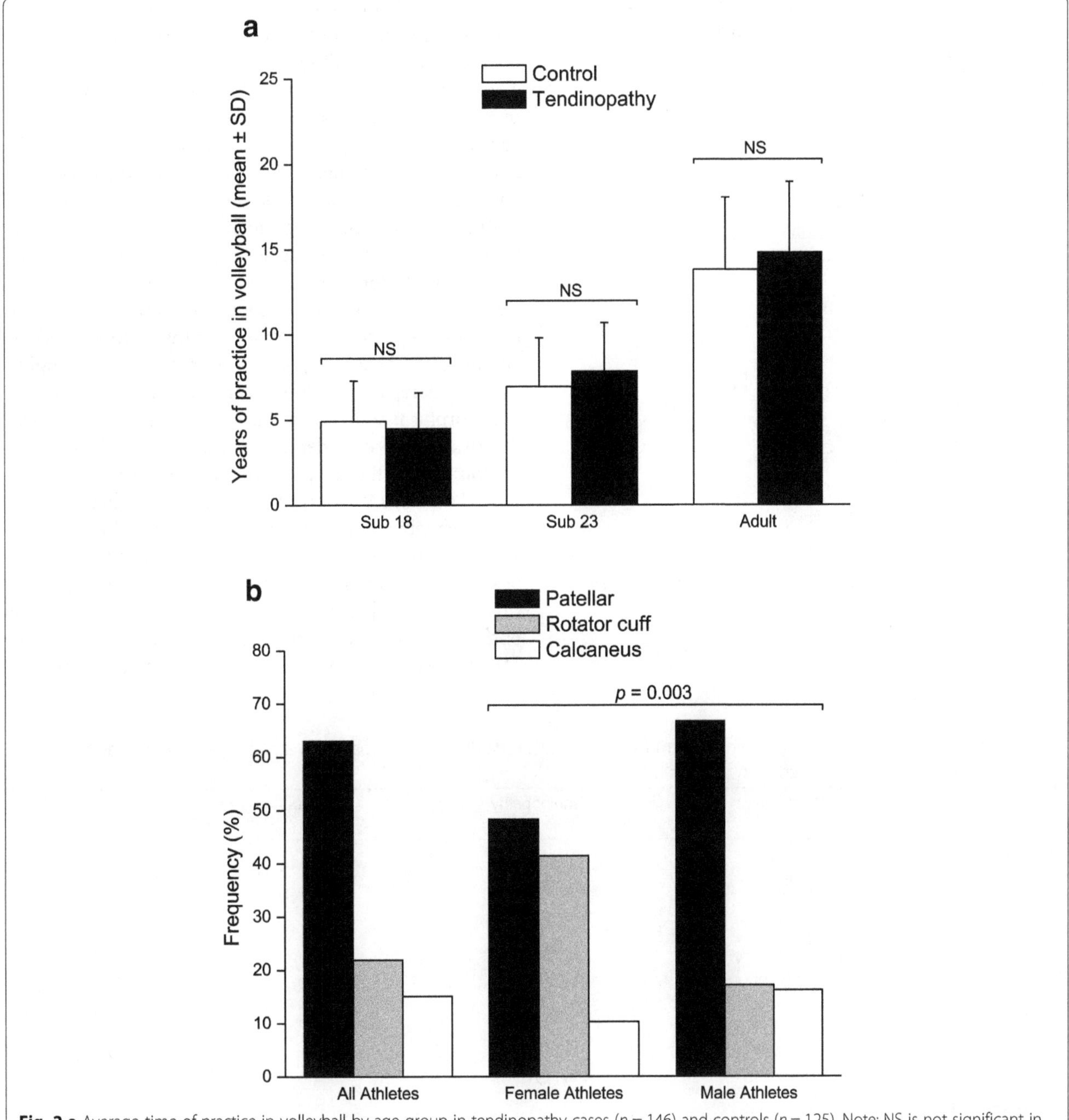

Fig. 2 **a** Average time of practice in volleyball by age group in tendinopathy cases ($n = 146$) and controls ($n = 125$). Note: NS is not significant in Student T test ($p > 0.05$). **b** Distribution of the sites most affected by tendinopathy in Brazilian volleyball athletes ($n = 146$). $p < 0.05$ was obtained through the Chi-squared Test (Pearson p-value)

20% of the injuries occurring in the shoulder [33] and nearly 45% of injuries in volleyball athletes are identified as patellar tendinopathy [34, 35]. In present study, tendinopathy in Brazilian volleyball athletes was more frequent in the knee (63% patellar) followed by the shoulder (22%). Moreover, female athletes presented a higher frequency of tendinopathy in the shoulder (41% in female versus 17% in male), corroborating the findings of a study unrelated to sport that the female gender was a risk factor for the development of rotator cuff disease [36]. Furthermore, Reeser and colleagues investigated risk factors for volleyball-related shoulder pain and dysfunction, and observed that female players showed lower simple shoulder test scores than male athletes [33].

Repetitive and strong physical activity, characteristic of elite athletes, contributes to excessive loading of tendons, promoting inflammation and pathological degeneration [4, 37]. Despite the development of physical

Table 2 Association analyses of the *FCRL3 −169T>C* and *FOXP3 −2383C>T* polymorphisms in tendinopathy cases compared with controls

SNP	Controls n (%)	Tendinopathy	p-value[a]	OR (95% CI)[b]
FCRL3 -169T>C	(n = 123)	(n = 142)		
TT	48 (39.0)	40 (28.2)		1[c]
TC	56 (45.6)	70 (49.3)	0.19	1.50 (0.86–2.59)
CC	19 (15.4)	32 (22.5)	0.04	2.02 (0.10–4.09)
TC + CC	75 (61.0)	102 (71.8)	0.08	1.63 (0.97–2.73)
T	152 (61.8)	150 (52.8)	0.04	1[c]
C	94 (38.2)	134 (47.2)		1.44 (1.02–2.04)
FOXP3 -2383C>T	(n = 123)	(n = 138)		
CC	86 (69.9)	97 (70.3)		1[c]
CT	30 (24.4)	37 (26.8)	0.86	1.09 (0.62–1.92)
TT	7 (5.7)	4 (2.9)	0.45	0.51 (0.14–1.79)
CT + TT	37 (30.1)	41 (29.7)	1.0	0.98 (0.58–1.67)
C	202 (82.1)	231 (83.7)	0.71	1[c]
T	44 (17.9)	45 (16.3)		0.89 (0.57–1.41)

Note: *SNP* single nucleotide polymorphism, *OR* odds ratio, *CI* confidence interval
[a]Chi-Square Test or Fisher's exact test
[b]Adjusted by age, years of practice in volleyball, gender and pain
[c]Reference group

qualities in high performance teams to reduce the tendinopathy risk, no standard that sufficiently compensates for the demands of the training has yet been established. Therefore, considering the high costs involved with overuse injuries in athletes, new strategies should be considered for the prevention of these injuries. Recently, studies based on identifying the DNA polymorphisms have been relevant in sports medicine investigation with the purpose of identifying the athletes most likely to develop lesions and thus suggesting individualized training to improve performance in sports [28, 29, 38–42].

As far as we know, the present study is the first study to focus on the possible contribution of the *FCRL3 −169T>C* and *FOXP3 −2383C>T* polymorphisms to the susceptibility to tendinopathy in elite athletes. The *FCRL3 −169T>C* polymorphism was associated with increased tendinopathy risk, either considering all cases, only athletes with tendon pain or those who were away from training due to pain. The *FCRL3 −169T>C* polymorphism changes promoter activity and consequently alters NFκB binding [27]. Therefore, the *FCRL3 −169T>C* polymorphism has previously been reported in association with rheumatoid arthritis [27, 43, 44], psoriasis vulgaris [22], neuromyelitis optica [45], multiple sclerosis [46] and endometriosis [21, 47]. Furthermore, in present study the combined

Table 3 Analysis of *FCRL3 −169 T > C* polymorphism frequency with regards to tendon pain and athletes who were away from training due pain in cases compared with controls

FCRL3 -169T>C	Controls n (%)	Tendinopathy n (%)	p-value[a]	OR (95% CI)
Tendon pain[b]				
	(n = 77)	(n = 128)		
TT	38 (49.3)	34 (26.6)		1[d]
TC	29 (37.7)	65 (50.8)	0.007	2.5 (1.32–4.74)
CC	10 (13.0)	29 (22.6)	0.010	3.24 (1.38–7.62)
TC + CC	39 (50.7)	94 (73.4)	0.002	2.69 (1.49–4.88)
T	105 (68.2)	133 (51.9)	0.002	1[d]
C	49 (31.8)	123 (48.1)		1.98 (1.30–3.01)
Away from training due pain[c]				
	(n = 33)	(n = 63)		
TT	15 (45.5)	15 (23.8)		1[d]
TC	15 (45.5)	37 (58.7)	0.09	2.47 (0.97–6.28)
CC	3 (9.0)	11 (17.5)	0.14	3.66 (0.85–15.90)
TC + CC	18 (54.5)	48 (76.2)	0.05	2.67 (1.09–6.54)
T	45 (68.2)	67 (53.2)	0.03	1[d]
C	21 (31.8)	59 (46.8)		1.89 (1.01–3.53)

Differences in sample sizes are due to available data from PCR amplification for each polymorphism
Note: *OR* odds ratio, *CI* confidence interval
[a]Chi-Squared Test or Fisher's exact test
[b]The analysis for tendon pain was adjusted by age, years of practice in volleyball and gender
[c]The analysis for away from training due pain was adjusted by age, years of practice in volleyball, gender and pain
[d]Reference group

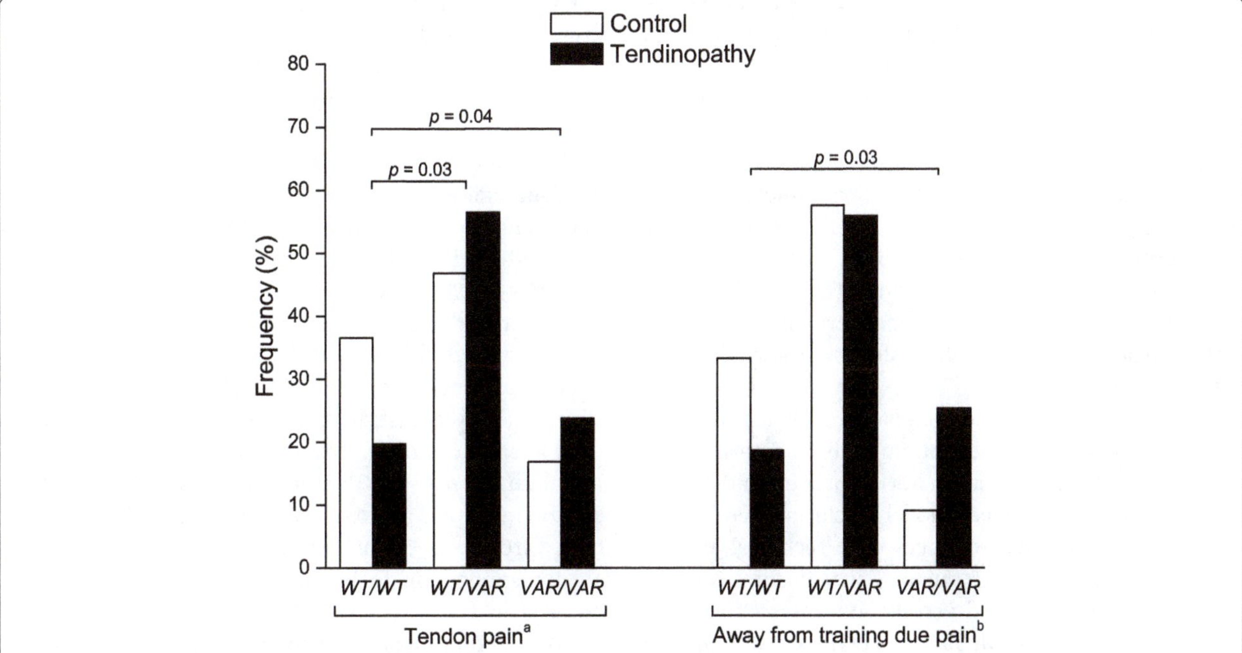

Fig. 3 Combined analysis of the *FCRL3 −169T>C* and *FOXP3 −2383C>T* polymorphisms and the risk of developing of tendinopathy among athletes who present pain or who were away from training due pain. Notes: *WT/WT: FCRL3 -169TT and FOXP3 -2383CC. WT/VAR: FCRL3 -169TT* and *FOXP3 -2383CT; FCRL3 -169TT* and *FOXP3 -2383TT; FCRL3 -169TC* and *FOXP3 -2383CC* or *FCRL3 -169CC* and *FOXP3 -2383CC. VAR/VAR: FCRL3 -169TC* and *FOXP3 -2383CT; FCRL3 -169TC* and *FOXP3 -2383TT; FCRL3 -169CC* and *FOXP3 -2383CT* or *FCRL3 -169CC* and *FOXP3 -2383TT.* $p < 0.05$ was obtained through the Chi-squared Test (Pearson *p*-value) or Fisher's exact test. [a]The analysis for tendon pain was adjusted by age, years of practice in volleyball and gender. [b]The analysis for away from training due pain was adjusted by age, years of practice in volleyball, gender and pain

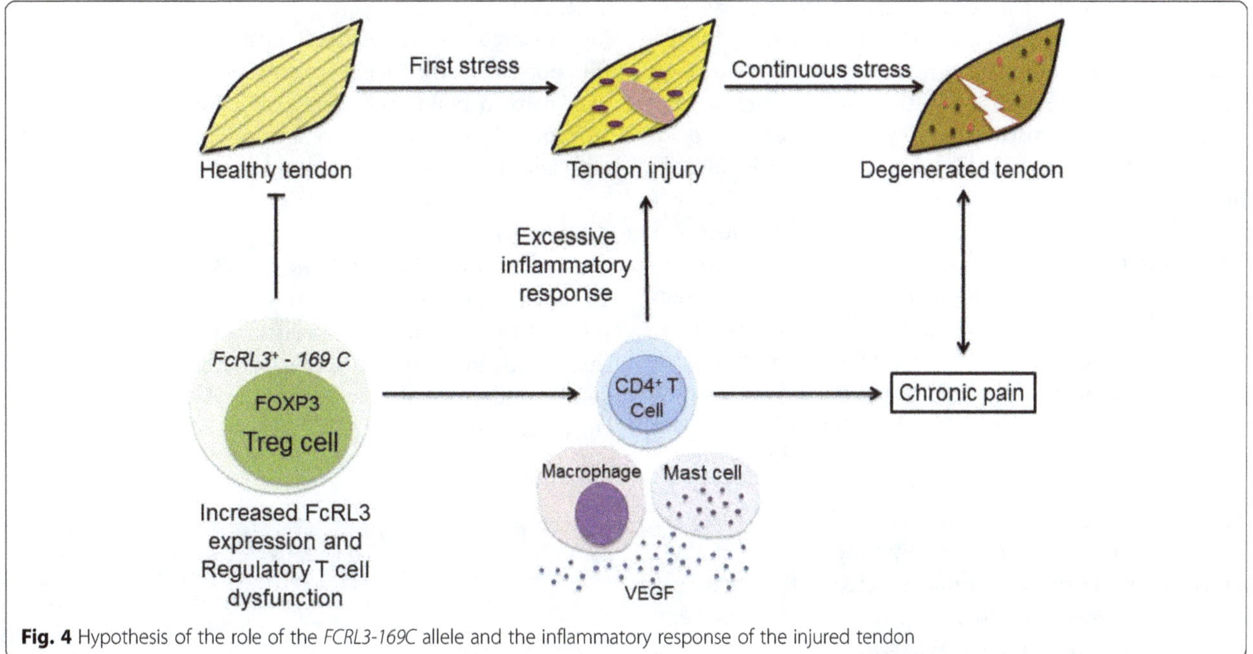

Fig. 4 Hypothesis of the role of the *FCRL3-169C* allele and the inflammatory response of the injured tendon

variant genotypes of *FCRL3 –169T>C* and *FOXP3 –2383C>T* were also associated with an increased risk for developing tendinopathy among athletes who presented tendon pain or were away from training due to pain. The combined analysis of *FCRL3 –169T>C* and *FOXP3 –2383C>T* suggested a gene-gene interaction in the susceptibility to tendinopathy. The cumulative effect of interaction of *FCRL3 –169T>C* and *FOXP3 –2383C>T* polymorphisms has previously been demonstrated in the development of endometriosis [47]. The *FOXP3 –2383C>T* polymorphism may interfere in the FOXP3 factor, promoting Treg cell dysfunction and development of diseases [48].

In the early stages of tendinopathy, changes in tissue microenvironment and activation of the innate immune system contribute to inflammatory repair in tendons [4]. In an experimental animal model of chronic tendinopathy, mast cells and macrophages were recruited and released angiogenic growth factors, which stimulate the proliferation of new blood vessels [49]. Interestingly, the major angiogenic growth factor VEGF is not found in healthy tendons [50], but it is expressed in tendons in chronic degeneration [51]. Recently, our group investigated whether polymorphisms in *VEGF* and its receptor *KDR* genes could be correlated with susceptibility to tendinopathy. We described evidences that the polymorphisms in *KDR* might alter receptor activity, influence the angiogenic process and consequently contribute to inter-individual variation in the development of tendinopathy in volleyball athletes [29].

In addition to the recruitment of macrophages and mast cells, and increase in angiogenesis signals in the tendon injury microenvironment, the CD4+ T cell also migrated into tissue and released pro-inflammatory cytokines, including interleukin 2 (IL-2), enhancing the innate immune response for tendon repair [11]. However, the persistence of stimuli in the tendon over a long period may cause tissue degeneration by excessive inflammatory responses and lead to chronic pain [37]. In this context, we suggest that CD4 + Foxp3+ regulatory T cells (Treg) could modulate the function of effector T cells during tendon repair by regulating the expression of target genes in the inflammatory response. As already described in other pathological conditions, polymorphisms can modulate the function of Tregs, harming the immune response [24, 52]. In present study, we found that *FCRL3 -169C* allele was associated with increased tendinopathy risk. This allele increased *FCRL3* gene expression in Treg cells and promoted inflammatory response to a greater extent in by the CD4+ T cell generating higher levels of immune activation [24]. Thus, we proposed a hypothesis relative to the role of the *FCRL3 -169C* allele in Treg cell dysfunction preventing the tendon regeneration (Fig. 4).

The main limitation of this approach was that the present study did not collect information on ethnicity of all athletes. The high degree of admixture of different ethnic backgrounds (mostly Europeans, Africans and Amerindians) in the Brazilian population, poses special challenges to ethnic classification. The Instituto Brasileiro de Geografia e Estatística (IBGE) responsible for the official census of Brazil, has used only few pre-established color categories, which are based on self-classification (see Methods). However, there is poor correlation of self-reported race/color with genetic ancestry among Brazilians and this is based on a complex subjective phenotypic evaluation [53]. Therefore, it was not possible to apply adjustments for population stratification [54], in spite of no significant difference in ethnicity being observed between the tendinopathy athletes and the control group. The extrapolation of genetic data obtained from well-defined ethnic groups is not appropriate for application to Brazilians [53] and our data can be used in future studies to improve understanding of the risk factors involved in the development of tendinopathy in athletes.

Finally, our group has been developing studies with the purpose of identifying genetic characteristics that may clarify new therapeutic targets or personalized training programs to treat the disease or to avoid the development of tendinopathy in athletes. However, the information about magnitude of each variable is necessary to determine if the effect has an important role in practical and clinical decisions about applicability of the outcome [55]. In this study, *FCRL3* and *FOXP3* polymorphisms and male gender were associated with a moderate risk (approximate 2-fold), whereas athlete older age and higher years of practice in volleyball were associated with a higher risk (approximate 8-fold) of tendinopathy. The knowledge of the potential risk factors associated with tendinopathy may help to build models to use for diagnosing athletes susceptible to tendon injury and providing these athletes with additional personalized support.

Conclusion

The cumulative effect of *FCRL3 –169T>C* and *FOXP3 –2383C>T* polymorphisms was associated with development of tendinopathy in Brazilian volleyball athletes, and this genetic knowledge together potential risk factors (age, gender and years of practice in volleyball) could improve the personalized training or treatment of athletes.

Abbreviations

95% CI: 95% Confidence interval; FCRL3: FC-receptor-like 3; FOXP3: Forkhead box P3; HWE: Hardy-Weinberg equilibrium; IBGE: Instituto Brasileiro de Geografia e Estatística; IL2: Interleukin 2; KDR: Kinase insert domain receptor; MRI: Magnetic resonance image examination; NFκB: Nuclear factor-κB; OR: Odds ratios; PCR: Polymerase chain reaction; SD: Standard deviation; SNPs: Single nucleotide polymorphisms; Treg: Regulator T cells; VAR: Variant; VEGF: Vascular endothelial growth factor; WT: Wild-type; $\chi 2$: Chi-square

Authors' contributions

JAP participated in conception and design of study. JIS and MBM collated the data and developed the database. LRL and JAP helped to experiments. LRL, DEM and JAP analysis, interpretation of data and wrote the manuscript. JMG, DM and MELD critical revision of the manuscript for important intellectual content. All authors read and approved the final manuscript.

Competing interests

The authors declare that they have no competing interests.

Author details

[1]Research Division, National Institute of Traumatology and Orthopaedics, Avenida Brasil, 500, Rio de Janeiro, RJ 20940-070, Brazil. [2]Federation International de Volleyball (FIVB) - Coach Commission, Rio de Janeiro, Brazil. [3]Research Laboratory of Pharmaceutical Sciences, West Zone State University, Rio de Janeiro, Brazil. [4]Centre for Sports Exercise Medicine, Queen Mary University of London, London, UK. [5]Program of Post-graduation in Public Health and Environment, National School of Public Health, Oswald Cruz Foundation, Rio de Janeiro, Brazil.

References

1. van der Worp H, van Ark M, Roerink S, Pepping GJ, van den Akker-Scheek I, Zwerver J. Risk factors for patellar tendinopathy: a systematic review of the literature. Br J Sports Med. 2011;45(5):446–52.
2. Eerkes K. Volleyball injuries. Curr Sports Med Rep. 2012;11(5):251–6.
3. Rees J, Maffulli N, Cook J. Management of tendinopathy. Am J Sports Med. 2009;37:1855–67.
4. Millar NL, Murrell GAC, McInnes IB. Inflammatory mechanisms in tendinopathy – towards translation. Nat Rev Rheumatol. 2017;13(2):110–22.
5. Astrom M, Rausing A. Chronic Achilles tendinopathy. A survey of surgical and histopathologic findings. Clin Orthop Relat Res. 1995;316:151–64.
6. Khan KM, Maffulli N. Tendinopathy: an Achilles' heel for athletes and clinicians. Clin J Sport Med. 1998;8(3):151–4.
7. Jelinsky SA, Rodeo SA, Li J, Gulotta LV, Archambault JM, Seeherman HJ. Regulation of gene expression in human tendinopathy. BMC Musculoskelet Disord. 2011;12:86.
8. Lories RJ, McInnes IB. Primed for inflammation: enthesis-resident T cells. Nat Med. 2012;18(7):1018–9.
9. Marsolais D, Cote CH, Frenette J. Neutrophils and macrophages accumulate sequentially following Achilles tendon injury. J Orthop Res. 2001;19(6):1203–9.
10. Dean BJ, Gettings P, Dakin SG, Carr AJ. Are inflammatory cells increased in painful human tendinopathy? A systematic review. Br J Sports Med. 2016; 50(4):216–20.
11. Millar NL, Hueber AJ, Reilly JH, Xu Y, Fazzi UG, Murrell GA, et al. Inflammation is present in early human tendinopathy. Am J Sports Med. 2010;38(10):2085–91.
12. Kragsnaes MS, Fredberg U, Stribolt K, Kjaer SG, Bendix K, Ellingsen T. Stereological quantification of immune-competent cells in baseline biopsy specimens from achilles tendons: results from patients with chronic tendinopathy followed for more than 4 years. Am J Sports Med. 2014;42(10): 2435–45.
13. Schubert TE, Weidler C, Lerch K, Hofstadter F, Straub RH. Achilles tendinosis is associated with sprouting of substance P positive nerve fibres. Ann Rheum Dis. 2005;64(7):1083–6.
14. Brusko TM, Putnam AL, Bluestone JA. Human regulatory T cells: role in autoimmune disease and therapeutic opportunities. Immunol Rev. 2008; 223:371–90.
15. Oh S, Rankin AL, Caton AJ. CD4+CD25+ regulatory T cells in autoimmune arthritis. Immunol Rev. 2010;233:97–111.
16. Fontenot JD, Gavin MA, Rudensky AY. Foxp3 programs the development and function of CD4 + CD25+ regulatory T cells. Nat Immunol. 2003;4:330–6.
17. Brunkow ME, Jeffery EW, Hjerrild KA, Paeper B, Clark LB, Yasayko SA, et al. Disruption of a new forkhead/winged-helix protein, scurfin, results in the fatal lymphoproliferative disorder of the scurfy mouse. Nat Genet. 2001; 27(1):68–73.
18. Oda JM, Hirata BK, Guembarovski RL, Watanabe MA. Genetic polymorphism in FOXP3 gene: imbalance in regulatory T-cell role and development of human diseases. J Genet. 2013;92(1):163–71.
19. Jiang LL, Ruan LW. Association between FOXP3 promoter polymorphisms and cancer risk: a meta-analysis. Oncol Lett. 2014;8(6):2795–9.
20. Burton PR, Clayton DG, Cardon LR, Craddock N, Deloukas P, Duncanson A, et al. Association scan of 14,500 nonsynonymous SNPs in four diseases identifies autoimmunity variants. Nat Genet. 2007;39(11):1329–37.
21. Bianco B, Teles JS, Lerner TG, Vilarino FL, Christofolini DM, Barbosa CP. Association of FCRL3 -169T/C polymorphism with endometriosis and identification of a protective haplotype against the development of the disease in Brazilian population. Hum Immunol. 2011;72(9):774–8.
22. Song QH, Shen Z, Xing XJ, Yin R, Wu YZ, You Y, et al. An association study of single nucleotide polymorphismsof the FOXP3 intron-1 and the risk of psoriasis vulgaris. Indian J Biochem Biophys. 2012;49(1):25–35.
23. Bajpai UD, Swainson LA, Mold JE, Graf JD, Imboden JB, McCune JM. A functional variant in FCRL3 is associated with higher FcRL3 expression on T cell subsets and rheumatoid arthritis disease activity. Arthritis Rheum. 2012; 64(8):2451–9.
24. Swainson LA, Mold JE, Bajpai UD, McCune JM. Expression of the autoimmune susceptibility gene FcRL3 on human regulatory T cells is associated with dysfunction and high levels of programmed cell death-1. J Immunol. 2010; 184(7):3639–47.
25. Chistiakov DA, Chistiakov AP. Is FCRL3 a new general autoimmunity gene? Hum Immunol. 2007;68:375–83.
26. Nagata S, Ise T, Pastan I. Fc receptor-like 3 protein expressed on IL-2 nonresponsive subset of human regulatory T cells. J Immunol. 2009; 182(12):7518–26.
27. Kochi Y, Yamada R, Suzuki A, Harley JB, Shirasawa S, Sawada T, et al. A functional variant in FCRL3, encoding Fc receptor-like 3, is associated with rheumatoid arthritis and several autoimmunities. Nat Genet. 2005;37(5): 478–85.
28. Salles JI, Amaral MV, Aguiar DP, Lira DA, Quinelato V, Bonato LL, et al. BMP4 and FGF3 haplotypes increase the risk of tendinopathy in volleyball athletes. J Sci Med Sport. 2015;18(2):150–5.
29. Salles JI, Duarte ME, Guimarães JM, Lopes LR, Vilarinho Cardoso J, Aguiar DP, et al. Vascular endothelial growth factor Receptor-2 polymorphisms have protective effect against the development of tendinopathy in volleyball athletes. PLoS One. 2016;11(12):e0167717.
30. Seminati E, Minetti AE. Overuse in volleyball training/practice: review on shoulder and spine-related injuries. Eur J Sport Sci. 2013;13(6):732–43.
31. Chan KM, Yuan Y, Li CK, Chien P, Tsang G. Sports causing most injuries in Hong Kong. Br J Sports Med. 1993;27(4):263–7.
32. Challoumas D, Artemiou A, Dimitrakakis G. Dominant vs. non-dominant shoulder morphology in volleyball players and associations with shoulder pain and spike speed. J Sports Sci. 2017;35(1):65–73.
33. Reeser JC, Joy EA, Porucznik CA, Berg RL, Colliver EB, Willick SE. Risk factors for volleyball-related shoulder pain and dysfunction. PM R. 2010;2(1):27–36.
34. Lian OB, Engebretsen L, Bahr R. Prevalence of jumper's knee among elite athletes from different sports: a cross-sectional study. Am J Sports Med. 2005;33(4):561–7.
35. Zwerver J, Bredeweg SW, van den Akker-Scheek I. Prevalence of Jumper's knee among nonelite athletes from different sports: a cross-sectional survey. Am J Sports Med. 2011;39(9):1984–8.
36. Motta Gda R, Amaral MV, Rezende E, Pitta R, Vieira TC, Duarte ME, et al. Evidence of genetic variations associated with rotator cuff disease. J Shoulder Elb Surg. 2014;23(2):227–35.
37. Browne GJ, Barnett PLJ. Common sports-related musculoskeletal injuries presenting to the emergency department. J Paediatr Child Health. 2016; 52(2):231–6.
38. Maffulli N, Margiotti K, Longo UG, Loppini M, Fazio VM, Denaro V. The genetics of sports injuries and athletic performance. Muscles Ligaments Tendons J. 2013;3(3):173–89.
39. Pruna R, Artells R, Ribas J, Montoro B, Cos F, Muñoz C, et al. Single nucleotide polymorphisms associated with non-contact soft tissue injuries in elite professional soccer players: influence on degree of injury and recovery time. BMC Musculoskelet Disord. 2013;14:221.
40. Cauci S, Migliozzi F, Trombetta CS, Venuto I, Saccheri P, Travan L, et al. Low back pain and FokI (rs2228570) polymorphism of vitamin D receptor in athletes. BMC Sports Sci Med Rehabil. 2017;9:4.
41. Li YC, Wang LQ, Yi LY, Liu JH, Hu Y, Lu YF, et al. ACTN3 R577X genotype and performance of elite middle-long distance swimmers in China. Biol Sport. 2017;34(1):39–43.
42. Orysiak J, Mazur-Różycka J, Busko K, Gajewski J, Szczepanska B, Malczewska-Lenczowska J. Individual and combined influence of ACE and ACTN3 genes on muscle phenotypes in Polish athletes. J Strength Cond Res. 2017; https://doi.org/10.1519/JSC.0000000000001839

43. Maehlen MT, Nordang GB, Syversen SW, van der Heijde DM, Kvien TK, Uhlig T, et al. FCRL3 -169C/C genotype is associated with anti-citrullinated protein antibody-positive rheumatoid arthritis and with radiographic progression. J Rheumatol. 2011;38(11):2329–35.
44. Lin X, Zhang Y, Chen Q. FCRL3 gene polymorphisms as risk factors for rheumatoid arthritis. Hum Immunol. 2016;77(2):223–9.
45. Lan W, Fang S, Zhang H, Wang DT, Wu J. The Fc receptor-like 3 polymorphisms (rs7528684, rs945635, rs3761959 and rs2282284) and the risk of Neuromyelitis Optica in a Chinese population. Medicine (Baltimore). 2015;94(38):e1320.
46. Yuan M, Wei L, Zhou R, Bai Q, Wei Y, Zhang W, et al. Four FCRL3 gene polymorphisms (FCRL3_3, _5, _6, _8) confer susceptibility to multiple sclerosis: results from a case-control study. Mol Neurobiol. 2016;53(3):2029–35.
47. Barbosa CP, Teles JS, Lerner TG, Peluso C, Mafra FA, Vilarino FL, et al. Genetic association study of polymorphisms FOXP3 and FCRL3 in women with endometriosis. Fertil Steril. 2012;97(5):1124–8.
48. Wildin RS, Smyk-Pearson S, Filipovich AH. Clinical and molecular features of the immunodysregulation, polyendocrinopathy, enteropathy, X linked (IPEX) syndrome. J Med Genet. 2002;39(8):537–45.
49. de Oliveira RR, Martins CS, Rocha YR, Braga AB, Mattos RM, Hecht F, et al. Experimental diabetes induces structural, inflammatory and vascular changes of Achilles tendons. PLoS One. 2013;8(10):e74942.
50. Karsten K. The role of tendon microcirculation in Achilles and patellar tendinopathy. J Orthop Surg Res. 2008;3:18.
51. Nakama LH, King KB, Abrahamsson S, Rempel DM. VEGF, VEGFR-1, and CTGF cell densities in tendon are increased with cyclical loading: an in vivo tendinopathy model. J Orthop Res. 2006;24(3):393–400.
52. Ben Jmaa M, Abida O, Bahloul E, Toumi A, Khlif S, Fakhfakh R, et al. Role of FOXP3 gene polymorphism in the susceptibility to Tunisian endemic pemphigus Foliaceus. Immunol Lett. 2017;184:105–11.
53. Pena SD, Di Pietro G, Fuchshuber-Moraes M, Genro JP, Hutz MH, Kehdy Fde S, et al. The genomic ancestry of individuals from different geographical regions of Brazil is more uniform than expected. PLoS One. 2011;6(2):e17063.
54. Price AL, Patterson NJ, Plenge RM, Weinblatt ME, Shadick NA, Reich D. Principal components analysis corrects for stratification in genome-wide association studies. Nat Genet. 2006;38(8):904–9.
55. Hopkins WG. Linear models and effect magnitudes for research, clinical, and practical applications. Sportscience. 2010;14(1):49–58.

3

Novel digenic inheritance of *PCDH15* and *USH1G* underlies profound non-syndromic hearing impairment

Isabelle Schrauwen[1], Imen Chakchouk[1], Anushree Acharya[1], Khurram Liaqat[2], Irfanullah[3], University of Washington Center for Mendelian Genomics, Deborah A. Nickerson[4], Michael J. Bamshad[4,5], Khadim Shah[3], Wasim Ahmad[3] and Suzanne M. Leal[1*]

Abstract

Background: Digenic inheritance is the simplest model of oligenic disease. It can be observed when there is a strong epistatic interaction between two loci. For both syndromic and non-syndromic hearing impairment, several forms of digenic inheritance have been reported.

Methods: We performed exome sequencing in a Pakistani family with profound non-syndromic hereditary hearing impairment to identify the genetic cause of disease.

Results: We found that this family displays digenic inheritance for two *trans* heterozygous missense mutations, one in *PCDH15* [p.(Arg1034His)] and another in *USH1G* [p.(Asp365Asn)]. Both of these genes are known to cause autosomal recessive non-syndromic hearing impairment and Usher syndrome. The protein products of *PCDH15* and *USH1G* function together at the stereocilia tips in the hair cells and are necessary for proper mechanotransduction. Epistasis between Pcdh15 and Ush1G has been previously reported in digenic heterozygous mice. The digenic mice displayed a significant decrease in hearing compared to age-matched heterozygous animals. Until now no human examples have been reported.

Conclusions: The discovery of novel digenic inheritance mechanisms in hereditary hearing impairment will aid in understanding the interaction between defective proteins and further define inner ear function and its interactome.

Keywords: Digenic inheritance, Hearing impairment, Deafness, *PCDH15*, *USH1G*

Background

Over the last decade, genetic studies have taught us that there is a continuous spectrum of genetic influences between monogenic and oligogenic diseases. The simplest model of multifactorial inheritance is digenic, where in its original definition, two loci are necessary to express or extremely modify the severity of a phenotype. Compared to monogenic disease inheritance, digenic inheritance does not follow Mendelian segregation and is probably underdiagnosed due to the difficulty in verifying true digenic effects. However, several convincing cases of digenic inheritance have been found in genetically heterogeneous disorders including hearing impairment (HI) [1–4]. These findings encouraged researchers when analyzing exome and genome sequence data to consider variants in related genes or similar pathways that fit a digenic disease model as candidates, which has led to additional promising reports [5–9].

Several putative digenic recessive interactions causing non-syndromic (NS) HI and syndromic HI, e.g. Usher and Pendred syndromes have been described [1–9]. Digenic *GJB2* (Cx26) and *GJB6* (Cx30) heterozygous variants are an often observed cause of HI in humans [4, 5]. A 309-kb deletion, also referred to as del (GJB6-D13S1830), which involves *GJB6*, causes HI in the homozygous state, or in the compound heterozygous state with a large variety of *GJB2* mutations. However,

* Correspondence: sleal@bcm.edu
[1]Center for Statistical Genetics, Department of Molecular and Human Genetics, Baylor College of Medicine, One Baylor Plaza 700D, Houston, TX 77030, USA
Full list of author information is available at the end of the article

this example should be considered as monogenic *GJB2* autosomal recessive NSHI and not truly digenic in its underlying molecular nature, since the *GJB6* deletion inactivates *GJB2* [10, 11], which is its neighboring gene on chromosome 13.

There are several examples of true digenic inheritance for HI. For example, digenic inheritance of *CDH23* and *PCDH15* is well established [1], and has been shown to cause age-related HI in mice, and Usher Syndrome Type I in humans. Both proteins interact closely and are crucial for the normal organization of the stereocilia bundle. Digenic heterozygous mice showed degeneration of the stereocilia and a base-apex loss of hair cells and spiral ganglion cells [1]. Other described digenic cases include *SLC26A4* and *FOXI* [2], which causes Pendred syndrome or HI associated with enlarged vestibular aqueducts (EVA) in humans or EVA in the mouse mutant, and *SLC26A4* and *KCNJ10* [3], which have been observed to cause HI and EVA in humans. In addition, some putative digenic inheritances have been suggested but still require further evidence or need to be replicated, such as *GJB2* and *TMPRSS3* [7] and *MYO7A* and *PCDH15* [8], amongst others.

For HI, dominant 'digenic' additive effects of two genes have also been described, which leads to a more severe hearing loss than the effect of a single variant. For example, for a Swedish family, an additive effect of linked loci *DFNA2* and *DFNA11,* resulted in a more severe phenotype for which the causative variants and genes have yet to be identified [12].

Digenic inheritance can refer to different scenarios [13, 14], and there is currently no clear consensus regarding the definition of digenic inheritance. The most commonly used definition, requires two loci for expression or extreme modification of the severity of a similar phenotype. There is a thin line between the digenic modification definition and genetic modifiers, as both are often used in a similar context.

The Digenic Diseases Database (DIDA) [13] classifies digenic cases into two classes which are simplifications of the original definitions provided by Schäffer [15]: 1) The first class is referred to as the 'true digenic' class, i.e. variants at both loci are required for expression of the disease, and neither variant alone displays a phenotype. 2) The second class is a composite class as it includes different possibilities, such as Mendelian variants plus modifiers that vary the phenotype, or dual molecular diagnoses, wherein Mendelian variants at each of the two loci segregate independently and results in a combination of both phenotypes [13]. However, there are a spectrum of scenarios possible that can blur these defined borders [14]. In *OMIM* (Online Mendelian Inheritance in Man), digenic inheritance is classified into two categories: Digenic dominant inheritance is defined as heterozygous mutations in two genes, while digenic recessive inheritance signifies a homozygous or compound heterozygous mutation in one gene and a heterozygous mutation in a second gene.

The digenic inheritance described in this article entails a true digenic model, in which two *trans* heterozygous mutations in two genes (on different chromosomes) whose protein products function closely together at the stereocilia tips in the hair cells (*PCDH15* and *USH1G*) are required for the expression of a phenotype.

Methods

The study was approved by the Institutional Review Boards of the Quaid-i-Azam University and the Baylor College of Medicine and Affiliated Hospitals (H-17566). Written informed consent was obtained from all participating members.

DNA samples were collected from five family members of a consanguineous family with hereditary non-syndromic hearing loss (Family 4667; Fig. 1a) from the Khyber Pakhtunkhwa province in Pakistan. These samples include DNA from two affected siblings (IV:3 and IV:4), two unaffected siblings (IV:1 and IV:2) and their mother (III:2) (Fig. 1a).

Genomic DNA was extracted from peripheral blood using a phenol chloroform procedure [16]. Exomic libraries were prepared from one affected individual (IV:4) with the Roche NimbleGen SeqCap EZ Human Exome Library v.2.0 (~ 37 Mb target), following the manufacturer's protocol. Sequencing was performed by 70 bp paired-end sequencing on a HiSeq2500/4000 instrument (Illumina Inc., San Diego, CA, USA). Reads were aligned to the Human genome (Hg19/GRC37) using the Burrows-Wheeler transform (BWA-MEM), PCR duplicates were removed with Picard MarkDuplicates, and indel realignment was performed (GATK IndelRealigner). Single nucleotide polymorphisms (SNP) s and small insertions/deletions (Indels) variants were recalibrated with BaseRecalibrator and called jointly with HaplotypeCaller (GATK), annotated with dbNSFP and ANNOVAR for further filtering and interpretation [17]. Copy number variants (CNVs) were called using CoNIFER [18] and XHMM [19].

Variants were further filtered based on location (coding region and splice region +/– 12 bp), and frequency [minor allele frequency (MAF) Genome Aggregation Database (gnomAD) < 0.005 in all populations]. Variants with a predicted damaging functional effect were identified (e.g., splice-site, non-synonymous, nonsense, etc.), and conservation scores (e.g., PhastCons, GERP), and the Combined Annotation Dependent Depletion (CADD) score were evaluated prior to testing for segregation within the pedigree. We selected both heterozygous and homozygous variants for segregation testing in the pedigree, assuming several modes of

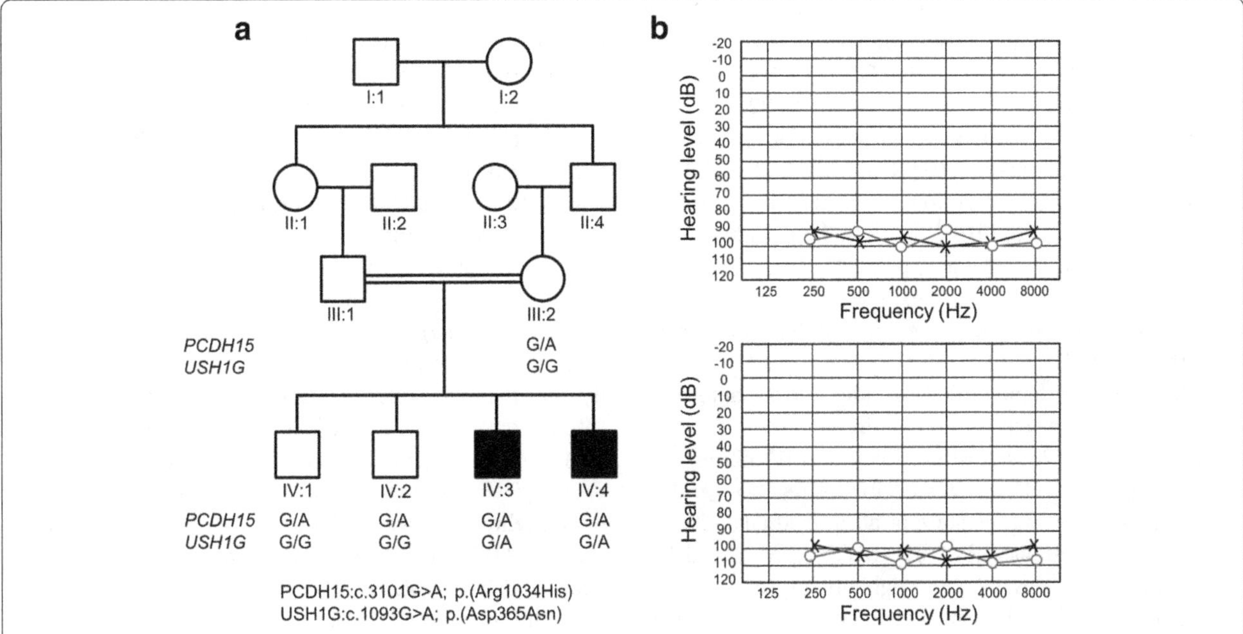

Fig. 1 Pedigree drawing for family 4667 and audiograms for the affected family members. Panel **a** Pedigree drawing displaying family members with NSHI as filled symbols and unaffected family members as clear symbols. Males are represented by squares and females by circles. For the three unaffected and two affected family members genotypes for the *PCDH15* variant NM_033056:c.3101G > A and *USH1G* variant NM_173477:c.1093G > A are shown under each family member and demonstrate digenic inheritance. The DNA sample from Individual IV:4 was exome sequenced. Panel **b** Audiograms for affected family members IV:3 (top) and IV:4 (bottom). Pure-tone audiometry was performed between 250 and 8000 Hz and x represents the results for the left ear and o for the right ear. Affected individual IV:3 was 34 years old, and affected individual IV:4 was 22 years old at the time of pure-tone audiometry and physical examination

inheritance possible in this pedigree: autosomal recessive (homozygous or compound heterozygous), X-linked, germline mosaicism or parental mosaicism, and digenic.

Sanger sequencing was used to validate variants and verify segregation with the HI phenotype in the family. Primers surrounding region of interest were designed using primer3 software [20]. PCR amplified products were treated with ExoSAP-IT™ PCR Product Cleanup Reagent (ThermoFisher Scientific, Sugerland, TX) and sequenced using the BigDye terminator v3.1 cycle sequencing kit (Applied Biosystems, Foster City, CA) on an ABI 3130 Genetic Analyzer (Applied Biosystems, Foster City, CA).

Results

Clinical evaluation

Pure-tone audiometry showed bilateral profound HI in both affected persons (Fig. 1b). An external eye exam, visual acuity and ophthalmoscopy, showed no vision problems. Other causes of HI, including infections, trauma and ototoxic medications were evaluated and excluded. Tandem gait and Romberg tests were performed to evaluate for gross vestibular deficits. No vestibular problems were identified. Careful physical examinations revealed no other problems in addition to HI in the family members, supporting that the HI is non-syndromic.

Exome and Sanger sequencing

Exome sequencing revealed several variants of interest (Additional file 1: Table S1), which were all tested for segregation by performing Sanger sequencing using DNA from all available family members. None of the variants in genes previously associated with HI segregated with the HI phenotype with the exception of the *PCDH15* [GRCh37/hg19; chr10:55719513C > T; NM_033056: c.3101G > A; p.(Arg1034His)] and *USH1G* [GRCh37/hg19; chr17:72915838C > T; NM_173477:c.1093G > A; p.(Asp365Asn)] variants which displayed digenic inheritance (Fig. 1a).

The *PCDH15* variant [NM_033056: c.3101G > A; p.(Arg1034His)] has a CADD score of 23.9, is predicted damaging according to MutationTaster, and is conserved amongst species (GERP++ RS 4.53 and PhyloP20way 0.892). The variant is not present in the gnomAD database of 123,136 exomes and 15,496 whole-genomes of unrelated individuals, which includes 15,391 South Asian exomes [21]. In addition, the variant is not present in the Greater Middle East (GME) Variome Project that contains 1111 unrelated individuals from the Greater Middle East, including 168 Iranian and Pakistani individuals [22]. The variant was not observed in 81 in-house Pakistani exomes which had other Mendelian Traits but not NSHI or syndromic HI. This variant, in the homozygous state, was previously been described as pathogenic in an Iranian family with NSHI [23].

The *USH1G* [NM_173477:c.1093G > A; p.(Asp365Asn); rs538983393] variant has a CADD score of 22.9, is predicted damaging according to MutationTaster, and is conserved amongst species (GERP++ RS 4.53 and PhyloP20way 1.000). It has a low frequency in gnomAD (3.3×10^{-5} overall; 2.3×10^{-4} South Asian), with no homozygotes reported, and is not present in the GME Variome Project nor our in-house exomes. The *PCDH15* and *USH1G* variants are available in ClinVar (accession SCV000608345) [24].

Additionally for family 4667, we identified a heterozygous variant in *CDH23* [NM_022124:c.C2263T:p.(His755Tyr); rs181255269] via exome sequencing. It was tested for segregation and is present in a heterozygous state in all individuals with an available DNA sample (III: 2, IV: 1, IV: 2, IV: 3 and IV: 4). Although this variant was originally suggested to be pathogenic [25], based upon recent evidence in ClinVar, and a high population frequency in certain populations (2.2% MAF in the Turkish Peninsula [22]; Additional file 1: Table S1), this variant is likely benign. This variant also does not fit a digenic inheritance model with known digenic partner *PCDH15* in this family.

To find any other potentially missed pathogenic variants in this family, we examined the BAM files for individual IV:4 using Integrative Genomics Viewer (IGV2.3.97) to try to detect any variants that were not called and/or regions with no reads or low read depth (<= 8× coverage). All low and/or uncovered exonic and splice regions of *USH1G* and *PCDH15* were Sanger sequenced, and no additional variants were found. We also performed a CNV analysis on the exome data, and only one heterozygous deletion was called in the sequenced exome of individual IV: 4 by both CoNIFER and XHMM (GRCh37/hg19; chr13:100511115–100,915,087). This region does not contain any known HI genes. Additionally, no other CNVs in this region have been reported in the Database of Genomic Variants (DVG) associated with any disease [26].

Discussion

Hair cells of the inner ear are mechanosensors for the detection of sound and balance/movement. At the apical surface of each hair cell is its mechanically sensitive organelle, the hair bundle, which consists of dozens of stereocilia. Mechanotransduction channels are located near stereociliary tips and open or close on deflection of the stereocilia. Tip-links stretch from the tips of stereocilia in the short and middle rows to the sides of neighboring, taller stereocilia. These Tip-links on stereocilia are made of cdh23 and pcdh15 [27]. In the Ames waltzer mice, recessive mutations of *Pcdh15* cause deafness due to disorganized stereocilia bundles and degeneration of inner ear neuroepithelia [28].

Sans, the protein coded by *Ush1g*, interacts with the cytoplasmic domains of cdh23 and pcdh15 in vitro and is absent from the hair bundle in mice defective for either of the two cadherins [27]. Sans *(Ush1g)* localizes mainly to the tips of short- and middle-row stereocilia in vivo, and plays a critical role in the maintenance of molecular complex at the lower end of the tip-link [27]. Thus, Sans locates at stereocilia tips, near the location of Pcdh15. In *Ush1g*$^{-/-}$ mice, the cohesion of stereocilia is also disrupted, and both the amplitude and the sensitivity of the transduction currents are reduced [27]. Interaction between USH1G and PCDH15 is further demonstrated in digenic heterozygous mice. +/*Pcdh15*$^{av\text{-}3J}$ +/*Ush1g*^{js} double heterozygous mice display hearing loss, with highly significant elevated auditory brainstem response (ABR) thresholds at 3–4 months [29], suggesting Pcdh15-Ush1g epistasis [29].

In the traditional definition, epistasis describes the interaction of two or more genetic loci, which can substantially modify disease severity or result in an entirely new phenotype. In the literature within and between different fields, there are contradictions in the definitions and interpretations of epistasis [30]. Adopting the original definition of epistasis, a non-linear interaction, we describe a family where the hearing impaired members carry *trans* heterozygous variants in *PCDH15* and *USH1G* and have profound HI and single variant carriers have normal hearing (Fig. 1). We cannot, confirm epistasis in vitro, i.e. biochemical epistasis [31]. We hypothesize that the biochemical function of their network is severely affected by these two variants and results in a profound HI, because both proteins function together at the stereocilia tips in the hair cells and are necessary for proper mechanotransduction. Since each gene separately is known to cause autosomal recessive HI, reduced activity/functioning of both proteins in the same close interacting network is a likely disease model.

Conclusions

In this study, we suggest epistasis between PCDH15 and USH1G in humans, through the study of a consanguineous family with profound hereditary HI, segregating a heterozygous and predicted damaging mutation in both *PCDH15* and *USH1G* (Fig. 1). Digenic inheritance of hearing impairment in mice and humans suggest that the proteins interact or perform co-dependent functions in hair cells. The study of digenic diseases can help us understand more about the complex interaction within the inner ear and is an initial step towards the understanding of more complex oligogenic diseases, such as age-related hearing loss.

Abbreviations

ABR: Auditory Brainstem Response; CADD: Combined Annotation Dependent Depletion; CNV: Copy Number Variant; CoNIFER: Copy number inference from exome reads; DGV: Database of Genomic Variants; DIDA: Digenic Diseases Database; EVA: Enlarged vestibular aqueducts; ExAC: Exome Aggregation Consortium; GATK: Genome Analysis Toolkit; GERP: Genomic Evolutionary Rate Profiling; GME: Greater Middle East Variome Project; GnomAD: Genome Aggregation Database; HI: Hearing Impairment; MAF: Minor Allele Frequency; NSHI: Non-syndromic Hearing Impairment; OMIM: Online Mendelian Inheritance of Man; PCR: Polymerase Chain Reaction; XHMM: eXome-Hidden Markov Model

Acknowledgements

We are very grateful to the families that participated in this study. Sequencing was provided by the University of Washington Center for Mendelian Genomics (UW-CMG) and was funded by the National Human Genome Research Institute and the National Heart, Lung and Blood Institute grant HG006493 to Drs. DAB, MJB, and SML. The University of Washington Center for Mendelian Genomics (UW-CMG) contains:
Michael J. Bamshad[1,2], Suzanne M. Leal[3], and Deborah A. Nickerson[1].
Peter Anderson[1], Marcus Annable[1], Elizabeth E. Blue[1], Kati J. Buckingham[1], Imen Chakchouk[3], Jennifer Chin[1], Jessica X Chong[1], Rodolfo Cornejo Jr.[1], Colleen P. Davis[1], Christopher Frazar[1], Martha Horike-Pyne[1], Gail P. Jarvik[1], Eric Johanson[1], Ashley N. Kang[1], Tom Kolar[1], Stephanie A. Krauter[1], Colby T. Marvin[1], Sean McGee[1], Daniel J. McGoldrick[1], Karynne Patterson[1], Sam W. Phillips[1], Jessica Pijoan[1], Matthew A. Richardson[1], Peggy D. Robertson[1], Isabelle Schrauwen[3], Krystal Slattery[1], Kathryn M. Shively[1], Joshua D. Smith[1], Monica Tackett[1], Alice E. Tattersall[1], Marc Wegener[1], Jeffrey M. Weiss[1], Marsha M. Wheeler[1], Qian Yi[1], and Di Zhang[3][1]University of Washington [2]Seattle Children's Hospital [3]Baylor College of Medicine.

Funding

This work was supported by the Higher Education Commission of Pakistan (to W.A.) and National Institutes of Health (NIH)-National Institute of Deafness and other Disorders grants R01 DC011651 and R01 DC003594 (to S.M.L). Exome sequencing performed at the University of Washington Center for Mendelian Genomics was funded by the NIH–National Human Genome Research Institute and National Heart, Lung, and Blood Institute grant UM1 HG006493 (to D.A.N., M.J.B. and S.M.L.).

Web resources

ANNOVAR, http://annovar.openbioinformatics.org/.
Burrows-Wheeler Aligner, http://bio-bwa.sourceforge.net/.
Clinvar, https://www.ncbi.nlm.nih.gov/clinvar/
Combined Annotation Dependent Depletion (CADD), http://cadd.gs.washington.edu/.
Copy number inference from exome reads (CoNIFER), http://conifer.sourceforge.net/.
Database of Genomic Variants (DGV), http://dgv.tcag.ca/dgv/app/home
dbNSFP, https://sites.google.com/site/jpopgen/dbNSFP
dbSNP, https://www.ncbi.nlm.nih.gov/projects/SNP/
Digenic Diseases Database (DIDA), http://dida.ibsquare.be/.
Exome Aggregation Consortium (ExAC), http://exac.broadinstitute.org/.
Genome Aggregation Database (gnomAD), http://gnomad.broadinstitute.org/.
Genome Analysis Toolkit (GATK), https://software.broadinstitute.org/gatk/
Genomic Evolutionary Rate Profiling (GERP), http://mendel.stanford.edu/SidowLab/downloads/gerp/

Greater Middle East (GME) Variome Project, http://igm.ucsd.edu/gme
MutationTaster, http://www.mutationtaster.org/.
Online Mendelian Inheritance of Man (OMIM), https://www.omim.org/.
PhastCons and PhyloP, http://compgen.cshl.edu/phast/
Picard, http://broadinstitute.github.io/picard/
eXome-Hidden Markov Model (XHMM), https://atgu.mgh.harvard.edu/xhmm/

Author's contributions

Exome sequencing was performed at the UW-CMG, under supervision of DAN, MJB and SML. AA performed Sanger sequencing and sample handling. Data analysis was done by IS, IC and the UW-CMG. KL, I, KS, WA were involved in sample collection, DNA extraction and clinical evaluation. IS and SML prepared the manuscript, all authors reviewed, read and approved the final manuscript.

Competing interests

I.S. and W.A. are members of the BMC Medical Genetics editorial board. All other authors declare that they have no competing interests.

Author details

[1]Center for Statistical Genetics, Department of Molecular and Human Genetics, Baylor College of Medicine, One Baylor Plaza 700D, Houston, TX 77030, USA. [2]Department of Biotechnology, Faculty of Biological Sciences, Quaid-i-Azam University, Islamabad, Pakistan. [3]Department of Biochemistry, Faculty of Biological Sciences, Quaid-i-Azam University, Islamabad, Pakistan. [4]Department of Genome Sciences, University of Washington, Seattle, Washington, USA. [5]Department of Pediatrics, University of Washington, Seattle, Washington, USA.

References

1. Zheng QY, Yan D, Ouyang XM, Du LL, Yu H, Chang B, et al. Digenic inheritance of deafness caused by mutations in genes encoding cadherin 23 and protocadherin 15 in mice and humans. Hum Mol Genet. 2005;14:103–11.
2. Yang T, Vidarsson H, Rodrigo-Blomqvist S, Rosengren SS, Enerbäck S, Smith RJH. Transcriptional control of SLC26A4 is involved in Pendred syndrome and nonsyndromic enlargement of vestibular aqueduct (DFNB4). Am J Hum Genet. 2007;80:1055–63.
3. Yang T, Gurrola JG, Wu H, Chiu SM, Wangemann P, Snyder PM, et al. Mutations of KCNJ10 together with mutations of SLC26A4 cause digenic nonsyndromic hearing loss associated with enlarged vestibular aqueduct syndrome. Am J Hum Genet. 2009;84:651–7.
4. del Castillo I, Villamar M, Moreno-Pelayo MA, del Castillo FJ, Álvarez A, Tellería D, et al. A deletion involving the Connexin 30 gene in nonsyndromic hearing impairment. N Engl J Med. 2002;346:243–9.
5. Mei L, Chen J, Zong L, Zhu Y, Liang C, Jones RO, et al. A deafness mechanism of digenic Cx26 (GJB2) and Cx30 (GJB6) mutations: reduction of endocochlear potential by impairment of heterogeneous gap junctional function in the cochlear lateral wall. Neurobiol Dis. 2017;108:195–203.
6. Liu X-Z, Yuan Y, Yan D, Ding EH, Ouyang XM, Fei Y, et al. Digenic inheritance of non-syndromic deafness caused by mutations at the gap junction proteins Cx26 and Cx31. Hum Genet. 2009;125:53–62.
7. Leone MP, Palumbo P, Ortore R, Castellana S, Palumbo O, Melchionda S, et al. Putative TMPRSS3/GJB2 digenic inheritance of hearing loss detected by targeted resequencing. Mol Cell Probes. 2017;33:24–7.
8. Yoshimura H, Iwasaki S, Nishio S, Kumakawa K, Tono T, Kobayashi Y, et al. Massively parallel DNA sequencing facilitates diagnosis of patients with usher syndrome type 1. PLoS One. 2014;9:e90688.
9. Ebermann I, Phillips JB, Liebau MC, Koenekoop RK, Schermer B, Lopez I, et al. PDZD7 is a modifier of retinal disease and a contributor to digenic usher syndrome. J Clin Invest. 2010;120:1812–23.
10. Rodriguez-Paris J, Schrijver I. The digenic hypothesis unraveled: the GJB6 del (GJB6-D13S1830) mutation causes allele-specific loss of GJB2 expression in cis. Biochem Biophys Res Commun. 2009;389:354–9.
11. Rodriguez-Paris J, Tamayo ML, Gelvez N, Schrijver I. Allele-specific impairment of GJB2 expression by GJB6 deletion del (GJB6-D13S1854). PLoS One. 2011;6:e21665.
12. Balciuniene J, Dahl N, Borg E, Samuelsson E, Koisti MJ, Pettersson U, et al. Evidence for digenic inheritance of nonsyndromic hereditary hearing loss in a Swedish family. Am J Hum Genet. 1998;63:786–93.
13. Gazzo A, Raimondi D, Daneels D, Moreau Y, Smits G, Van Dooren S, et al. Understanding mutational effects in digenic diseases. Nucleic Acids Res. 2017;45:e140.
14. Deltas C. Digenic inheritance and genetic modifiers. Clin Genet. 2018;93:429–38.
15. Schäffer AA. Digenic inheritance in medical genetics. J Med Genet. 2013;50:641–52.
16. Sambrook J, Russell DW. Purification of nucleic acids by extraction with phenol:chloroform. Cold Spring Harb Protoc. 2006;2006:pdb.prot4455.
17. Wang K, Li M, Hakonarson H. ANNOVAR: functional annotation of genetic variants from high-throughput sequencing data. Nucleic Acids Res. 2010;38:e164.

18. Krumm N, Sudmant PH, Ko A, O'Roak BJ, Malig M, Coe BP, et al. Copy number variation detection and genotyping from exome sequence data. Genome Res. 2012;22:1525–32.
19. Fromer M, Purcell SM. Using XHMM Software to Detect Copy Number Variation in Whole-Exome Sequencing Data. Curr Protoc Hum Genet. 2014; 81:7.23.1–21.
20. Koressaar T, Remm M. Enhancements and modifications of primer design program Primer3. Bioinformatics. 2007;23:1289–91.
21. Lek M, Karczewski KJ, Minikel EV, Samocha KE, Banks E, Fennell T, et al. Analysis of protein-coding genetic variation in 60,706 humans. Nature. 2016; 536:285–91.
22. Scott EM, Halees A, Itan Y, Spencer EG, He Y, Azab MA, et al. Characterization of greater middle eastern genetic variation for enhanced disease gene discovery. Nat Genet. 2016;48:1071–6.
23. Bademci G, Foster J, Mahdieh N, Bonyadi M, Duman D, Cengiz FB, et al. Comprehensive analysis via exome sequencing uncovers genetic etiology in autosomal recessive nonsyndromic deafness in a large multiethnic cohort. Genet Med. 2016;18:364–71.
24. Landrum MJ, Lee JM, Benson M, Brown G, Chao C, Chitipiralla S, et al. ClinVar: public archive of interpretations of clinically relevant variants. Nucleic Acids Res. 2016;44:D862–8.
25. Oshima A, Jaijo T, Aller E, Millan JM, Carney C, Usami S, et al. Mutation profile of the CDH23 gene in 56 probands with usher syndrome type I. Hum Mutat. 2008;29:E37–46.
26. MacDonald JR, Ziman R, Yuen RKC, Feuk L, Scherer SW. The database of genomic variants: a curated collection of structural variation in the human genome. Nucleic Acids Res. 2014;42:D986–92.
27. Caberlotto E, Michel V, Foucher I, Bahloul A, Goodyear RJ, Pepermans E, et al. Usher type 1G protein sans is a critical component of the tip-link complex, a structure controlling actin polymerization in stereocilia. Proc Natl Acad Sci U S A. 2011;108:5825–30.
28. Woychik RP, Alagramam KN, Murcia CL, Kwon HY, Pawlowski KS, Wright CG. The mouse Ames waltzer hearing-loss mutant is caused by mutation of Pcdh15, a novel protocadherin gene. Nat Genet. 2001;27:99–102.
29. Zheng QY, Scarborough JD, Zheng Y, Yu H, Choi D, Gillespie PG. Digenic inheritance of deafness caused by 8J allele of myosin-VIIA and mutations in other usher I genes. Hum Mol Genet. 2012;21:2588–98.
30. Cordell HJ. Epistasis: what it means, what it doesn't mean, and statistical methods to detect it in humans. Hum Mol Genet. 2002;11:2463–8.
31. Ameratunga R, Woon S-T, Bryant VL, Steele R, Slade C, Leung EY, et al. Clinical implications of Digenic inheritance and epistasis in primary immunodeficiency disorders. Front Immunol. 2017;8:1965.

4

The altered activity of P53 signaling pathway by *STK11* gene mutations and its cancer phenotype in Peutz-Jeghers syndrome

Yu-Liang Jiang[1,2†], Zi-Ye Zhao[3,4†], Bai-Rong Li[2†], Fu Yang[3], Jing Li[2], Xiao-Wei Jin[2], Hao Wang[4], En-Da Yu[4], Shu-Han Sun[3*] and Shou-Bin Ning[2*]

Abstract

Background: Peutz-Jeghers syndrome (PJS) is caused by mutations in serine/threonine kinase 11 (*STK11*) gene. The increased cancer risk has been connected to P53 pathway.

Methods: PJS probands with *STK11* mutation were included in the function analysis. P53 activity elevated by *STK11* mutants was investigated using dual-luciferase reporter assay in vitro after constructing expression vectors of *STK11* wild type and mutants generated by site-directed substitution. The association between the P53 activity and clinicopathological factors was analysis, especially the cancer history.

Results: Thirteen probands with *STK11* mutations were involved, and within the mutations, c.G924A was novel. P53 activity elevation caused by 6 truncating mutations were significantly lower than that of *STK11* wild type ($P < 0.05$). Family history of cancer was observed in 5 families. Within them, P53 activity was reduced and cancer occurred before 40 in 2 families, while it was not significantly changed and cancers happened after 45 in the other 3 families.

Conclusions: The affected P53 activity caused by *STK11* mutations in PJS patients is significantly associated with protein truncation, while cancer risk in PJS can be elevated through pathways rather than P53 pathway. P53 activity test is probably a useful supporting method to predict cancer risk in PJS, which could be helpful in clinical practice.

Keywords: Peutz-Jeghers syndrome (PJS), *STK11* gene, *P53* gene, Cancer risk, Reporter gene technique

Backgroud

Peutz-Jeghers syndrome (PJS; OMIM #175200) is an autosomal dominant disorder characterised by mucocutaneous melanin pigmentation (MP), gastrointestinal(GI) hamartomatous polyposis, and an increased risk for the development of various neoplasms [1, 2], which is rare with a low incidence of 1/50,000 [3]. The cumulative lifetime risk is 20, 43, 71, and 89% at ages of 40, 50, 60 and 65 years, respectively [4].

* Correspondence: shsun@vip.sina.com; ningshoubin@126.com
†Yu-Liang Jiang, Zi-Ye Zhao and Bai-Rong Li contributed equally to this work.
[3]Department of Medical Genetics, Naval Medical University, Shanghai 200433, China
[2]Department of Gastroenterology, Airforce General Hospital of PLA, Beijing 100142, China
Full list of author information is available at the end of the article

Germline mutations in the serine–threonine kinase 11 (*STK11*) gene on chromosome 19p13.3 were identified as a major genetic cause of PJS in 1998 [5, 6]. This gene is divided into 9 coding exons that encode a 433 amino-acid protein, which acts as a tumor suppressor. The STK11 protein is mainly comprised of 3 major domains: an N-terminal regulatory domain, a catalytic kinase domain, and a C terminal regulatory domain [7]. Amino acids 49–309 of STK11 are the catalytic kinase domain, which can form a complex with STRAD and scaffold protein 25 (MO25) to maintain kinase activation [8]. Several studies have described a role of STK11 in cell cycle arrest [9], P53 mediated apoptosis [10], Wnt signaling [11, 12], TGF-β signaling [13], Ras induced cell transformation [14], and cell polarity [15–18].

P53, the most widely studied tumor suppressor gene, regulates of the expression of various genes that are related to cell cycle arrest, DNA damage repair and apoptosis [19], and furtherly controls the cell proliferation and apoptosis. *P53* gene mutations have been found in about 50% of human cancers, suggesting the important role of *P53* inactivation in tumorigenesis [20]. *STK11* has been reported to play a critical role in P53-mediated cell apoptosis [10]. $STK11^{+/-}/P53^{+/-}$ mice showed a dramatically reduced life span and increased tumor incidence compared to the mice with either *STK11* or *P53* single gene knockout, indicating that *P53* and *STK11* gene mutations cooperate in tumor progression [21].

In this study, we identified mutations in *STK11* gene from Chinese PJS probands, and observed the changes in P53 activity brought by different *STK11* mutants and their association with the canceration in PJS.

Methods

Patient and sample collection

Materials in this study were collected retrospectively. A total of 154 PJS patients were ascertained in Airforce General Hospital of PLA between May 2013 and April 2016. Blood samples of the probands and all available family members were collected after obtaining informed consent. This study was approved by the Medical Ethics Committee, Airforce General Hospital of PLA. Only PJS patients with both complete information and mutation detected and successfully constructed were included in final analysis.

Clinical diagnosis for PJS was based on the presence of any one of the following clinical findings which was recommended by WHO [22]: (1) three or more histologically confirmed PJ polyps (PJP) in the gastrointestinal tract, (2) any number of PJPs detected with a positive family history of PJS, (3) characteristic mucocutaneous pigmentation with a positive family history of PJS, and (4) any number of PJPs together with characteristic mucocutaneous pigmentation (MP).

Genomic DNA isolation and mutation analysis

Genomic DNA of peripheral blood leucocytes was extracted routinely by animal genomic DNA kit (TSP201, TsingKe Biotech, Beijing, China) according to the manufacturer's instructions. All 9 coding exons and their flanking sequences of the *STK11* gene were amplified by the use of primers listed in Additional file 1: Table. S1. Polymerase chain reactions (PCR) of *STK11* exons were performed in a 50-ul reaction which contained 0.4 uM of each primer, 50 ng genomic DNA, and 25ul 2 × modified DNA polymerase mix (TSE004, TsingKe Biotech, Beijing, China). The PCRs were performed under the following conditions: denaturation at 95 °C for 4 min, followed by 35 thermal cycles, each composed of 95 °C for 30 s, 58 °C for 30 s, and 72 °C for 45 s.

All available family members underwent *STK11* germline mutation test to confirm cosegregation of the mutation with the disease. For frameshift mutation, T vector assay (pClone007 Vector Kit, TSV-007, TsingKe Biotech, Beijing, China) was used to identify each haplotype by constructing monoclonal cells [23]. In order to rule out polymorphisms and to confirm the pathogenic effects of the variations, 100 chromosomes from 50 unrelated ethnicity-matched healthy individuals were also screened for the presence of the mutations. Allele frequency of each mutation in ExAC was checked [24].

The PCR products were gel- and column-purified and directly sequenced. The purified PCR fragments were then sequenced using BigDye Terminator on an ABI Prism 3100 genetic analyzer (Applied Biosystems, Foster City, CA, USA) by Majorbio Co. Ltd. (Shanghai, China). The results were used to performance sequence alignment according to *STK11* gene sequence (NP_000446.1 and NM_000455.4 in GRCh38.p7). All experiment details above had been reported previously [23, 25].

Function prediction and analysis, and association with Clinicopathological features

To predict the effects of mutations in *STK11*, PolyPhen-2 (http://genetics.bwh.harvard.edu/pph2) and SIFT (http://sift.jcvi.org/) were used for specific mutations.

To investigate the impact on P53 activity, we employed dual-luciferase reporter gene technique. Human *STK11* cDNA was amplified from the HEK293T cells, and cloned into pcDNA3.1 (+) (V790–20, Carlsbad, CA) vector to create expression vectors of wild type (wt) and mutant (mu) of *STK11* gene. The mutant site was generated by site-directed substitution (D0206, Beyotime, Nantong, Jiangsu, China).

The luciferase reporter plasmid pp53-TA-luc which contained a P53-responsive element (D2223, Beyotime, Nantong, Jiangsu, China) was transfected into the cells, together with pRL-TK vector (E2241, Promega, Madison, WI) and pcDNA3.1(+)-*STK11* expression vector, using the Lipo6000 transfection reagent (C0526, Beyotime, Nantong, Jiangsu, China). pRL-TK vector expresses wild-type Renilla luciferase reporter and is used as internal control by cotransfected with pp53-TA-luc. Twenty-four hours after transfection, cells were lysed in a passive lysis buffer, which was a component of Dual-Luciferase® Reporter Assay Systems (E1910, Promega, Madison, WI) [26]. According to the manufacturer's protocol, luciferase activity was measured with the Synergy 2 modular multi-mode reader (BioTek Instruments, Winooski, VT). The ratio of pp53 to pRL-TK was calculated in each assay. Each experiment was repeated triple times from cell seeding to luciferase activity measurement. Data were showed as mean ± standard deviation. Student's t test was used to test the significance, and $p < 0.05$ was considered as significant.

Factors related to cancer history including sex, family history and P53 activity change were compared using the Fisher exact test, and $p < 0.05$ was considered as significant.

Results

During the period investigated, 154 PJS patients were diagnosed in our department, among whom, 89 declined to participant in mutation test, and 26 had inadequate information. Finally, 39 patients from 31 unrelated families had blood samples collected and received mutation detection. A total of 17 disease-specific mutations in *STK11* were detected in 31 probands. Since 3 mutations concerning splicing site (c.290 + 1G > A, c.734-1G > A, c.863-8_870del16bp) could not be investigated by reporter gene assay, and one mutation (c.426_448del23bp) was hard to be generated by site-directed mutagenesis, there were 13 mutants involved in the final analysis (Additional file 2: Figure S1). Expression vectors of the wild-type and the 13 mutant *STK11* gene were constructed for function analysis, and the corresponding PJS families and individuals were included in analysis.

Clinical features

As shown in Table 1, the 13 probands from unrelated families were 7 familial and 6 sporadic patients, and their native places were various in China (Additional file 1: Table S2). The median age of diagnosis, first polypectomy and at present was 25, 28 and 33 years. Seven of these families (PJS03, 05, 06, 07, 09, 10 and 12) showed autosomal dominant pattern and the remaining 6 cases (PJS01, 02, 04, 08, 11 and 13) are sporadic (Fig. 1a). MP on the lips, buccal mucosa, and digits were observed at all patients (Fig. 1b). Twelve probands in these families underwent laparotomy or polypectomy due to intussusception or intestinal obstruction (Fig. 1c and d). Three probands of these families (PJS03, 06 and 11) in this study had developed colon cancer before 40 years old (Fig. 1e), and cancer history existed in 3 families (PJS06, 09 and 12). Detail information is showed in Table 2.

Table 1 Characteristics of the cohort with PJS

Characteristics		Number (percentage)	
Probands with mutation test		31	
Mutation detected		17	54.8%
Probands enrolled in the luciferase analysis		13	
Age[a] Median (range)	D	25 (12–37) years	
	F	28 (11–39) years	
	P	33 (24–51) years	
Gender			
Male		7	51.8%
Female		6	48.2%
Family history			
Familial		7	51.8%
Sporadic		6	48.2%
Cancer history		5	38.5%

[a] D, diagnosis; F, first polypectomy or laparotomy; P, present. There were 12 probands having polypectomy

Mutation analysis

Sequencing analysis identified 13 mutations of *STK11* gene in the 13 probands which were included in the function analysis (Table 2, Fig. 2a). Most of the mutations have been previously reported [25, 27–29] except for c.924G > A (Fig. 3). The 13 mutations included 8 truncating mutations (4 frameshift and 4 nonsense) and 5 missense mutations. Regarding frameshift mutations, those of PJS05, 06 and 07 (p.P281Rfs*6, p.P281Pfs*4 and p.L285Lfs*2) led to a partial loss of the kinase domain and a completed loss of the C-terminal, and the one in PJS11 (p.P321Hfs*38) led to a partial loss of the α-helix of the C-terminus. PJS02, 03, 04 and 10 possessed nonsense mutations of *STK11* that resulted in the production of truncated proteins (p.E65*, p.K84*, p.Y118* and p.W308*) (Additional file 2: Figure S2A). Among the PJS cases owning the 13 mutations, 7 were familial and 6 were sporadic, and 5 of them were associated with cancer history. Tested in 100 chromosomes from control individuals, 16 of the detected mutations were not discovered and only c.1062C > G was detected in 5/100 controls. c.1062C > G and c.1225C > T were recorded in ExAC database with allele frequencies of 0.005757 and 0.000147, and all other mutations were not recorded (Table 2).

Function analysis and association with Clinicopathological features

Analyzed using PolyPhen-2, missense mutation c.911 was predicted as probably damaging, mutations c.56, c.862 and c.1225 were predicted as possible damaging, while c.1062 was benign (Table 2).

Analyzed using SIFT, missense mutation c.56 and c.1225 were predicted as intolerated, and mutations c.862, c.911 and c.1062 were tolerated (Table 2).

P53 activity was measured using dual-luciferase reporter gene technique after cotransfection of pp53-TA-luc, pRL-TK vector, and pcDNA3.1 (+)-*STK11*-wt or -mu. Luciferase activity was significantly elevated when *STK11*-wt was transfected into HEK293T cells. Using the elevation caused by *STK11*-wt as control, elevations by mutants c.193, c.250, c.354, c.842, c.843 and c.855 were significantly reduced, while those by mutants c.56, c.862, c.911,

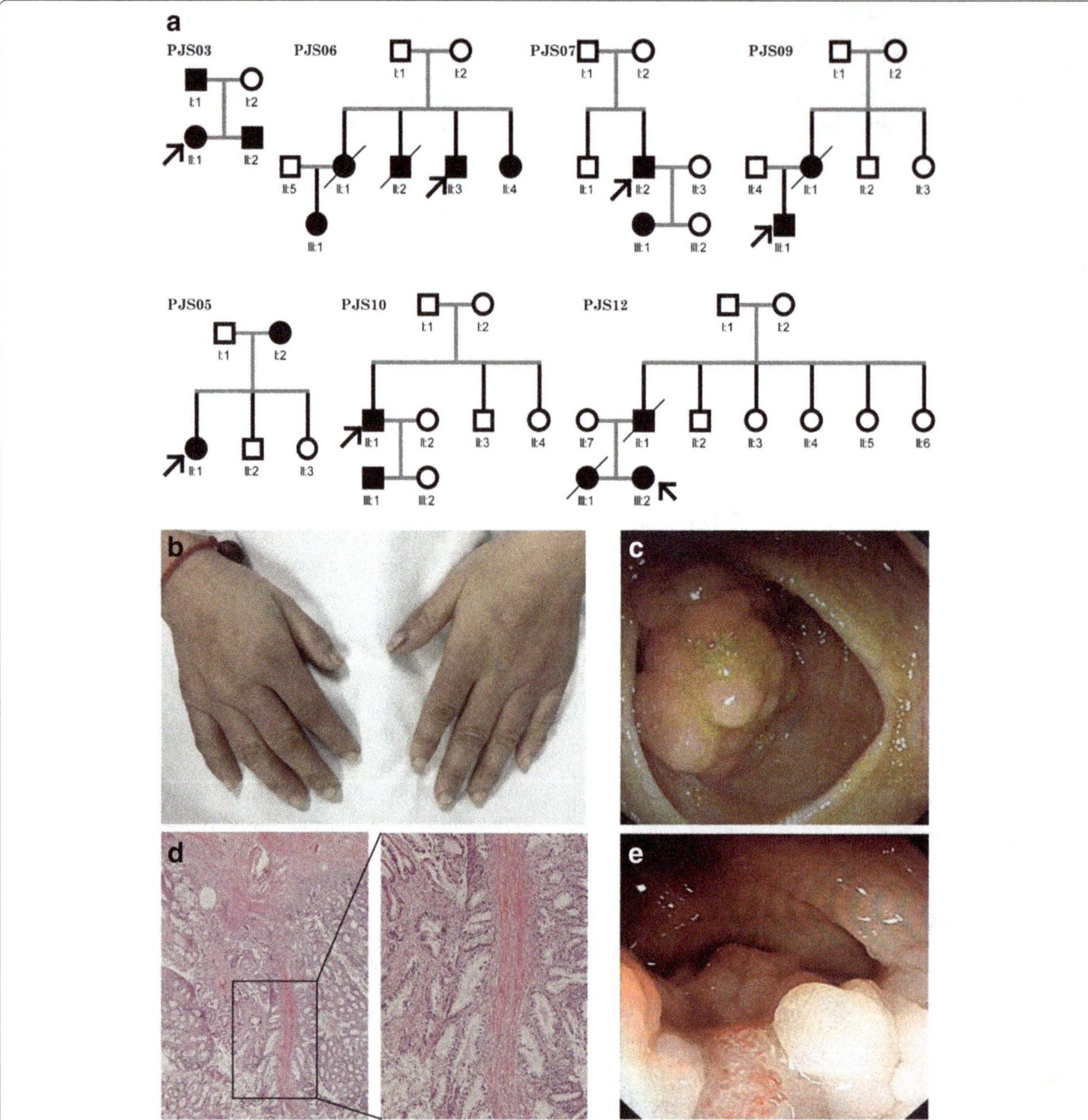

Fig. 1 Genogram and Clinicopathological feature of PJS patients. **a** Pedigrees of the 7 PJS cases with positive family history. Roman numerals indicate generations and Arabic numbers indicate individuals. Squares = males, circles = females. Affected individuals are denoted by solid symbols and unaffected individuals are denoted by open symbols. The probands are indicated by arrows. **b** and **c**. Melanin pigmentation spots of the fingers, endoscopic view of the recurrent polyp near the anastomotic stoma after the radical surgery of colon cancer and were observed in the proband of PJS03. **d** Hematoxylin-eosin-stained tissue slices of the polyp specimens above confirm hamartomatous. Left, × 40 magnification; right, × 100 magnification. **e** Endoscopic view of the polyps in PJS11, one of which had cancerogenesis

c.924, c.962_963, c.1062 and c.1225 were not changed significantly (Fig. 2b).

There were total 5 families with cancer history (PJS03, 06, 09, 11 and 12). Within the 5 cancer families, P53 activity was reduced and cancer occurred before 40 in 2 families (PJS03 and 06), while in the other 3 families, P53 activity was not significantly changed and cancers happened after 45 years old (PJS09, 11 and 12) (Table 3).

Through Fisher exact test, none of the factors (sex, family history and P53 activity change) was significantly associated with cancer in PJS (Additional file 1: Table S3).

Table 2 Clinical characteristics and function analysis of *STK11* mutations in PJS patients

ID	FH[a]	Sex[b]	Age[c]			Polyp location	Int	Mutation	Exon	Function domain	Effect	Function Prediction		ExAC allele frequency	P53 activity	Index cancer	Cancers in family
			D	F	P							PolyPhen-2	SIFT				
PJS01	S	M	12	11	24	SB, C	Yes	c.56C > G	1	N	p.S19 W	0.663	0.00	0	Normal		
PJS02	S	F	15	15	29	SB	Yes	c.193G > T	1	I	p.E65[a]	NA	NA	0	Decreased		
PJS03	F	F	31	27	33	SB, C	Yes	c.250A > T	1	II	p.K84[a]	NA	NA	0	Decreased	colon	
PJS04	S	F	17	12	28	SB	Yes	c.354C > G	2	IV	p.Y118[a]	NA	NA	0	Decreased		
PJS05	F	F	23	23	27	SB, C	Yes	c.842delC	6	XI	p.P281Rfs[a]6	NA	NA	0	Decreased		
PJS06	F	M	21	21	45	SB, C	Yes	c.843insC	6	XI	p.P281Pfs[a]4	NA	NA	0	Decreased	colon	lung, lymphoma
PJS07	F	M	32	32	38	SB, C	Yes	c.855delG	6	XI	p.L285Lfs[a]2	NA	NA	0	Decreased		
PJS08	S	F	31	15	35	G, SB, C	Yes	c.862G > A	6	XI	p.G288S	0.0.573	0.10	0	Normal		
PJS09	F	M	30	30	51	SB, C	No	c.911G > C	7	XI	p.R304P	0.0.987	0.05	0	Normal		stomach
PJS10	F	M	24	39	43	SB, C	Yes	c.924G > A	8	XI	p.W308[a]	NA	NA	0	Normal		
PJS11	S	M	37	37	47	C	Yes	c.962_963delCC	8	C	p.P321Hfs[a]38	NA	NA	0	Normal	colon	
PJS12	F	F	12	12	29	G, SB, C	Yes	c.1062C > G	8	C	p.F354 L	0.022	0.36	0.005757	Normal		colon
PJS13	S	M	24	23	30	G	Yes	c.1225C > T	9	C	p.R409W	0.549	0.00	0.000147	Normal		

[a]Family history. S = sporadic, F = familial. [b] M = male, F = female. [c]D, diagnosis; F, first polypectomy or laparotomy; P, present. If a patient is dead, the present age with a underline refers to the age of death. G = stomach, SB = small bowel, C = colon. Int = intussusception. NA = not available

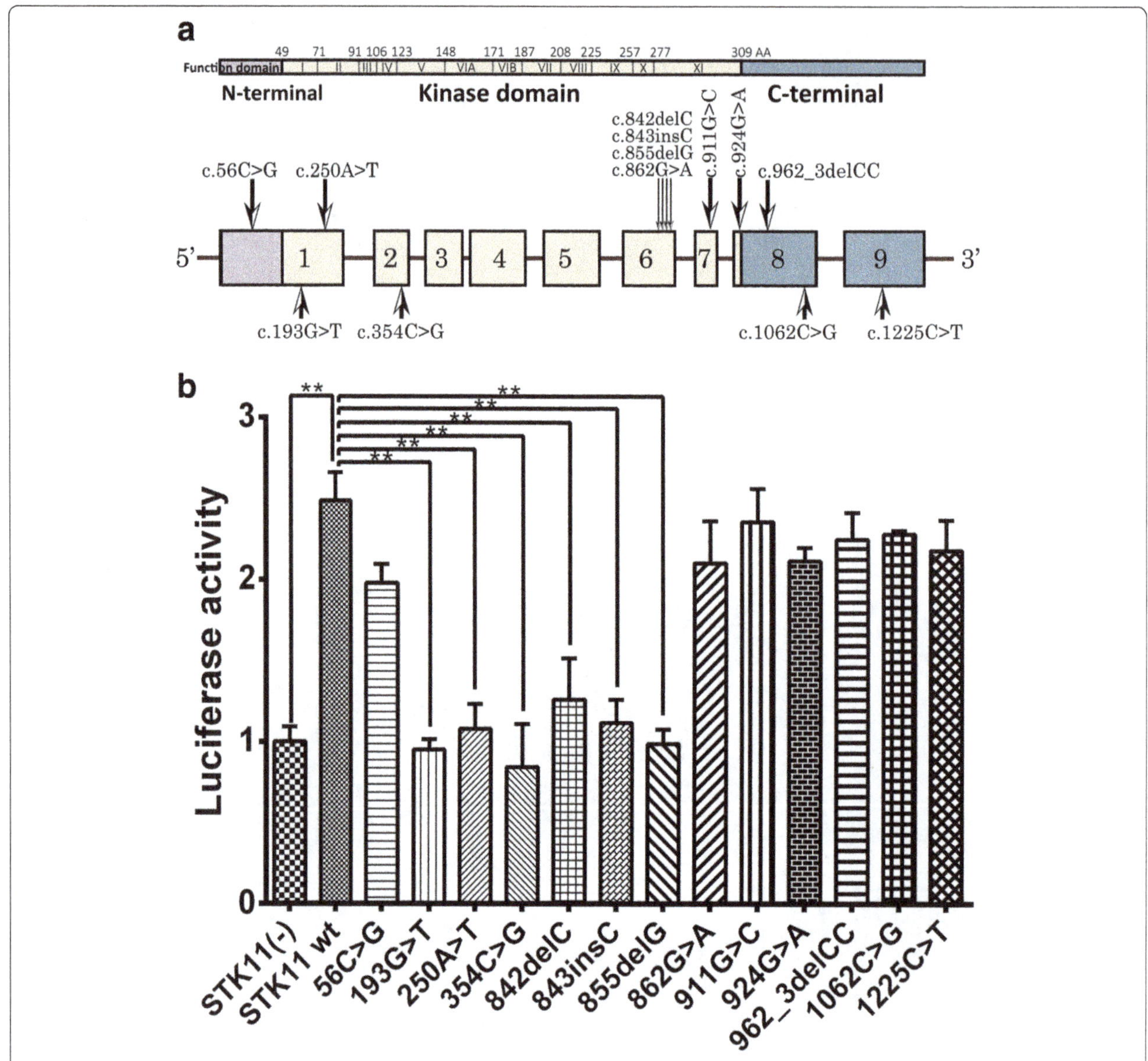

Fig. 2 Distribution of all the *STK11* mutations detected (**a**) and P53 pathway activity tested by dual-luciferase reporter gene technique in HEK293T cells transfected with these mutants (3 replicates) (**b**). Double-asterisks present significant ($p < 0.05$)

Discussion

Peutz-Jeghers syndrome (PJS) has various manifestations related to GI polyps, such as abdominal pain, rectal blood loss, chronic anemia, prolapsed rectal polyp, bowel obstruction and clinical intussusception [30–32]. Beyond these symptoms, PJS patients also have an increased risk of cancer at multiple sites, including the GI tract, breast, ovary, testis, and lung [33]. As the only validated and the major pathogenic gene in PJS, *STK11* is involved in cell cycle regulation and apoptosis, whose abnormality can induce and promote tumorigenesis. It has been proven that *STK11*-mediated cell cycle regulation has been shown to be regulated via P53-dependent and P53-independent mechanisms [34–39]. STK11 can directly interact with and phosphorylate P53, and to mediate P53-induced apoptosis [40]. What's more, PJS-associated *STK11* mutants can diminish P53 activity [41].

In our study, we investigated the effect of *STK11* mutations on the transcriptional activity of P53, and we found that six of them inhibited the activity significantly compared with the wild-type. All of the 6 mutations resulted in protein truncation, and all the truncated protein lost partial kinase domain and completed C-terminal. The other seven mutations which didn't significantly decrease P53 activity located in the margin of or outside the kinase domain, and they caused only single amino acid change in the margin of or outside the kinase domain or loss of C-terminal regulatory domain. So we suspected the main part of the kinase domain or

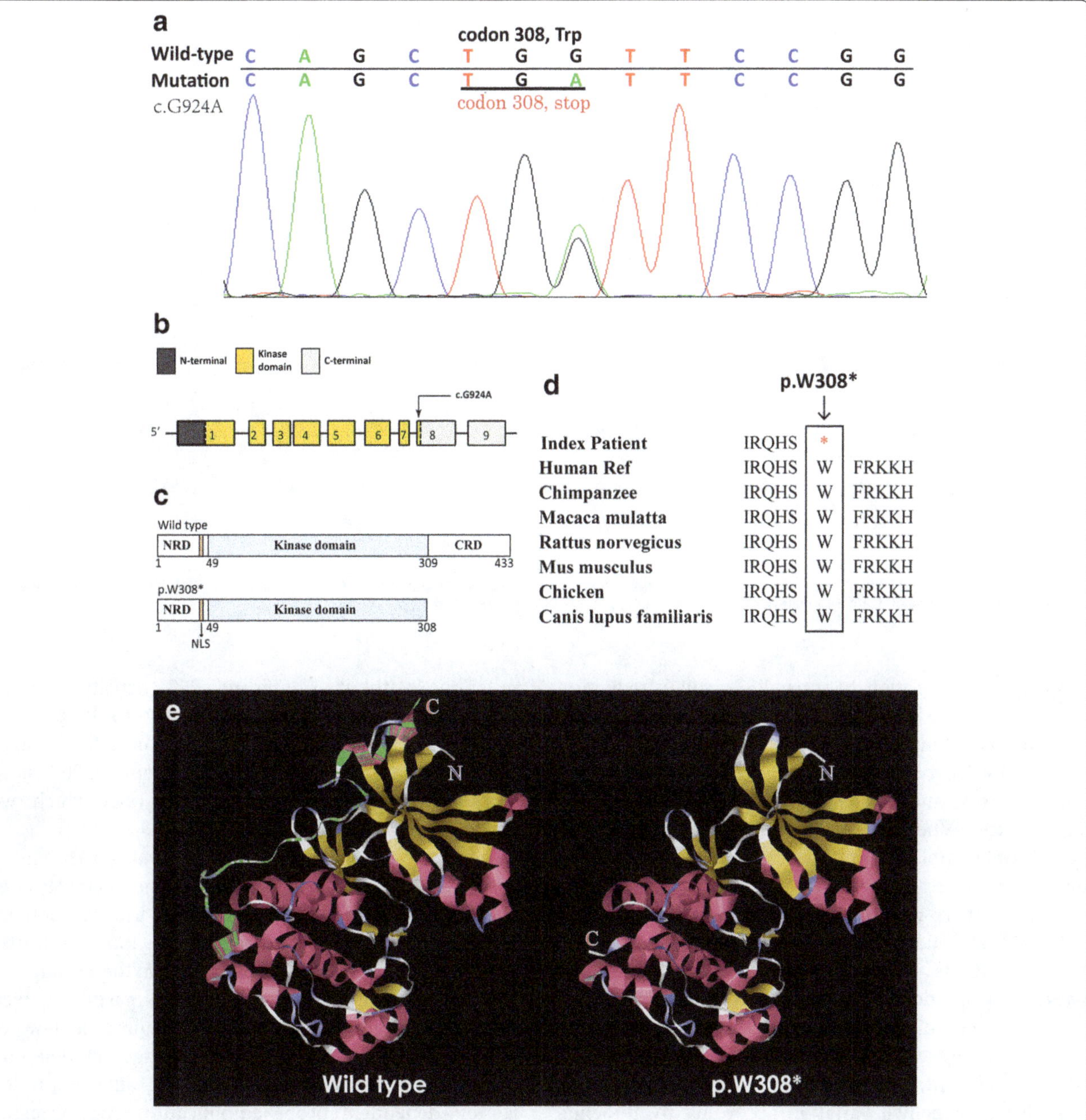

Fig. 3 Details about the novel mutation c.G924A (p.W308*). **a** Sanger sequencing showed a heterozygous mutation. **b** The structure of STK11 gene. The mutation is located in exon 8. **c** Schematics of the secondary structure or functional domains of the STK11 protein. The mutant protein results in a partial loss of kinase domain and a complete loss of the C-terminal domain compared to the wild type. NLS, Nuclear localization signal, NRD or CRD, N- or C-terminal regulatory domain. **d** Evolutionary conservation of amino acid residues altered across different species. **e** The mutant proteins was predicted to result in partial loss of the kinase domain and complete loss of the C-terminal domain of the a-helix (which is labelled using green gaps in the wild type protein) by Swiss-Model online software (http://swissmodel.expasy.org/) compared to the wild type (for which the 3D template model used was 2wtk.2.C) [46]

some key points within it was key for STK11 depended P53 activity rather than the boundary of it or regulatory parts, and truncating mutations were easier to cause the change since they usually resulted in large-scale loss of the amino acid residues. We also encountered three splice site mutations, which cannot be investigated by the luciferase assay. Since splicing errors usually cause exon skipping or abnormal mRNA processing and mRNA degradation, the large-scale changes may also result in P53 activity decrease. But due to the limitation of patient number, the assumption cannot be justified at the present.

Table 3 Characteristics of affected individuals in PJS families with cancer history

Family	Individual	Sex	Age[b]					Cause of death	Mutation	Prediction		P53 activity
			MP	D	F	C	P			PolyPhen	SIFT	
PJS03	I:1	M	NR	NR	NR	60	60	Colon cancer	c.250A > T/ p.K84[a]	NA	NA	Decreased
	II:1[a]	F	5	31	27	27	33	Colon cancer				
	II:2	M	6	19	26	–	28	–				
PJS06	II:1	F	NR	NR	NR	NR	40	Lung cancer	c.843insC/ p.P281Pfs[a]4	NA	NA	Decreased
	II:2	M	NR	NR	NR	NR	39	Lymphoma				
	II:3[a]	M	3	21	21	39	45	Colon cancer				
	II:4	F	3	20	20	–	39	–				
	III:1	F	3	11	18	–	30	–				
PJS09	II:1	F	NR	55	NR	65	65	Stomach cancer	c.911G > C/ p.R304P	Probable damaging	Tolerated	Normal
	III:1[a]	M	7	30	30	–	51	–				
PJS11	Index[a]	M	6	37	37	47	47	Colon cancer	c.962_963delCC/ p.P321Hfs[a]38	NA	NA	Normal
PJS12	II:1	M	NR	43	43	48	52	Colon cancer	c.1062C > G/ p.F354 L	Benign	Tolerated	Normal
	III:1	F	4	15	–	–	16	Bowel obstruction				
	III:2[a]	F	4	12	12	–	29	–				

[a] Probands. [b] MP, melanin pigmentation; D, diagnosis; F, first polypectomy or laparotomy; C, canceration; P, present. If a patient is dead, the present age with a underline refers to the age of death. M = male, F = female. NA = not applicable. NR = not reported

As to the association between P53 activity reduction and cancerogenesis, there is no significance under statistical analysis. One of the reasons is the limited number of cases involved in analysis, just like another two analyses (sex and family history) without statistical significance. When analysed one by one, we can discover some implications from them. Early onset is a distinguishing feature of inherited cancer, and among our cases, there are cancers patients younger than 40 in PJS03 and 06 whose P53 activity is reduced by their mutations. While in PJS09, 11 and 12, cancer patients are older than 45, which means they are more like sporadic ones. Though there is a death case of youth in PJS12, it is not a certain case of cancer. More important, the mutation c.1062C > G is now regarded as a benign variation according to guideline from American College of Medical Genetics and Genomics (ACMG) [42, 43]. So most likely there is a large scale deletion rather than point mutation like c.1062C > G which is to blame. Another possibility is that P53 pathway is not the key one taking part in these three PJS families' cancerogenesis, and some non-P53 pathways leads to the occurrence of tumors.

There are still four families without cancer diagnosed, whose mutations were tested to impact P53 activity. The four mutation carriers are still young (29, 28, 27 and 38 years), so it is important to carry out a more rigorous and comprehensive follow-up as cancer prevention before any advanced methods come up. As to the other four PJS families carrying *STK11* mutations without significant P53 activity change, routine surveillance is still necessary to keep them uneventful. The recommendations for PJS management produced by Mallorca conference 2007 is a comprehensive and widely accepted one, which we can refer to [44, 45].

There are several important limitations to note. First, here we try to elucidate the pathways of tumorigenesis in PJS by investigating the P53 activity change caused by *STK11* mutations, but the mutations are not evenly distributed within the coding sequence and the limited number of cases involved largely limits the results. Second, quite a few of *STK11* mutations in PJS are large fragment deletion, so it is necessary to perform test like multiplex ligation–dependent probe amplification (MLPA) assay to make a more comprehensive analysis in the future. Finally, this is a single center study, and the data here may not be the whole picture of PJS in China. It will be very helpful if there is a national database of PJS patients.

Conclusions

The affected P53 activity caused by STK11 mutations in PJS patients is significantly associated with protein truncation, while cancer risk in PJS can be elevated through pathways rather than P53 pathway. P53 activity test is probably a useful supporting method to predict cancer risk in PJS, which could be helpful in clinical practice.

Abbreviations

DBE: Double-balloon enteroscopy; GI: Gastrointestinal; MLPA: Multiplex ligation–dependent probe amplification; MP: Melanin pigmentation; PCR: Polymerase chain reaction; PJP: Peutz-Jeghers syndrome polyp; PJS: Peutz-Jeghers syndrome; *STK11*: Serine/threonine kinase 11

Acknowledgements

We thank the subjects for their participation. We appreciate very much for Dr. Wen-Sheng LIN and Dr. Hong-Yu CHEN's kindly help with the pathologic and endoscopic pictures of the polyps.

Funding

This work was supported by National Natural Science Foundation of China (81500490), Application Research of Capital Clinical Character (Z151100004015215), Annual Project of Airforce General Hospital of PLA (KZ2015026 and KZ2016021), Discipline Construction Project - 1255 of Changhai Hospital (CH125530800) and National Key R&D Program of China (2017YFC1308802).

Authors' contributions

HW, JL and XWJ collected the samples and did the follow-up. YLJ and ZYZ performed experiments and did the analysis. EDY, BRL and FY designed the study and supervised the study. ZYZ wrote the manuscript. SHS and SBN supervised the study and revised the manuscript. All of the co-authors have read this manuscript and support this submission. All authors read and approved the final manuscript.

Competing interests

The authors declare that they have no competing interests.

Author details

[1]Hebei North University, Zhangjiakou 075061, Hebei Province, China. [2]Department of Gastroenterology, Airforce General Hospital of PLA, Beijing 100142, China. [3]Department of Medical Genetics, Naval Medical University, Shanghai 200433, China. [4]Department of Colorectal Surgery, Changhai Hospital, Shanghai 200433, China.

References

1. Giardiello FM, Brensinger JD, Tersmette AC, Goodman SN, Petersen GM, Booker SV, Cruz-Correa M, Offerhaus JA. Very high risk of cancer in familial Peutz-Jeghers syndrome. Gastroenterology. 2000;119(6):1447–53.
2. Boardman LA, Thibodeau SN, Schaid DJ, Lindor NM, McDonnell SK, Burgart LJ, Ahlquist DA, Podratz KC, Pittelkow M, Hartmann LC. Increased risk for cancer in patients with the Peutz-Jeghers syndrome. Ann Intern Med. 1998; 128(11):896–9.
3. Giardiello FM, Trimbath JD. Peutz-Jeghers syndrome and management recommendations. Clin Gastroenterol Hepatol. 2006;4(4):408–15.
4. Resta N, Pierannunzio D, Lenato GM, Stella A, Capocaccia R, Bagnulo R, Lastella P, Susca FC, Bozzao C, Loconte DC, et al. Cancer risk associated with STK11/LKB1 germline mutations in Peutz-Jeghers syndrome patients: results of an Italian multicenter study. Dig Liver Dis. 2013;45(7):606–11.
5. Jenne DE, Reimann H, Nezu J, Friedel W, Loff S, Jeschke R, Muller O, Back W, Zimmer M. Peutz-Jeghers syndrome is caused by mutations in a novel serine threonine kinase. Nat Genet. 1998;18(1):38–43.
6. Hemminki A, Markie D, Tomlinson I, Avizienyte E, Roth S, Loukola A, Bignell G, Warren W, Aminoff M, Hoglund P, et al. A serine/threonine kinase gene defective in Peutz-Jeghers syndrome. Nature. 1998;391(6663):184–7.
7. Hanks SK, Quinn AM, Hunter T. The protein kinase family: conserved features and deduced phylogeny of the catalytic domains. Science. 1988; 241(4861):42–52.
8. Boudeau J, Baas AF, Deak M, Morrice NA, Kieloch A, Schutkowski M, Prescott AR, Clevers HC, Alessi DR. MO25alpha/beta interact with STRADalpha/beta enhancing their ability to bind, activate and localize LKB1 in the cytoplasm. EMBO J. 2003;22(19):5102–14.
9. Tiainen M, Ylikorkala A, Makela TP. Growth suppression by Lkb1 is mediated by a G(1) cell cycle arrest. Proc Natl Acad Sci U S A. 1999;96(16):9248 51.
10. Karuman P, Gozani O, Odze RD, Zhou XC, Zhu H, Shaw R, Brien TP, Bozzuto CD, Ooi D, Cantley LC, et al. The Peutz-Jegher gene product LKB1 is a mediator of p53-dependent cell death. Mol Cell. 2001;7(6):1307–19.
11. Spicer J, Rayter S, Young N, Elliott R, Ashworth A, Smith D. Regulation of the Wnt signalling component PAR1A by the Peutz-Jeghers syndrome kinase LKB1. Oncogene. 2003;22(30):4752–6.
12. Ossipova O, Bardeesy N, DePinho RA, Green JB. LKB1 (XEEK1) regulates Wnt signalling in vertebrate development. Nat Cell Biol. 2003;5(10):889–94.
13. Smith DP, Rayter SI, Niederlander C, Spicer J, Jones CM, Ashworth A. LIP1, a cytoplasmic protein functionally linked to the Peutz-Jeghers syndrome kinase LKB1. Hum Mol Genet. 2001;10(25):2869–77.
14. Bardeesy N, Sinha M, Hezel AF, Signoretti S, Hathaway NA, Sharpless NE, Loda M, Carrasco DR, DePinho RA. Loss of the Lkb1 tumour suppressor provokes intestinal polyposis but resistance to transformation. Nat. 2002; 419(6903):162–7.
15. Watts JL, Morton DG, Bestman J, Kemphues KJ. The C. elegans par-4 gene encodes a putative serine-threonine kinase required for establishing embryonic asymmetry. Dev (Cambridge, England). 2000;127(7):1467–75.
16. Boudeau J, Sapkota G, Alessi DR. LKB1, a protein kinase regulating cell proliferation and polarity. FEBS Lett. 2003;546(1):159–65.
17. Martin SG, St Johnston D. A role for Drosophila LKB1 in anterior-posterior axis formation and epithelial polarity. Nature. 2003;421(6921):379–84.
18. Baas AF, Kuipers J, van der Wel NN, Batlle E, Koerten HK, Peters PJ, Clevers HC. Complete polarization of single intestinal epithelial cells upon activation of LKB1 by STRAD. Cell. 2004;116(3):457–66.
19. Vogelstein B, Lane D, Levine AJ. Surfing the p53 network. Nat. 2000; 408(6810):307–10.
20. Donehower LA, Harvey M, Slagle BL, McArthur MJ, Montgomery CA Jr, Butel JS, Bradley A. Mice deficient for p53 are developmentally normal but susceptible to spontaneous tumours. Nat. 1992;356(6366):215–21.
21. Wei C, Amos CI, Stephens LC, Campos I, Deng JM, Behringer RR, Rashid A, Frazier ML. Mutation of Lkb1 and p53 genes exert a cooperative effect on tumorigenesis. Cancer Res. 2005;65(24):11297–303.
22. Aaltonen LA, Hamilton SR. Pathology and genetics of Tumours of the digestive system. Lyon: IARC Press; 2010.
23. Zhao ZY, Jiang YL, Li BR, Yang F, Li J, Jin XW, Ning SB, Sun SH. A 23-nucleotide deletion in STK11 gene causes Peutz-Jeghers syndrome and malignancy in a Chinese patient without a positive family history. Dig Dis Sci. 2017;62(11):3014–20.
24. Lek M, Karczewski KJ, Minikel EV, Samocha KE, Banks E, Fennell T, O'Donnell-Luria AH, Ware JS, Hill AJ, Cummings BB, et al. Analysis of protein-coding genetic variation in 60,706 humans. Nat. 2016;536(7616):285–91.
25. Zhao ZY, Jiang YL, Li BR, Yang F, Li J, Jin XW, Ning SB, Sun SH. Sanger sequencing in exonic regions of STK11 gene uncovers a novel de-novo germline mutation (c.962_963delCC) associated with Peutz-Jeghers syndrome and elevated cancer risk: case report of a Chinese patient. BMC Med Genet. 2017;18(1):130.
26. Yu J, Xu QG, Wang ZG, Yang Y, Zhang L, Ma JZ, Sun SH, Yang F, Zhou WP. Circular RNA cSMARCA5 inhibits growth and metastasis in hepatocellular carcinoma. J Hepatol. 2018;68(6):1214–27.
27. Mao X, Zhang Y, Wang H, Mao G, Ning S. Mutations of the STK11 and FHIT genes among patients with Peutz-Jeghers syndrome. Zhonghua Yi Xue Yi Chuan Xue Za Zhi. 2016;33(2):186–90.
28. Mao X, Zhang Y, Mao G, Wang H, Ning S. STK11 gene mutations in patients with Peutz-Jeghers syndrom. World Chin J Digestol. 2015;23(2):332.
29. Zhao ZY, Jiang YL, Li BR, Yu ED, Ning SB. A novel mutation (c.855delG) in STK11 gene is associated with Peutz-Jeghers syndrome in a Chinese family. Dig Liver Dis. 2018;50(3):312–4.
30. Rufener SL, Koujok K, McKenna BJ, Walsh M. Small bowel intussusception secondary to Peutz-Jeghers polyp. Radiographics. 2008;28(1):284–8.
31. Harned RK, Buck JL, Sobin LH. The hamartomatous polyposis syndromes: clinical and radiologic features. AJR Am J Roentgenol. 1995;164(3):565–71.
32. Latchford A, Greenhalf W, Vitone LJ, Neoptolemos JP, Lancaster GA, Phillips RK. Peutz-Jeghers syndrome and screening for pancreatic cancer. Br J Surg. 2006;93(12):1446–55.
33. van Lier MG, Wagner A, Mathus-Vliegen EM, Kuipers EJ, Steyerberg EW, van Leerdam ME. High cancer risk in Peutz-Jeghers syndrome: a systematic review and surveillance recommendations. Am J Gastroenterol. 2010;105(6): 1258 64. author reply 1265

34. Zeng PY, Berger SL. LKB1 is recruited to the p21/WAF1 promoter by p53 to mediate transcriptional activation. Cancer Res. 2006;66(22):10701–8.
35. Tiainen M, Vaahtomeri K, Ylikorkala A, Makela TP. Growth arrest by the LKB1 tumor suppressor: induction of p21(WAF1/CIP1). Hum Mol Genet. 2002; 11(13):1497–504.
36. Gurumurthy S, Hezel AF, Sahin E, Berger JH, Bosenberg MW, Bardeesy N. LKB1 deficiency sensitizes mice to carcinogen-induced tumorigenesis. Cancer Res. 2008;68(1):55–63.
37. Scott KD, Nath-Sain S, Agnew MD, Marignani PA. LKB1 catalytically deficient mutants enhance cyclin D1 expression. Cancer Res. 2007;67(12):5622–7.
38. Setogawa T, Shinozaki-Yabana S, Masuda T, Matsuura K, Akiyama T. The tumor suppressor LKB1 induces p21 expression in collaboration with LMO4, GATA-6, and Ldb1. Biochem Biophys Res Commun. 2006;343(4):1186–90.
39. Liang J, Shao SH, Xu ZX, Hennessy B, Ding Z, Larrea M, Kondo S, Dumont DJ, Gutterman JU, Walker CL, et al. The energy sensing LKB1-AMPK pathway regulates p27(kip1) phosphorylation mediating the decision to enter autophagy or apoptosis. Nat Cell Biol. 2007;9(2):218–24.
40. Cheng H, Liu P, Wang ZC, Zou L, Santiago S, Garbitt V, Gjoerup OV, Iglehart JD, Miron A, Richardson AL, et al. SIK1 couples LKB1 to p53-dependent anoikis and suppresses metastasis. Sci Signal. 2009;2(80):ra35.
41. Dai L, Fu L, Liu D, Zhang K, Wu Y, Meng H, Zhang B, Guan X, Guo H, Bai Y. Novel and recurrent mutations of STK11 gene in six Chinese cases with Peutz-Jeghers syndrome. Dig Dis Sci. 2014;59(8):1856–61.
42. Hampel H, Bennett RL, Buchanan A, Pearlman R, Wiesner GL. A practice guideline from the American College of Medical Genetics and Genomics and the National Society of genetic counselors: referral indications for cancer predisposition assessment. Genet Med. 2015;17(1):70–87.
43. Tan H, Wei X, Yang P, Huang Y, Li H, Liang D, Wu L. A lesson from a reported pathogenic variant in Peutz-Jeghers syndrome: a case report. Familial Cancer. 2017;16(3):417–22.
44. Beggs AD, Latchford AR, Vasen HF, Moslein G, Alonso A, Aretz S, Bertario L, Blanco I, Bulow S, Burn J, et al. Peutz-Jeghers syndrome: a systematic review and recommendations for management. Gut. 2010;59(7):975–86.
45. Syngal S, Brand RE, Church JM, Giardiello FM, Hampel HL, Burt RW, American College of G. ACG clinical guideline: genetic testing and management of hereditary gastrointestinal cancer syndromes. Am J Gastroenterol. 2015;110(2):223–62. quiz 263
46. Biasini M, Bienert S, Waterhouse A, Arnold K, Studer G, Schmidt T, Kiefer F, Gallo Cassarino T, Bertoni M, Bordoli L, et al. SWISS-MODEL: modelling protein tertiary and quaternary structure using evolutionary information. Nucleic Acids Res. 2014;42(Web Server issue):W252–8.

5

Functional study on new *FOXL2* mutations found in Chinese patients with blepharophimosis, ptosis, epicanthus inversus syndrome

Lu Zhou, Jiaqi Wang and Tailing Wang*

Abstract

Background: Blepharophimosis, ptosis, epicanthus inversus syndrome (BPES) is a rare inheritable disease that mainly affects eyelid development associated with (type I) or without (type II) ovarian dysfunction, resulting in premature ovarian failure (POF). Mutations in the gene forkhead box L2 (*FOXL2*) have been shown to be responsible for BPES. The aim of this study was to determine and functionally validate the *FOXL2* mutation in a Chinese BPES family.

Methods: Twelve individuals including five BPES patients from a Chinese family were enrolled. Genomic DNA was extracted from peripheral blood of enrolled subjects. The coding region of the *FOXL2* gene was amplified and mutations were determined by sequencing analyses. Functional analysis was carried out to study changes in expression and transcriptional activity of the mutant FOXL2 protein.

Results: A novel mutation in the *FOXL2* gene (c.931C > T) was detected in all five BPES patients, which converts a histidine residue into a tyrosine (p.H311Y) in the FOXL2 protein. Functional analysis revealed that this point mutation reduces FOXL2 protein expression, concomitant with decreased transcriptional activity on the steroidogenic acute regulatory (StAR) gene promotor.

Conclusions: Our results expand the mutational spectrum of the *FOXL2* gene and provide additional insights to the research on the molecular pathogenesis of *FOXL2* in BPES.

Keywords: BPES, FOXL2, Gene mutation

Background

Blepharophimosis, ptosis, epicanthus inversus syndrome (BPES, OMIM # 110100) is a rare genetic disorder with an estimated incidence of 1 in 50,000 births [1]. It can occur sporadically or associate with autosomal dominant mutations. The characteristic clinical presentations of this disease include a complex eyelid/ocular malformation characterized by blepharophimosis, ptosis, epicanthus inversus and telecanthus. The horizontal shortening of the palpebral aperture can lead to amblyopia in one or both eyes [2]. Depending on the occurrence of premature ovarian failure (POF) or not, female BPES patients are classified into two different groups, with type I patients having POF while type II referring to those with normal ovarian function [3]. However, both types of BPES are widely recognized to result predominantly from mutations in the forkhead transcriptional factor-2 (*FOXL2*) gene that is involved in palpebral and ovarian development [4].

The *FOXL2* gene in human is approximately 2.7-kb long located on chromosome 3q22.3, which encodes a protein with 376 residues. The FOXL2 protein contains a characteristic 100 amino-acid DNA-binding forkhead domain, which categorizes the FOXL2 protein into the superfamily of Forkhead transcription factors [5]. An alanine-rich domain, also known as a polyalanine (poly-Ala) tract highly conserved across various mammals, lies downstream of the forkhead domain and is responsible

* Correspondence: tailing.cn.wang@gmail.com
The 3rd Department, Plastic Surgery Hospital of the Chinese Academy of Medical Sciences, Peking Union Medical College, Badachu Road, Shijingshan District, No. 33, Beijing 100041, China

for negatively regulating its transcriptional activity [5]. FOXL2 localizes in the nucleus and transcriptionally modulates genetic programs required for early eyelid development and ovary differentiation and maintenance, at the same time, represses components essential for somatic testis determination [6]. FOXL2 acts as a transcriptional repressor for multiple genes, including the human steroidogenic acute regulatory (StAR) gene. StAR mediates the transports of cholesterol across mitochondrial membrane, and controls the rate-limiting step in steroidogenesis [7]. Mutations in *FOXL2* may contribute to de-repression of the StAR promoter and cause increased differentiation of granulosa cells, leading to the onset of POF [8].

A collection of more than 100 genetic alternations affecting the *FOXL2* locus have been identified in patients with BPES, including frameshifts, insertions, nonsense as well as missense mutations [9, 10], with intragenic mutations accounting for the majority (71%) [11]. Although there are some claims about the correlations between different mutations in FOXL2 and BPES types, direct genotype-phenotype association remains to be further demonstrated because of the lack of de novo genetic study using animal model and the clinical heterogeneity among patients with BPES [12]. Furthermore, the mechanisms underlying individual mutations causing the development of BPES are largely unknown and could be complicated. It is likely that some mutant FOXL2 might collaborate with other cellular alternations to promote disease progression, as exemplified by the coexistence of the FOXL2 deletion and BMP15 in some BPES patients [13]. Therefore, identification of novel *FOXL2* mutations and further characterization of their contributions to the pathogenesis of BPES will provide not only biomarkers for early detection of BPES but also potential implications for therapeutic intervention.

Here, we report a novel FOXL2 mutation identified in a Chinese family with BPES. Functional studies of this missense mutation (c.931C > T, p.H311Y) revealed a reduction in both FOXL2 protein expression and its transcriptional repression activity on the promoter of StAR gene, underscoring the significance of this mutation in the pathogenesis of BPES.

Methods

Patients

A Chinese family with BPES was ascertained at the Plastic Surgery Hospital of Chinese Academy of Medical Sciences (Fig. 1a). A total of 12 individuals, including five with BPES were enrolled in this study. Clinical examinations of the patients were performed by ophthalmologists, following the criteria listed below to diagnose BPES [14]: blepharophimosis, ptosis, epicanthus inversus, and telecanthus. POF was determined if the patients underwent ovarian failure under the age of 40 and they presented features including amenorrhoea, hypoestrogenism and elevated serum gonadotrophin concentrations. This study was approved by the Ethics Committee

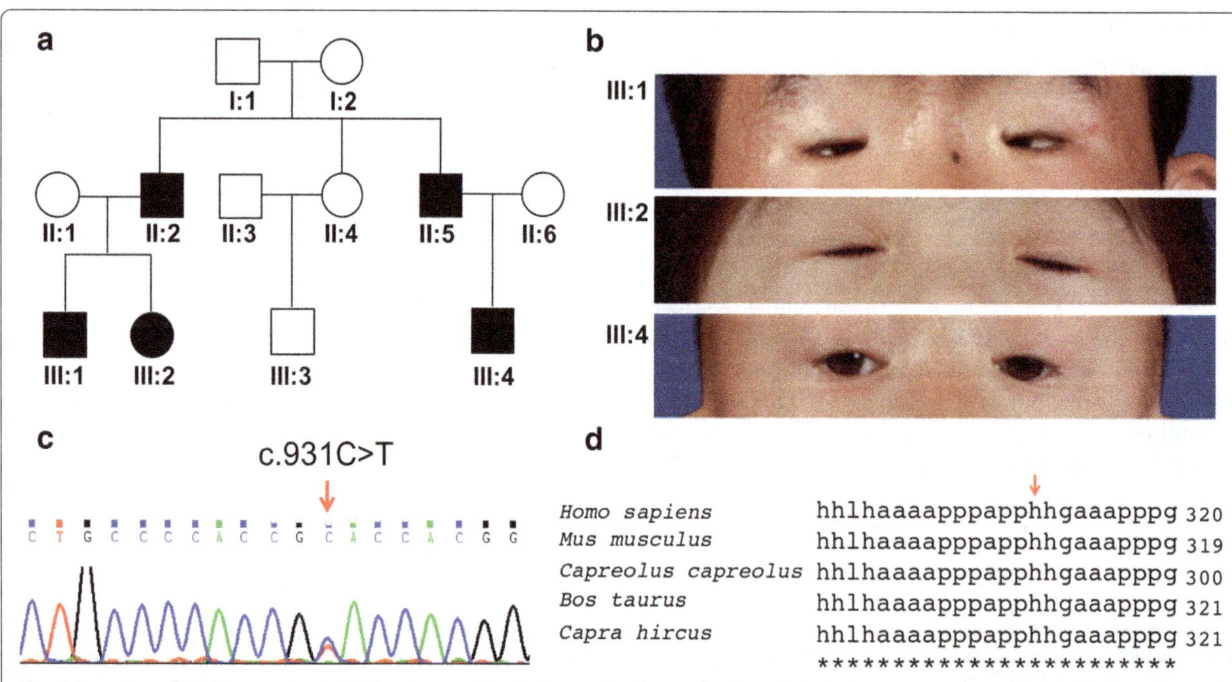

Fig. 1 Detection of *FOXL2* mutation in BPES patients. **a**. The Pedigree of a Chinese family with BPES. **b**. Representative images of BPES patients. **c**. Sequencing result indicating the c.931C > T mutation in the *FOXL2* gene. **d**. Alignment of FOXL2 proteins from different species showing the conserved site of H311

of our institute, and informed consent was obtained from all participants or their guardians for research.

DNA extraction and sequencing

Blood samples were collected from peripheral vein, followed by leukocytes enrichment and genomic DNA isolation using phenol and chloroform. The full-length FOXL2 open reading frame (ORF) was amplified by touch-down PCR with High-Fidelity Taq Polymerase (Invitrogen). After gel analysis to confirm the success of PCR, the amplicons were subjected to Sanger sequencing (Applied Biosystems), followed by nucleotide blasting to determine any mutation. Primers are available upon request.

Tissue culture and DNA vectors

HEK293T cells and HeLa cells were obtained from ATCC and maintained in DMEM (Sigma-Aldrich) with 10% fetal bovine serum (FBS), 2 mM L-glutamine, 100 U/ml penicillin and 100 mg/ml streptomycin. The ovarian granulosa cell tumor KGN cells were cultured in DMEM-F12 medium with 10% FBS, 100 U/ml penicillin and 100 mg/ml streptomycin. All cells were cultured in humidified incubator at 37 °C with 5% CO_2. Transfection was performed using Lipofectamine 2000 (Invitrogen) according to the manufacturer's instruction. WT and mutant *FOXL2* (NM_023067) expression constructs are based on a pcDNA3.1 plasmid backbone. The FOXL2-H311Y expression vector was obtained using junction-PCR according to method as previously described [15].

Cellular fractionation and immunoblotting

Cytosolic/nuclear fraction from cells transfected with different expression vectors was performed with Cell Fractionation Kit (Abcam), according to the manufacturer's instruction. For whole cell lysate, cells were lysed in a buffer containing 1% IGEPAL, 150 mM NaCl, 20 mM HEPES (pH 7.9), 10 mM NaF, 0.1 mM EDTA, 1 mM sodium orthovanadate and 1× protease inhibitor cocktail. Protein concentration was quantified using BCA protein concentration assay kit (Pierce). Lysates were electrophoresed on SDS-polyacrylamide (SDS-PAGE) gels and proteins were then transferred to nitrocellulose membrane (Millipore). Membranes were incubated with primary antibodies (FOXL2, actin, Lamin B1) in 5% bovine serum albumin containing 0.05% Tween-20 at 4 °C overnight, followed by incubation with HRP-conjugated secondary antibody at room temperature for 1 h, and visualization by an ECL or ECL Prime (GE Healthcare) [16].

Luciferase assay

For luciferase assays, HeLa cells and KGN cells were seeded in 24-well plates. Transient co-transfection was carried out with indicated combinations of luciferase reporter vectors (pGL2-basic, pGL2-StAR:– 1300 bp-luciferase [17] and RSV-Renilla) and the control pcDNA 3.1 expression vector. A Renilla reporter driven by an RSV promoter (Promega) was used as a control for transfection efficiency. After incubation for 24 h at 37 °C, the transfected cells were washed 3 times with phosphate buffered saline (PBS) and lysed by passive lysis buffer, followed by Dual-luciferase assay according to manufacturer's instructions (Promega). Transfection was conducted in triplicate and experiments were performed at least three times. Relative luciferase unit is the ratio of Firefly over Renilla luciferase read. Statistical significance was determined by non-parametric Mann-Whitney test.

Quantitative real-time PCR

RNA was prepared using Trizol reagent (Agilent Technologies) and Direct-zol RNA MiniPrep Kit (Zymo Research) according to the manufacturer's instructions and cDNA was generated using high capacity cDNA reverse transcription kit (Applied Biosystems) with random primers [18]. RT-qPCR was performed with SYBR Green (Qiagen) using primers as described previously [19].

Statistics

Graph Pad Prism 5.0 was used to perform non-parametric Mann-Whitney test to compare all interval variables. Error bars express +/– standard error of the mean.

Results

Clinical findings

All five patients from the affected family in this study demonstrated the typical features of BPES, including small palpebral fissures, ptosis of the eyelids, telecanthus and epicanthus inversus (Fig. 1a, b). Only one female patient was identified, with no sign of POF, probably due to the young age.

Genetic findings

Sequencing analysis of the *FOXL2* locus from the affected individuals revealed a heterozygous missense mutation c.931C > T (p.H311Y) (Fig. 1c), which has never been reported in familial BPES and is absent in the 100 ethnically matched control chromosomes. The C > T mutation causes a single amino acid substitution at the residue 311, converting a histidine residue into a tyrosine (p.H311Y). Interestingly, the histidine 311 residue of FOXL2 protein is highly conserved across species (Fig. 1d) while the Grantham distance score (83) between histidine and tyrosine is high [20], suggesting this amino acid substitution might have a functional impact on FOXL2 protein and subsequently the pathogenesis of BPES.

Expression level of mutant FOXL2

To test whether the c.931C > T (p.H311Y) mutation influences the functions of FOXL2 protein, we generated expression vectors for both wild-type (WT) and mutant (p.H311Y) FOXL2. Upon transfection into HEK293T cells, the expression of FOXL2 can be detected at both mRNA and protein levels (Fig. 2). Whereas the transcription of FOXL2 was comparable between cells transfected with WT and mutant constructs (Fig. 2a), the WT FOXL2 protein was more abundant than the mutant one (Fig. 2b), suggesting that this point mutation affects the stability of the FOXL2 protein.

Subcellular localization of mutant FOXL2

Given that FOXL2 functions as a transcription factor predominantly localizing in the nucleus, we continued to examine whether p.H311Y mutation influences the subcellular localization of the FOXL2 protein. Both WT and mutant FOXL2 localized exclusively in the nucleus (Fig. 3), suggesting that the p.H311Y mutation does not alter the cellular distribution pattern of FOXL2.

Transcriptional activity on StAR promoter

To confirm whether the missense mutation alters the transcriptional activity of FOXL2, we performed luciferase-based reporter assays to assess their transactivation capacity on promoter of StAR, a well-characterized target of FOXL2 [8, 21]. Given that the mutant FOXL2 is less stable than its WT counterpart, we first titrated the amount of DNA for transfection so as to obtain similar protein level (Fig. 4a). As expected, WT FOXL2 repressed the StAR promoter activity as reflected by decreased luciferase intensity (Fig. 4b). In contrast, cells transfected with the same amount of mutant FOXL2 construct (p.H311Y) did not show significant inhibition of the StAR promoter activity (Fig. 4b), suggesting the loss of FOXL2 function upon p.H311Y mutation.

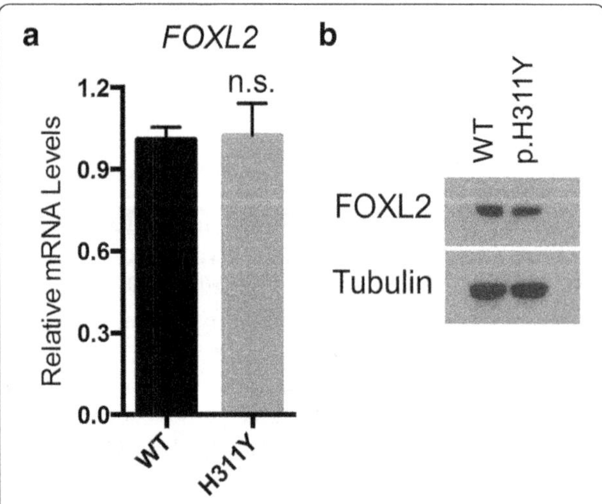

Fig. 2 Expression levels of WT and p.H311Y mutant *FOXL2*. **a**. mRNA expression level of *FOXL2*, as measured by qPCR, was comparable between WT and p.H311Y mutant. **b**. Protein level of *FOXL2*, as determined by Western Blot, showed lower p.H311Y expression when compared to WT. n.s.: not significant

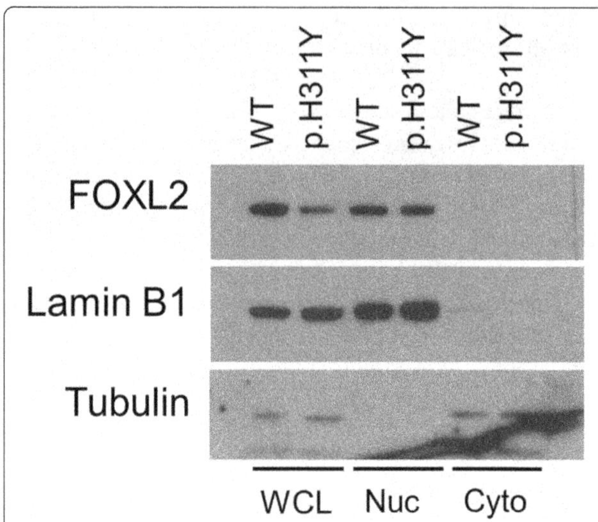

Fig. 3 Subcellular distribution of WT and p.H311Y mutant *FOXL2*. Nuclear (Nuc) and cytosolic (Cyto) extracts, as well as whole cell lysate (WCL) of cells transfected with WT or p.H311Y FOXL2 were subjected to Western blotting. Both WT and mutant FOXL2 showed nuclear localization. Lamin B1 and tubulin were used as markers of nuclear and cytoplasmic fractions, respectively

Discussion

In this study, we report a novel missense mutation in the *FOXL2* gene from a Chinese family with BPES. Additionally, we functionally characterized the effects of this mutation on FOXL2 activity, experimentally validating the relevance of this mutation to the pathogenesis of BPES.

Genetic alternation in *FOXL2* locus has been long appreciated as an important causal factor for the pathogenesis of BPES. The highly conserved FOXL2 protein is a transcription regulator containing a DNA-binding forkhead domain and a poly-Ala tract, both of which host the vast majority of BPES-associated mutations identified to date [9]. The novel mutation c.931C > T causes a single amino acid substitution at the residue 311, converting a histidine residue into a tyrosine (p.H311Y). Although located outside the forkhead domain and poly-Ala tract, the histidine 311 residue of FOXL2 protein is highly conserved across species (Fig. 1c). Given that a histidine residue is nucleophilic and usually serves a role in stabilizing the folded structures of proteins while a tyrosine residue is hydrophobic and can make a protein exceedingly unstable when ionized, the replacement of histidine by tyrosine is likely to alter the functional property of FOXL2 protein. Indeed, further tests

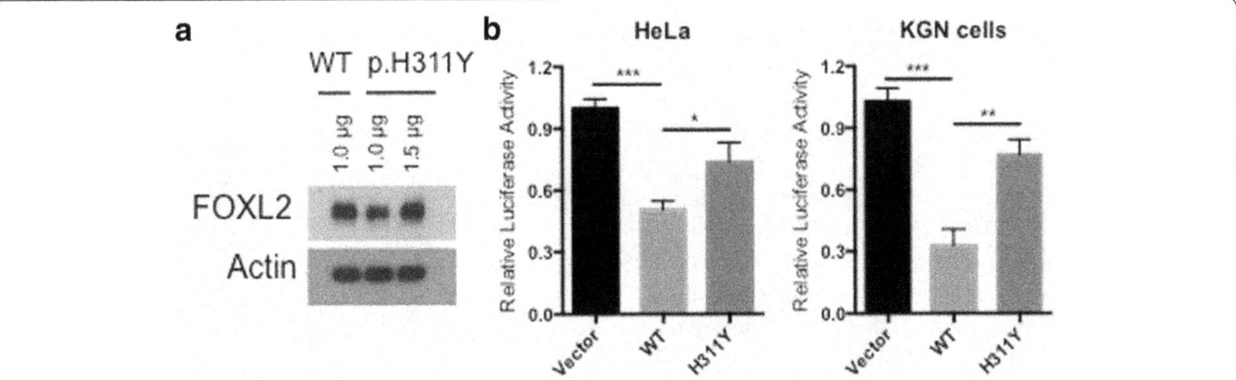

Fig. 4 Transcriptional repression activity of WT and p.H311Y mutant *FOXL2*. **a**. Expression level of WT and p.H311Y mutant FOXL2. **b**. Transcriptional repression activity of WT and p.H311Y mutant FOXL2 as measured by luciferase assay in both HeLa and KGN cells. Luciferase vector driven by the StAR promoter was cotransfected with empty vector, WT or p.H311Y mutant FOXL2 plasmids, followed by luciferase activity measurement. $*p < 0.05$, $**p < 0.01$

showed that although the c.931C > T (p.H311Y) mutation does not alter mRNA levels of FOXL2; it greatly decreases its protein expressions, probably by reducing the stability of FOXL2 protein.

Both WT and mutant FOXL2 localized exclusively in the nucleus, suggesting that the p.H311Y mutation does not affect the protein's nuclear localization signal or disturb interactions with nuclear transporters. A previous study has reported that mutations in the forkhead domain of FOXL2 are more likely to cause cytoplasmic mislocalization and aggregation of the protein [22]. The c.931C > T (p.H311Y) mutation occurs outside the forkhead and the poly-Ala domains, and does not seem to alter the subcellular localization and aggregation pattern of FOXL2. This is confirmed by another report by Beysen et al. that a missense mutation located outside the forkhead domain (p.S217F) had no effect on intracellular protein distribution [23]. Interestingly, luciferase assay of the StAR gene showed loss of FOXL2 repressor function upon p.H311Y mutation as compared to the WT FOXL2. This could be due to a decrease of total available FOXL2 in the nucleus. It is also possible that the mutation may decrease intranuclear mobility, as well as binding affinity of FOXL2 to the StAR gene. Further studies are required to corroborate these assumptions.

Given the critical roles of FOXL2 mutations in the development and progression of BPES, enormous efforts have been made in the correlations between genotypes and phenotypes. Initial studies have been focused more on the FOXL2 structural alternations and ended with a preliminary genotype-phenotype correlation, that is, mutations resulting in truncated FOXL2 proteins without the poly-Ala tract are likely associated with BPES type I, whereas poly-Ala expansions might preferentially give rise to BPES type II [12]. However, clear correlation seems difficult for the mutations contributing to mutant proteins but with an intact forkhead domain and poly-Ala tract. Therefore, the functional properties of the affected FOXL2 proteins, including their transactivation capacity, subcellular localization, aggregation as well as protein 3D structure, are taken into account when classifying pathogenic FOXL2 mutations [23–25]. For example, using luciferase reporter systems, Dipietromaria et al. were able to demonstrate that loss-of-function FOXL2 mutants are likely BPES type I mutations [24]. Based on this theory, it is speculated that mutations outside the forkhead domain without affecting the FOXL2 transactivation are possibly associated with BEPS type II. Indeed, this seems true when analyzing all the known non-forkhead missense mutations. Including this novel one reported by our study, there are six different non-forkhead missense FOXL2 mutations: p.K193C, p.Y215C, p.S217C, p.S217F, p.Y258N and p.H311Y. Among these mutations, p.K193C was identified in a type II family [9]; p.Y215C, p.S217C and p.S217F have been experimentally validated using the dual 4xFLRE-luc and SIRT1-luc reporter systems and classified as BPES type II [24]. Although the individual carrying the p.Y258N mutation displayed POF, she was not a BPES patient [26]. As for our novel p.H311Y mutation, we are not able to tell its phenotype association at this point. On one hand, the single female patient in this affected family is still too young to pathologically classify the BPES subtype; on the other hand, the experimental approach we employed in this study was completely different than those used by Dipietromaria et al. (StAR-luciferase construct rather than the dual 4xFLRE-luc/SIRT1-luc reporters) [24], making it impossible to compare the transactivation capacity of p.H311Y. Therefore, whether or not our novel p.H311Y belongs to the BEPS type II still deserves further experimental investigation and clinical follow-up.

Furthermore, the severe phenotype associated with p.H311Y mutation is somehow consistent with other published missense mutations located outside the forkhead domain. For example, a heterozygous *FOXL2* missense mutation c.C650G (p.S217C) identified in an Iranian family with BPES gives rise to a striking phenotype with bilateral amblyopia [27]. Interestingly, the same mutation (p.S217C) has also been reported in an Indian family with mild eyelid phenotype [22], implying that additional genetic and/or epigenetic variations between these two p.S217C families might underlie the discrepancy in disease presentation. Despite that *FOXL2* located on 3q23 is the only gene known to cause BPES, considering the previous reports that the whole segment of 3q21–24 contributes to BPES [28], and that FOXL2 deletion coexists with BMP15 variants in a BPES patient [13], it is reasonable to speculate that other genetic and/or epigenetic factors synergize mutant FOXL2, especially those with intact transactivation capacity, to cause and/or exacerbate BPES. Further investigation on this aspect will be of interest, as it might reveal some novel components that are therapeutically targetable.

Conclusions

In summary, we not only identified a novel mutation, c.931C > T (p.H311Y), in the *FOXL2* gene in a Chinese family with BPES, but also confirmed that this missense mutation causes a reduction in both the expression and the activity of FOXL2 protein. The novel mutation reported here further expands the mutation spectrum of the *FOXL2* gene and contributes to the understanding of the molecular pathogenesis of BPES.

Abbreviations

BPES: Blepharophimosis-ptosis-epicanthus inversus syndrome; FOXL2: Forkhead box L2; ORF: Open reading frame; PCR: Polymerase chain reaction; POF: Premature ovarian failure; Poly-Ala: Poly-alanine; StAR: Steroidogenic acute regulatory; WT: Wildtype

Funding

This work is partially supported by funding from the National Natural Science Foundation of China and the PUMC Youth Fund No. 3332016044. The funders had no role in study design, data collection and analysis, decision to publish, or preparation of the manuscript.

Authors' contributions

LZ and JW conducted the experiments, analyzed data; LZ and TW wrote the manuscript. All authors read and approved the final manuscript.

Competing interests

The authors declare that they have no competing interests.

References

1. Oley C, Baraitser M. Blepharophimosis, ptosis, epicanthus inversus syndrome (BPES syndrome). J Med Genet. 1988;25(1):47–51.
2. Dawson EL, Hardy TG, Collin JR, Lee JP. The incidence of strabismus and refractive error in patients with blepharophimosis, ptosis and epicanthus inversus syndrome (BPES). Strabismus. 2003;11(3):173–7.
3. Zlotogora J, Sagi M, Cohen T. The blepharophimosis, ptosis, and epicanthus inversus syndrome: delineation of two types. Am J Hum Genet. 1983;35(5):1020–7.
4. Crisponi L, Deiana M, Loi A, Chiappe F, Uda M, Amati P, Bisceglia L, Zelante L, Nagaraja R, Porcu S, et al. The putative forkhead transcription factor FOXL2 is mutated in blepharophimosis/ptosis/epicanthus inversus syndrome. Nat Genet. 2001;27(2):159–66.
5. De Baere E, Dixon MJ, Small KW, Jabs EW, Leroy BP, Devriendt K, Gillerot Y, Mortier G, Meire F, Van Maldergem L, et al. Spectrum of FOXL2 gene mutations in blepharophimosis-ptosis-epicanthus inversus (BPES) families demonstrates a genotype–phenotype correlation. Hum Mol Genet. 2001; 10(15):1591–600.
6. Georges A, Auguste A, Bessiere L, Vanet A, Todeschini AL, Veitia RA. FOXL2: a central transcription factor of the ovary. J Mol Endocrinol. 2014;52(1):R17–33.
7. Stocco DM. StAR protein and the regulation of steroid hormone biosynthesis. Annu Rev Physiol. 2001;63:193–213.
8. Pisarska MD, Bae J, Klein C, Hsueh AJ. Forkhead l2 is expressed in the ovary and represses the promoter activity of the steroidogenic acute regulatory gene. Endocrinology. 2004;145(7):3424–33.
9. Beysen D, De Paepe A, De Baere E. FOXL2 mutations and genomic rearrangements in BPES. Hum Mutat. 2009;30(2):158–69.
10. Beysen D, Vandesompele J, Messiaen L, De Paepe A, De Baere E. The human FOXL2 mutation database. Hum Mutat. 2004;24(3):189–93.
11. Verdin H, De Baere E. FOXL2 impairment in human disease. Horm Res Paediatr. 2012;77(1):2–11.
12. De Baere E, Beysen D, Oley C, Lorenz B, Cocquet J, De Sutter P, Devriendt K, Dixon M, Fellous M, Fryns JP, et al. FOXL2 and BPES: mutational hotspots, phenotypic variability, and revision of the genotype-phenotype correlation. Am J Hum Genet. 2003;72(2):478–87.
13. Settas N, Anapliotou M, Kanavakis E, Fryssira H, Sofocleous C, Dacou-Voutetakis C, Chrousos GP, Voutetakis A. A novel FOXL2 gene mutation and BMP15 variants in a woman with primary ovarian insufficiency and blepharophimosis-ptosis-epicanthus inversus syndrome. Menopause. 2015; 22(11):1264–8.
14. Beysen D, De Jaegere S, Amor D, Bouchard P, Christin-Maitre S, Fellous M, Touraine P, Grix AW, Hennekam R, Meire F, et al. Identification of 34 novel and 56 known FOXL2 mutations in patients with Blepharophimosis syndrome. Hum Mutat. 2008;29(11):E205–19.
15. Moumne L, Dipietromaria A, Batista F, Kocer A, Fellous M, Pailhoux E, Veitia RA. Differential aggregation and functional impairment induced by polyalanine expansions in FOXL2, a transcription factor involved in cranio-facial and ovarian development. Hum Mol Genet. 2008;17(7):1010–9.
16. Luo C, Pietruska JR, Sheng J, Bronson RT, Hu MG, Cui R, Hinds PW. Expression of oncogenic BRAFV600E in melanocytes induces Schwannian differentiation in vivo. Pigment Cell Melanoma Res. 2015;28(5):603–6.
17. Sugawara T, Holt JA, Kiriakidou M, Strauss JF 3rd. Steroidogenic factor 1-dependent promoter activity of the human steroidogenic acute regulatory protein (StAR) gene. Biochemistry. 1996;35(28):9052–9.
18. Luo C, Lim JH, Lee Y, Granter SR, Thomas A, Vazquez F, Widlund HR, Puigserver P. A PGC1alpha-mediated transcriptional axis suppresses melanoma metastasis. Nature. 2016;537(7620):422–6.
19. Shah SP, Kobel M, Senz J, Morin RD, Clarke BA, Wiegand KC, Leung G, Zayed A, Mehl E, Kalloger SE, et al. Mutation of FOXL2 in granulosa-cell tumors of the ovary. N Engl J Med. 2009;360(26):2719–29.
20. Grantham R. Amino acid difference formula to help explain protein evolution. Science. 1974;185(4154):862–4.
21. Fleming NI, Knower KC, Lazarus KA, Fuller PJ, Simpson ER, Clyne CD. Aromatase is a direct target of FOXL2: C134W in granulosa cell tumors via a single highly conserved binding site in the ovarian specific promoter. PLoS One. 2010;5(12):e14389.
22. Nallathambi J, Laissue P, Batista F, Benayoun BA, Lesaffre C, Moumne L, Pandaranayaka PE, Usha K, Krishnaswamy S, Sundaresan P, et al. Differential functional effects of novel mutations of the transcription factor FOXL2 in BPES patients. Hum Mutat. 2008;29(8):E123–31.
23. Beysen D, Moumne L, Veitia R, Peters H, Leroy BP, De Paepe A, De Baere E. Missense mutations in the forkhead domain of FOXL2 lead to subcellular mislocalization, protein aggregation and impaired transactivation. Hum Mol Genet. 2008;17(13):2030–8.
24. Dipietromaria A, Benayoun BA, Todeschini AL, Rivals I, Bazin C, Veitia RA. Towards a functional classification of pathogenic FOXL2 mutations using transactivation reporter systems. Hum Mol Genet. 2009;18(17):3324–33.
25. Todeschini AL, Dipietromaria A, L'Hote D, Boucham FZ, Georges AB, Pandaranayaka PJ, Krishnaswamy S, Rivals I, Bazin C, Veitia RA. Mutational probing of the forkhead domain of the transcription factor FOXL2 provides insights into the pathogenicity of naturally occurring mutations. Hum Mol Genet. 2011;20(17):3376–85.
26. Harris SE, Chand AL, Winship IM, Gersak K, Aittomaki K, Shelling AN. Identification of novel mutations in FOXL2 associated with premature ovarian failure. Mol Hum Reprod. 2002;8(8):729–33.

Role of DFNB1 mutations in hereditary hearing loss among assortative mating hearing impaired families from South India

Pavithra Amritkumar[1,2], Justin Margret Jeffrey[1], Jayasankaran Chandru[1], Paridhy Vanniya S[1], M. Kalaimathi[1], Rajagopalan Ramakrishnan[3], N. P. Karthikeyen[4] and C. R. Srikumari Srisailapathy[1*]

Abstract

Background: DFNB1, the first locus to have been associated with deafness, has two major genes *GJB2* & *GJB6,* whose mutations have played vital role in hearing impairment across many ethnicities in the world. In our present study we have focused on the role of these mutations in assortative mating hearing impaired families from south India.

Methods: One hundred and six assortatively mating hearing impaired (HI) families of south Indian origin comprising of two subsets: 60 deaf marrying deaf (DXD) families and 46 deaf marrying normal hearing (DXN) families were recruited for this study. In the 60 DXD families, 335 members comprising of 118 HI mates, 63 other HI members and 154 normal hearing members and in the 46 DXN families, 281 members comprising of 46 HI and their 43 normal hearing partners, 50 other HI members and 142 normal hearing family members, participated in the molecular study. One hundred and sixty five (165) healthy normal hearing volunteers were recruited as controls for this study. All the participating members were screened for variants in *GJB2* and *GJB6* genes and the outcome of gene mutations were compared in the subsequent generation in begetting deaf offspring.

Results: The DFNB1 allele frequencies for DXD mates and their offspring were 36.98 and 38.67%, respectively and for the DXN mates and their offspring were 22.84 and 24.38%, respectively. There was a 4.6% increase in the subsequent generation in the DXD families, while a 6.75% increase in the DXN families, which demonstrates the role of assortative mating along with consanguinity in the increase of DFNB1 mutations in consecutive generations. Four novel variants, p.E42D (in *GJB2* gene), p.Q57R, p.E101Q, p.R104H (in *GJB6* gene) were also identified in this study.

Conclusion: This is the first study from an Indian subcontinent reporting novel variants in the coding region of *GJB6* gene. This is perhaps the first study in the world to test real-time, the hypothesis proposed by Nance et al. in 2000 (intense phenotypic assortative mating mechanism can double the frequency of the commonest forms of recessive deafness [DFNB1]) in assortative mating HI parental generation and their offspring.

Keywords: Assortative mating, *GJB2* mutations, *GJB6* mutations, DFNB1, Deafness, South India

Background

Hearing is one of the vital sensations, which keeps humans connected with each other and the world around. Consequently, hearing loss can have a profound impact on cognitive, psychosocial and educational development of an individual. Greater part of our present day knowledge on the physiology of hearing has come from various studies on hearing loss.

Till date, nearly 80 genes in over 142 deafness loci are associated with non-syndromic hearing loss (NSHL) reflecting the heterogenic and complex nature of the mechanism of hearing. Approximately 1200 different deafness-causing mutations are identified across the human genome. However, mutations do not occur at same frequencies across ethnicities. Eleven autosomal recessive loci (DFNB1, DFNB3, DFNB4, DFNB5, DFNB6, DFNB7/11, DFNB12, DFNB15, DFNB17, DFNB18 and

* Correspondence: crsrikumari@gmail.com; srikumaripavithra@gmail.com
[1]Department of Genetics, Dr. ALM Post Graduate Institute of Basic Medical Sciences, University of Madras, Taramani, Chennai 600113, India
Full list of author information is available at the end of the article

DFNB95) and one autosomal dominant locus (DFNA59) are currently known to be associated with hearing loss in India (Hereditary hearing loss homepage, http://hereditaryhearingloss.org/). Despite this genetic heterogeneity across ethnicities, DFNB1 locus on chromosome 13q11–12, accounts for up to 50% of NSHL [1, 2]. The first deafness associated gene in the DFNB1 locus, the *GJB2* gene (GenBank M86849, MIM 121011) coding the gap junction protein, Connexin 26 (Cx26), was reported in 1997 [3]. Connexin 26 protein is found in the cochlea of the inner ear and is a major regulator of K^+ homeostasis. In the absence of K^+ circulation, the hair cells are unable to generate action potential in response to sound. Recent studies have suggested that they play an important role in inter and intracellular signaling pathways of the inner ear [4]. Over 220 mutations, polymorphisms and unknown variants in the *GJB2* gene have been reported worldwide ([5]; Connexins and deafness homepage, http://davinci.crg.es/deafness/).High prevalence of *GJB2* mutations among many populations has made it necessary to depend on molecular testing for diagnosis. However, nearly 10–50% of deaf subjects in many studies showing only one *GJB2* mutant allele, further complicated the molecular diagnosis of DFNB1 deafness [6]. This led to the hypothesis that there could be other mutations in the DFNB1 locus but outside the *GJB2* gene. Subsequently, two large deletions occurring in the *GJB6* gene, which encodes connexin 30 (Cx30) protein and lying ~ 35 kb telomeric to *GJB2* on chromosome 13, were reported [6, 7]. Cx30 protein is of size 30 kDa, having 261 amino acids and shares 77% identity with Cx26. Cx26/Cx30 cochlear gap junctions forming heteromeric channels have been implicated in the maintenance of K+ homeostasis in the inner ear and contributing to the inner ear homeostasis [8, 9]. The *GJB6* gene was first described as a causative in a rare dominant form of deafness, DFNA3, and its implication in NSHL were ascertained through the identification of two large deletions, del(GJB6-D13S1830) of size 309 kb and del(GJB6-D13S1854) of size 232 kb, which truncate the *GJB6* gene [6, 7]. Till date, only four point mutations and four deletions in the *GJB6* gene or the region upstream have been reported (http://hereditaryhearingloss.org/). Studies on common mutations in assortative mating families have not been accomplished in the Indian subcontinent till date, except for our preliminary findings from this study [10–12].

In the hearing impaired (HI) population, assortative mating refers to the preference of a HI individual to marry another HI individual (deaf marrying deaf, or DXD) or a HI individual opting for a normal hearing individual as a partner (deaf marrying normal hearing, or DXN), with hearing impairment forming the basis for selection or non-selection. Segregation analysis with respect to the distribution of deaf and hearing offspring in such mating scan provide estimation of the proportion of such marriages that can have only deaf children (non-complementary matings), only hearing children (complementary matings), and those capable of producing both deaf and hearing children. A non-complementary mating is when both the deaf mates are homozygous for recessive alleles at the same locus, and can therefore produce only deaf offspring, while a complementary mating could be when mates either have non-genetic deafness or a combination of non-genetic deafness and recessive deafness, or both the mates having different forms of recessive deafness [13–15].

There are very few reports available on the mutational dynamics of assortative mating among the HI. The available reports state that between nineteenth and twentieth centuries, the frequency of HI children in the US with one or two HI parents increased by 38% from 0.064 to 0.089 [15]. These reports have focused only on assortative mating HI families as consanguinity as a practice was absent in these regions. Consanguineous marriage is a tradition that is commonly practiced among many parts of the world especially in North and Sub-Saharan Africa, Latin American communities, West, Central and South Asia where there is 10–50% prevalence of consanguinity among their general population [16]. In India, especially Tamil Nadu, Andhra Pradesh, and Karnataka overwhelmingly prefer and practice consanguineous marriages across all major religious groups and ethnic entities. There have been studies on hereditary hearing loss from south India reporting parental consanguinity of deaf subjects screened ranging between 32.55 and 54.10% [17–19] In Tamil Nadu, the studies on childhood hearing impaired have shown parental consanguinity ranging from 28 to 50% [20].

Consanguinity leads to an increase in identity by decent for all loci, indiscriminately. In contrast, once recessive genes are expressed phenotypically, assortative mating creates "gametic phase disequilibrium" [21], or the non-random association and gametic transmission of potentially very rare alleles at unlinked loci (genocopies) that have similar effects on the phenotype. Thus genetic heterogeneity and consanguinity add further complexity to the genetic studies on assortative mating deaf families. There are no genetic studies till date that have addressed the genetic and socio demographic dynamics simultaneously, on assortatively mating HI families from India.

Deaf marrying deaf is an increasing trend with sign language being the preferred mode of communication. Despite their preferential choice of a HI mate, the preferential desire for offspring's hearing status has largely been only normal hearing. The HI mates consider their deafness as a disability, which is a sharp deviation from 'Deaf culture' prevalent in the western HI population.

With more than 50% of hearing loss having genetic predisposition, it is very important to systematically analyze the role of genetic mutations in such matings. Therefore, screening for common mutations associated with hearing loss among assortatively mating HI couples and their families in Indian population would be essential to understand the role of incidence of hearing impairment in the subsequent generation, which forms the basis for this study.

Methods

Recruitment of participants and clinical data collection

One hundred and six (106) assortatively mating hearing impaired families comprising of **60 deaf marrying deaf, or DXD families** and **46 deaf marrying normal hearing, or DXN families**, predominantly from south India, with no familial interconnectivity, were recruited for this study. All international standards for ethical research were met and the Institutional Human Ethical Committee of the University of Madras, Post Graduate Institute of Basic Medical Sciences, Chennai, India, approved the study (Ref Nos: PGIBMS/CO/Human Ethical/2010–11/1458, PGIBMS/CO/Human Ethical/2011–12/546, IHEC Approval No: UM/IHEC/11–2013-I). Assortatively mating hearing impaired (HI) families were primarily identified through adult deaf organizations and associations for the HI, Alumni and Parent-Teacher associations of deaf schools in the four states (Andhra Pradesh, Karnataka, Kerala and Tamil Nadu) of south India. Some families were also referred by ENT surgeons, audiologists, gynecologists and neonatologists wherein the family members were seeking genetic counseling pertaining to the incidence of hearing loss in the family. Only those families in which the proband was prelingual HI and married to a partner who was either of normal hearing status (DXN) or was also prelingual HI (DXD), with at least two generations of family members available for the study, were included. Written informed consent was obtained from all participants in every family. Detailed family pedigrees were drawn. Information on demography, nativity, consanguinity, age at onset of hearing loss, detailed prenatal and perinatal history, use of ototoxic drugs (aminoglycosides), etc. was documented through a structured schedule. Attitudinal preferences of the HI mates as well as the hearing partner in each of the family towards choice of mate, parental choice, preference towards hearing status of their child/ children, mode of communication and genetic testing were also documented. Where both the mates were HI, information was obtained from at least two speaking relatives well informed about the family. Pre-test genetic counseling was provided to each of these families with the help of a sign language expert in our team. The degree of hearing loss for the participating members was evaluated through pure tone audiometry by measuring the air and bone conduction thresholds.

A total of 621 members comprising of hearing impaired and normal hearing from these 106 assortative mating families were recruited for this study (Table 1).

GJB2 and *GJB6* mutation analysis

Genomic DNA was extracted by standard PCI method [22]. The coding region of GJB2 gene (exon 2) was PCR-amplified using primer pair GJB2-EX2-1F (5′ -TCT CCC TGT TCT GTC CTA GC-30) and GJB2-EX2-1R (50-GAC AGC ATG AGA GGG ATG AG-3′) with annealing temperature of 62 °C. Amplification of the non-coding first exon and the flanking donor splicing site was carried out using Advantage-GC Genomic PCR kit (Clontech, Mountain View, USA) and PCR primers EXON 1A (5′-TCC GTA ACT TTC CCA GTC TCC GAG GGA AGA GG-3′) and EXON 1 M (5′ -CCC AAG GAC GTG TGT TGG TCC AGC CCC-3′) with conditions previously described by Ramshanker et al. [17], for all the HI members. Coding exon (exon 6) of *GJB6* gene was amplified by hot-start PCR using overlapping primer pairs: GJB6-1F (5′- AGA CTA GCA GGG CAG GGA GT- 3′) and GJB6-1R (5′- AGG GGT CAA TCC CAC ATT TC -3′) measuring 676 bp; GJB6-2F (5′ -GAT AGA GGG GTC GCT GTG GT -3′) and GJB6-2R (5′- GGC TAC AGA AGG AAC TTT CAG G -3′) measuring 494 bp with annealing temperature of 63 °C for both.

The amplified products were purified using QIAquick® PCR purification kit (Qiagen, Valencia, CA, USA). Bidirectional sequencing of the purified PCR products were carried out applying the same set of primers and ABI Prism Big-Dye Terminator 3.1 cycle sequencing reaction kit on an ABI 3730 automated sequencer (Applied Biosystems, Foster City, USA). The chromatogram sequences obtained were compared with the reference sequences of *GJB2* and *GJB6* in National Center for

Table 1 Distribution of hearing impaired and normal hearing members in the assortative mating families

Type of Mating	No. of hearing impaired mates	No. of hearing partners	Other hearing impaired members in the family	Other hearing members in the family	Total
Deaf marrying deaf (DXD)	120	0	63	154	337
Deaf marrying normal hearing (DXN)	46	46	50	142	284
TOTAL	166	46	113	296	621

Biotechnology Information (NCBI: http://www.ncbi.nlm.nih.gov/) to identify any nucleotide base-pair changes.

Additionally, the affected members were screened for the presence of two large deletions in the *GJB6* gene, del (GJB6-D13S1830) and del (GJB6-D13S1854) by amplifying the regions containing the breakpoint fragments [6, 7].

In silico analysis of novel variants

The bioinformatics tools used in this study to analyze the novel variants observed in the *GJB2* and *GJB6* genes were (i) Sorting Intolerant From Tolerant (SIFT), a sequence homology-based tool that predicts the phenotypic effect of amino acid substitution in a protein by scoring the substitution as tolerant or intolerant on the basis of sequence homology and physical properties of amino acids [23] and (ii) PolyPhen (Polymorphism Phenotyping), a tool which predicts possible impact of an amino acid substitution on the structure and function of a human protein using straight forward physical and comparative considerations [24]. The amino acid sequences of the native and variant proteins were then individually analyzed for physicochemical characteristics by Expasy's online ProtParam tool available at http://web.expasy.org/protparam/ [25], and the results were compared.

Homology modeling

The three dimensional structure of human *GJB6* was modeled from its protein sequence using the *automatic modelling mode* SWISS MODEL repository (http://swissmodel.expasy.org/). This resultant model was based on the template 2zw3 (*GJB2*), which shared 74.42% sequence identity with *GJB6*. It should be noted that the modeled residue range for *GJB6* was from amino acid 2 to 216 for a single chain. The protein structures were then minimized energetically using Swiss-PdbViewer [26]. The energy of the minimized protein was recorded. The native model was then mutated at the specified amino acid position using the "mutate" option in Swiss-PdbViewer, energy-minimized and the layer was saved as a ".pdb" file. The native and mutated proteins were crosschecked for alterations using Ramachandran plot at RAMPAGE portal available at http://mordred.bioc.cam.ac.uk/~rapper/rampage.php [27].

Control study

One hundred and sixty five (165) healthy and normal hearing volunteers aged 19 to 66 years, belonging to different castes and states of south India were recruited as controls for this study and were screened for the most common variants in *GJB2* and *GJB6* genes. All the controls were subjected to audiological profiling to record their normal hearing status.

Results

In the present study, consanguinity was recorded at two levels, parental consanguinity of the hearing impaired partners and consanguinity among the assortative mating partners in the 106 HI families. It was observed that consanguinity was conspicuously high among the normal hearing parents of the 120 DXD mates (45%), compared to that observed in the DXD mating (3.33%) (Table 2). Parental consanguinity of affected partners of 46 DXN mating was lower (32.61%) than the consanguinity observed in the DXN mating (39.13%) (Table 3). Additionally, the parental consanguinity of normal hearing mates in DXN mating (10.87%) was comparable with the parental consanguinity of the control group (11.51%), both reflecting the consanguinity trend in the general population.

In the first subgroup of 60 DXD families, 335 members comprising of 118 HI mates, 63 other HI members and 154 normal hearing members participated in the molecular study. In the second subgroup of 46 DXN families, 281 members comprising of 46 HI and their 43 normal hearing partners, 50 other HI members and 142 normal hearing family members, participated in the molecular study. Two HI mates in DXD families and three normal hearing partners in DXN families did not consent for blood sampling.

Outcome of *GJB2* mutation screening

Twenty three *GJB2* variants were observed; 11 pathogenic, one novel variant and 11 polymorphisms (Table 4). Out of the 118 HI mates, 63.79% (37/58) of the deaf husbands and 66.67% (40/60) of the deaf wives had at least one nucleotide change in the *GJB2* gene. Fifteen different mutations/ variants in the *GJB2* gene were observed among the 118 HI mates (Table 5). **A novel mutation, p.E42D** hitherto unreported was observed in this study (Fig. 1).

Two dominant mutations, p.R75Q [11] and p.R184Q [12] were recorded for the first time in the Indian population through our study. The variants, p.V37I, p.T55 T and p.R165W were represented only once in this cohort.

Among the 46 DXN families, 46 HI individuals and 43 normal hearing mates were included in the molecular

Table 2 Consanguinity in parents of DXD mating and in DXD mating

Type of marriage based on consanguinity	PARENTAL CONSANGUINITY			In DXD mating
	In husbands' parents (%)	In wives' parents (%)	Combined (%)	
Consanguineous	24 (40%)	30 (50%)	54 (45%)	2 (3.33%)
Non Consanguineous	36 (60%)	30 (50%)	66 (55%)	58 (96.67%)
TOTAL	60	60	120	60

Table 3 Consanguinity in parents of DXN mating and in DXN mating

Type of marriage based on consanguinity	PARENTAL CONSANGUINITY			In DXN mating
	In husbands' parents (%)	In wives' parents (%)	Combined (%)	
Consanguineous	17 (36.96%)	13 (28.26%)	30 (32.61%)	18 (39.13%)
Non Consanguineous	29 (63.04%)	33 (71.74%)	62 (67.39%)	28 (60.87%)
TOTAL	46	46	92	46

analysis. On *GJB2* mutation screening, 56.52% (26/46) of the HI partners and 41.86% (18/43) of the normal hearing partners had at least one nucleotide change in the *GJB2* gene. The *GJB2* mutations/variants observed among the affected and normal partners in DXN mating has been tabulated separately in Table 6. Ten different mutations/ variants in the *GJB2* gene were observed among the participating mates of 46 DXN families. A rare variant p.T86M was observed for the first time in the Indian population. The mutations/ variants, p.W77X, p.A88A, p.V153I, p.R165W, p.M195I and p.P225P were represented only once in this cohort. The overall allelic frequency of *GJB2* variants among the HI partners was 45.65%, which was lower than the frequency observed in DXD mates. Interestingly, the allelic frequency of *GJB2* variants in HI individuals with parental consanguinity (33.33%) was much lower than those without parental consanguinity (59.09%). The allelic frequency of *GJB2* variants in the normal hearing partners was 22.09%, is comparable with that observed in the normal hearing controls (24.85%). The allelic frequency is higher in normal hearing mates with parental consanguinity (30%) than those without parental consanguinity (21.05%), similar to that observed in DXD mates.

The frequency of pathogenic *GJB2* mutations was 33.90% in DXD mating (Table 5) and 35.86% in DXN mating (Table 6) with a combined frequency of 34.45%. Among them, p.W24X was the most common mutation at a frequency of 25.42% in DXD mates and 30.43% in the affected members of DXN mating with a combined frequency of 27.93%. More than 75% of the pathogenic alleles in this study had p.W24X mutation.

Outcome of *GJB6* mutation screening

Hearing impaired individuals from both the types of mating, DXD and DXN, who were homozygous or compound heterozygous for pathogenic mutations in the coding and non-coding region of *GJB2* gene were excluded for further screening. Thus, 33 HI DXD mates and 14 affected partners of DXN mating were excluded. One hundred and seventeen HI individuals comprising of 85 DXD mates and 32 affected DXN mates were included for further screening for mutations in the *GJB6* gene. These included individuals with novel variants in the *GJB2* gene, heterozygous carriers of pathogenic mutations in the *GJB2* gene or negative for pathogenic *GJB2* mutations. In addition, 110 normal hearing controls were also included for the study of *GJB6* gene mutations.

Large deletions- 309 kb deletion (GJB6-D13S1830) & 232 kb deletion (GJB6-D13S1854) in GJB6 gene

All the 117 HI individuals (85 DXD mates and 32 HI mates of DXN mating) and 110 normal hearing controls were negative for both the deletions, D13S1830 and D13S1854 in the *GJB6* gene, checked by multiplex PCR method [6, 7].

Point mutations in GJB6 gene

Table 7 lists the *GJB6* variants observed in the 85 DXD mates and 32 HI partners of DXN mating by direct sequencing of the coding exon 6 of *GJB6* gene. Three novel variants, p.Q57R, p.E101Q and p.R104H were observed in heterozygous condition in 4 individuals. These three novel variants were found in heterozygous condition in three DXD mating individuals and one DXN affected member. These novel variants are reported for the first time ever in the HI population. Figure 1 shows the partial chromatograms of novel variants observed in *GJB6* gene.

Genotypes of *GJB2* & *GJB6* mutations

The various *GJB2* genotypes observed among the affected partners of 60 DXD families are listed in Table 8. Two mutations, p.W24X and p.W77X, a novel variant p.E42D, and polymorphisms, p.R127H and p.V153I, were found in homozygous state. Homozygous p.W24X was the most common pathogenic genotype observed with an overall frequency of 22.03%. Two HI individuals showed triallelic combinations, with one having a rare triallelic combination R184Q/Q124X/ IVS1 + 1G > A, involving a dominant mutation p.R184Q [12] and another having a combination of W24X/T55T/R127H. In one individual, the novel variant p.E42D was also found in combination with another novel variant, p.R104H in the second auditory gene analyzed, *GJB6*, showing digenic inheritance.

The various *GJB2 & GJB6* genotypes observed among the affected partners and the normal hearing partners of 46 DXN families have been listed in Table 9. Three mutations, p.W24X, p.Q124X and p.T86M, have been found in homozygous state. Homozygous p.W24X is the

Table 4 Summary of mutations/ variants in *GJB2* gene observed among the DXD, DXN mates and normal hearing controls

S. No.	GJB2 VARIANTS		DOMAIN/ LOCATION	No. of alleles in DXD mates (n=236)	Frequency in DXD mating (%)	No of alleles in affected partners of DXN mating (n=92)	Frequency in HI partners of DXN mating (%)	No of alleles in normal partners of DXN mating (n=86)	Frequency in normal hearing partners of DXN (%)	No. of alleles in normal hearing control (n=330)	Frequency in Normal hearing controls (%)
	CODON	PROTEIN									
1	c.71 G>A	p.W24X	TM1	60	25.42	28	30.43	6	6.98	6	1.82
2	c.79 G>A	p.V27I	TM1	2	0.85	0	0	0	0	0	0
3	c.104 T>G	p.I35S	TM1	2	0.85	0	0	0	0	0	0
4	c. 109 G>A	p.V37I	TM1	1	0.42	0	0	0	0	0	0
5	c. 126 G>T	p.E42D	EC1	3	1.27	0	0	0	0	0	0
6	c.135 A>G	p.G45G	EC1	0	0	0	0	0	0	1	0.3
7	c.165 C>A	p.T55T	EC1	1	0.42	0	0	0	0	3	0.91
8	c. 185 A>G	p.N62S	EC1	0	0	0	0	0	0	1	0.3
9	c. 224 G>A	p. R75Q	TM2	1	0.42	0	0	0	0	0	0
10	c.231 G>A	p.W77X	TM2	5	2.12	1	1.09	0	0	0	0
11	c.240 G>A	p.Q80Q	TM2	0	0	0	0	0	0	2	0.61
12	c.257C>T	p.T86M	TM2	0	0	2	2.17	1	1.16	0	0
13	c.262 G>A	p.A88A	TM2	0	0	2	2.17	1	1.16	0	0
14	c.341 A>G	p.E114G	IC2	2	0.85	0	0	0	0	0	0
15	c. 370 C>T	p.Q124X	IC2	3	1.27	2	2.17	1	1.16	0	0
16	c.380 G>A	p.R127H	IC2	25	10.59	4	4.35	6	6.98	57	17.27
17	c.439 G>A	p.E147K	TM3	0	0	0	0	0	0	1	0.3
18	c.457 G>A	p.V153I	TM3	14	5.93	1	1.09	3	3.49	6	1.82
19	c.493 C>T	p.R165W	EC2	1	0.42	0	0	1	1.16	3	0.91
20	c. 551G>A	p.R184Q	EC2	1	0.42	0	0	0	0	0	0
21	c.585 G>A	p.M195I	TM4	0	0	1	1.09	0	0	1	0.3
22	c.675 A>T	p.P225P	IC3	0	0	1	1.09	0	0	1	0.3
23	c.IVS 1+1 G>A (-3172 G>A)		Intronic Splice site region	4	1.7	0	0	0	0	0	0
TOTAL				125	52.96	42	45.65	19	22.09	82	24.85

TM1-4 – Transmembrane domain 1 -4; EC1 & EC2 – extracellular domains 1 & 2; IC – cytoplasmic domain

Table 5 Summary of pathogenic mutations/ variants in the *GJB2* gene observed among the HI mates of 60 DXD families

S No	GJB2 VARIANTS		DOMAIN/ LOCATION	EFFECT	No of alleles in husbands (116)*	Frequency (%)	No. of alleles in wives (120)	Frequency (%)	TOTAL ALLELES (n=236)	OVERALL FREQUENCY (%)	With parental consanguinity (n=106)	Without parental consanguinity (n=130)
	CODON	PROTEIN										
1	c.71 G>A	p.W24X	TM1	Nonsense mutation (Transition); Pathogenic	31	26.72	29	24.17	60	**25.42**	31	29
2	c.79 G>A	p.V27I	TM1	Missense mutation (Transition); Polymorphism	1	0.86	1	0.83	2	0.85	1	1
3	c.104 T>G	p.I35S	TM1	Missense mutation (Transversion); Pathogenic	0	0	2	1.67	2	0.85	1	1
4	c. 109 G>A	p.V37I	TM1	Missense mutation (Transition); Pathogenic	1	0.86	0	0	1	0.42	0	1
5	c. 126 G>T	p.E42D	EC1	Missense mutation (Transversion);NOVEL	1	0.86	2	1.67	3	1.27	3	0
6	c.165 C>A	p.T55T	EC1	Missense mutation (Transversion); Polymorphism	1	0.86	0	0	1	0.42	0	1
7	c. 224 G>A	p. R75Q#	TM2	Missense mutation (Transition); Pathogenic	0	0	1	0.83	1	0.42	0	1
8	c.231 G>A	p.W77X	TM2	Nonsense mutation (Transition); Pathogenic	2	1.72	3	2.5	5	2.12	2	3
9	c.341 A>G	p.E114G	IC2	Missense mutation (Transition); Polymorphism	1	0.86	1	0.83	2	0.85	1	1
10	c. 370 C>T	p.Q124X	IC2	Nonsense mutation (Transition); Pathogenic	1	0.86	2	1.67	3	1.27	0	3
11	c.380 G>A	p.R127H	IC2	Missense mutation (Transition); Polymorphism	13	11.21	12	10	25	**10.59**	13	12
12	c.457 G>A	p.V153I	TM3	Missense mutation (Transition); Polymorphism	6	5.17	8	5.83	14	5.93	5	9
13	c.493 C>T	p.R165W	EC2	Missense mutation (Transversion); Polymorphism	0	0	1	0.83	1	0.42	1	0
14	c. 551G>A	p.R184Q#	EC2	Missense mutation (Transition); Pathogenic	1	0.86	0	0	1	0.42	0	1
15	c.IVS 1+1 G>A (-3172 G>A)		EXON 1	Splice site mutation (Transition); Pathogenic	1	0.86	3	2.5	4	1.7	0	4
TOTAL					60	51.72	65	54.17	125	52.96	58 (54.72%)	67 (51.54%)

* Out of the 60 DXD couples comprising of 120 individuals, 2 HI males did not participate in the molecular study, of which one had parental consanguinity and other did not have.

#Autosomal dominant mutations

Red color – Pathogenic; Green – polymorphism; Blue – Novel Variants; TM1-3 – Transmembrane domain 1 - 3; EC1 & EC2 – extracellular domains 1 & 2; IC – cytoplasmic domain

most common pathogenic genotype observed in this sub group also with a frequency of 23.91%, which is marginally higher than in DXD mating. The *GJB2* genotypes observed among the control group have been listed out in Table 10 No *GJB6* variants were observed among the normal hearing controls.

The overall carrier frequency for *GJB2* pathogenic mutations, including the novel variants, among the HI mates, in both the sub groups included (DXD and affected partners of DXN mating), was 4.88%, which was twice the frequency observed in the normal hearing controls (2.42%). The carrier frequency of normal hearing partners of DXN mating was as high as 9.30%.

Novel variants in *GJB2* and *GJB6* genes

Four novel variants, p.E42D (in *GJB2* gene), p.Q57R, p.E101Q, p.R104H (in *GJB6* gene) were identified in this study. This is the first study from Indian subcontinent reporting novel variants in the coding region of *GJB6* gene.

p.E42D was observed at a frequency of 1.27% among the DXD mates. It is a missense mutation due to G > T transversion at 126th nucleotide, resulting in a change from glutamic acid to aspartic acid at 42nd codon in the EC1 domain of the protein. It was observed in two DXD families, in homozygous, heterozygous as well as in compound heterozygous state along with a novel *GJB6* mutation and variable phenotypes. In the first DXD family (DXD BND19, Fig. 2a) it was observed in homozygous state (E42D/E42D) in the female DXD mate & in heterozygous state among her two siblings and her mother, all of whom showed variable phenotypes ranging from mild to profound, conductive, sensorineural and mixed type of hearing losses (Fig. 2b). The affected members did not have any other associated clinical features. The members with mild and moderate hearing losses were not aware of their hearing status until our audiometric evaluation.

In the second DXD family (DXD BLR47, Fig. 3a), the novel mutation was observed in compound heterozygous state (E42D/+) along with a novel *GJB6* gene mutation (R104H/+) in the HI husband, suggesting a digenic interaction between the two. The affected elder sister showed a similar genotype involving the two novel variants in the *GJB2* and *GJB6* genes. The affected elder brother did not have any changes in the *GJB2* gene and had only the novel variant in heterozygous condition (R104H/+) in the *GJB6* gene. Audiological evaluation of the affected husband, affected wife and affected elder brother showed them to have bilateral, profound, sensorineural hearing loss, while the affected elder sister had bilateral, moderately severe, sensorineural hearing loss (Fig. 3b). The affected elder brother had goiter, which appeared in the second decade of his life. The affected members did not have any other associated clinical features. p.R104H is a G > A transition at 311th nucleotide resulting in a change from arginine to histidine at the 104th codon in the IC2 domain of the connexin 30 protein (Fig. 1).

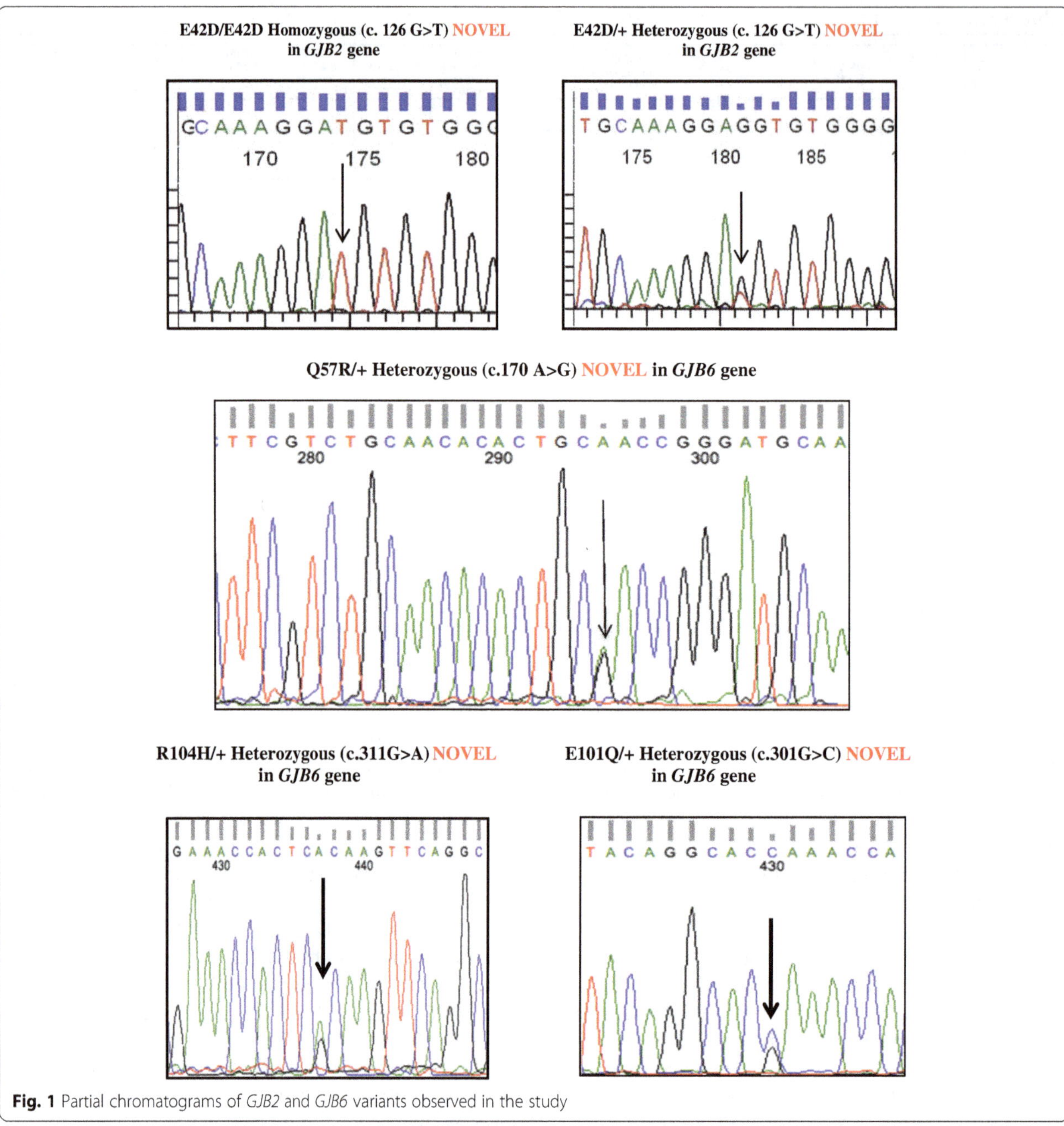

Fig. 1 Partial chromatograms of *GJB2* and *GJB6* variants observed in the study

The novel missense variant p.R104H in the *GJB6* gene was observed at a frequency of 1.71% in the 117 HI individuals selected for the second level screening, in this study.

p.Q57R variant (in GJB6 gene)

p.Q57R, a **novel missense variant**, was observed in the *GJB6* gene at a frequency of 0.85% in the 117 HI individuals. This variant was observed in only one DXD mate in a heterozygous condition (Q57R/+) with no associated *GJB2* gene mutations (Fig. 4). The DXD couple did not have any changes in the *GJB2* gene. The affected husband, his affected brother and sister had a novel variant p.Q57R in heterozygous condition (Q57R/+) in the *GJB6* gene. The affected wife did not have any changes in the *GJB6* gene. This novel mutation was not observed in the selected DXN mates and the normal hearing controls. p.Q57R is an A > G transition at 170th nucleotide resulting in a change from glutamine to arginine at the 57th codon in the EC1 domain of the connexin 30 protein (Fig. 1).

p.E101Q variant (in GJB6gene)

p.E101Q is a G > C transition at the 301st nucleotide resulting in a change from glutamic acid to glutamine at

Table 6 Summary of pathogenic mutations/ variants in the *GJB2* gene observed among the HI and Normal hearing partners of 46 DXN families

S. No	GJB2 VARIANTS		EFFECT	HI partners (n=46)				Normal Hearing partners (n=43*)			
	CODON	PROTEIN		ALLELES (n=92)	FREQUENCY (%)	With parental consanguinity (n=48)	Without parental consanguinity (n=44)	ALLELES (n=86)	FREQUENCY (%)	With parental consanguinity (n=10)	Without parental consanguinity (n=76)
1	c.71 G>A	p.W24X	Nonsense mutation (Transition); Pathogenic	28	30.43	11	17	6	6.98	0	6
2	c.231 G>A	p.W77X	Nonsense mutation (Transition); Pathogenic	1	1.09	0	1	0	0	0	0
3	c.257 C>T	p.T86M	Missense mutation (Transition); Pathogenic	2	2.17	2	0	1	1.16	1	0
4	c.262 G>A	p.A88A	Missense mutation (Transition); Polymorphism	2	2.17	1	1	1	1.16	0	1
5	c. 370 C>T	p.Q124X	Nonsense mutation (Transition); Pathogenic	2	2.17	0	2	1	1.16	0	1
6	c.380 G>A	p.R127H	Missense mutation (Transition); Polymorphism	4	4.35	1	3	6	6.98	2	4
7	c.457 G>A	p.V153I	Missense mutation (Transition); Polymorphism	1	1.09	1	0	3	3.49	0	3
8	c.493 C>T	p.R165W	Missense mutation (Transversion); Polymorphism	0	0	0	0	1	1.16	0	1
9	c.585 G>A	p.M195I	Missense mutation (Transition); Polymorphism	1	1.09	0	1	0	0	0	0
10	c.675 A>T	p.P225P	Missense mutation (Transversion); Polymorphism	1	1.09	0	1	0	0	0	0
TOTAL				42	45.65	16 (33.33%)	26 (59.09%)	19	22.09	3 (30%)	16 (21.05%)

*** Out of the 46 normal hearing partners, three did not participate in the molecular study. All the three did not have any parental consanguinity;**
Red color - Pathogenic; Green - polymorphism

the 101st codon in the IC2 cytoplasmic domain of the connexin 30 protein (Fig. 1). This novel missense variant in the *GJB6* gene was observed at a frequency of 0.85% in 117 HI individuals. It was observed in only one affected female partner of a DXN family in a heterozygous condition (E101Q/+) with no associated *GJB2* mutations (Fig. 5).There was no parental consanguinity in both the sides, but the wife's side had history of deafness with four siblings affected. The couple had two affected monozygotic twins, but one of them died due to unspecified illness. The couple also had a normal hearing daughter, who did not participate in the study. The DXN couple, two affected siblings of the proband and the surviving affected son participated in the study. Audiological evaluation of the four affected members showed them to have bilateral, profound, sensorineural hearing loss. The affected members did not have any other associated clinical features. The HI wife, her HI son and her two HI siblings did not have any changes in the *GJB2* gene. They all had the novel variant p.E101Q in the *GJB6* gene in heterozygous condition (E101Q/+).It was absent in the 85 DXD mating individuals and the normal hearing controls. The normal hearing husband of the deaf mate in this DXN family was a carrier of the common polymorphism p.R127H in the *GJB2* gene in heterozygous condition (R127H/+), which was also present in the affected son.

In silico analysis of novel variants observed in *GJB2* and *GJB6* genes

We predicted the functional significance of the novel variant p.E42D identified in *GJB2* and the 3 novel variants, p.Q57R, p.E101Q and p.R104H, identified in *GJB6* using two in silico tools namely SIFT and PolyPhen2. Predictions by the former tool is based on the alignment of orthologous and/or paralogous protein sequences while the latter considers evolutionary conservation, the physiochemical differences, and the proximity of the substitution to predicted functional domains and/or structural features. The outputs of both tools show that p.Q57R and p.R104H may affect or damage the structure and functioning of the Cx30 protein, but p.E101Q is tolerable or benign. Also, p.E42D in *GJB2* was predicted to be tolerable or benign (Table 11).

To further gain insight on the effect of these mutations on the physicochemical parameters of Cx26 or Cx30 protein, we analysed their native and mutant

Table 7 Novel *GJB6* variants observed in DXD and DXN families

S. No.	*GJB6* Variants		Domain/ Location	Effect	Alleles in DXD (n=170)*	Alleles in DXN (n=64)*	Overall Allelic Frequency (%)
	Codon	Protein					
1	c.311 G>A	p.R104H	IC2	Missense mutation; Transition; NOVEL; Possibly pathogenic	2 (1.18%)	0	0.85%
2	c.170 A>G	p.Q57R	EC1	Missense mutation; Transition; NOVEL; Possibly pathogenic	1 (0.59%)	0	0.43%
3	c.301 G>C	p.E101Q	IC2	Missense mutation; Transversion; NOVEL; Possibly pathogenic	0	1 (1.56%)	0.43%

* HI mates with novel variants in the *GJB2* gene, heterozygous carriers of pathogenic mutations in the *GJB2* gene or negative for pathogenic *GJB2* mutations were included for *GJB6* mutation screening

Table 8 Frequency and distribution of *GJB2* and *GJB6* genotypes observed among the 118 hearing impaired mates of DXD mating

S. No.	*GJB2* and *GJB6* genotypes	HI Husband (n=58)*	Frequency %	HI Wife (n=60)	Frequency %	Total (n=118)	Combined Frequency (%)
I	*GJB2*-Biallelic & Triallelic						
1	W24X/W24X	13	22.41	13	21.67	26	22.03
2	V153I/V153I	1	1.72	2	3.33	3	2.54
3	W77X/W77X	1	1.72	1	1.67	2	1.7
4	R127H/R127H	1	1.72	1	1.67	2	1.7
5	R127H/V153I	1	1.72	1	1.67	2	1.7
6	V27I/E114G	1	1.72	1	1.67	2	1.7
7	E42D/E42D	0	0	1	1.67	1	0.85
8	W77X/Q124X	0	0	1	1.67	1	0.85
9	W24X/I35S	0	0	1	1.67	1	0.85
10	Q124X/IVS1+1G>A	0	0	1	1.67	1	0.85
11	R75Q[#]/V153I	0	0	1	1.67	1	0.85
12	V37I/V153I	1	1.72	0	0	1	0.85
13	V153I/R165W	0	0	1	1.67	1	0.85
14	R184Q[#]/Q124X/IVS1+1G>A	1	1.72	0	0	1	0.85
15	W24X/T55T/R127H	1	1.72	0	0	1	0.85
II	*GJB2*-Monoallelic						
1	R127H/+	9	15.52	9	15	18	15.25
2	W24X/+	4	6.9	2	3.33	6	5.08
3	V153I/+	2	3.45	1	1.67	3	2.54
4	IVS1+1G>A/+	0		2	1.67	2	1.7
5	I35S/+	0		1	1.67	1	0.85
III	*GJB6*-Monoallelic						
1	R104H/+	1	1.72	0	0	1	0.85
2	Q57R/+	1	1.72	0	0	1	0.85
IV	*GJB2/GJB6*-Digenic						
1	E42D/+; R104H/+	1	1.72	0	0	1	0.85

* Out of the 60 DXD couples comprising of 120 individuals, 2 individuals did not participate in the molecular study
[#]Autosomal dominant mutations

structures individually in Expasy's ProtParam tool and compared the results (Table 12).

The native and the mutant proteins differ in their molecular weight and the number of atoms they are composed of. Moreover, the total number of positively charged residues increases from 29 to 30 in case of p.Q57R. On the other hand, p.R104H decreases the positively charged residues from 29 to 28. The mutation p.E101Q reduces the number of negatively charged residues from 23 to 22. The instability index of p.Q57R and p.R104H, shows a slight variation when compared to that of the native protein. p.Q57R tends to slightly increase the stability of the protein and in contrast p.R104H makes the protein more unstable. However, an instability value > 40 suggests that the mutant forms as well as the native form are quite unstable since they are membrane channels. Moreover, a shift was observed in the GRAVY score for the mutants p.Q57R and p.R104H. Positive scores of GRAVY indicate the hydrophobic nature of the protein. p.Q57R reduces the hydrophobicity while p.R104H increases this property. There is no change in the aliphatic index and this high score (91.07) suggests that the native and the mutant proteins may retain their conformation over a wider range of temperatures.

The function of a protein not only relies on its properties but also on its three dimensional structure. Hence we queried RCSB Protein Data Bank for the 3-dimensional structures of Cx26 and Cx30 proteins. Only the crystal structure of Cx26 was available, which was downloaded and used for analyzing the effect of p.E42D mutation. The model was viewed with the help of Swiss-PdbViewer. The Glutamic acid at position 42 was found to be a part of an alpha helix and it was mutated to Aspartic acid in all 6 chains of the hexameric protein. Both the mutated and the native structures were subjected to Ramachandran Plot analysis through RAMPAGE

Table 9 Frequency and distribution of *GJB2* and *GJB6* genotypes observed among the mates of DXN mating

S. No.	Genotypes	Affected Partner (n= 46)	Frequency (%)	Normal hearing partner (n=43)*	Frequency (%)
I	*GJB2*-Biallelic				
1	W24X/W24X	11	23.91	0	0
2	Q124X/Q124X	1	2.17	0	0
3	T86M/T86M	1	2.17	0	0
4	W24X/W77X	1	2.17	0	0
5	W24X/A88A	1	2.17	0	0
6	R153I/R165W	0		1	2.33
6	M195I/P225P	1	2.17	0	0
II	*GJB2*-Monoallelic				
1	W24X/+	4	8.7	6	13.95
	T86M/+	0	0	1	2.33
	Q124X/+	0	0	1	2.33
2	R127H/+	4	8.7	6	13.95
3	V153I/+	1	2.17	2	4.65
4	A88A/+	1	2.17	1	2.33
III	*GJB6*-Monoallelic				
1	E101Q/+	1	2.17	0	0

* Out of the 46 normal hearing partners, three did not participate in the molecular study. All the three did not have any parental consanguinity

Table 10 Frequency and distribution of *GJB2* genotypes observed among the 165 normal hearing controls

S.No.	*GJB2* genotype	Normal hearing control population (n=165)	Frequency %
1	W24X/+	5	3.02
2	N62S/+	1	0.61
3	E147K/T55T	1	0.61
4	W24X/M195I/P225P	1	0.61
1	R127H/R127H	5	3.02
2	R127H/R165W	1	0.61
3	R127H/T55T	1	0.61
4	V153I/R165W	2	1.21
5	Q80Q/R127H	1	0.61
6	R127H/+	44	26.67
7	V153I/+	4	2.41
8	Q80Q/+	1	0.61
9	T55T/+	1	0.61
10	G45G/+	1	0.61
		69	41.82

Online portal. The results showed that the mutation p.E42D did not alter the percentage of amino acid residues in the favorable, allowed and outlier regions of the plot (Fig. 6).

Connexin 30 structure was also modeled using SWISS MODEL repository. As expected, the QMEAN Z-score of the model was low (– 6.59), reinforcing the fact that it is a membrane protein. The predicted structure of Cx30 protein is shown in Fig. 7a and b with 7 Helices, 8 Strands and 13 Turns. In this model, Glutamic Acid (E) at position 101 and Arginine (R) at position 104 are part of alpha helices, while Glutamine (Q) at position 57 was found in the loop region that connects a beta sheet with alpha helix.

The mutant structures of Cx30 with the substituting amino acid at the above mentioned positions (p.Q57R, p.E101Q and p.R104H) were created with the help of Swiss-PdbViewer and saved as separate files. These structures were energy minimized and submitted to RAMPAGE online portal. Computation of Ramachandran plot showed that only p.Q57R is capable of changing the conformation of the protein, since the substitution decreased the number of residues in the favored region and increased the number of residues in the allowed region (Fig. 6).

Genotype-phenotype correlation of *GJB2/GJB6* mutations in the incidence of hearing loss in DXD families

The 60 DXD families are further classified based on the genotype-phenotype correlation in the offspring with respect to the *GJB2* and *GJB6* mutations, as listed in Table 13. The table divides the 60 DXD mating families further into four groups: Group-I: Non-complementary mating families with all affected offspring only Group-II: Complementary mating families with all hearing offspring only Group-III: Segregating type families with both affected and normal hearing offspring Group-IV: Families with no offspring.

Group I

Seventeen families (28.33%) belonged to this group where all offspring were affected. In 8 out of these 17 families, both the affected partners had *GJB2* mutations in either homozygous condition or in compound heterozygous condition. In other words, 47.06% of the non-complementary matings were caused by *GJB2* mutations. Overall, 13.33% of the DXD families were affected by *GJB2* mutations. One among these 8 families had a unique triallelic pattern involving both a dominant mutation as well as recessive mutations of *GJB2* gene (R184Q/ Q124X/ IVS1 + 1G > A), observed for the first time in the world [12].

In 3 other families, only one of the two deaf partners had either a homozygous, or heterozygous *GJB2* mutation or a heterozygous *GJB6* mutation, but had HI

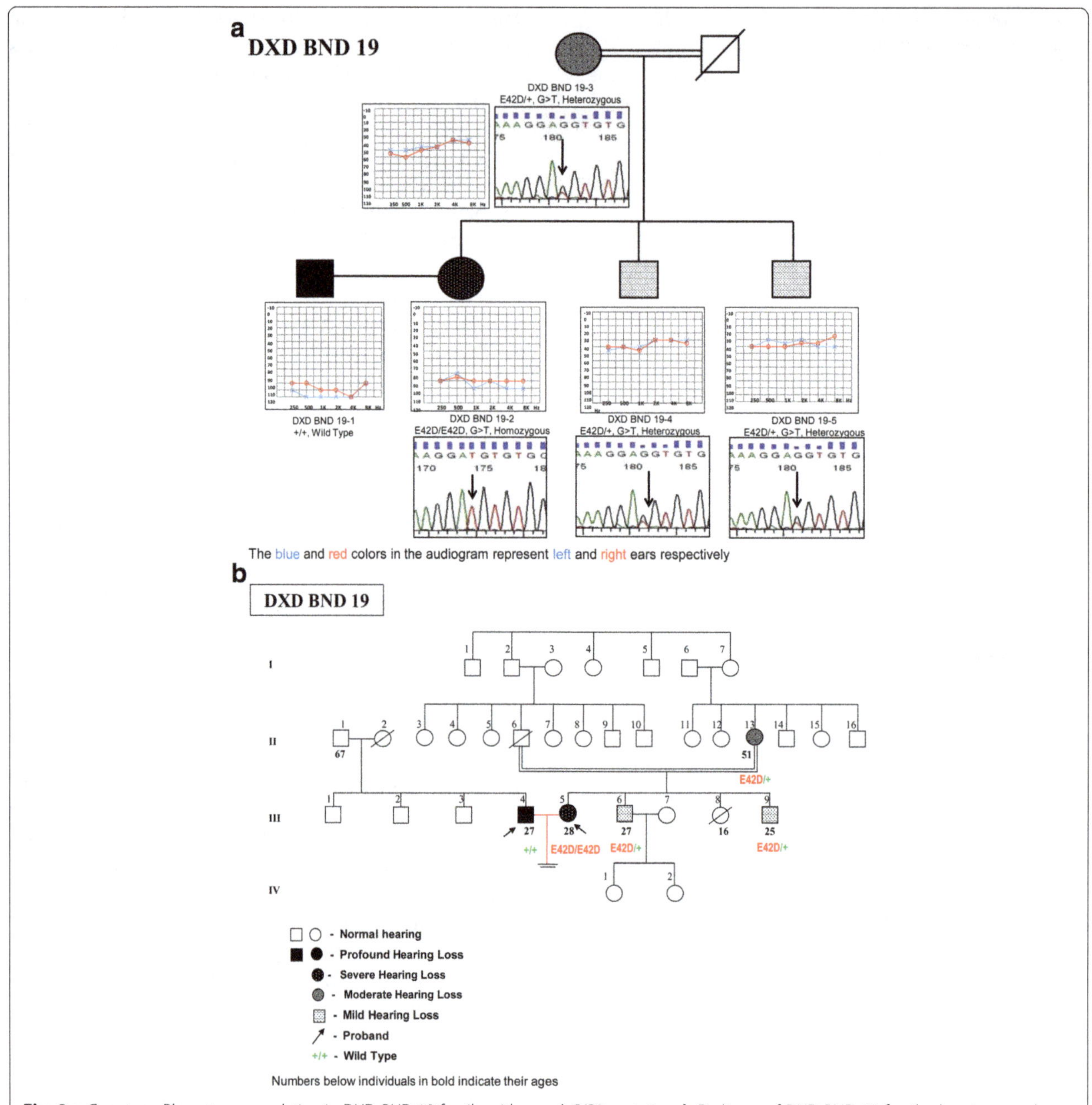

Fig. 2 a Genotype-Phenotype correlation in DXD BND 19 family with novel *GJB2* mutation. **b** Pedigree of DXD BND 19 family showing novel mutation p.E42D in *GJB2* gene

offspring. In the remaining 6 families, none of the partners had any *GJB2*/*GJB6* mutations.

Group II

Thirty families (50%) in this group had all normal hearing offspring. Eleven out of these families did not have any *GJB2* or *GJB6* mutations. In the remaining 19 families (63.33%), one family had a combination of one deaf partner having *GJB2* mutation in homozygous condition and other partner having a *GJB2* mutation in heterozygous condition, but having normal hearing offspring. In the remaining 18 families, only one partner had a single *GJB2* mutation in homozygous condition or heterozygous condition, or a *GJB6* mutation in heterozygous condition.

Group III

Two families (3.33%) out of the 60 DXD families had one normal hearing and one affected offspring each. One family was a non-*GJB2* family with both the HI

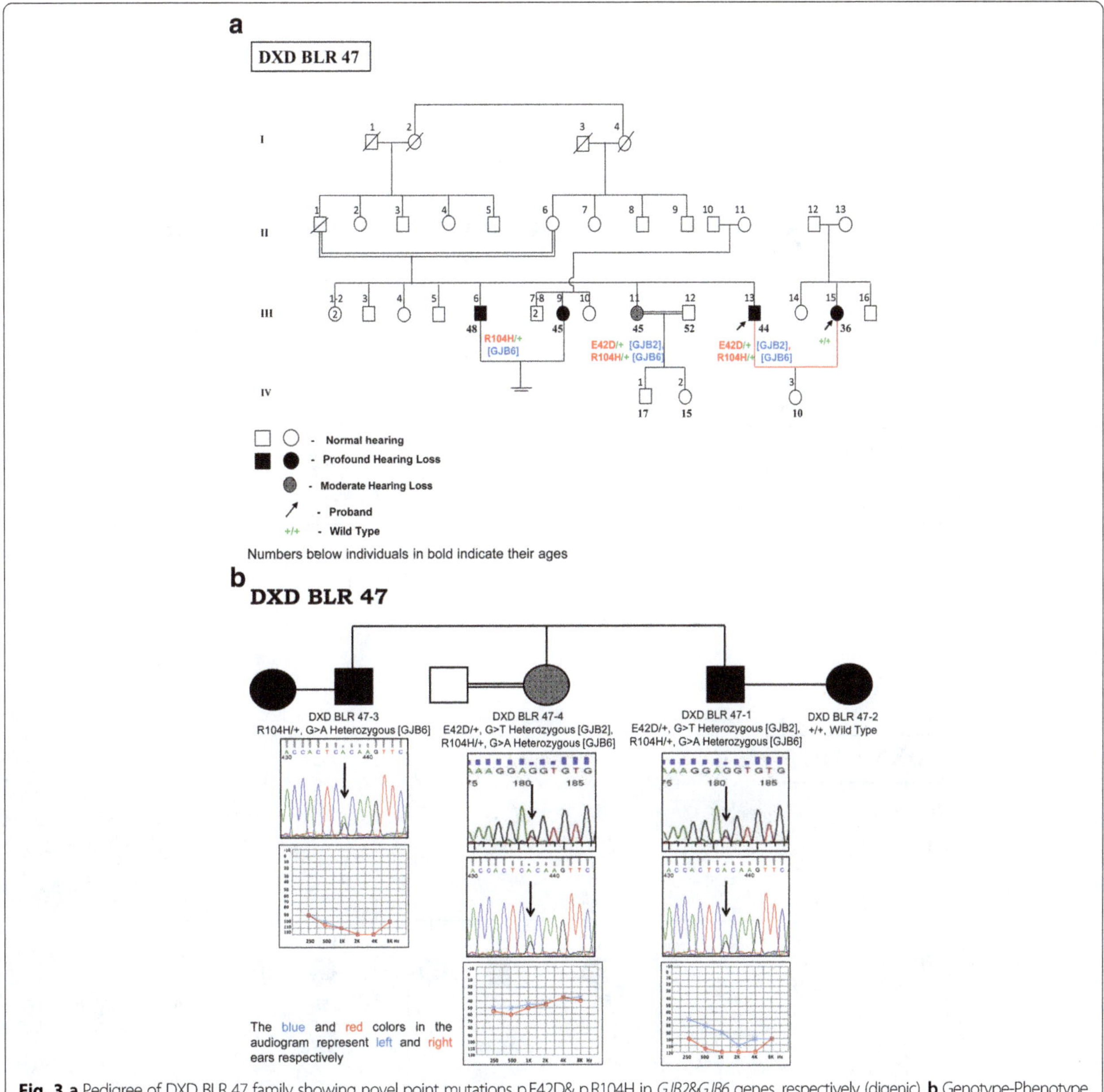

Fig. 3 a Pedigree of DXD BLR 47 family showing novel point mutations p.E42D& p.R104H in *GJB2&GJB6* genes, respectively (digenic). **b** Genotype-Phenotype correlation in DXD BLR 47 family with novel *GJB2/GJB6* mutations

partners not having any *GJB2* mutations. In the second family in this group, one of the deaf partners had an autosomal dominant *GJB2* mutation in heterozygous condition (R75Q/+) with the affected offspring also inheriting the same from the parent [11].

Group IV

Eleven families (18.33%) out of the 60 DXD families did not have any offspring. Five out of these families did not have any *GJB2* or *GJB6* mutations. In 1 out of the remaining 6 families, one deaf partner had homozygous *GJB2* mutation while the other had in heterozygous condition. In the remaining 5 families, 4 families had one partner with a homozygous *GJB2* mutation and the remaining one had one partner with novel *GJB6* mutation in heterozygous condition (Q57R/+).

Role of *GJB2/GJB6* mutations in the incidence of hearing loss in DXN families

The 46 DXN families were further classified based on consanguinity and the role of *GJB2/ GJB6* mutations in the incidence of hearing loss, as the principle of complementarity cannot be applied to this subgroup at the phenotypic level.

DXD TN 46
I
II
III
70
+/+
+/+
Q57R/+
Q57R/+
Q57R/+
- Normal hearing
- Profound Hearing Loss
- Proband
+/+ - Wild Type

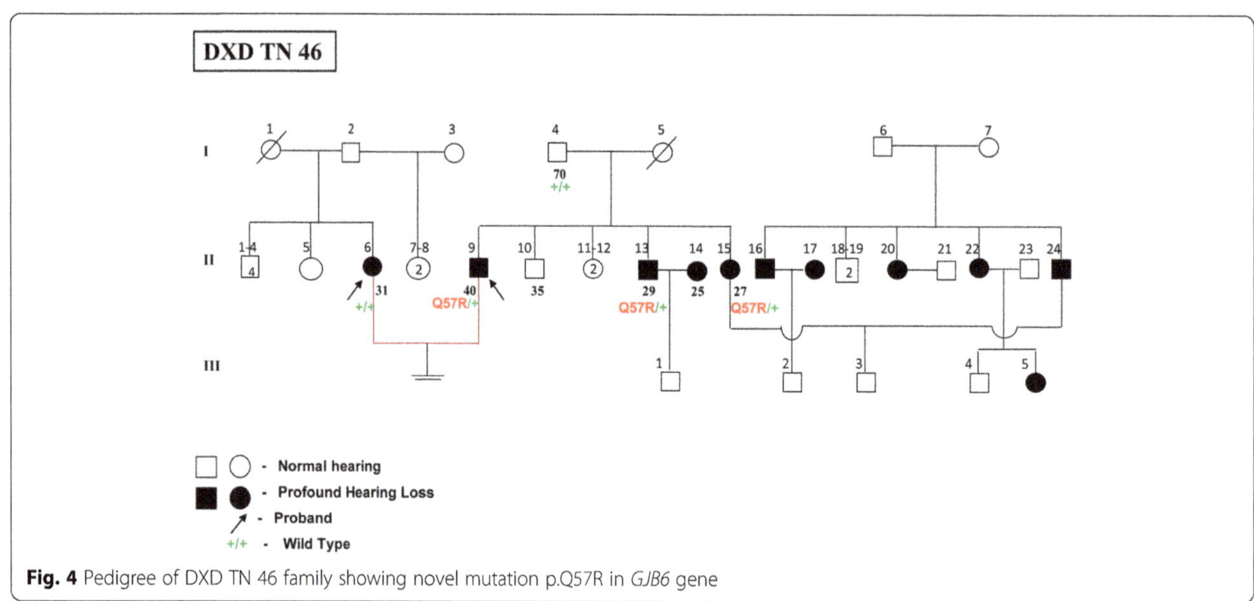

Fig. 4 Pedigree of DXD TN 46 family showing novel mutation p.Q57R in *GJB6* gene

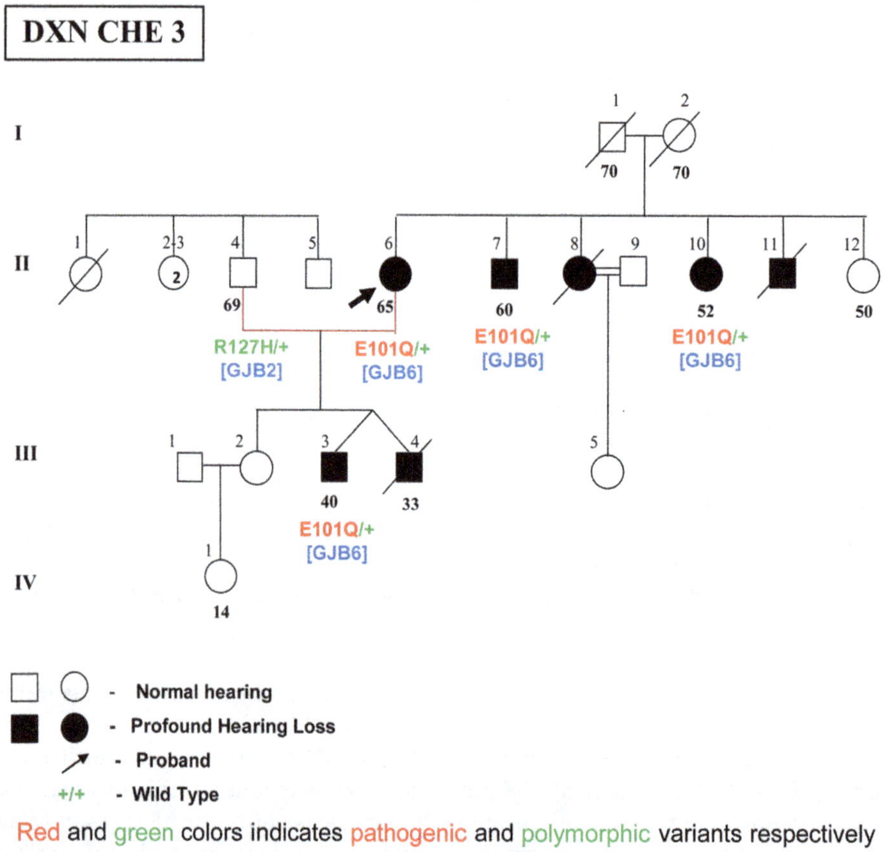

DXN CHE 3
I
II
III
IV
R127H/+
[GJB2]
E101Q/+
[GJB6]
E101Q/+
[GJB6]
E101Q/+
[GJB6]
E101Q/+
[GJB6]
- Normal hearing
- Profound Hearing Loss
- Proband
+/+ - Wild Type
Red and green colors indicates pathogenic and polymorphic variants respectively

Fig. 5 Pedigree of DXNCHE3 family showing novel mutation p.E101Q in *GJB6* gene

Table 11 Comparative analysis of the SIFT predictions for the novel variants in *GJB2* and *GJB6* genes

Mutation	SIFT				PolyPhen-2					
					HumDiv			HumVar		
	Score	Median Sequence conservation	Sequences represented at position	Comment	Score	Sensitivity, Specificity	Comment	Score	Sensitivity, Specificity	Comment
p.E42D (*GJB2*)	0.57	3.05	42	Tolerated	0.038	0.94, 0.82	Benign	0.052	0.93, 0.63	Benign
p.Q57R (*GJB6*)	0.00	3.09	35	Affect protein function	1.000	0.00, 1.00	Probably damaging	1.000	0.00, 1.00	Probably damaging
p.E101Q (*GJB6*)	0.48	3.10	29	Tolerated	0.183	0.92, 0.87	Benign	0.114	0.90, 0.69	Benign
p.R104H (*GJB6*)	0.01	3.09	35	Affect protein function	0.990	0.41, 0.98	Probably damaging	0.749	0.77, 0.86	Possibly damaging

Group-I families: Consanguineously mating DXN families with and without GJB2/GJB6 mutation affliction

This group consisted of 18 DXN families (39.13%), with consanguineous marriages. Twelve families (66.67%) had affected offspring, indicating the role of consanguinity in the incidence of hearing loss. Eight families (44.44%) had *GJB2*/*GJB6* mutations in one or both the partners in homozygous or heterozygous conditions (Table 14). Five out of these 8 families had affected offspring, two had normal hearing offspring and in one family there was no offspring.

Group II families: Non-consanguineously mating DXN families with and without GJB2/GJB6 mutation affliction

This group consisted of 28 DXN families (61.87%), with non-consanguineous mating. Seven out of the 28 families (25%) had affected offspring while 71.43% of these families had only normal hearing offspring (20/28). One family did not have offspring. Twelve out of the 28 families (42.86%) had *GJB2*/*GJB6* mutations in one or both the partners in homozygous or heterozygous conditions (Table 15). Out of these 12 families, two families (16.67%) had affected offspring, one of whom had a novel variant p.E101Q in the *GJB6* gene in heterozygous condition, reported for the first time through this study. In 7 families, the affected partners have the most common mutation p.W24X in homozygous condition (W24X/W24X), five of whom have normal hearing offspring and one does not have any offspring.

Statistical analysis for significance

The *GJB2* mutation frequency observed among the four study groups, (DXD mating, affected partners in DXN mating, normal hearing partners in DXN mating and the normal hearing controls) was compared using chi-square test, with the assumption that the differences if observed may be only due to chance. We observed that the chi-square value, which compares the differences between the observed and the expected values across the three groups, to be 58.21, with a p- value < 0.001, which is highly significant (Table 16).

Table 12 Comparison of native and the mutant structure with p.E42D variant in Cx26 protein using Expasy's ProtParam tool

	GJB2		*GJB6*			
Property	Native	p.E42D	Native	p.Q57R	p.E101Q	p.R104H
Number of amino acids	226	226	261	261	261	261
Molecular weight	26215	26201	30387.4	30415.5	30386.4	30368.4
Theoretical pI (Isoelectric point)	9.11	9.11	8.81	8.92	8.92	8.68
Total number of negatively charged residues (Asp + Glu)	18	18	23	23	22	23
Total number of positively charged residues (Arg + Lys)	27	27	29	30	29	28
Total number of atoms	3721	3718	4274	4280	4275	4268
Ext. coefficient assuming all pairs of Cys residues form cystines	52410	52410	52410	52410	52410	52410
Ext. coefficient assuming all Cys residues are reduced	51910	51910	51910	51910	51910	51910
Estimated half life (mammalian reticulocytes, in vitro)	30 hrs	30 hrs	30 hrs	30 hrs	30 hrs	30 hrs
Instability index	42.8	42.8	43.11	42.60	43.11	44.01
Aliphatic index	98.67	98.67	91.07	91.07	91.07	91.07
Grand average of hydropathicity (GRAVY)	0.288	0.288	0.055	0.051	0.055	0.06

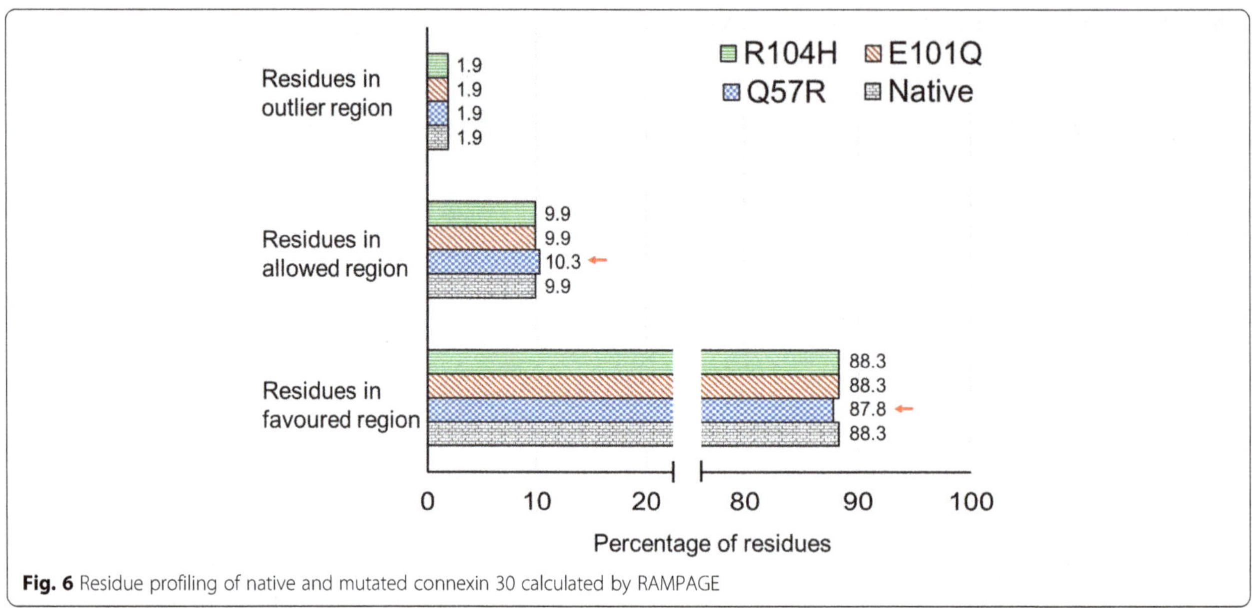

Fig. 6 Residue profiling of native and mutated connexin 30 calculated by RAMPAGE

Discussion

Assortative mating as a form of non-random mating has the potential to act as an evolutionary agent. Assortative mating is capable of bringing together rare, non-allelic genes for the same phenotype, creating a non-random distribution of genes that has been termed "gametic-phase disequilibrium." It also increases the population variance. However, as the number of genes involved in creating a particular trait increases, assortative mating has a reduced capability to increase homozygosity at any one locus. There have been several studies on assortative mating among the deaf in the US. Edward Allen Fay [28], through his monumental work "Marriages among the Deaf in America", observed that marriages of the deaf had rapidly increased in America in that century, attributing largely to the establishment of schools for the deaf. Deaf marrying deaf constituted 72.5% of the married deaf population. Analysis of the DXD matings showed that 79% were "complementary" matings (i.e., only hearing offspring), 4.2% were "non-complementary" matings (capable of producing only deaf offspring), and the remaining 16.8% were "segregating" matings, in which the parents were capable of producing both deaf and hearing offspring.

This work was followed by another landmark work by Rose [29, 30] in which the data generated by Fay was compared with the contemporary data generated through a 1969 survey. Rose's results showed that between the 19th and 20th centuries, the frequency of deaf children with one or two deaf parents increased by 38%. Among the deaf children through DXD mating, the estimated proportion of non-complementary marriages also increased by 23%. Based on these observations and using computer simulations, Nance et al. proposed that the introduction of sign language 400 years ago in many Western countries and subsequent establishment of residential schools for the deaf could have favored assortative mating among deaf and relaxed genetic selection against deafness, leading to doubling of frequency of DFNB1 deafness in the United States in the last 200 years [13, 14]. In a study on living deaf alumni of Gallaudet University, Arnos et al. [15] collected pedigree data on 311 marriages among deaf individuals. On the basis of segregation analysis on these 311 matings between deaf individuals, the authors reported that 23% were non-complementary, an increase of more than fivefold over the previous century's data of 4.2%, as reported by Fay. Mutational analysis within these non-complementary mating individuals showed a statistically significant linear increase in the prevalence of pathologic *GJB2* mutations. In addition to this, 199 probands with one or both parents deaf were also screened for *GJB2* mutations and they too showed similar significant linear increase. In both these studies, c.35delG was the most common mutation in the *GJB2* gene, ranging from 69 to 73%. These data were consistent with the increase in the frequency of DFNB1 predicted by the previous simulation studies and provided convincing evidence over the influence of assortative mating on the frequency of common genes for deafness.

DFNB1 dynamics in DXD families

In our present study, we observed 17 families out of the 60 DXD families (28.33%) to be non-complementary, i.e. with *all affected offspring*. This is higher than the Arnos et al.'s observation of 23%. While Arnos' sampling was restricted to Gallaudet University alumni and not to a particular ethnicity or population, our study represents the south Indian HI population belonging to the four

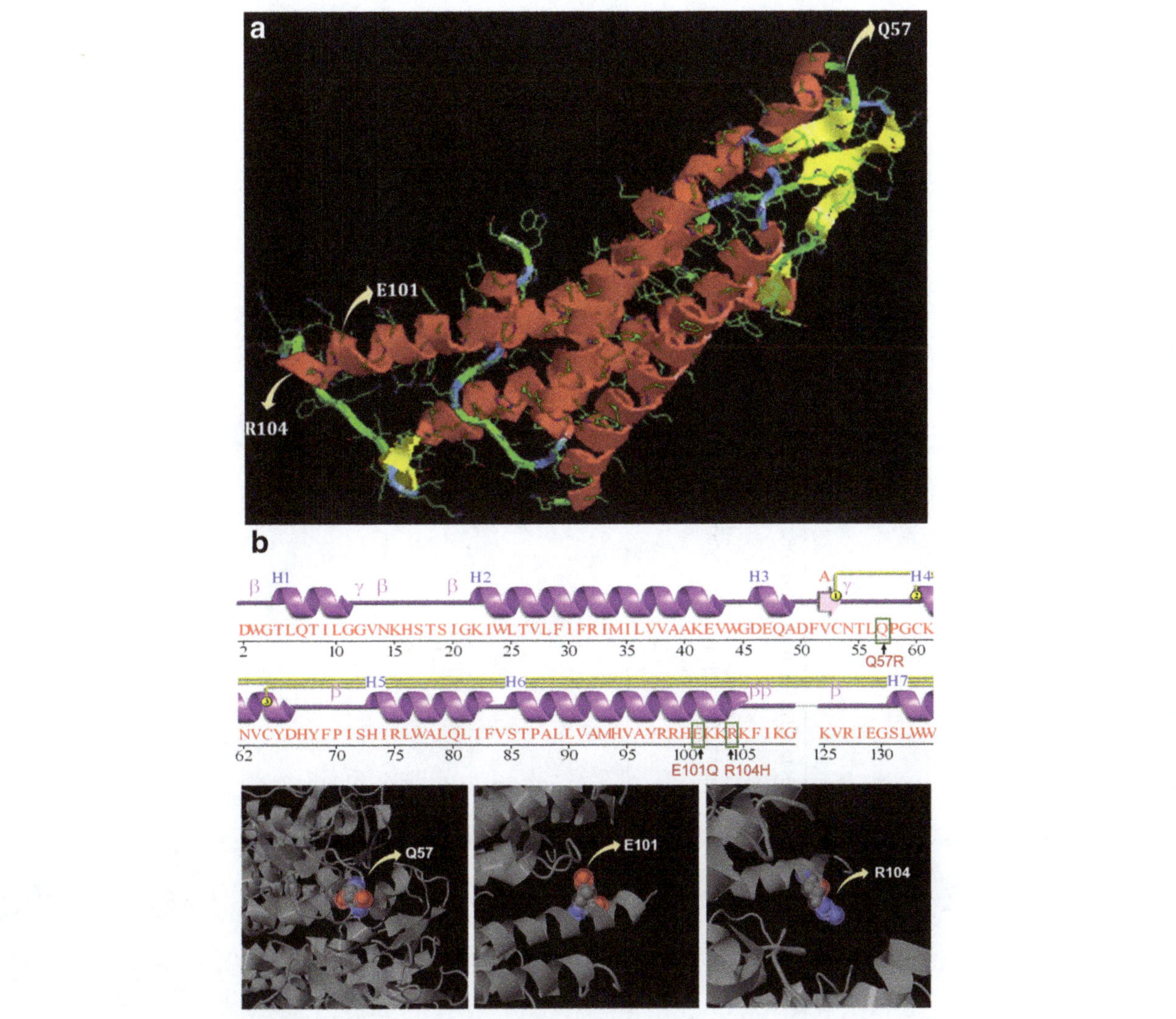

Fig. 7 **a** Predicted model of connexin 30 protein single chain indicating the positions of the variants, Q57, E101 & R104 observed in this study. **b**: Wiring diagram and 3-D structure of connexin 30 protein showing the position of Q57, E101 and R104

southern states-Andhra Pradesh, Karnataka, Kerala and Tamil Nadu. In 8 families out of the 17 non-complementary mating families, both the affected partners had *GJB2* mutations in either homozygous condition or in compound heterozygous condition (Table 8). Biallelic *GJB2* mutations accounted for 13.33% of the DXD families and 47.06% of the non-complementary families.

In three other families from our 17, only one of the two deaf partners had either a homozygous, or heterozygous *GJB2* mutation or a heterozygous *GJB6* mutation, but with HI offspring. In two of these families, the affected offspring had one copy of the pathogenic DFNB1 allele indicating the possibility of probable role of these mutations in the incidence of hearing loss. This phenomenon has been explained by Arnos et al. [15] through their observation on *GJB2* mutations among DXD families and their pedigree analysis. In their study, the pedigree analysis of such families suggested that many of the additional segregating matings reflect pseudo-dominant transmission in families when one parent with deafness resulting from *GJB2* and/or *GJB6* mutations married a partner who is deaf for reasons yet to be determined but was also a heterozygous carrier of a single *GJB2* or *GJB6* mutation. One of the important effect of assortative mating is the bringing together of rare, non-allelic genes (on different gene loci) for the same phenotype, creating a non-random distribution of genes that has been termed "gametic-phase disequilibrium." In our study the possibility of co-occurrence of non-allelic genes in the affected offspring in at least two families (Fig. 8a and b) may be due to gametic phase disequilibrium.

One of the most important observations from this study is out of these eight biallelic *GJB2* mutation

Table 13 Genotype-phenotype correlation of *GJB2/GJB6* mutations in the offspring of DXD mating

		BOTH PARTNERS HAVING *GJB2*			ONLY ONE PARTNER WITH *GJB2*		ONLY ONE PARTNER WITH *GJB6*	ONLY ONE PARTNER WITH *GJB2/GJB6*		
S. No.	SUBGROUPS IN DXD MATING BASED ON PHENOTYPE OF OFFSPRING	BOTH HOMOZYGOUS OR COMPOUND HETEROZYGOUS	BOTH HETEROZYGOUS	ONE HOMOZYGOUS, ONE HETEROZYGOUS	HOMOZYGOUS	HETEROZYGOUS	ONE HETEROZYGOUS	DIGENIC	NON-*GJB2* & NON-*GJB6*	TOTAL (%)
1	Non-complementary with all deaf offspring	8	0	0	1	1	1	0	6*	17 (28.33%)
2	Complementary with all hearing offspring	0	1	1	11	6	0	1	10#	30 (50%)
3	Mixed offspring (hearing and hearing impaired)	0	0	0	0	1	0	0	1	2 (3.33%)
4	NO OFFSPRING	0	0	1	4	0	1	0	5	11 (18.33%)
5	TOTAL	8	1	2	16	8	2	1	22	60

*One HI male partner did not participate in the study, but his offspring did not carry any *GJB2* mutations

#One HI male partner expired, but his offspring did not carry any *GJB2* mutations

Table 14 Consanguineously mating DXN Families (Group I) with *GJB2/GJB6* mutations

S No.	Family ID	*GJB2/GJB6** genotype in Affected Partner	*GJB2/GJB6** Genotype in Normal hearing partner	Offspring hearing status	Consanguinity type
1	DXN NLR 9	W24X/W77X	W24X/+	One affected and one normal hearing	First Cousin type
2	DXN TVC 18	Q124X/Q124X	Q124X/+	One affected and one normal hearing	First Cousin type
3	DXN CHE 24	T86M/T86M	T86M/+	One affected and one normal hearing	Uncle-Niece type
4	DXN CHE 32	W24X/W24X	W24X/+	One affected and three normal hearing	Uncle-Niece type
5	DXN CHE 35	W24X/W24X	W24X/+	One affected and one normal hearing	Uncle-Niece type
6	DXN NLR 8	W24X/W24X	+/+	Normal hearing	Uncle-Niece type
7	DXN CHE 30	W24X/W24X	W24X/R127H	Normal hearing	Distantly related
8	DXN CHE 38	W24X/A88A	A88A/+	NO OFFSPRING	First Cousin type

******GJB6* **mutations were absent in this group**
The genotypes in column 3 refer to compound heterozygosity.
Red and Green colors indicate pathogenic and polymorphic variants respectively

carrying non-complementary mating DXD families, 50% of them have p.W24X mutation in homozygous condition in both the partners. While one of these eight DXD pairs was related as first cousins, the remaining seven pairs were unrelated. This high prevalence of p.W24X mutations among the south Indian DXD families could be attributed to the high carrier rate (1.82%) and high parental consanguinity (45%) as observed in our study.

In our study, 50% of the 60 DXD families had *only normal hearing offspring* (complementary mating DXD families). In 19 of these DXD families, one of the mates had a *GJB2/GJB6* mutation in homozygous or heterozygous condition. p.W24X mutation was the most common mutation, with 11 out of these 19 mates having it in homozygous condition and 7 of them having in heterozygous condition. In these 11 matings, the non-*GJB2* partner possibly had mutations in genes that did not contribute towards an affected phenotype in the offspring in combination with the *GJB2* mutation. The remaining 7 mates with heterozygous condition could simply be carriers of p.W24X mutation but with cause

Table 15 Non-consanguineously mating DXN families (Group II) with *GJB2/GJB6* mutations

S.No.	Family ID	*GJB2/GJB6* genotype in Affected Partner	*GJB2/GJB6* Genotype in Normal hearing partner	Offspring hearing status
1	DXN MDY 43	W24X/W24X	W24X/+	Two affected
2	DXN CHE 3	E101Q/+ (*GJB6*)	R127H/+	Two affected and one normal hearing
3	DXN CHE 20	W24X/W24X	+/+	Normal hearing
4	DXN CHE 21	W24X/W24X	+/+	Normal hearing
5	DXN TVC 22	W24X/W24X	+/+	Normal hearing
6	DXN CHE 36	W24X/W24X	+/+	Normal hearing
7	DXN HSR 41	W24X/W24X	V153I/+	Normal hearing
8	DXN NLR 7	W24X/+	+/+	Normal hearing
9	DXN NLR 10	W24X/+	+/+	Normal hearing
10	DXN TVC 28	W24X/+	+/+	Normal hearing
11	DXN HSR 40	W24X/+	+/+	Normal hearing
12	DXN CHE 48	W24X/W24X	+/+	NO Offspring

The genotypes in column 3 refer to compound heterozygosity.
Red and Green colors indicate pathogenic and polymorphic variants respectively.

Table 16 Chi-square analysis of *GJB2* variants among the four groups in our study

S. No.	Group		*GJB2* Positive Alleles	*GJB2* Negative Alleles	Total Alleles	Percentage (%)
1	DXD-Both Affected Partners	Observed (O)	125	111	236	52.96
		Expected (E)	85.01	150.99		
2	DXN- Affected Partners	Observed (O)	42	50	92	45.65
		Expected (E)	33.14	58.86		
3	DXN-Normal Hearing Partners	Observed (O)	19	67	86	22.09
		Expected (E)	30.98	55.02		
4	Control	Observed (O)	82	248	330	24.85
		Expected (E)	124.88	205.12		
	TOTAL		268	476	744	
	Chi-Square Value ($\Sigma(O-E)^2/E$)		58.21 (P< 0.001)			

for deafness lying in mutation or mutations in genes not associated with the DFNB1 locus. In the remaining one member, two novel *GJB2* and *GJB6* variants were observed in heterozygous condition showing digenic interaction, but his partner could be having a gene with no interaction with DFNB1 deafness causative factors.

In our study, 3.33% of 60 DXD families were of *segregating type* with one affected and one normal hearing offspring. One of these families had a dominant *GJB2* mutation, p.R75Q, in one partner and the affected offspring. This dominant mutation p.R75Q was observed for the first time in this study from India with non-syndromic presentation [11].

Interestingly, 11/60 DXD families (18.33%) had no offspring and hence could not be classically categorized as complementary/ non-complementary mating. This group too demonstrated a high frequency of *GJB2* mutations. In 6 of these families one of the mates carried *GJB2/GJB6* mutations, both novel and known, in homozygous or heterozygous condition. In one particular childless DXD family, the husband was a p.W24X carrier while the wife was W24X homozygous. Further analysis of these 11 families for deafness associated infertility genes such as *FOXI1, CATSPER2* and *STRC* could possibly throw more light on the etiology of this phenotype.

DFNB1 dynamics in DXN families

In our other study group of 46 DXN mating, we observed a higher rate of consanguinity (39.13%) in their marriages compared to their parental consanguinity (32.61%). Nearly 50% of the consanguineous DXN families had *GJB2* mutations. Once again, p.W24X mutation was the most common mutation in this subgroup also, with one-third of the families having this mutation in homozygous or heterozygous condition. More than 60% of these consanguineous families have affected offspring and p.W24X mutation is implicated in 60% of them. The same factor has perhaps resulted in the surfacing of a rare pathogenic variant like p.T86 M (observed for the first time in India), persistently in two consecutive generations as a result of continuous inbreeding for three generations (Fig. 9). Our findings present consanguinity as an important and additional dimension to assortative mating contributing to hearing impairment in the Indian subcontinent. It also further reiterates that consanguinity factor along with genetic drift plays an important role in the survival and initial phenotypic expression of such rare *GJB2* mutations.

Considering the non-consanguineous DXN mating families, only 7% were implicated with DFNB1 mutations. One-fourth of these families had affected offspring. Nearly 40% of the affected mates did have p.W24X mutation in homozygous or heterozygous condition. The presence of this mutation in this subgroup once again reiterates the high prevalence as well as high carrier rate of p.W24X mutation in south Indian population.

The overall allele frequency for DFNB1 mutations (*GJB2* and *GJB6* mutations) among the affected members in both the subgroups of assortatively mating was 35.67%while the carrier frequency for same among the affected members was 5.8%. The carrier frequency in the normal hearing partners of the DXN subgroup was 9.30% while among the normal hearing control group was 2.42%.

Role of novel variants in DFNB1 loci in assortative mating

Four novel variants, p.E42D (in *GJB2* gene), p.Q57R, p.E101Q, p.R104H (in *GJB6* gene) were identified in this study. This is the first study from Indian subcontinent reporting novel variants in the coding region of *GJB6* gene. In silico analysis of these variants using popular tools such as SIFT and PolyPhen2 revealed that p.Q57R and p.R104H may affect or damage the structure and functioning of Cx30 protein coded by *GJB6*, but p.E101Q in *GJB6* and p.E42D in the *GJB2* gene are tolerable or benign to the integrity of the protein structure.

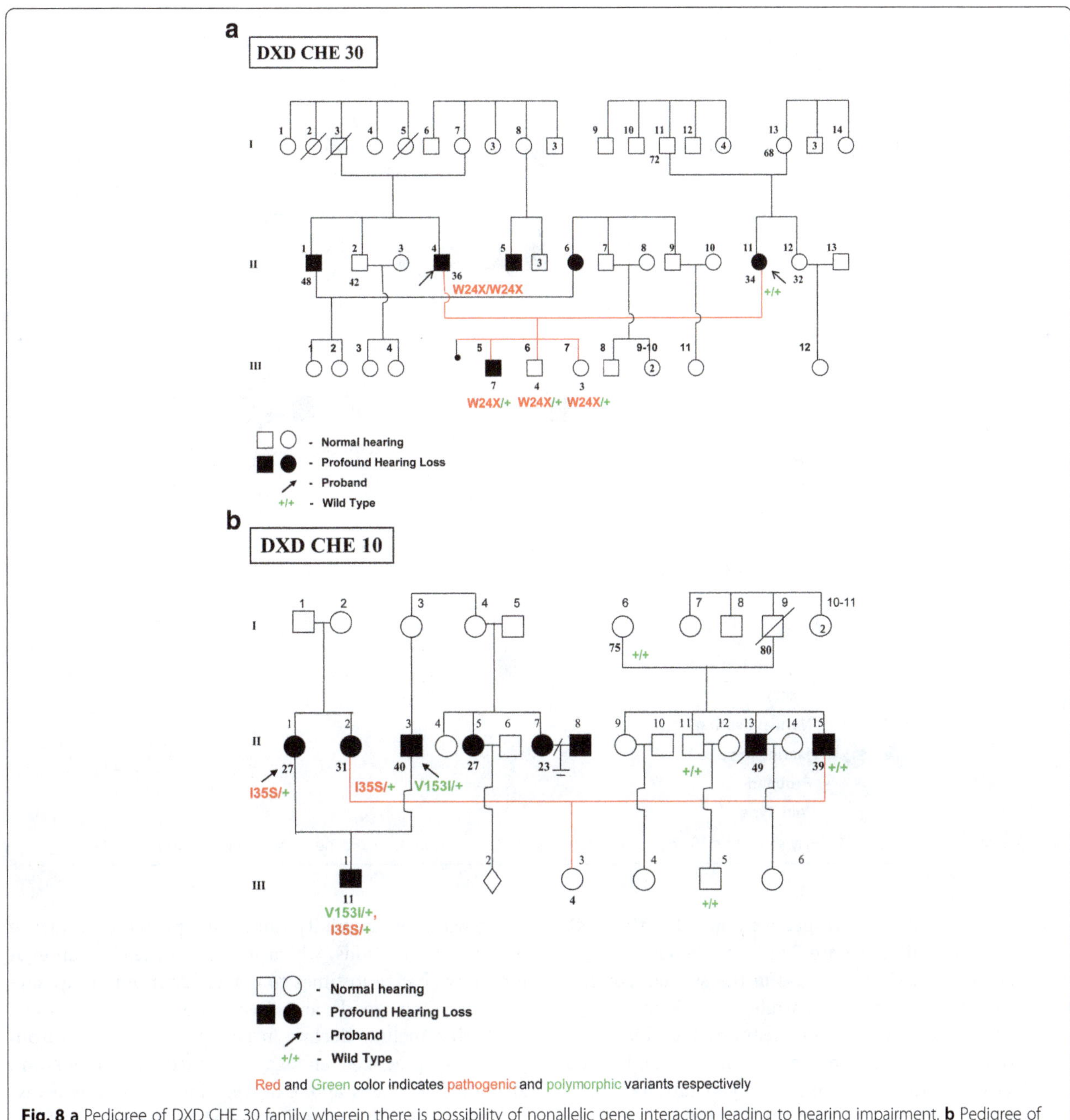

Fig. 8 a Pedigree of DXD CHE 30 family wherein there is possibility of nonallelic gene interaction leading to hearing impairment. **b** Pedigree of DXD CHE 10 family wherein there is possibility of non-allelic gene interaction leading to hearing impairment

However, p.E42D mutation was observed in both homozygous and heterozygous conditions in two unrelated HI individuals from different geographic and linguistic regions and with variable phenotypes in the family members ranging from mild to profound, conductive, sensorineural and mixed type of hearing losses. The individuals with other three *GJB6* novel variants in heterozygous condition have also shown profound SNHL phenotype. These variants, perhaps contribute, in association with mutations in either unrelated or yet-to-be determined loci through unknown interactive pathways, for the observed phenotype. Further investigation of these samples through whole exome sequencing and functional analysis could perhaps throw more light into their mode of action.

We calculated the allele frequency of DFNB1 pathogenic mutations, including the novel variants, in two generations of our study group, the assortative mating partners forming one generation and their offspring forming the next generation. Only families in both the subgroups that had offspring were included. The DFNB1 allele frequencies for DXD mates and their offspring

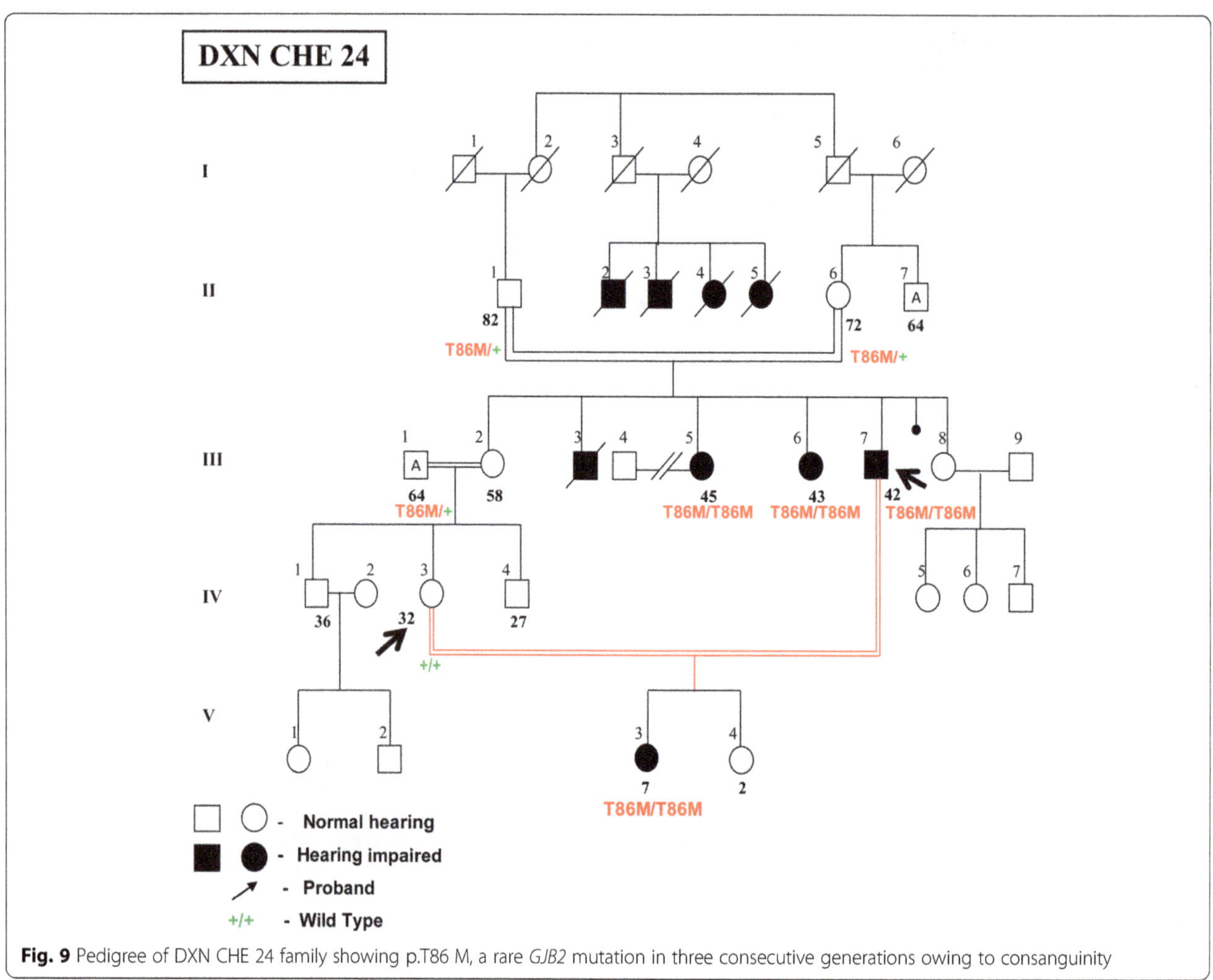

Fig. 9 Pedigree of DXN CHE 24 family showing p.T86 M, a rare *GJB2* mutation in three consecutive generations owing to consanguinity

were 36.98 and 38.67%, respectively and for the DXN mates and their offspring are 22.84 and 24.38%, respectively. There was a 4.6% increase in the subsequent generation in the DXD families, while a 6.75% increase in the DXN families, which demonstrates the role of assortative mating along with consanguinity in the increase of DFNB1 mutations in consecutive generations. This is perhaps the first study in the world to test real-time, the hypothesis proposed by Nance et al. in 2000 (intense phenotypic assortative mating mechanism can double the frequency of the commonest forms of recessive deafness [DFNB1]) on assortative mating HI parental generation and their offspring.

Human populations are shaped not only by the usual forces of natural selection like famine, disease or climate but also through genetic variations. A new force is emerging with surprising implications wherein people themselves have started shaping their own evolution. This new force is the human culture, broadly defined as any learned behavior including technology. Assortative mating among the deaf is one such cultural force, which along with consanguinity can have a profound influence on genetic variations, which in turn can lead to an evolutionary change in times to come. From our study, several changing trends are already noticeable at various levels that include decline in family size, deviation from previously practiced endogamous caste limitations and attitudinal changes about hearing impairment as a disability. If the preference for a deaf to marry a deaf becomes a norm in future with the advent of rampant technological advancements that empower the deaf to be better educated and economically independent, the impact on the auditory gene pool/ phenotype has several outcomes like:

1. Increase in DFNB1 mutation frequencies from existing ~ 35% as observed in our study to several folds, both in the deaf and in the normal population.
2. Deafness being a heterogeneous disorder, the remaining ~ 65% of unresolved group of gene mutations (known and unknown) will also contribute further to the gene pool and alter this equation.

3. As the genetic testing picks up gradually with cost-effective rapid multi-gene search in terms of whole genome, the knowledge may empower the prospective mates to choose partners of complementary type. This relaxed selection would again lead to simultaneous carrier status for a number of rare genes in normal hearing offspring of these mates. These normal hearing offspring may, in future, even develop variable levels of hearing losses as the proteins associated with mechanism of hearing tend to express variably.
4. Throwing newer combinations of unlinked multi-genic interactions and producing a deaf phenotype, confounding the research on the mechanism of hearing loss, there by complicating the path of unraveling the mystery of hearing.

Conclusion

This is the first study from an Indian subcontinent reporting novel variants p.Q57R, p.E101Q, p.R104H in the coding region of *GJB6* gene. This is also the first study in the world to test real-time, the hypothesis proposed by Nance et al. in 2000 (intense phenotypic assortative mating mechanism can double the frequency of the commonest forms of recessive deafness [DFNB1]) in assortative mating HI parental generation and their offspring. The DFNB1 allele frequencies for DXD mates and their offspring were 36.98 and 38.67%, respectively and for the DXN mates and their offspring are 22.84 and 24.38%, respectively. There was a 4.6% increase in the subsequent generation in the DXD families, while a 6.75% increase in the DXN families, which demonstrated the role of assortative mating along with consanguinity in the increase of DFNB1 mutations in consecutive generations. This study has revealed that assortative mating among the deaf may well be a cultural force, which along with consanguinity can have a profound influence on genetic variations, which in turn can lead to an evolutionary change in times to come.

Abbreviations

Cx26: Connexin 26; Cx30: Connexin 30; DFNB: Deafness, autosomal recessive; DXD: Deaf marrying deaf; DXN: Deaf marrying normal hearing; EC1: Extracellular loop 1; *GJB2*: Gap Junction *beta* 2; *GJB6*: Gap Junction *beta* 6; HI: Hearing Impaired; IC2: Intracellular domain 2; NSHL: Non-syndromic hearing loss; PCR: Polymerase Chain Reaction; SNHL: Sensory neural hearing loss

Acknowledgements

We are grateful to the deaf families for their cooperation and participation in this study. We appreciate the support in Bioinformatic analysis provided by Dr. M. Manikandan, PGIBMS. We are thankful for the financial assistance provided through University Grants Commission (UGC) Major Grant (F.No.37-443/2009 (SR)) and Ad hoc Research Project (5/8/10-17(Oto)/CFP/2011-NCD-I) of the Indian Council of Medical Research (ICMR), Government of India, to CRS. AP was ICMR-SRF & MK was ICMR-FA; JMJ was a UGC-UPE Phase II fellow and is currently CSIR-SRF; JC was supported by UGC-BSR; PVS was a JRF-TNPCB and is currently ICMR-SRF.

Funding

This study was funded by University Grants Commission (UGC) Major Grant (F.No.37–443/2009(SR)) and Ad hoc Research Project (5/8/10–17(Oto)/CFP/2011-NCD-I) of the Indian Council of Medical Research (ICMR), Government of India, to CRS.

Authors' contributions

CRS, AP, JC, JMJ, RR and NPK contributed to the conceptualisation of this study and obtained funding. CRS, AP, JC, JMJ, SPV and MK recruited deaf families and controls for the study from four different states, collected detailed clinical data, family history and pedigrees, and isolated DNA from blood samples. AP and JMJ carried out all molecular analysis associated with DFNB1 mutations; RR & NPK carried out the clinical investigations and audiometric profile for the subjects and controls; CRS & AP prepared the original draft and all authors contributed to editing and review and provided intellectual input to the final manuscript. All authors read and approved the final manuscript.

Competing interests

The authors declare that they have no competing interests.

Author details

[1]Department of Genetics, Dr. ALM Post Graduate Institute of Basic Medical Sciences, University of Madras, Taramani, Chennai 600113, India. [2]Current affiliation: PG and Research Department of Biotechnology, Women's Christian College, Chennai, India. [3]Department of ENT, SRM Medical College Hospital and Research Centre, SRM Institute of Science and Technology, Kattankulathur, India. [4]DOAST Hearing Care Center, Anna Nagar, Chennai 600040, India.

Reference

1. Kenneson A, Van Naarden Braun K, Boyle C. GJB2 (connexin 26) variants and nonsyndromic sensorineural hearing loss: a HuGE review. Genet Med. 2002;4:258–74.
2. Snoeckx RL, Huygen PL, Feldmann D, Marlin S, Denoyelle F, Waligora J, et al. GJB2 mutations and degree of hearing loss: a multicenter study. Am J Hum Genet. 2005;77:945–57.
3. Kelsell DP, Dunlop J, Stevens HP, Lench NJ, Liang JN, Parry G, et al. Connexin 26 mutations in hereditary non-syndromic sensorineural deafness. Nature. 1997;387:80–3.
4. Dror AA, Avraham KB. Hearing loss: mechanisms revealed by genetics and cell biology. Annu Rev Genet. 2009;43:411–37.
5. Hilgert N, Smith RJH, Van Camp G. Forty-six genes causing nonsyndromic hearing impairment: which ones should be analyzed in DNA diagnostics? Mutat Res Rev Mutat Res. 2009;681(2):189–96.
6. Del Castillo FJ, Rodríguez-Ballesteros M, Álvarez A, Hutchin T, Leonardi E, De Oliveira CA, et al. A novel deletion involving the connexin-30 gene, del(GJB6-d13s1854), found in trans with mutations in the GJB2 gene (connexin-26) in subjects with DFNB1 non-syndromic hearing impairment. J Med Genet. 2005;42:588–94.
7. del Castillo I, Villamar M, Moreno-Pelayo MA, del Castillo FJ, Álvarez A, Tellería D, et al. A deletion involving the Connexin 30 gene in nonsyndromic hearing impairment. N Engl J Med. 2002;346:243–9.
8. Ahmad S, Chen S, Sun J, Lin X. Connexins 26 and 30 are co-assembled to form gap junctions in the cochlea of mice. Biochem Biophys Res Commun. 2003;307:362–8.
9. Marlin S, Feldmann D, Blons H, Loundon N, Rouillon I, Albert S, et al. GJB2 and GJB6 mutations: genotypic and phenotypic correlations in a large cohort of hearing-impaired patients. Arch Otolaryngol - Head Neck Surg. 2005;131:481–7.
10. Pavithra A, Jeffrey JM, Chandru J, Ramesh A, Srikumari Srisailapathy CR. High incidence of GJB2 gene mutations among assortatively mating hearing impaired families in Kerala: future implications. J Genet. 2014;93:207–13.
11. Pavithra A, Selvakumari M, Nityaa V, Sharanya N, Ramakrishnan R, Narasimhan M, et al. Autosomal dominant hearing loss resulting from p. R75Q mutation in the GJB2 gene: nonsyndromic presentation in a south Indian family. Ann Hum Genet. 2015;79:76–82.

12. Pavithra A, Chandru J, Jeffrey JM, Karthikeyen NP, Srisailapathy CRS. Rare compound heterozygosity involving dominant and recessive mutations of GJB2 gene in an assortative mating hearing impaired Indian family. Eur Arch Oto-Rhino-Laryngology. 2017;274:119–25.
13. Nance WE, Kearsey MJ. Relevance of Connexin deafness (DFNB1) to human evolution. Am J Hum Genet. 2004;74:1081–7.
14. Nance WE, Liu XZ, Pandya A. Relation between choice of partner and high frequency of connexin-26 deafness. Lancet. 2000;356:500–1.
15. Arnos KS, Welch KO, Tekin M, Norris VW, Blanton SH, Pandya A, et al. A comparative analysis of the genetic epidemiology of deafness in the United States in two sets of pedigrees collected more than a century apart. Am J Hum Genet. 2008;83:200–7.
16. Consanguinity BA. Its relevance to clinical genetics. Clin Genet. 2001;60:89–98.
17. RamShankar M, Girirajan S, Dagan O, Shankar HR, Jalvi R, Rangasayee R, Avraham KBAA. Contribution of connexin26 (GJB2) mutations and founder effect to non-syndromic hearing loss in India. J Med Genet. 2003;40:e68.
18. Padma G, Ramchander PV, Nandur UV, Padma T. GJB2 and GJB6 gene mutations found in Indian probands with congenital hearing impairment. J Genet. 2010;88:267–72.
19. Godbole K, Hemavathi J, Vaid N, Pandit AN, Sandeep MN, Chandak GR. Low prevalence of GJB2 mutations in non-syndromic hearing loss in western India. Indian J Otolaryngol Head Neck Surg. 2010;62:60–3.
20. Subathra M, Ramesh A, Selvakumari M, Karthikeyen NP, Srisailapathy CRS. Genetic epidemiology of mitochondrial pathogenic variants causing nonsyndromic hearing loss in a large cohort of south Indian hearing impaired individuals. Ann Hum Genet. 2016;80:257–73.
21. Denniston C. Equivalence by descent: pedigree analysis with inbreeding and gametic phase disequilibrium. Ann Hum Genet. 2000;64:61–82.
22. Sambrook J, Fritsch EF, Maniatis T. Molecular cloning: a laboratory manual. Cold Spring Harb Lab Press. 1989;1:626.
23. Ng PC, Henikoff SSIFT. Predicting amino acid changes that affect protein function. Nucleic Acids Res. 2003;31:3812–4.
24. Ramensky V. Human non-synonymous SNPs: server and survey. Nucleic Acids Res. 2002;30:3894–900.
25. Gasteiger E, Hoogland C, Gattiker A, Duvaud S, Wilkins MR, Appel RD, et al. Protein identification and analysis tools on the ExPASy server. In: Walker JM, editor. The Proteomics Protocols Handbook. Humana Press; 2005. p. 571–607.
26. Guex N, SWISS-MODEL PMC. The Swiss-PdbViewer: an environment for comparative protein modeling. Electrophoresis. 1997;18:2714–23.
27. Lovell SC, Davis IW, Arendall WB, de Bakker PIW, Word JM, Prisant MG, et al. Structure validation by Calpha geometry: phi,psi and Cbeta deviation. Proteins. 2003;50:437–50.
28. Fay E. Marriages of the deaf in America. Washington, DC: Volta Bureau; 1898.
29. Rose S. Genetic studies of profound prelingual deafness (PhD dissertation). Bloomington: Indiana University; 1975.
30. Rose SP, Conneally PM, NW. Genetic analysis of childhood deafness. Child Deaf New York Grune Strat. 1977:19–35.

7

Novel mutations in *HSF4* cause congenital cataracts in Chinese families

Zongfu Cao[2,3,4†], Yihua Zhu[5†], Lijuan Liu[6†], Shuangqing Wu[7], Bing Liu[5], Jianfu Zhuang[8], Yi Tong[5], Xiaole Chen[1], Yongqing Xie[1], Kaimei Nie[1], Cailing Lu[2,4], Xu Ma[2,3,4*] and Juhua Yang[1*]

Abstract

Background: Congenital cataract, a kind of cataract presenting at birth or during early childhood, is a leading cause of childhood blindness. To date, more than 30 genes on different chromosomes are known to cause this disorder. This study aimed to identify the *HSF4* mutations in a cohort from Chinese families affected with congenital cataracts.

Methods: Forty-two unrelated non-syndromic congenital cataract families and 112 ethnically matched controls from southeast China were recruited from the southeast of China. We employed Sanger sequencing method to discover the variants. To confirm the novel mutations, STR haplotypes were constructed to check the co-segregation with congenital cataract. The pathogenic potential of the novel mutations were assessed using bioinformatics tools including SIFT, Polyphen2, and Human Splicing Finder. The pathogenicity of all the mutations was evaluated by the guidelines of American College of Medical Genetics and InterVar software.

Results: No previously reported *HSF4* mutations were found in all the congenital cataract families. Five novel *HSF4* mutations including c.187 T > C (p.Phe63Leu), c.218G > T (p.Arg73Leu), c.233A > G (p.Tyr78Cys), IVS5 c.233-1G > A and c.314G > C (p.Ser105Thr) were identified in five unrelated families with congenital cataracts, respectively. These mutations co-segregated with all affected individuals in each family were not observed in the unaffected family members or in 112 unrelated controls. All five mutations were categorized to be the disease "pathogenic" according to ACMG guidelines and using InterVar software. Mutations in the *HSF4* were responsible for 11.90% Chinese families with congenital cataracts in our cohort.

Conclusions: In the study, we identified five novel *HSF4* mutations in Chinese families with congenital cataracts. Our results expand the spectrum of *HSF4* mutations causing congenital cataracts, which may be helpful for the molecular diagnosis of congenital cataracts in the era of precision medicine.

Keywords: Congenital cataracts, Mutation, *HSF4*, Chinese

Background

Congenital cataracts (CC) are a kind of cataracts that present at birth or during early childhood, which account for the most important causes of severe visual impairment in the children especially in infants [1]. More than 1 million childhood blindness is resulted from congenital cataracts in Asia, while around 400,000 of whom probably in China. In the developing countries, 7.4–15.3% of childhood blindness results from congenital cataracts. The prevalence of congenital cataracts in children has been estimated about 1–15/10,000 [2]. Prevention of visual impairment caused by congenital cataracts is an important component of the World Health Organization's (WHO) international program for the elimination of avoidable blindness by 2020 [3].

Genetic factors play key roles in the development of congenital cataracts. With the genetic heterogeneity of congenital cataracts, more than 30 genes on different chromosomes are known to cause the disorder, which include crystallins genes, lens specific connexins genes, major intrinsic protein or aquaporine genes, cytoskeletal

* Correspondence: genetic88@126.com; julian_yang@fjmu.edu.cn
†Zongfu Cao, Yihua Zhu and Lijuan Liu contributed equally to this work.
[2]Graduate School of Peking Union Medical College, Beijing, China
[1]Biomedical Engineering Center, Fujian Medical University, Fuzhou, Fujian, China
Full list of author information is available at the end of the article

structural proteins genes, paired-like homeodomain transcription factor 3 genes, avian musculoaponeurotic fibrosarcoma, and heat shock transcription factor 4 [4]. The most frequent modes of inheritance are autosomal dominant (AD), autosomal recessive (AR), and then X-linked recessive. Based on our survey in Chinese population, the eighteen genes, containing *CRYAA*, *CRYAB*, *CRYBA1*, *CRYBA4*, *CRYBB1*, *CRYBB2*, *CRYBB3*, *CRYGC*, *CRYGD*, *CRYGS*, *GJA8*, *GJA3*, *HSF4*, *MIP*, *BFSP2*, *EPHA2*, *FYCO1* and *PITX3*, can be chosen as the candidate genes to screen congenital cataracts.

In this study, 42 unrelated families with congenital cataracts were recruited from Southeast China, and five mutations in the *HSF4* (MIM# 602438, heat shock transcription factor 4) cause congenital cataracts were reported.

Methods

Subjects and DNA specimens

As part of a genetic screening program for genetic eye disorders, we collected peripheral blood from 42 families with congenital cataracts and 225 related individuals from the southeast China. All the affected individuals and unaffected relatives in their family were performed ophthalmological examinations by slit lamp photography. The study followed the tenets of the Declaration of Helsinki. Informed consents were obtained from each participant except for the children. For any participants that are under the age of 16, the consent to participate was obtained from their parents or legal guardians. 112 samples from ethnically matched control individuals were obtained prior to the study. The experiments were approved by the Ethics Committee of Fujian Medical University. Total genomic DNA was extracted from whole blood using the Wizard Genomic DNA Purification Kit (Promega, Beijing, China) according to the manufacturer's instructions.

Mutation screening

Before this study, we had compiled hot-spot regions of cataract-causing mutations. Briefly, 72 mutant exons of 31 pathogenic genes associated with 299 congenital cataract families or sporadic cases have been reported in 210 selected articles. The 72 exons, account for 34.62% of all the 208 exons in the 31 genes, were ordered by the summary frequency of disease-causing mutations decreasingly across each gene exons, and the top 26 exons in 18 pathogenic genes were selected as the hot-spot mutation regions. The hot-spot regions covered about 80 percentages of mutations in the compiled mutations with only 36.11 percentages (26/72) of all the mutant exons, and 12.5 percentages (26/208) of all the exons.

All the mutations in the 18 common genes causing congenital cataracts were screened for all the probands of 42 families. These genes including *CRYAA*, *CRYAB*, *CRYBA1*, *CRYBA4*, *CRYBB1*, *CRYBB2*, *CRYBB3*, *CRYGC*, *CRYGD*, *CRYGS*, *GJA8*, *GJA3*, *HSF4*, *MIP*, *BFSP2*, *EPHA2*, *FYCO1* and *PITX3*. The selected hot spot exons and splice junctions of these genes were amplified by PCR from genomic DNA. The PCR primers and conditions for HSF4 were listed in Table 1, and that for other genes listed in Additional file 1: Table S1. PCR products were purified and directly sequenced on an ABI 3730XL Automated Sequencer (PE Biosystems, Foster City, CA) using the same PCR primers. Intra-familial segregation analysis was performed after identification of *HSF4* mutations in probands. The identified *HSF4* mutations were also checked in 112 normal unrelated individuals from the same ethnic background.

Haplotyping analysis

To validate the co-segregation of the novel mutations, the genotyping was performed with three selected microsatellite markers flanking each corresponding pathogenic gene in available family members. Three microsatellites in *HSF4* include D16S3043, D16S3067 and D16S496. Briefly, PCR products from each DNA sample were separated by gel electrophoresis with a fluoresence-based on ABI 3730 automated sequencer (Applied Biosystems) using ROX-500 as the internal lane size standard. The amplified DNA fragment lengths were assigned to allelic sizes with GeneMarker Version 2.4.0 software (SoftGenetics, State College, Pennsylvania, USA). Cyrillic (version 2.1) software was employed to manage the Pedigree and haplotype data.

Bioinformatics analysis

Mutations description followed the recommendation of the Human Genomic Variation Society (HGVS). The effects of novel missense mutations on the encoded proteins were further evaluated by Polymorphism Phenotyping [5] v2 (PolyPhen-2) and Sorting Intolerant From Tolerant [6] v5.1.1 (SIFT), and the effects of intronic variants on splicing site changes were predicted by the Human Splicing Finder [7] v2.4.1 (HSF). The pathogenicity of all the mutations was evaluated by the standards and guidelines of American College of Medical Genetics and Genomics [8] (ACMG) using InterVar [9] software.

Table 1 The PCR primers and conditions for *HSF4* primers

Exon	Primer name	Primer sequence(5'-3')	Amplicon size (bp)	PCR condition
4, 5	HSF4e4/5F	GGACCCAAGAGTGAGCATGA	481	58 °C/GC Buffer1
	HSF4e4/5R	CCCTCCTCCTCTTTGCTCAT		

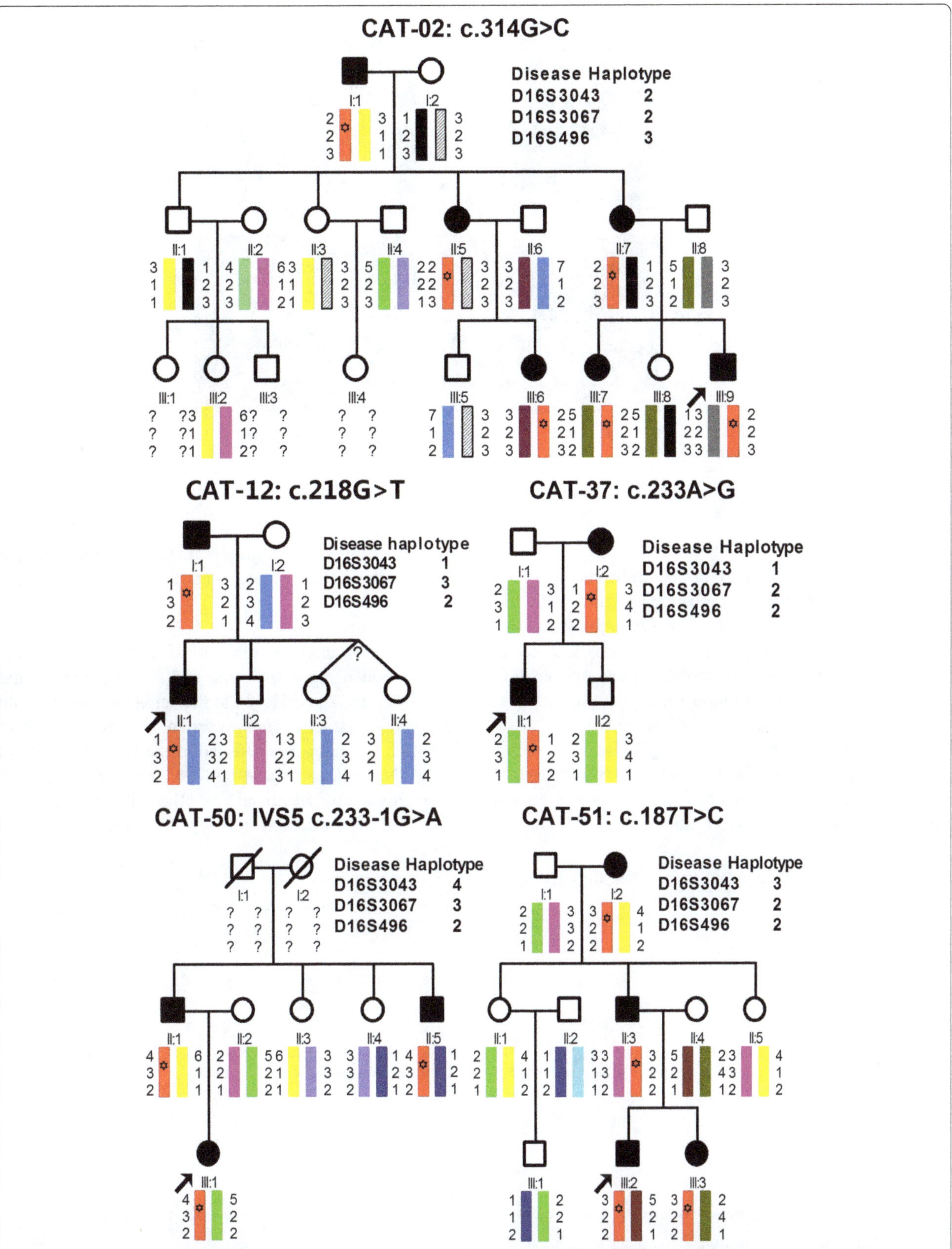

Fig. 1 Haplotypes of gene *HSF4* in each family. All the pathogenic haplotypes (red color) indicate that segregation of the haplotypes in affected individuals in each family but not in the unaffected family members. The mutations were labeled with hexagrams in the haplotypes

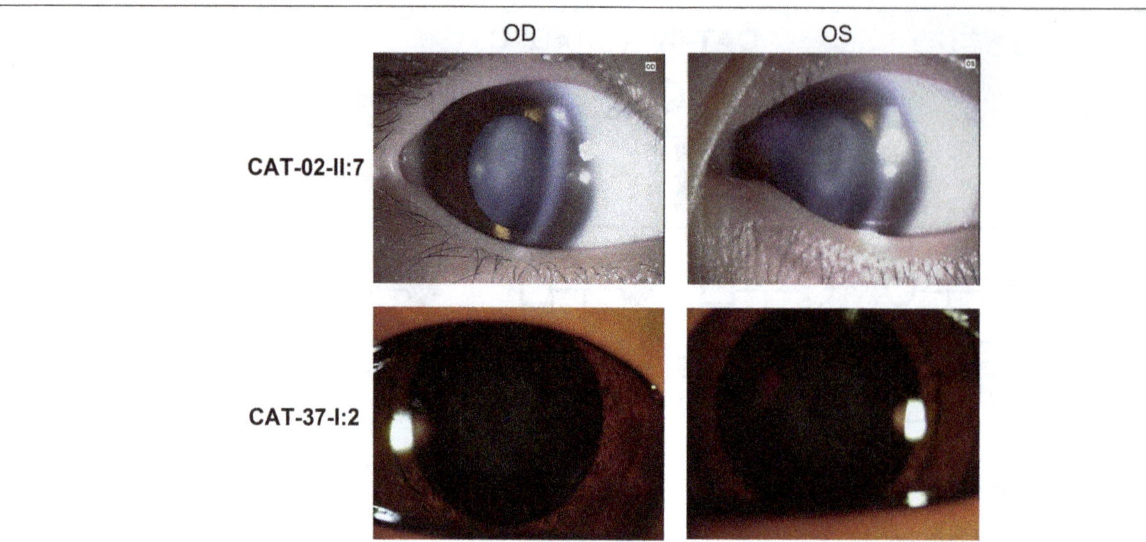

Fig. 2 The slit-lamp photographs in two families. The slit-lamp photographs shows congenital nuclear cataract for CAT-37 family, and congenital perinuclear cataract for CAT-02 family

Results

Clinical description

The 42 probands are composed of 30 probands from autosomal dominant families, 8 probands with no family history, and 4 isolated cases. In total, 379 individuals were recruited in this study. All the probands were diagnosed as bilateral cataracts at early childhood. No other ophthalmic or systemic diseases were found for all the patients. Five unrelated families were identified *HSF4* mutations. The inheritance pattern of those families is AD (Fig. 1). Based on clinical descriptions, family CAT-02 and family CAT-37 have been diagnosed as congenital perinuclear and nuclear cataracts, respectively`. Other three families including CAT-12, CAT-50 and CAT-51 with congenital total cataracts. The slit-lamp photographs of the patients in two families also showed the phenotype of cataracts (Fig. 2).

Mutation analysis

In total, five mutations were identified respectively using directly sequencing of the exons and flanking splicing sites of *HSF4* (Table 2 and Fig. 3), in five unrelated families with congenital cataracts. There were no variants on other seventeen causing genes detected in these five families. All of the five mutations have not been previously reported. Some mutations identified in other 17 families with congenital cataracts were not reported here. The clinical

Table 2 Classification of *HSF4* mutations in this study according to ACMG guideline

Family ID	Inheritance	Cataract Phenotype	Variation					PVS1	PM	PP			Classification
			gDNA change (hg19)	cDNA change	p.change	Status	type	PVS1	PM1	PM2	PP1	PP3	
CAT-02	AD	Perinuclear	g.67199703G > C	c.314G > C	p.Ser105Thr	Hetero	missense		Y	Y	*Y*	Y	Likely pathogenic
CAT-12	AD	Total	g.67199519G > T	c.218G > T	p.Arg73Leu	Hetero	missense		Y	Y	*Y*	Y	Likely pathogenic
CAT-37	AD	Nuclear	g.67199622A > G	c.233A > G	p.Tyr78Cys	Hetero	missense		Y	Y	*Y*	Y	Likely pathogenic
CAT-50	AD	Total	g.67199621G > A	IVS5 c.233-1G > A	/	Hetero	canonical splice sites	*Y*	*Y*	*Y*	*Y*	*Y*	Pathogenic
CAT-51	AD	Total	g.67199488 T > C	c.187 T > C	p.Phe63Leu	Hetero	missense		Y	Y	*Y*	Y	Likely pathogenic

AD autosomal dominant, *Hetero* heterozygosity, Manually adjustments (italic) were performed for the PP3 criteria for all the mutations and all the criteria for c.233-1G > A

PVS1 = The prevalence of the variant in affected individuals is significantly increased compared with the prevalence in controls;

PM1 = Located in a mutational hot spot and/or critical and well-established functional domain (e.g., active site of an enzyme) without benign variation;

PM2 = Absent from controls (or at extremely low frequency if recessive) in Exome Sequencing Project, 1000 Genomes Project, or Exome Aggregation Consortium;

PP1 = Cosegregation with disease in multiple affected family members in a gene definitively known to cause the disease;

PP3 = Multiple lines of computational evidence support a deleterious effect on the gene or gene product (conservation, evolutionary, splicing impact, etc.)

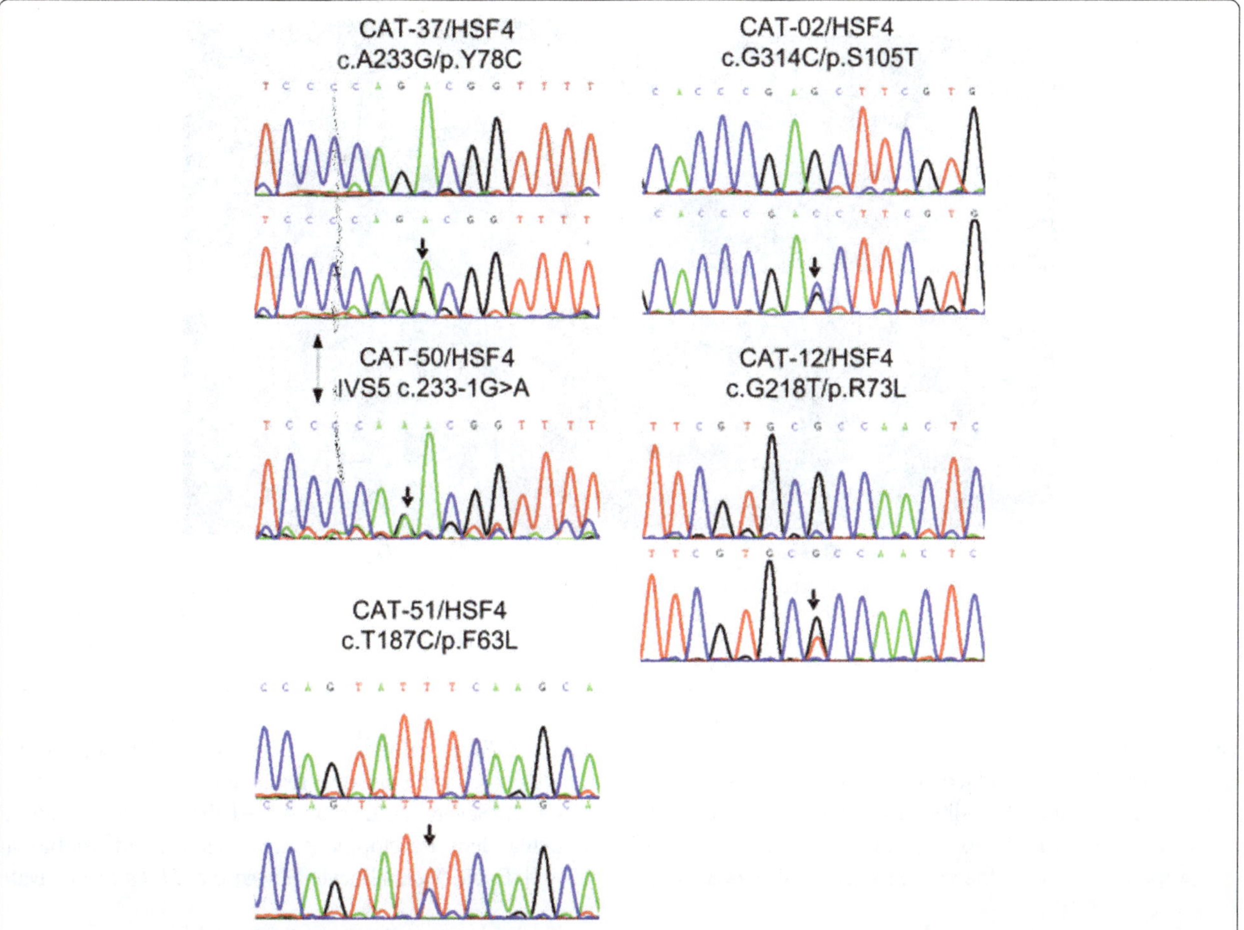

Fig. 3 The 5 novel mutations in *HSF4* identified by direct sequencing. The black arrows indicate the mutations in the probands, and the wild type can be seen in the corresponding sequences from normal control

significances of the five mutations were generated by InterVar [9] software on the basis of the criteria recommended by ACMG/AMP guidelines. The process is automatically done firstly, and then follows a manual adjustment to reclassify the mutations for the criteria that InterVar recommends. These five mutations match the criterion of pathogenic moderate 1 (PM1) since all of them are in the hot spot regions. The five mutations were absent in the public databases including 1000 Genomes, ExAC and Genome Aggregation Database, which indicates they match the criterion of pathogenic moderate 2 (PM2). These five mutations were cosegregation with congenital cataracts in each affected family members (Figs. 1 and 3), indicating that they match the criterion of pathogenic supporting 1 (PP1).

In Family CAT-02, the mutation was identified as a c.314G > C missense mutation, where a Serine was replaced by a Threonine at codon 105 (p.Ser105Thr). In Family CAT-12, a c.218G > T substitution was identified, which result in the replacement of an Arginine at position 73 by Leucine (p.Arg73Leu). In Family CAT-37, a c.233A > G missense mutation was identified, which led to Tyrosine at position 78 replaced by Cysteine (p.Tyr78Cys). In Family CAT-51, a c.187 T > C substitution led to Phenylalanine at position 63 replaced by Leucine (p.Phe63Leu). PolyPhen-2 predicted "probably damaging" of all the four variants except for c.233A > G (benign); while the SIFT method predicted "deleterious" for all the four variants except for c.314G > C (tolerated). These predictions indicated that the four variants may have effect on protein function. In Family CAT-50, a IVS5 c.233-1G > A mutation at 1 bp splice sites of the codon 78 is predicted to alter the WT acceptor site and most probably affect splicing by Human Splicing Finder software, which meet the criterion of pathogenic very strong (PVS1).

Finally, all five novel mutations were classified as "likely pathogenic" for congenital cataracts except for IVS5 c.233-1G > A mutation "pathogenic" using InterVar [9] software in accordance with ACMG standards. PM1, PM2 and PP3 were automated for the four missense mutations. The details of each mutation can be seen in the Table 2.

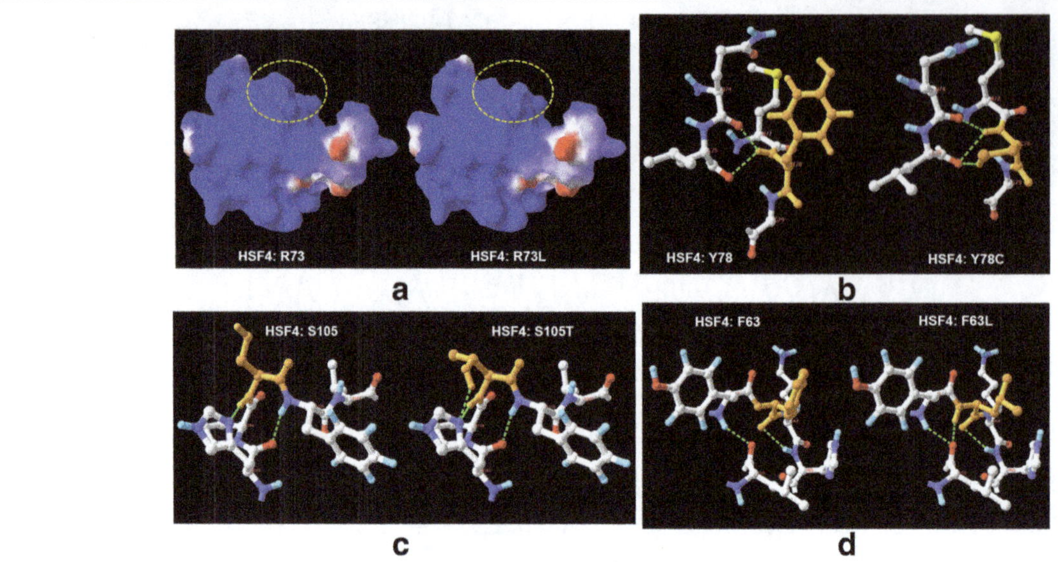

Fig. 4 The structural changes of the missense mutations. **a** Surface change of *HSF4*:p.R73L. The molecular surface is colored according to electrostatic potential with Swiss-PdbViewer, with red-white-blue corresponding to acidic-neutral-basic potential. **b** *HSF4*:p.Y78C gains an H-bond with L75. **c** *HSF4*:p.S105 T gains an H-bond with P104. **d** *HSF4*:p.F63 L gains an H-bond with L59. Yellow dotted circle represents the region of significant alteration. Green dotted lines indicate potential strong H-bonds

Discussion

Heat-shock transcription factors (HSFs) activate heat-shock response genes under conditions of elevated temperature and other stress stimuli [10, 11]. All vertebrate HSFs share the property of lacking the carboxyl-terminal hydrophobic repeat. *HSF4*, a member of the HSF family, has been found to participate in the negative regulation of DNA binding activity [12]. Several studies presented that *HSF4* is required for ocular lens development and fiber cell differentiation [13–15]. Enoki Y et., al have showed that *HSF4* can activate

Table 3 Summary of reported mutations in *HSF4* associated with congenital cataracts

Exon/Intron	DNAChange	CodingChange	Inheritance	Origin	Reference
Ex3	c.56C > A	p.A19D	AD	China	Bu et al. 2002[18]; ClinVar
Ex3	c.69G > T	p.K23 N	AD	China	Lv et al. 2014[19]
Ex3	c.89delA	p.D30Afs	/	US	ClinVar
Ex4	c.187 T > C	p.F63 L	AD	China	This study
Ex4	c.218G > A	p.R73H	AD	China	Ke et al. 2006[20]
Ex4	c.218G > T	p.R73L	AD	China	This study
IVS5	c.233-1G > A	/	AD	China	This study
Ex5	c.233A > G	p.Y78C	AD	China	This study
Ex5	c.256A > G	p.I86V	AD	China	Bu et al. 2002[18]; ClinVar
Ex5	c.314G > C	p.S105 T	AD	China	This study
Ex5	c.341 T > C	p.L114P	AD	China	Bu et al. 2002[18]; Clinvar
Ex5	c.341 T > C	p.L114P	AD	Denmark	Hansen et al. 2009[21]
Ex5	c.355C > T	p.R119C	AD	Denmark	Bu et al. 2002[18]; ClinVar
Ex5	c.355C > T	p.R119C	AD	Denmark	Hansen et al. 2009[21]
Ex7	c.524G > C	p.R175P	AR	Pakistan	Forshew et al. 2005[22]
Ex8	c.595-599del5bp	p.G199EfsX15	AR	Pakistan	Forshew et al. 2005[22]
IVS11	c.1165-2A > G	/	/	US	ClinVar
Ex12	c.1213C > T	p.R405X	AR	Pakistan	Sajjad et al. 2008[23]
IVS12	c.1327 + 4A > G	p.M419GfsX29(delEx14)	AR	Tunisia	Smaoui et al. 2004[24]

transcription of genes encoding crystallins and beaded filament structural proteins in lens epithelial cells [16], whereas the mutations in *HSF4* gene may inhibit DNA-binding of *HSF4*, which may result in the loss of lens protein gene expression and cataractogenesis. Mutations in the human *HSF4* gene have been reported in both autosomal dominant and recessive cataracts.

In this study, we compiled hot-spot regions of cataract-causing mutations to sequence. All the five mutation reported here are in the hot-spot regions of cataract-causing mutations. Meanwhile, InterVar automatically reported that all the mutations match the criterion of pathogenic moderate 1 (PM1) because all of them are in the hot spot regions. The four missense mutations cause amino acid changes, which maybe eventually result in structural changes of the Heat-shock factor protein 4. Swiss-PdbViewer predicted that the molecular surface may be changed by R73L mutation, while an H-bond is probably obtained to connect Y78C with L75, S105 T with P104, and F63 L with L59, respectively (Fig. 4). The splicing mutation IVS5 c.233-1G > A, was predicted to be broken wild-type acceptor of *HSF4* protein, and most probably affecting splicing.

To date, ten mutations of *HSF4* gene have been reported to cause congenital cataract and additional two from ClinVar [17] (Table 3), including seven missense mutations (p.A19D, p.K23 N, p.R73H, p.I86V, p.L114P, p.L114P, p.R119C, p.R119C, p.R175P) [18–22], one nonsense mutations (p.R405X) [23], one splice mutation (c.1165-2A > G), and three frame shift mutations (p.D30Afs, p.G199EfsX15, p.M419GfsX29(delEx14) [24]).

Together with five *HSF4* mutations reported here, Table 3 showed that *HSF4* mutations may be more requent in Chinese than in other world populations. These results suggest that direct screening *HSF4* mutations with one pair of primers, co-segregation and bioinformatics analyses, and mutation evaluation based on ACMG guidelines, might be a cost-effective, comprehensive and reliable method for molecular diagnosis of congenital cataracts.

Conclusions

In summary, we identified five novel mutations in *HSF4* causing autosomal dominant congenital cataracts in Chinese families. *HSF4* mutations are responsible for 11.9% (five out of 42) of the families with congenital cataracts in our cohort. Our report extends the spectrum of *HSF4* mutations and may be helpful for the genetic diagnosis of congenital cataracts in the era of precision medicine.

Abbreviations

ACMG: American College of Medical Genetics and Genomics; AD: Autosomal dominant; AR: Autosomal recessive; CC: Congenital cataracts; HGVS: Human Genomic Variation Society; HSF: Human splicing finder v2.4.1; HSF4: Heat shock transcription factor 4; HSFs: Heat-shock transcription factors (HSFs); PolyPhen-2: Polymorphism phenotyping v2; SIFT: Sorting intolerant from tolerant

Acknowledgements

We are grateful to the patients and their families for participating in this study.

Funding

The study was supported by National Natural Science Foundation of China (81570870, 81270999), Natural Science Foundation of Fujian Province (2016 J01375), The National Key Research and Development Program of China (2016YFC1000307), Health Science and technology project of Hangzhou (2015A26), and Youth Science and Technology Innovation Grant (2016GJM06).

Authors' contributions

JY, CL, and XM conceived, designed and supervised the study. YZ, LL and SW rescuited patients and performed clinical examination. YZ, LL, SW, BL, JZ, YT, XC, YX and KN acquisition of data, conducted the experiments, performed genetic analysis, provided intellectual input and assisted with the preparation of the manuscript. JY and ZC analyzed and interpreted the data. JY and ZC wrote the manuscript. JY, XM and ZC revised the manuscript. All authors reviewed the manuscript. All authors have read and approved the final manuscript.

Competing interests

The authors declare that they have no competing interests.

Author details

[1]Biomedical Engineering Center, Fujian Medical University, Fuzhou, Fujian, China. [2]Graduate School of Peking Union Medical College, Beijing, China. [3]National Center for Human Genetics, Beijing, China. [4]National Human Genetic Resources Center, National Research Institute for Family Planning, Peking Union Medical College, 12 Da-hui-si, Hai Dian, Beijing 100081, China. [5]Department of Ophthalmology, the First Affiliated Hospital of Fujian Medical University, Fuzhou, Fujian, China. [6]Fuzhou Southeast Eye Hospital, Fuzhou, Fujian, China. [7]Department of Ophthalmology, Hangzhou Red-cross hospital, Zhejiang, Hangzhou, China. [8]Xiamen Eye Center of Xiamen University, Xiamen, Fujian, China.

References

1. Deng H, Yuan L. Molecular genetics of congenital nuclear cataract. Eur J Med Genet. 2014;57:113–22.
2. Yi J, Yun J, Li ZK, Xu CT, Pan BR. Epidemiology and molecular genetics of congenital cataracts. Int J Ophthalmol. 2011;4:422–32.
3. Ackland P. The accomplishments of the global initiative VISION 2020: the right to sight and the focus for the next 8 years of the campaign. Indian J Ophthalmol. 2012;60:380–6.
4. Santana A, Waiswo M. The genetic and molecular basis of congenital cataract. Arq Bras Oftalmol. 2011;74:136–42.
5. Adzhubei IA, Schmidt S, Peshkin L, et al. A method and server for predicting damaging missense mutations. Nat Methods. 2010;7:248–9.
6. Ng PC, Henikoff S. SIFT: predicting amino acid changes that affect protein function. Nucleic Acids Res. 2003;3:3812–4.
7. Desmet FO, Hamroun D, Lalande M, et al. Human splicing finder: an online bioinformatics tool to predict splicing signals. Nucleic Acids Res. 2009;37:e67.
8. Richards S, Aziz N, Bale S, et al. Standards and guidelines for the interpretation of sequence variants: a joint consensus recommendation of the American College of Medical Genetics and Genomics and the Association for Molecular Pathology. Genet Med. 2015;17:405–24.
9. Li Q, Wang K. InterVar: clinical interpretation of genetic variants by the 2015 ACMG-AMP guidelines. Am J Hum Genet. 2017;100:267–80.
10. Akerfelt M, Morimoto RI, Sistonen L. Heat shock factors: integrators of cell stress, development and lifespan. Nat Rev Mol Cell Biol. 2010;11:545–55.
11. Liang L, Liegel R, Endres B, et al. Functional analysis of the Hsf4(lop11) allele responsible for cataracts in lop11 mice. Mol Vis. 2011;17:3062–71.
12. Nakai A, Tanabe M, Kawazoe Y, et al. HSF4, a new member of the human heat shock factor family which lacks properties of a transcriptional activator. Mol Cell Biol. 1997 Jan;17(1):469–81.

13. Fujimoto M, Izu H, Seki K, et al. HSF4 is required for normal cell growth and differentiation during mouse lens development. EMBO J. 2004;23(21):4297–306.
14. Min JN, Zhang Y, Moskophidis D, Mivechi NF. Unique contribution of heat shock transcription factor 4 in ocular lens development and fiber cell differentiation. Genesis. 2004;40(4):205–17.
15. Gao M, Huang Y, Wang L, et al. HSF4 regulates lens fiber cell differentiation by activating p53 and its downstream regulators. Cell Death Dis. 2017;8(10):e3082.
16. Enoki Y, Mukoda Y, Furutani C, Sakurai H. DNA-binding and transcriptional activities of human HSF4 containing mutations that associate with congenital and age-related cataracts. Biochim Biophys Acta. 2010;1802(9):749–53.
17. Landrum MJ, Lee JM, Benson M, et al. ClinVar: public archive of interpretations of clinically relevant variants. Nucleic Acids Res. 2016;44(D1):D862–8.
18. Bu L, Jin Y, Shi Y, et al. Mutant DNA-binding domain of HSF4 is associated with autosomal dominant lamellar and Marner cataract. Nat Genet. 2002;31:276–8.
19. Lv H, Huang C, Zhang J, et al. A novel HSF4 gene mutation causes autosomal-dominant cataracts in a Chinese family. G3 (Bethesda). 2014;4:823–8.
20. Ke T, Wang QK, Ji B, et al. Novel HSF4 mutation causes congenital total white cataract in a Chinese family. Am J Ophthalmol. 2006;142(2):298–303.
21. Hansen L, Mikkelsen A, Nürnberg P, et al. Comprehensive mutational screening in a cohort of Danish families with hereditary congenital cataract. Invest Ophthalmol Vis Sci. 2009;50:3291–303.
22. Forshew T, Johnson CA, Khaliq S, et al. Locus heterogeneity in autosomal recessive congenital cataracts: linkage to 9q and germline HSF4 mutations. Hum Genet. 2005;117:452–9.
23. Sajjad N, Goebel I, Kakar N, et al. A novel HSF4 gene mutation (p.R405X) causing autosomal recessive congenital cataracts in a large consanguineous family from Pakistan. BMC Med Genet. 2008;9:99.
24. Smaoui N, Beltaief O, BenHamed S, et al. A homozygous splice mutation in the HSF4 gene is associated with an autosomal recessive congenital cataract. Invest Ophthalmol Vis Sci. 2004;45:2716–21.

8

Clinical and molecular characterization of *POU3F4* mutations in multiple DFNX2 Chinese families

Yu Su[1,2†], Xue Gao[1,4†], Sha-Sha Huang[1†], Jing-Ning Mao[3], Bang-Qing Huang[2], Jian-Dong Zhao[1], Dong-Yang Kang[1], Xin Zhang[1] and Pu Dai[1*]

Abstract

Background: Many X-linked non-syndromic hearing loss (HL) cases are caused by various mutations in the POU domain class 3 transcription factor 4 (*POU3F4*) gene. This study aimed to identify allelic variants of this gene in two Chinese families displaying X-linked inheritance deafness-2 (DFNX2) and one sporadic case with indefinite inheritance pattern.

Methods: Direct DNA sequencing of the *POU3F4* gene was performed in these families and in 100 Chinese individuals with normal hearing.

Results: There are characteristic imaging findings in DFNX2 Chinese families with *POU3F4* mutations. The temporal bone computed tomography (CT) images of patients with DFNX2 are characterized by a thickened stapes footplate, hypoplasia of the cochlear base, absence of the bony modiolus, and dilated internal acoustic meatus (IAM) as well as by abnormally wide communication between the IAM and the basal turn of the cochlea. We identified three causative mutations in *POU3F4* for three probands and their extended families. In family 1468, we observed a novel deletion mutation, c.973delT, which is predicted to result in a p.Trp325Gly amino acid frameshift. In family 2741, the mutation c. 927delCTC was identified, which is predicted to result in the deletion of serine at position 310. In both families, the mutations were located in the POU homeodomain and are predicted to truncate the C-terminus of the POU domain. In the third family, a novel de novo transversion mutation (c.669 T > A) was identified in a 5-year-old boy that resulted in a nonsense mutation (p.Tyr223*). The mutation created a new stop codon and is predicted to result in a truncated POU3F4 protein.

Conclusions: Based on characteristic radiological findings and clinical features, *POU3F4* gene mutation analysis will increase the success rate of stapes operations and cochlear implantations, and improve molecular diagnosis, genetic counseling, and knowledge of the molecular epidemiology of HL among patients with DFNX2.

Keywords: *POU3F4*, DFNX2, X-linked deafness, Mutation

Background

Hearing loss (HL) affects 1–3 per 1000 newborns, and the majority of congenital cases of HL are attributable to genetic factors [1]. Previous studies have indicated that deafness is transmitted with an inheritance pattern consistent with autosomal recessive transmission in 75–77% of cases and with autosomal dominant transmission in 15–20% of cases; 2–3% of human hereditary HL is caused by X-linked mutations [2, 3].To date, six deafness loci (DFNX1–6) have been mapped to chromosome X, with five of the corresponding genes identified: *PRPS1* for DFNX1 [4], *POU3F4* for DFNX2 [5], *SMPX* for DFNX4, AIFM1 for DFNX5 [6] and *COL4A6* for DFNX6 [7–9] . *PRPS1* on Xq22 encodes phosphoribosyl pyrophosphate synthetase 1; *POU3F4* on Xq21 encodes a member of a transcription factor family that contains a POU domain; *SMPX* on Xp22 encodes the small muscle

* Correspondence: daipu301@vip.sina.com
†Yu Su, Xue Gao and Sha-Sha Huang contributed equally to this work.
[1]Department of Otorhinolaryngology, Head and Neck Surgery, PLA General Hospital, Beijing 100853, People's Republic of China
Full list of author information is available at the end of the article

protein; and the recently identified gene *COL4A6* encodes the alpha-6 chain of collagen type IV at Xp21.

DFNX2, X-linked deafness type 2, is the most common type of X-linked HL in humans. Mutations in the *POU3F4* gene were first found in 1995 [5] following its chromosomal localization to the X chromosome in 1988 [10]. In fact, deafness caused by *POU3F4* mutation accounts for nearly 50% of all cases of X-linked non-syndromic HL [5, 11]. Clinical features of DFNX2 often include mixed, progressive HL, temporal bone anomalies, and stapes fixation [12, 13]. Affected males exhibit either mixed deafness or, less commonly, only sensorineural deafness. The temporal bone computed tomography (CT) image is characterized by a thickened stapes footplate, hypoplasia of the cochlear base, absence of the bony modiolus, and dilated internal acoustic meatus (IAM), as well as abnormally wide communication between the IAM and the basal turn of the cochlea [14]. Nance et al. first reported X-linked mixed deafness with congenital stapes fixation and a perilymphatic gusher [15]. Sennaroglu et al. suggested that the radiologic phenotype "X-linked deafness with stapes gusher" be called "incomplete partition type III" (IP- III) [16].

To date, nearly 60 different mutations in the coding region of the *POU3F4* gene, including deletions, inversions, and duplications, have been reported to be associated with non-syndromic HL in families with DFNX2 (Table 1). Several reports have described mutations of *POU3F4* in patients with HL and temporal bone abnormalities. In this report, we describe the clinical features and genetic analysis of two Chinese families displaying X-linked inheritance HL and one sporadic case with indefinite inheritance pattern. Moreover, two novel mutations (including a de novo mutation) were identified in the POU-specific and homeodomains of *POU3F4*, coinciding with familial HL.

Methods

Clinical evaluation

Patients were enrolled from families 1486, 2741, and ZSJ (three ethnic Han Chinese families) through the Department of Otolaryngology of the General Hospital of the People's Liberation Army, Beijing, China which collected data and DNA samples from more than 10,000 patients. We chose three families with specific manifestation of temporal bone CT from this cohort. Clinical evaluations, temporal bone imaging results, audiograms, and other relevant clinical information were collected for each family member. The probands had no obvious syndromic symptoms, and *GJB2*, *SLC26A4*, and m.1555A > G and m.1494C > T mutations in mtDNA *12S rRNA* were excluded. Genomic DNA was extracted from peripheral blood using a blood DNA extraction kit according to the protocol provided by the manufacturer (Tiangen Biotech, Beijing, China).

Families 1486, 2741, and ZSJ

Family 1486 is a four-generation Chinese family, and the pedigree of this family is consistent with an X-linked inheritance pattern (Fig. 1b). Fifteen family members, including four patients (4 males: II:1, II:2, IV:3, and IV:4) with HL and 11 individuals (5 males: II:5, III:1, III:4, III:6, and IV:1, and 6 females: II:4, III:3, III:5, IV:2, IV:5, and IV:6) with normal hearing participated. The medical histories of the participants were obtained through structured questionnaires, otological examinations, and systematic assessments for signs of syndromic deafness. The proband underwent temporal bone CT scans and auditory brainstem responses. Pure tone audiometry was not available for the proband because of his young age.

Family 2741 is also a four-generation Chinese family, and the pedigree of this family showed a typical X-linked recessive inheritance pattern of HL (Fig. 2a). Ten family members were assessed: three patients (three males: II:3, III:9, and IV:2) with HL and seven individuals (two males: II:6 and III:13, and five females: II:5, II:7, II:12, III:10, and III:12) with normal hearing. The medical histories of the participants were obtained through structured questionnaires, otological examinations, and systematic assessments for signs of syndromic deafness. We obtained 10 blood samples (II:3, II:5, II:7, II:6, II:12, III:9, III:10, III:12, III:14, and IV:2) and the affected boy (IV:2) and his uncle (III:9) underwent temporal bone CT scans. Due to long distances, no temporal bone CT image was obtained from the affected boy's granduncle (II:3). The proband presented with mixed HL, his uncle had profound sensorineural HL, and the females presented with normal hearing.

In family ZSJ, the proband was a 5-year-old boy with congenital inner ear malformation and profound HL, but no one else in his family had HL, the inheritance pattern is unclear (Fig. 3e). Because of minimal progression in auditory ability after wearing hearing aid for 3 years and profound HL, the boy underwent cochlear implant surgery on his left ear at Chinese PLA General Hospital. A physical and otoscopic examination, temporal bone CT scans, and audiological studies were performed before surgery. According to the radiological and hearing findings, we suspected that he had DFNX2, and a mutation analysis of the *POU3F4* gene was performed.

Sequencing analysis of POU3F4

Genomic DNA was extracted from blood using a DNA Extraction Kit (Tiangen Biotech). Briefly, the entire coding region and splice sites of the single exon of *POU3F4* (NM_000307.1) were amplified in three overlapping

Table 1 Reported Mutations in the *POU3F4* Gene Resulting in DFNX2 Phenotypes

Nucleotide change	Amino acid change[a]	Protein domain[b]	Feature of deafness[c]	Defects on temporal bone CT	Location	References
del 2.6 kb, 6.5 kb, 7 kb, 4.4 kb	NA	U	NA	NA	Korea	[22]
del 8 kb	NA	U	Mixed	Yes	Korea	[22]
de30 kb	NA	U	Mixed	Yes	Korea	[22]
del 20 kb	NA	U	Mixed	Yes	Korea	[22]
del 130 kb	NA	U	Mixed	Yes	Korea	[22]
del 200 kb	NA	U	Mixed	Yes	Korea	[22]
del 220 kb	NA	U	Mixed	Yes	Korea	[22]
del530 kb	NA	U	SNHL	Yes	US	[23]
del 1200 kb	NA	U	SNHL	Yes	Spain	[24]
del entire gene	NA	Entire gene	Mixed	Yes	Korea	[22]
c.79C > T	p.Gln27*	U	SNHL	Yes	Poland,	[19]
c.293C > A	p.Ser98*	U	Mixed	Yes	France	[26]
c.341G > A	p.Trp114*	U	SNHL	Yes	Pakistan	[27]
c.346delG	p.Ala116Profs	U	SNHL, Mixed	Yes	Poland,Turkey	[19, 28]
c.383delG	p.Gly128 fs	U	SNHL	Yes	Korea	[29]
c.406C > T	p.Gln136*	U	SNHL	Yes	Pakistan	[27]
c.499 C > T	p.Arg167*	U	Mixed	Yes	Korea	[30]
c.530C > A	p.Ser177*	U	SNHL	Yes	China	[31]
c.559G > T	p.Glu187*	U	SNHL	Yes	Poland,	[19]
601–606delTTCAAA	p.Phe201/Lys202 del	S	Mixed	Yes	Japan	[32]
603-610delCAAA	p.Lys202 fs	S	SNHL	Yes	Netherlands	[5]
c.623 T > A	p. Leu208*	S	SNHL	Yes	Poland,Korea	[19, 29, 33]
c.632C > T	p.Thr211Met	S	Mixed	Yes	Korea	[33]
c.647G > A	p.Gly216 Glu	S	SNHL	Yes	China	[11]
c.648-651delG	p.Arg215 fs	S	Mixed	Yes	Netherlands	[5]
c.650 T > A	p.Leu217*	S	SNHL	Yes	Poland	[19]
c.669 T > A	p.Tyr223*	S	SNHL	Yes	China	Present study
c. 683C > T	p.Ser228Leu	S	SNHL	Yes	US	[23]
c.686A > G	p.Gln229Arg	S	SNHL	Yes	Korea	[33]
c.689C > T	p.Thr230Ile	S	Mixed	Yes	US	[34]
c.707A > C	p.Glu236Ala	S	SNHL	Yes	Turkey	[28]
NA	p.Glu236Asp	S	NA	No	France	[26]
c.727_728insA	p.Asn244Lysfs*26	S	SNHL	Yes	Japan	[18]
NA	p.Arg282Gln	H	NA	No	France	[26]
NA	p.Ile285Asn	H	NA	NA	France	[26]
c.772delG	p. Glu 258Argfs	H	SNHL	Yes	Turkey	[28]
c.823C > T	p.Gln275*	H	SNHL	Yes	Poland	[19]
c.862del4	p.Ser288Gln fs*37	H	Mixed	Yes	UK	[35]
NA	p.Ser288Cys fs*40	H	NA	No	France	[26]
c.895delA	p.Leu298 fs	H	Mixed	Yes	Netherlands	[5]
c.902C > T	p.Pro301Leu	H	SNHL	NA	Ecuador	[28]
c.907C > T	p.Pro303Ser	H	Mixed	Yes	UK	[25]
c.916C > T	p.Gln306*	H	SNHL	Yes	Poland,	[19]

Table 1 Reported Mutations in the *POU3F4* Gene Resulting in DFNX2 Phenotypes *(Continued)*

Nucleotide change	Amino acid change[a]	Protein domain[b]	Feature of deafness[c]	Defects on temporal bone CT	Location	References
c.923 T > A	p.Ile308Asn	H	Mixed	Yes	France	[26]
NA	p.Ile308 Ile fs*28	H	NA	No	France	[26]
c.925 T > C	p.Ser309Pro	H	SNHL	Yes	China	[36]
c.927delCTC	p.Ser310del	H	Mixed	Yes	Korea, China	[37] Present study
c.935C > T	p.Ala312Val	H	SNHL	Yes	UK	[35]
c.950 T > G	p.Leu317Trp	H	Mixed	Yes	Netherlands	[5]
c.950dupT	p. Leu317Phefs*12	H	SNHL	Yes	Korea	[33]
c.967C > G	p.Arg323Gly	H	Mixed	Yes	Korea	[38]
c.971 T > A	p.Val324Asp	H	SNHL	Yes	Poland,	[19]
c.973delT	p.Trp325Glyfs*12	H	Mixed	Yes	China	Present study
c.973 T > A	p.Trp325Arg	H	SNHL	Yes	Germany	[39]
c. 983A > C	p.Asn328Thr	H	Mixed	Yes	UK	[25]
c.985C > G	p.Arg329Gly	H	Mixed	Yes	US	[34]
c.986G > C	p.Arg329Pro	H	Mixed	Yes	Korea	[37]
c.987 T > C	p.Leu308Thr	H	SNHL	NA	Nigeria	[28]
c.990A > T	p.Arg330Ser	H	SNHL	Yes	Netherlands	[5]
c.1000A > G	p.Lys334Glu	H	Mixed	Yes	Netherlands	[5]
c.1069delA	p. Thr 354Glnfs*115	D	SNHL	Yes	Korea	[33]
c.1084 T > C	p.X362Argexf*113	D	SNHL	Yes	Korea	[33]

[a]*fs* frameshift, *NA* not available, [b]H and S indicate the POU-homeodomain and POU-specific domain respectively; *U* Upstream, *D* Downstream, [c]*SNHL* sensorineural HL, *Mixed* mixed HL

fragments using the following three pairs of forward (F) and reverse (R) primers: 5'-ACTTCCTGCTTGGGTC TCATTG (F1) and 5'-GGAGTGATCCTGGCAATGGT (R1), 5'-GGCACCGAACCCGTCTATC (F2) and 5'-TC CCCTGGCGGAGTCAT (R2), and 5'-TTGGAGAAG GAAGTGGTGCG (F3) and 5'-CCCAGCTTGGACTG CTTAATGTA (R3). Polymerase chain reaction (PCR) amplification was performed in a total volume of 20 μL: 2 μL of 10× buffer, 0.5 μL of primer L, 0.5 μL of primer R, 0.5 μL of deoxynucleotide triphosphates, 0.2 μL of Taq polymerase, 1 μL of DNA, and 15.3 μL of water. PCR began with incubation at 95 °C for 5 min, followed by nine cycles of denaturation for 45 s at 95 °C, annealing for 45 s at 58 °C, and extension for 30 s at 72 °C; this was followed by 34 cycles of denaturation for 45 s at 95 °C, annealing for 45 s at 55 °C, extension for 30 s at 72 °C, and a final 7-min extension at 72 °C. PCR products were resolved by gel electrophoresis to confirm product amplification. Sequencing was performed using the ABI 3100 Avant Capillary Electrophoresis System (Applied Biosystems, Foster City, CA, USA). We also sequenced 100 Chinese individuals with normal hearing to determine whether the mutations were present in the unaffected Chinese population.

Results

Clinical features of the family

In family 1486, the proband and the affected male members exhibited congenital severe-to-profound sensorineural hearing impairment. Auditory brainstem response thresholds with clicks were 70 dB in both ears of the proband. In family 2741, the proband exhibited typical audiometric features of mixed hearing impairment (Fig. 2b), while the maternal uncle of the proband was completely deaf (Fig. 2d). In family ZSJ, the proband exhibited profound sensorineural deafness (Fig. 3a).

Temporal bone computed tomography (CT) was performed in four patients from three families; identical findings were observed: an absent modiolus, and the basal turn of the cochlea was incompletely separated from the IAM and appeared to be a continuation of the IAM. Typically, a bulbous dilatation of the lateral end of the IAM was identified (Figs. 1a, 2c, e, and 3b: R) (arrow). All of the findings were symmetrical, except that the left cochlea of the affected boy in family ZSJ was not fully developed and smaller than the cochlea of the other side (Fig. 3e).

Cochlear implantation with the Nucleus® Slim Straight Electrode was performed in the proband from family

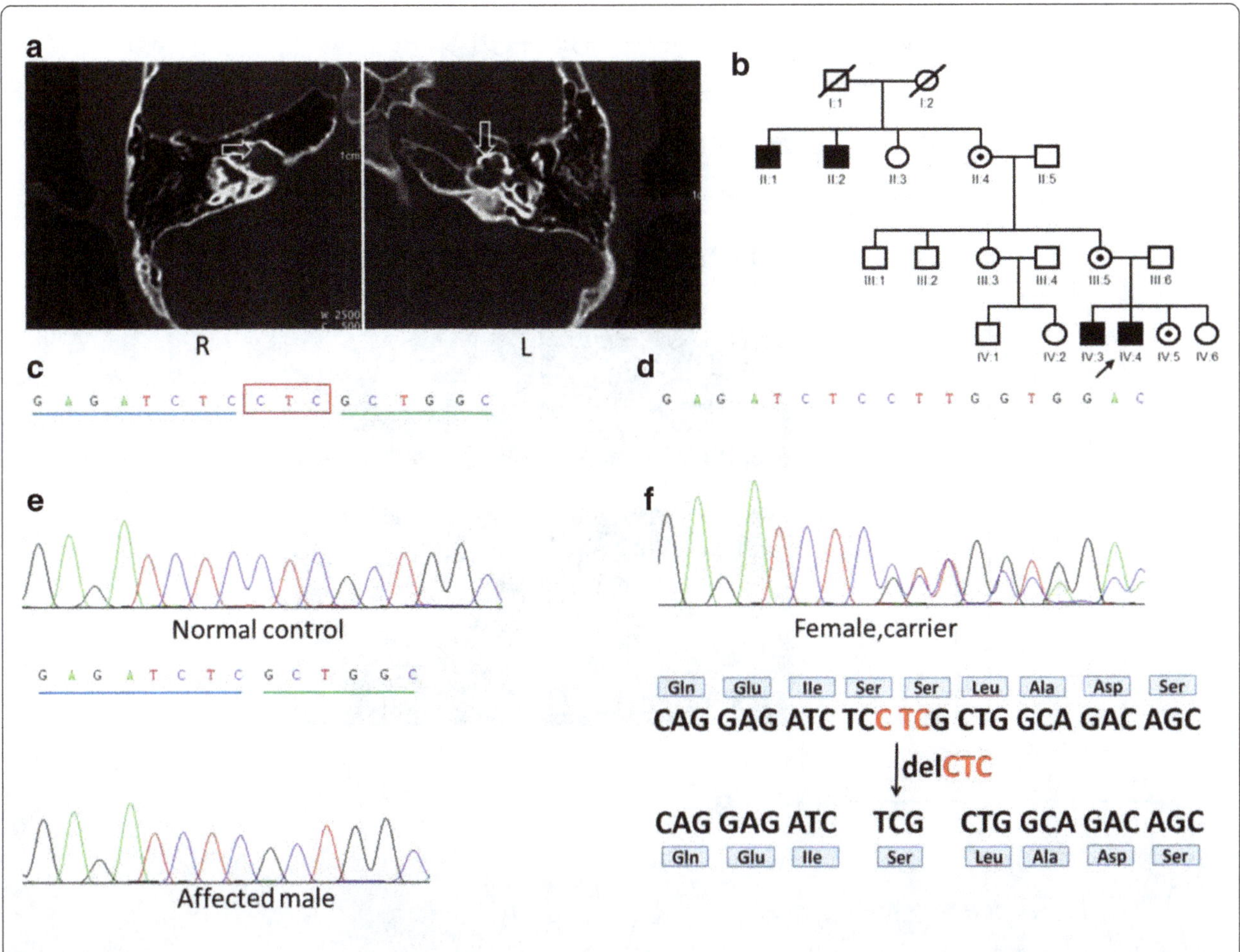

Fig. 1 Pedigree, clinical phenotypes, and mutation analysis in family 1486. **a** Temporal bone computed tomography (CT) images of the proband of family 1486 demonstrating dilation of the lateral end of the internal acoustic meatus (IAM) and a malformed cochlea; the basal turn of the cochlea was incompletely separated from the IAM (arrow); **b** Pedigree of Family 1486 with multiple congenital profound sensorineural hearing impairment cases (Affected subjects are denoted in black. Arrow indicates the proband. Mutation carrier are denoted with dot within a symbol); **c** Wild-type sequence of *POU3F4* including sites 927–929; **d** A heterozygous c.927delCTC mutation was found in the female carriers; **e** A hemizygotic c.927delCTC mutation was detected in the affected males; **f** Amino acid changes caused by changes in the DNA sequence. A three-nucleotide deletion (from position 927 to 929) in the coding region of *POU3F4* results in the deletion of serine at position 310

ZSJ. Due to widening of the bony IAM during cochlear implantation, cerebrospinal fluid (CSF) "gusher" was observed upon opening the round window, and a piece of prepared muscle tissue was used to block the leakage after inserting the electrodes. CSF leakage did not occur after surgery in this case. Intra-operative CT was utilized to ensure correct electrode positioning and to prevent the electrode from entering the IAM. The postoperative pure tone audiograms under aided conditions showed hearing thresholds of 60 dB.

Identification of POU3F4 mutations in families 1486, 2741, and ZSJ with DFNX2

In family 1486, the c.927delCTC (p.Ser310del) mutation was identified in the males (IV:3 and IV:4) with profound HL, consistent with X-linked inheritance. A three-nucleotide deletion (from position 927 to 929) in the coding region of *POU3F4* resulted in the deletion of a serine at position 310 within the POU homeodomain (Fig. 1e), without affecting the coding frame (Fig. 1f). The mother (III:5), grandmother (II:4), and sister (IV:5) were heterozygous for c.927delCTC (Fig. 1d).

In family 2741, the 10 family members were enrolled in the study, 3 of whom were classified as affected (consistent with X-linked inheritance) (Fig. 2a). The c.973delT (p.Trp325Glyfs*12) mutation was identified in these three male patients, leading to a predicted frameshift mutation and truncation of the protein. This mutant protein lacks part of the *POU3F4* protein, including the POU homeodomain, which is highly conserved across species (Fig. 2j). Sequence analysis of all family members revealed a deletion at nucleotide position 973

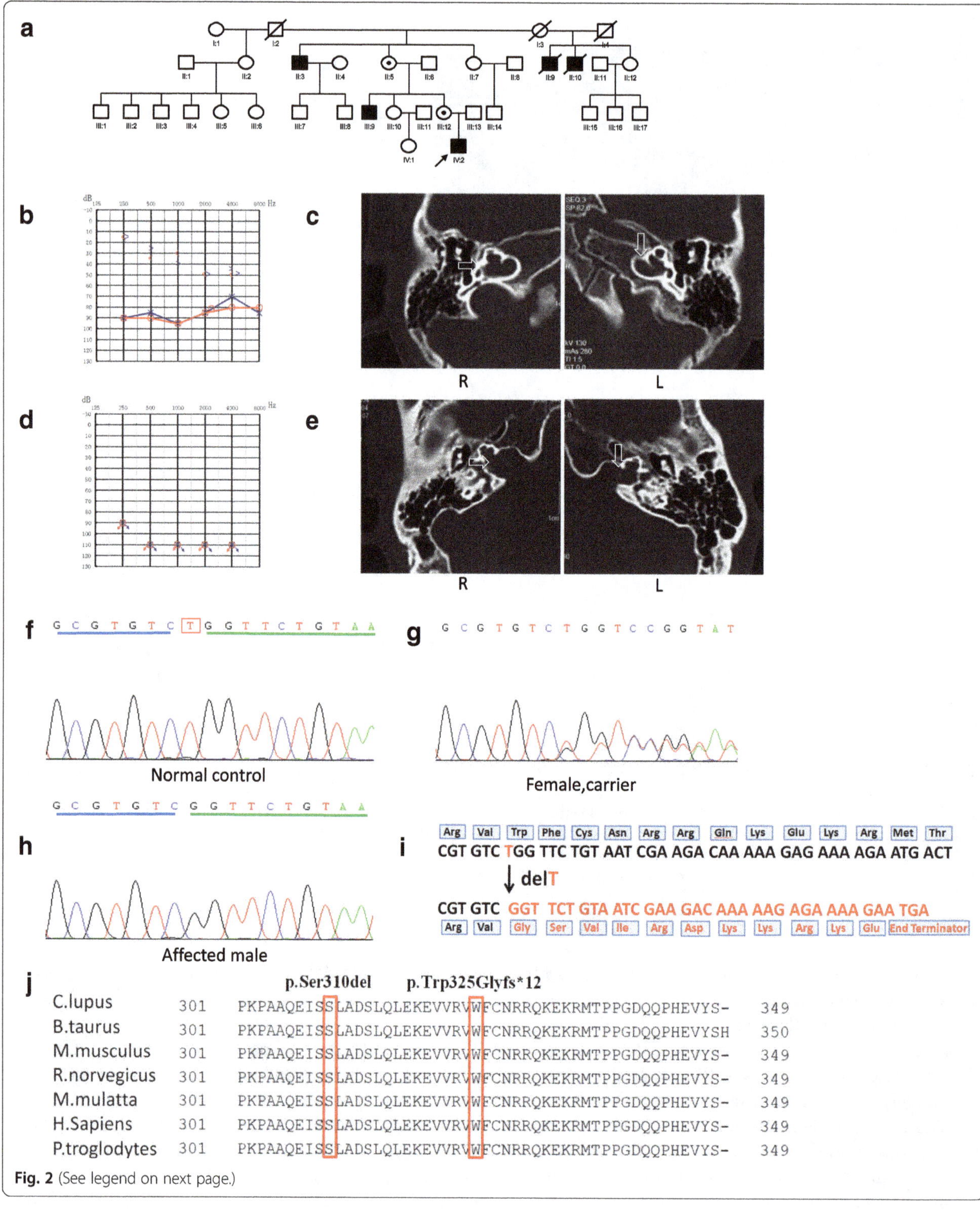

Fig. 2 (See legend on next page.)

(See figure on previous page.)
Fig. 2 Pedigree, clinical phenotypes and mutation analysis in family 2741. **a** Pedigree of family 2741 with congenital mixed hearing impairment and sensorineural hearing impairment cases (Affected subjects are denoted in black. Arrow indicates the proband. Mutation carrier are denoted with dot within a symbol); **b** Audiograms of both ears for the proband, who exhibited typical audiometric features of mixed hearing impairment; **c** Temporal bone CT images of the proband demonstrating dilation of the bottom of the IAM and a deficit in the bony plate, which separates the basal turn of the cochlea and the IAM (arrow); **d** Audiograms of both ears from the uncle of the proband, who shows profound sensorineural hearing impairment; **e** Temporal bone CT images of the uncle of the proband demonstrating dilation of the lateral end of the IAM and bone deficiency between the basal turn of the cochlea and the IAM (arrow). **f** Wild-type sequence of *POU3F4* including position 973; **g** A heterozygous c.973delT mutation was found in the female carriers; **h** A hemizygotic c.973delT mutation was detected in the affected males; **i** Amino acid change caused by changes in the DNA sequence leading to a predicted frameshift mutation and truncation of the POU3F4 protein; **j** Panel 1 marks the position of the c.973delT (p.Trp325Glyfs*12) mutation and panel 2 marks the position of the c.927delCTC (p.Ser310del) mutation. The POU homeodomain (from Gly276 to Arg335) is highly conserved in different species

in the patient (IV:2, II:3 and III:9; Fig. 2h), and the mother (III:12) and grandmother (II:5) were heterozygous for c.973delT (Fig. 2g). Mutation screening of *POU3F4* in families 2741 and 1486 showed that p.Trp325Glyfs*12 and p.Ser310del, respectively, co-segregated in all affected males examined. Heterozygous p.Trp325Glyfs*12 and p.Ser310del were also found in the female carriers, separately. Moreover, neither mutation was observed in any of the 100 unrelated controls with normal hearing by direct sequencing. According to the standards and guidance in

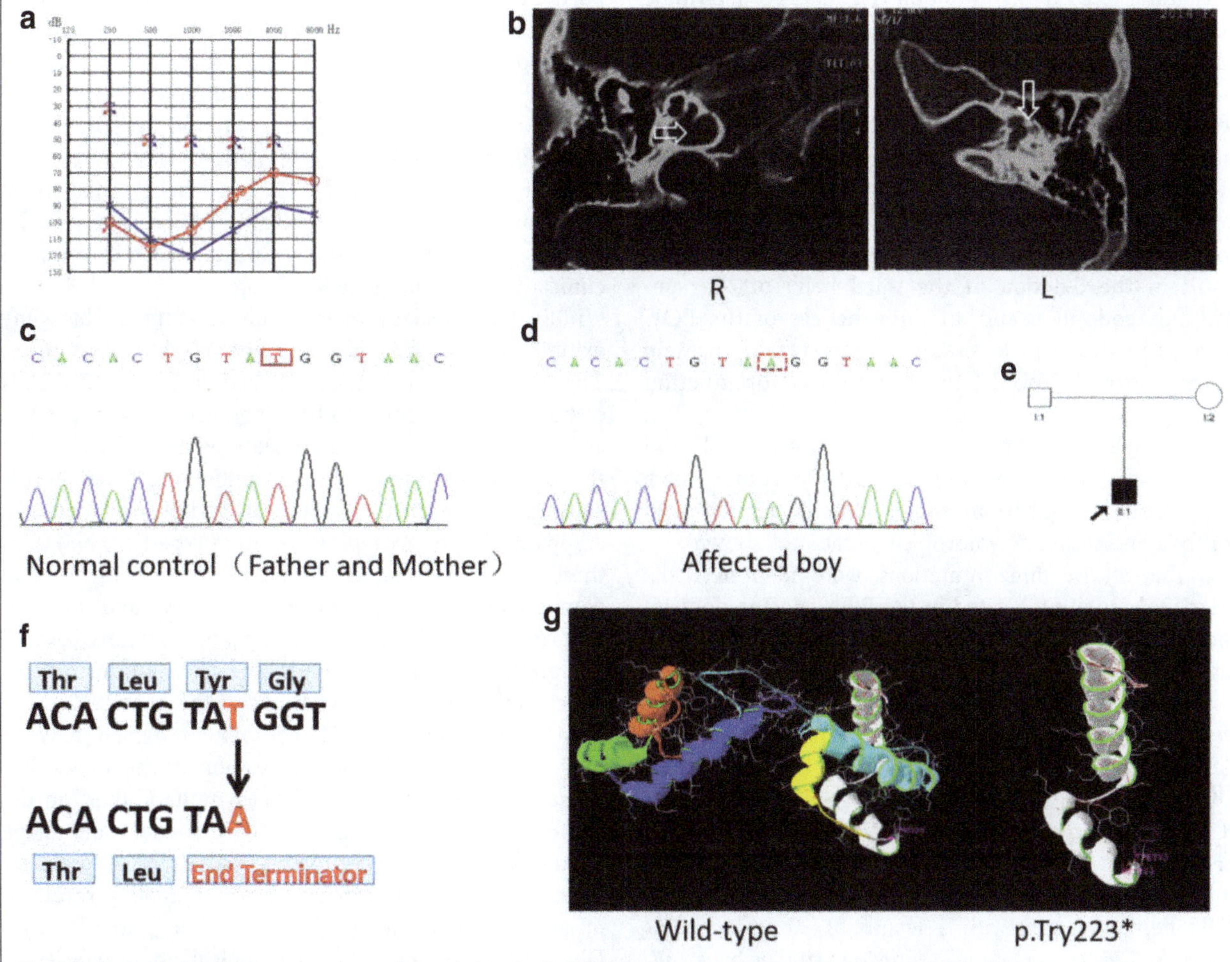

Fig. 3 Pedigree, clinical phenotypes and mutation analysis in family ZSJ. **a** Audiograms of both ears from the proband exhibited profound sensorineural hearing impairment; **b** Temporal bone CT images of the proband demonstrating dilation of the lateral end of the IAM and a deficit in the basal turn of the cochlea in the right ear (arrow) in addition to dilation of the lateral end of the IAM and an incompletely developed cochlea in the left ear (arrow); **c** Wild-type sequence of *POU3F4*, including site 669; **d** A hemizygotic c.669 T > A mutation was detected in the affected boy; **e** Pedigree of family ZSJ; **f** Stop codon caused by changes in the DNA sequence; **g** Molecular modeling of wild-type and mutant POU3F4 proteins. The c.669 T > A mutant creates a new stop codon and is predicted to result in a truncated protein lacking normal POU3F4 transcription factor function

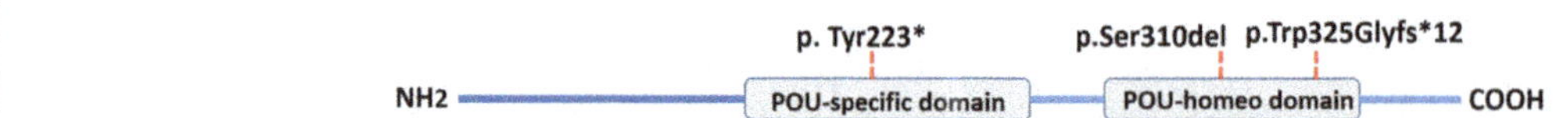

Fig. 4 Schematic illustration of the POU3F4 protein. In this study, three mutations were identified: the p.Tyr223*mutation located in the POU-specific domain, and the p.Trp325Glyfs*12 and p.Ser310del mutations located in the POU homeodomain

the 2015 American College of Medical Genetics and Genomics (ACMG), two variants identified in this study, c.973delT and c.927delCTC (p.Trp325Glyfs*12 and p.Ser310del), are pathogenic variants, not rare polymorphisms, and are among the most conserved amino acids in the POU homeodomain (Fig. 2j).

In family ZSJ, sequence analysis of *POU3F4* in the affected boy revealed a de novo transversion, c.669 T > A (Fig. 3d), resulting in a nonsense mutation (p.Tyr223*, Fig. 3f) and the creation of a new stop codon. Thus, it is predicted to result in a truncated protein lacking normal POU3F4 transcription factor function. Neither parent carried the c.669 T > A mutation (Fig. 3c). To determine the reliability of the de novo mutation, a paternity test was used to confirm the biological relationship between the parents and the boy. Moreover, the mutation was not found in any of the 100 unrelated controls with normal hearing by direct sequencing. Molecular modeling showed that the tyrosine residue at position 223 is located at the end of the second helix of the specific homeodomain. The c.669 T > A mutant is predicted to result in the deletion of the third helix of the specific homeodomain and all three helices of the POU homeodomain, which creates a truncated protein lacking normal POU3F4 transcription factor function (Fig. 3g).

Two single nucleotide polymorphisms, Ala708Gly and Gly710Cys (rs5921978 and rs5921979, respectively), were also observed in all subjects of the families and controls, indicating polymorphisms (data not shown).

In this study, three mutations were identified: the p.Tyr223* mutation located in the POU specific-domain, and the p.Trp325Glyfs*12 and p.Ser310del mutations located in the POU homeodomain (Fig. 4).

Discussion

Deafness segregating at the DFNX2 locus is associated with mutations in the *POU3F4* gene. The human POU3F4 protein contains a POU-specific domain, with a length of 67 amino acids (from Lys194 to Asp260), a linker of 15 residues (from Ser261 to Gln275), and a POU homeodomain, with a length of 60 amino acids (from Gly276 to Arg335) [17]. Previous studies have suggested that HL in DFNX2 is caused by loss-of-function of the POU3F4 protein rather than gain-of-ectopic functions in the mutant proteins.

Previous studies have identified more than 60 mutations invariably located in the POU- specific and homeodomains of *POU3F4*. In this study, we identified three mutations in the *POU3F4* gene in two Chinese families displaying X-linked inheritance HL and one sporadic case with indefinite inheritance pattern. Two of the mutations (p.Trp325Glyfs*12 and p.Ser310del) occurred in the POU homeodomain and the third mutation (p.Tyr223*) was identified as a de novo mutation occurring in the specific homeodomain, which caused a premature termination resulting in a protein lacking part of the specific homeodomain and the entire POU homeodomain. Usually, diagnosing the disorder in sporadic cases with inner ear malformation is difficult. In this report, *POU3F4* gene sequencing identified a "novel *de novo*" nonsense mutation (c.669 T > A). This is the third reported case in which such a disorder occurred in the affected individual due to a spontaneous de novo mutation not inherited from the parents. Two previously reported *POU3F4* de novo mutations were p.Asn244-Lysfs*26 [18] and p.Leu217* [19]. We believe that many more such patients with this disorder are likely to be diagnosed in the near future due to a combination of clinical features and genetic testing.

Individuals, usually males, with variants in this gene exhibit characteristic clinical and radiological features. The most frequent form of X-linked deafness, DFNX2, is characterized by temporal bone abnormalities, stapes fixation and, in most cases, a mixed type of deafness. All of the probands from the three families examined herein showed characteristic inner ear radiological features compatible with incomplete partition type III. The HL in these individuals can be mixed, with the sensorineural component usually presenting in infancy and showing progression with age. Temporal bone CT scans showed dilatation of the lateral end of the IAM and/or a bone deficiency between the basal turn of the cochlea and the IAM. The conductive HL component, which may or may not be present, is due to fixation of the stapes. Because of outward pressure of perilymphatic fluid on the oval window coupled with defects in the size and shape of the stapes footplate further compromise ossicular movement and, collectively, these anomalies result in progressive sensorineural deafness in patients with DFNX2. In patients with radiological abnormalities of the cochlea on CT scans like this, a perilymphatic flow (or "gusher") can occur during inner ear surgery [20], which will result in immediate deafness along with concomitant complaints of vertigo and tinnitus. Preoperative evaluation before stapes or cochlear implant surgery is very important. In our cases, an expected CSF gusher was seen in the patient (family ZSJ) when the round window was opened. Cochleostomy was sealed with muscle tissue, and there was no CSF leakage, meningitis, or facial stimulation after surgery. Saeed et al. encouraged additional surgical obliteration of the middle ear space and external auditory canal to avoid persistent CSF leakage and its associated complications [21]. However, in our cases, this was not necessary.

The management of patients with DFNX2 depends on the degree of the overall HL. If the HL is a milder conductive or sensorineural hearing impairment, hearing aids are often a first-line recommendation. Some patients with bilateral mixed HL but serviceable bone conduction thresholds benefit from bone-anchored hearing aid technologies. However, patients with severe-to-profound hearing impairment can benefit from cochlear implant surgery. Kang et al. compared the audiologic performance of patients with X-linked deafness after cochlear implantation to those with a normal inner ear structure after implantation and found no significant difference between the two groups. The patient who underwent cochlear implantation described in this article had postoperative hearing thresholds of approximately 60 dB at 12 and 24 months after activation of the cochlear implant. We believe that the limited auditory perception and language acquisition were due to serious malformation of the cochlea. Regardless, with thoughtful preparation and the assistance of intraoperative imaging, cochlear implantation in patients with DFNX2 can be performed safely.

Several studies have reported HL in female siblings or mothers of affected males with mutations in *POU3F4*. In 2009, Marlin et al. reported the phenotype of eight independent females from families which male carriers presenting with typical DFNX2 and carrying *POU3F4* variants, and in which three female carriers have hearing loss [35]. However, we did not observe HL in the heterozygous mothers in our two families (families 1486 and 2741).

Conclusions

The identification of pathogenic alleles causing X-linked recessive deafness will improve molecular diagnosis, genetic counseling, and knowledge of the molecular epidemiology of HL among Chinese individuals. Taking these results together, we recommend preoperative gene mutation analysis in patients who have DFNX2 diagnosed on the basis of characteristic radiological findings. If a genetic cause of HL is determined, families with hereditary HL can be provided with prognostic information, the risk of recurrence, and improved rehabilitation options.

Abbreviations

ACMG: American College of Medical Genetics and Genomics; CT: Computed tomography; DFNX2: X-linked inheritance deafness-2; HL: Hearing loss; IAM: Internal acoustic meatus; *POU3F4*: POU domain class 3 transcription factor 4

Acknowledgements

We sincerely thank all the family members for their participation and cooperation in this study.

Funding

These investigations were supported by funding from the National Natural Science Foundation of China (81730029 and 81371096) and the National Key Research and Development Project (2016YFC1000700 and 2016YFC1000704) to PD, the China Postdoctoral Granted Financial Support and Special Financial Grant (Nos. 20120481482 and 201104779) and the Chinese National Nature Science Foundation Research Grant (No. 81400471) to YS, the Chinese National Nature Science Foundation Research Grant (No. 81570929) to XG, and the Chinese National Natural Science Foundation of China (81200751) to SSH. Funders had no role in the study design, data collection and analysis, decision to publish, or preparation of the manuscript.

Authors' contributions

Conceived and designed the experiments: PD. Performed the experiments: YS, SSH, BQH, JDZ, and FY. Analyzed the data: YS, XG, and SSH. Contributed reagents/materials/analysis tools: XZ and DYK. Wrote the paper: YS and PD. All authors have read and approved the final manuscript.

Competing interests

The authors declare that they have no competing interests.

Author details

[1]Department of Otorhinolaryngology, Head and Neck Surgery, PLA General Hospital, Beijing 100853, People's Republic of China. [2]Department of Otorhinolaryngology, Hainan Branch of PLA General Hospital, Sanya 572000, People's Republic of China. [3]Department of Medical Imaging, PLA 307 Hospital, Beijing 100074, People's Republic of China. [4]Department of Otolaryngology, The General Hospital of the PLA Rocket Force, 16# Xi Wai Da Jie, Beijing 100088, People's Republic of China.

References

1. Morton CC, Nance WE. Newborn hearing screening–a silent revolution. N Engl J Med. 2006;354(20):2151–64.
2. Marazita ML, et al. Genetic epidemiological studies of early-onset deafness in the U.S. school-age population. Am J Med Genet. 1993;46(5):486–91.
3. Morton NE. Genetic epidemiology of hearing impairment. Ann N Y Acad Sci. 1991;630:16–31.
4. Liu X, et al. Loss-of-function mutations in the PRPS1 gene cause a type of nonsyndromic X-linked sensorineural deafness, DFN2. Am J Hum Genet. 2010;86(1):65–71.
5. de Kok YJ, et al. Association between X-linked mixed deafness and mutations in the POU domain gene POU3F4. Science. 1995;267(5198):685–8.
6. Zong L, et al. Mutations in apoptosis-inducing factor cause X-linked recessive auditory neuropathy spectrum disorder. J Med Genet. 2015;52(8): 523–31.
7. Huebner AK, et al. Nonsense mutations in SMPX, encoding a protein responsive to physical force, result in X-chromosomal hearing loss. Am J Hum Genet. 2011;88(5):621–7.
8. Schraders M, et al. Next-generation sequencing identifies mutations of SMPX, which encodes the small muscle protein, X-linked, as a cause of progressive hearing impairment. Am J Hum Genet. 2011;88(5):628–34.
9. Rost S, et al. Novel form of X-linked nonsyndromic hearing loss with cochlear malformation caused by a mutation in the type IV collagen gene COL4A6. Eur J Hum Genet. 2014;22(2):208–15.
10. Wallis C, et al. X-linked mixed deafness with stapes fixation in a Mauritian kindred: linkage to Xq probe pDP34. Genomics. 1988;3(4):299–301.
11. Li J, et al. Identification of a novel mutation in POU3F4 for prenatal diagnosis in a Chinese family with X-linked nonsyndromic hearing loss. J Genet Genomics. 2010;37(12):787–93.
12. Cremers CW, Huygen PL. Clinical features of female heterozygotes in the X-linked mixed deafness syndrome (with perilymphatic gusher during stapes surgery). Int J Pediatr Otorhinolaryngol. 1983;6(2):179–85.

13. Phelps PD, et al. X-linked deafness, stapes gushers and a distinctive defect of the inner ear. Neuroradiology. 1991;33(4):326–30.
14. Gong WX, Gong RZ, Zhao B. HRCT and MRI findings in X-linked non-syndromic deafness patients with a POU3F4 mutation. Int J Pediatr Otorhinolaryngol. 2014;78(10):1756–62.
15. Nance WE, et al. X-linked mixed deafness with congenital fixation of the stapedial footplate and perilymphatic gusher. Birth Defects Orig Artic Ser. 1971;07(4):64–9.
16. Sennaroglu L, Sarac S, Ergin T. Surgical results of cochlear implantation in malformed cochlea. Otol Neurotol. 2006;27(5):615–23.
17. Mathis JM, et al. Brain 4: a novel mammalian POU domain transcription factor exhibiting restricted brain-specific expression. EMBO J. 1992;11(7): 2551–61.
18. Moteki H, et al. De novo mutation in X-linked hearing loss-associated POU3F4 in a sporadic case of congenital hearing loss. Ann Otol Rhinol Laryngol. 2015;124(Suppl 1):169S–76S.
19. Pollak A, et al. Novel and De Novo Mutations Extend Association of POU3F4 with Distinct Clinical and Radiological Phenotype of Hearing Loss. PLoS One. 2016;11(12):e0166618.
20. Cremers CW, Hombergen GC, Wentges RT. Perilymphatic gusher and stapes surgery. A predictable complication? Clin Otolaryngol Allied Sci. 1983;8(4): 235–40.
21. Saeed H, Powell HR, Saeed SR. Cochlear implantation in X-linked deafness - How to manage the surgical challenges. Cochlear Implants Int. 2016;17(4): 178–83.
22. de Kok YJ, et al. Identification of a hot spot for microdeletions in patients with X-linked deafness type 3 (DFN3) 900 kb proximal to the DFN3 gene POU3F4. Hum Mol Genet. 1996;5(9):1229–35.
23. Vore AP, et al. Deletion of and novel missense mutation in POU3F4 in 2 families segregating X-linked nonsyndromic deafness. Arch Otolaryngol Head Neck Surg. 2005;131(12):1057–63.
24. Arellano B, et al. Sensorineural hearing loss and Mondini dysplasia caused by a deletion at locus DFN3. Arch Otolaryngol Head Neck Surg. 2000;126(9): 1065–9.
25. Cremers FP, Cremers CW, Ropers HH. The ins and outs of X-linked deafness type 3. Adv Otorhinolaryngol. 2000;56:184–95.
26. Marlin S, et al. Phenotype and genotype in females with POU3F4 mutations. Clin Genet. 2009;76(6):558–63.
27. Waryah AM, et al. Molecular and clinical studies of X-linked deafness among Pakistani families. J Hum Genet. 2011;56(7):534–40.
28. Bademci G, et al. Novel domain-specific POU3F4 mutations are associated with X-linked deafness: examples from different populations. BMC Med Genet. 2015;16:9.
29. Lee HK, et al. Novel POU3F4 mutations and clinical features of DFN3 patients with cochlear implants. Clin Genet. 2009;75(6):572–5.
30. Stankovic KM, et al. Cochlear implantation in children with congenital X-linked deafness due to novel mutations in POU3F4 gene. Ann Otol Rhinol Laryngol. 2010;119(12):815–22.
31. Huang B-q, Zeng J-l, Su Y, Dai P. A novel POU3F4 gene mutation for X-linked recessive hereditary hearing loss. Chinese J Otology. 2014;12(1):57–60.
32. Hagiwara H, et al. A new mutation in the POU3F4 gene in a Japanese family with X-linked mixed deafness (DFN3). Laryngoscope. 1998;108(10): 1544–7.
33. Choi BY, et al. Destabilization and mislocalization of POU3F4 by C-terminal frameshift truncation and extension mutation. Hum Mutat. 2013;34(2):309–16.
34. Friedman RA, et al. Molecular analysis of the POU3F4 gene in patients with clinical and radiographic evidence of X-linked mixed deafness with perilymphatic gusher. Ann Otol Rhinol Laryngol. 1997;106(4):320–5.
35. Bitner-Glindzicz M, et al. Further mutations in Brain 4 (POU3F4) clarify the phenotype in the X-linked deafness, DFN3. Hum Mol Genet. 1995;4(8):1467–9.
36. Wang QJ, et al. A novel mutation of POU3F4 causes congenital profound sensorineural hearing loss in a large Chinese family. Laryngoscope. 2006; 116(6):944–50.
37. Lee HK, et al. Clinical and molecular characterizations of novel POU3F4 mutations reveal that DFN3 is due to null function of POU3F4 protein. Physiol Genomics. 2009;39(3):195–201.
38. de Kok YJ, et al. The molecular basis of X-linked deafness type 3 (DFN3) in two sporadic cases: identification of a somatic mosaicism for a POU3F4 missense mutation. Hum Mutat. 1997;10(3):207–11.
39. Schild C, et al. Novel mutation in the homeobox domain of transcription factor POU3F4 associated with profound sensorineural hearing loss. Otol Neurotol. 2011;32(4):690–4.

9

Association of Catechol-O-methyltransferase (COMT Val^{158}Met) with future risk of cardiovascular disease in depressed individuals - a Swedish population-based cohort study

Aysha Almas[1,2*], Yvonne Forsell[1], Vincent Millischer[3,4], Jette Möller[1] and Catharina Lavebratt[3,4*]

Abstract

Background: Catechol-O-methyltransferase (COMT Val^{158}Met) has been implicated in both depression and cardiovascular disease. The purpose of this study was to assess if COMT Val^{158}Met, which influences the COMT enzyme activity, has an effect on the risk of cardiovascular disease (CVD) in individuals with a history of depression and also to determine if the risk differs depending on gender.

Methods: Data from a longitudinal cohort study of mental health among Swedish adults was used. Depression was assessed twice 3 years apart for each participant, in 1998–2001 and 2001–2003. Saliva DNA was contributed by 4349 (41.7%) of the participants and 3525 was successfully genotyped for COMT Val^{158}Met. Participants were followed up until December 2014 from the National Patient register with regard to cardiovascular outcomes (hypertensive or ischemic heart disease, and stroke).

Results: Those with depression and the high COMT enzyme activity genotype (Val/Val) had almost a three-fold increased risk of later CVD (OR 3.6; 95% CI: 2.0-6.6) compared to those non-depressed carrying the Val/Val allele. This effect on risk for CVD was higher in women compared to men (OR 7.0; 95% CI: 3.0-14.0 versus OR 2.1; 95% CI: 1.0-6.8). Both additive interaction (attributable proportion (AP) = 0.56; 95% CI: 0.24-0.90 and synergy index (SI) = 4.39; 1.0-18.7) and multiplicative interaction (log likelihood test $p = 0.1$) was present between depression and COMT Val^{158}Met in predicting risk of later CVD.

Conclusion: High COMT activity genotype Val^{158}Met increased the risk of CVD in depressed persons. The risk was higher in women compared to men.

Keywords: Genetic variation, Depression, Myocardial infarction, Stroke, Gender

Background

Epidemiological and family studies have repeatedly shown that genetic predisposition accounts for 40–60% of the risk for coronary artery disease. Correspondingly for depression, twin studies suggest a heritability of 40–50%, and family studies indicate a two- to threefold increase in lifetime risk of developing depression among first-degree relatives [1]. Multiple studies have shown that depression is a risk factor for cardiovascular diseases (CVD) including coronary heart disease and stroke [2]. Thus genetic vulnerability is important in both CVD and depression, and some of these genetic underpinnings may be shared between the disorders.

Catechol-O-methyltransferase (COMT) has previously been implicated in both depression and CVD. The enzyme COMT is expressed in several tissues and degrades not only dopamine but also other catecholamines and

* Correspondence: aysha.almas@aku.edu; catharina.lavebratt@ki.se
[1]Department of Public Health Sciences, Karolinska Institutet, 171 77 Stockholm, Sweden
[3]Department of Molecular Medicine and Surgery, Karolinska Institutet, Stockholm, Sweden
Full list of author information is available at the end of the article

sex steroids, like catechol estrogens and dietary polyphenols. Animal and human studies have shown that altered levels of dopamine neurotransmission contribute to depressive-like behavior and influence depressive symptoms [3, 4]. Dopamine, [5] catechol amines [6, 7] and estrogens [8] have well-known effects on the cardiovascular system, e.g. blood pressure regulation. The COMT enzymatic activity is dependent on genetic variations in the *COMT* gene. The Val^{158}Met has a large effect on the enzymatic activity and the minor allele is quite frequent in many human populations. COMT Val^{158}Met is a substitution of methionine (Met) for valine (Val) at codon 158 encoded by a single nucleotide polymorphism (SNP), rs4680. The Met allele has a lower enzymatic activity compared to the Val allele. The Val/Val genotype is associated with approximately 40% more effective degradation of dopamine compared to the Met/Met genotype, while those with Val/Met genotype display an intermediate COMT activity [9, 10].

Although COMT Val^{158}Met has not shown significance in genome-wide association studies (GWAS) on depression, a recent meta-analysis by Wang et al. suggested an effect on major depressive disorder depending on ethnicity, with Val being the vulnerability allele in Europeans [11, 12]. The COMT Val^{158}Met has also been reported to be associated with cardiovascular disease and metabolic disorder. COMT Val^{158}Met homozygosity for the low-activity allele (Met/Met), has been associated with myocardial infarction (n_{cases} = 69, $n_{controls}$ = 723) [13] and metabolic disorders like abdominal obesity and high blood pressure in men (*n* = 240) [14]. In contrast, in a larger cohort study in Swedes by Eriksson et al. (n_{cases} = 174, $n_{controls}$ = 348), Met/Met was reported to be protective against myocardial infarction [8]. The purpose of this study was to determine the effect of COMT Val^{158}Met on the risk of CVD among depressed persons. Based on the fact that the Val allele was the risk allele for depression in the meta analysis in Europeans [11], and Met/Met homozygosity had a protective effect on myocardial infarction in the large Swedish cohort [14], we hypothesized that the Val allele might increase the risk for depression leading to CVD. Because of previous gender-specific associations for COMT Val^{158}Met with depression and CVD [14–16] we performed gender-stratified analyses.

Methods

Cohort

This project utilized data from the PART study (In Swedish short for: Psykisk hälsa, Arbete och RelaTioner), a longitudinal cohort study of mental health, work and relations among randomly selected adults (20–64 years) residing in Stockholm County, Sweden. The Ethical Review Board at Karolinska Institutet, Stockholm, approved the study (case number: 96–260, 97–313, 01–218, 03–302, 2004–528/3, 2009/880–31, 2012/808–32. After a complete description of the study to the subjects, written informed consent was obtained. The PART study had three measurement points: wave 1 (W1) in 1998–2000, wave 2 (W2) in 2001–2003 and wave 3 (W3) in 2010. At each wave, participants answered a postal questionnaire. The questionnaire was divided into two parts, the first one comprised questions about childhood conditions, socio-economic and demographic factors, coping-strategies, financial status, working conditions, social network, life events, somatic disorders and use of medication. The second part included screening instruments for psychological wellbeing and psychiatric symptoms.

The PART study aimed to include 19,744 persons out of which 19,457 could be reached, and 10,443 individuals responded to the questionnaire at W1 (participation rate 53%). Non-response analyses were performed using available administrative registers, and participation was related to female gender, higher age, higher income and education, being born in the Nordic countries and having no previous psychiatric diagnosis in inpatient registers [17]. In the following two waves the participation rates were 83% (*n* = 8622) and 61% (*n* = 5228). Attrition in W2 was associated with similar factors as in W1 [18]. All respondents in W1 (*n* = 10,443) were invited to provide saliva for DNA and 4349 (42%) participated and were followed up for occurrence of cardiovascular disease event between 2001 and 2014 in the National Patient Register (NPR) [19] (Figure 1). Those with previous psychiatric illness were excluded from the non-depressed group (*n* = 206).

Definition of depression

A participant was assessed as 'Depressed' if scored with depression in W1 or W2 or both waves according to the Major Depression Inventory (MDI) [20]. The MDI has shown high validity in both clinical and non-clinical samples [21, 22]. The MDI scale comprises 10 questions on symptoms present nearly every day during the past 2 weeks. Each question has five response alternatives scored from 1 to 5 according to the presence of the symptom; all the time (5), most of the time (4), slightly more than half of the time (3), slightly less than half of the time (2) some of the time (1) and never (0). The sum score of all 10 questions ranges from 0 to 50. In both W1 and W2 of PART, a subsample was interviewed by psychiatrists using Schedules for Clinical Assessment in Neuropsychiatry to validate the MDI scale for diagnosis of depression. Using an MDI score cutoff > 20, the sensitivity was 78% and the specificity was 73% for Major depressive disorder, and 67 and 79%, respectively, for all depressive disorders [23]. In this current study we used cutoff MDI > 20 for defining depression.

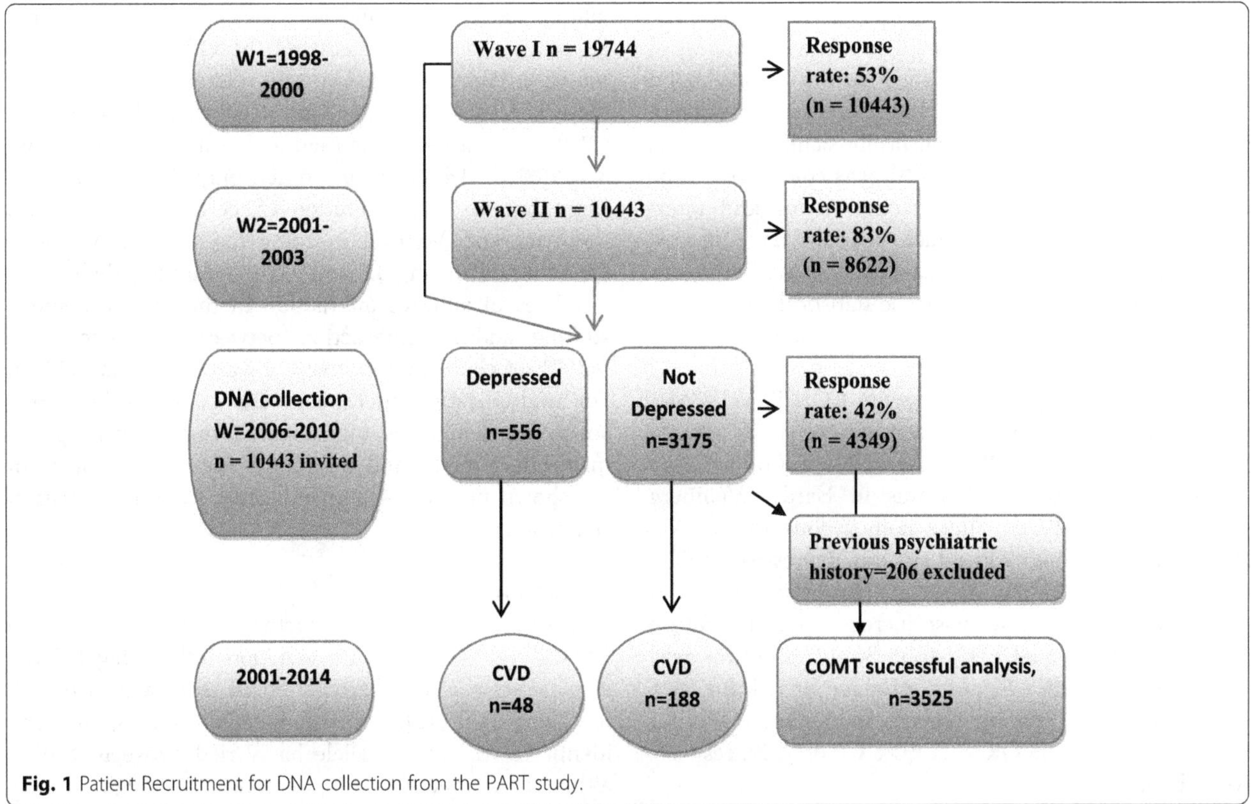

Fig. 1 Patient Recruitment for DNA collection from the PART study.

Definition of cardiovascular disease

Cardiovascular disease (CVD) was assessed by hospital discharge diagnoses from the Swedish National Patient Register (NPR) between 2001 and 2014 [24]. The following diagnoses according to the international classification of diseases (ICD10) were used and were grouped together as cardiovascular diseases: ischemic/hypertensive heart disease; hypertensive diseases (I11-I13), ischemic heart diseases (I20-I25), heart failure (I50), other peripheral vascular diseases, embolism and thrombosis (I73-I74); and stroke (I60-I67 and I69).

DNA sampling and genotyping

In 2006–2007 and 2010–2011, all participants who had responded in the first wave (W1) were invited to contribute DNA using a self-administered whole-saliva DNA sample collection kit (Oragene, DNA Genotek Inc., Ottawa, Canada) sent to their homes. Saliva was obtained from 4349 (42%) participants and genomic DNA was extracted using Oragene Purifier. The COMT Val^{158}Met (rs4680) genotype was successfully obtained for 3731 samples (91% of the randomly selected 4107 samples) using TaqMan SNP genotyping assays applying an ABI 7900 HT instrument (Applied Bio systems, Foster City, CA) [15]. Of 1443 samples run in duplicate plates, 96% had successful and identical result in both plates.

Statistical analyses

Logistic regression was used to calculate odds ratios (OR) and corresponding 95% confidence intervals (95% CI) for depression and CVD given COMT Val^{158}-Met, adjusting for age and body mass index (BMI). To determine the combined effect of Val^{158}Met and depression on later CVD, similar logistic regression analyses were performed using the four dummy variables; Met carriers (A/A plus A/G) with no depression (reference), Met carriers (A/A plus A/G) with depression, Val/Val (G/G) with no depression, and Val/Val (G/G) with depression. Additive interaction was estimated [25] by calculating the following indices [26, 27]: (i) the relative excess risk due to interaction (RERI), (ii) the attributable proportion due to interaction (AP) and (iii) the synergy index (S). RERI is the excess risk due to interaction relative to the risk without exposure. AP refers to the attributable proportion of disease that is due to interaction among individuals with both exposures. S is the excess risk from both exposures when the additive interaction, relative to the risk from both exposures without interaction. RERI $\neq 0$, AP $\neq 0$, or S $\neq 1$ are indicative of additive interaction [28]. Indices results over the null value indicate synergistic interactions; indices below the null value indicate antagonistic interactions [26]. Multiplicative interaction was estimated using a main effect model (depression and COMT Val^{158}Met as exposure) with and without multiplicative interaction term between depression and COMT Val^{158}Met. The relative goodness of fit among models was established by the Loglikelihood test using the main effect model as reference. A *p*-value of 0.05 was considered to be statistically significant for the main effects; and a p-value of 0.10 was considered to be statistically significant for interaction terms and interaction indices, since epidemiologic data have limited power to detect product terms [29, 30]. SPSS versions 19.11 and SAS 9.3 were used for the statistical analyses.

Results

Out of the 3525 participants with COMT Val^{158}Met data 1094 (31.0%) had Met/Met genotype, 1720 (48.0%) were Met/Val and 711 (20.2%) were Val/Val (Table 1).

The genotype distribution was in Hardy Weinberg equilibrium ($p = 0.31$). Those homozygous for Val/Val showed a borderline reduced risk for depression (OR = 0.70 (95% CI: 0.60-1.0), Table 2). However, those who were Val/Val had a point-wise increased risk for future CVD (OR = 1.3 (95% CI: 1.0-1.7)). Stratification on gender showed that the OR point estimate for risk for later CVD was higher among women than men (OR = 1.5 (95% CI: 0.8-2.4) and OR = 1.1 (95% CI: 0.7-1.7), respectively, Table 2).

Also, depression had a main effect increasing the risk for CVD in this cohort (OR = 1.9 (95% CI 1.4-2.5)) [31]. Considering both depression and Val^{158}Met genotype for future risk of CVD, the OR was 3.6 (95% CI: 2.0-6.6)) for those having both Val/Val and depression and 1.1 (95% CI: 0.8-1.6) for those having Val/Val and no depression (Table 3). The OR (95% CI) for those who were Met carriers and had depression was 1.5 (1.0-2.3). We also stratified the data by gender and found that the point-wise effect on risk of later CVD was higher in women compared to men among those having both Val/Val and depression; OR 7.0 (3.0-14) and 2.1 (1.0-6.8), respectively (Table 3). To explore the possibility of a dilution effect by having Met/Met plus Val/Met in the reference group, we calculated the OR for having Val/Val and depression using the reference group being those having Met/Met and no depression. This OR was 4.2 (95% CI 2.1-8.4) for men and women together, and 8.5 (95% CI 3.4-21.2) for women only. This indicated a slight but no major dilution effect by including both Met/Met and Met/Val in the reference group (corresponding ORs being 3.6 and 7.0, respectively, Table 3).

Indices of additive interaction in the sample demonstrating additive interaction between depression and Val^{158}Met genotype for later CVD are shown in Table 4. For multiplicative interaction, effect size of the interaction term and the loglikelihood test comparing the main effect model and the model with interaction term are shown in Table 4 and indicate borderline statistical significance.

Discussion

Depression is a known risk factor for CVD [31–33]. The COMT Val^{158}Met genetic variation influencing COMT enzyme activity has previously been associated with risk for depression [12], and risk for CVD [8, 13, 14]. The identity of the at risk allele has varied between studies, although a meta-analysis demonstrated high activity *COMT* Val allele as risk allele for depression. An influence of gender as well as childhood adversity on the Val^{158}Met association with depression has previously been reported [15], although a recent meta-analysis found no Val^{158}Met association to depression in any gender [16]. Using a large population-based Swedish cohort of adults we here show for the first time that the COMT Val^{158}Met genotype, corresponding to high COMT enzymatic activity, implies an increased risk of CVD especially for those who had depression up to 14 years earlier. Thus, both an additive and a multiplicative interaction between depression and COMT Val^{158}-Met for risk of CVD were detected. Additionally, this

Table 1 Distribution of COMT Val^{158}Met, depression and cardiovascular disease (CVD), stratified by gender

	All (n = 3525)	Men (n = 1495)	Women (n = 2030)
	n (%)		
Depression	556 (15.8)	157 (10.5)	399 (19.7)
Cardiovascular disease	236 (6.7)	152 (10.2)	84 (4.1)
COMT Val ^{158} Met[a]			
Met/Met	1094 (31.0)	457 (30.6)	637 (31.4)
Met/Val	1720 (48.0)	722 (48.3)	998 (49.2)
Val/Val	711 (20.2)	316 (21.1)	395 (19.5)
	Median (25th, 75th percentile)		
Age [years]	46 (34, 55)	47 (35, 55)	45 (33, 54)
BMI [kg/m2][b]	24.5 (22.5, 26.9)	25.3 (23.4, 27.4)	23.8 (22.0, 26.5)

[a]Met/Met (A/A), Met/Val (A/G), Val/Val (G/G)
[b]BMI: Body mass index

Table 2 Association of COMT $Val^{158}Met$ with depression and cardiovascular disease; stratified by gender

COMT $Val^{158}Met$	Depression			Cardiovascular disease (CVD)		
	All $n = 556$	Men $n = 157$	Women $n = 399$	All $n = 236$	Men $n = 152$	Womenn = 84
	$n_{Depressed}/n_{Non\text{-}depressed}$			$n_{CVD}/n_{Non\text{-}CVD}$		
Met/Met or Met/Val	463/2351	130/1049	333/1302	179/2635	117/1062	62/1573
Val/Val	93/618	27/289	66/329	57/654	35/281	22/373
	Odds ratio (95% confidence interval)[a]					
Met/Met or Met/Val	1 (ref)	1 (ref)	1 (ref)	1 (ref)	1 (ref)	1 (ref)
Val/Val	0.70 (0.60-1.0)	0.74 (0.50-1.1)	0.78 (0.60-1.0)	1.3 (1.0-1.7)	1.1 (0.7-1.7)	1.5 (0.8-2.4)
p value	0.02	0.20	0.11	0.13	0.60	0.13

[a]Odds ratio (OR) for Val/Val (G/G) was assessed relative to the reference: Met/Met (A/A) plus Met/Val (A/G), adjusted for age and body mass index

risk of CVD by high COMT activity genotype and depression was more pronounced in women compared to men. Both mild and severe depression were considered, scored at two time points for each participant, and the original cohort was randomly selected among Swedish nationals in the Stockholm County.

There are previous reports demonstrating a relationship between COMT $Val^{158}Met$ and acute coronary events, ischemic stroke and CVD risk factors like hypertension and lipid abnormalities [13, 14, 34]. The results from these studies are however not fully consistent with regard to which allele implies a disease risk and the influence of depression on the relationship was not previously assessed. Hagen and coworkers reported that high COMT activity (Val/Val genotype) is overrepresented in male and female Norwegians with systolic hypertension (≥140 mmHg) (n = 2591) [34]. This finding was confirmed in a Chinese population (n = 3079) showing that high activity COMT (Val/Val) was associated with cardio -metabolic risk factors including hypertension and high triglyceride levels [35]. Accordingly, Eriksson et al. reported a protective effect of low activity COMT (Met/Met or Val/Met) against myocardial infarction in Swedish and Finnish hypertensive men (n = 522) [8]. Contrary to this, low activity COMT (Met/Met or Val/Met) was associated with acute coronary events in Finnish men (n = 792) [13], and with high systolic and diastolic blood pressure and abdominal obesity in Swedish men (n = 1302) [14]. The reason for the discrepancy in risk allele identity between the aforementioned studies is unclear but could in part be related to different ranges of estrogen levels, and thereby different gender and age distributions. Accordingly, we found that high activity *COMT* (Val/Val)*depression was associated with increased CVD risk in women, but not in men. This sex-based difference might partially be explained by the difference in estrogen activity between men and women. Estrogen plays an important role in the cardiovascular system and COMT is key in the degradation of estrogens. Thus, the association between COMT Val/Val and CVD in females might reflect altered levels of estrogen and its metabolites [8, 36]. Moreover, estrogen signaling influences *COMT* transcription through estrogen response elements in the *COMT* promoter [37, 38]. The COMT enzyme metabolizes also dopamine and catecholamines which regulate both mood and cardiovascular functions through wide-spread expression of their receptors. Therefore, our Val/Val-CVD association finding may

Table 3 Interaction between COMT $Val^{158}Met$ and depression for later cardiovascular disease (CVD), stratified by gender

	All (n = 3525)		Men (n = 1495)		Women (n = 2030)	
	Met/Met or Met/Val	Val/Val	Met/Met or Met/Val	Val/Val	Met/Met or Met/Val	Val/Val
	n = 2814	n = 711	n = 1179	n = 316	n = 1635	n = 395
Depression	$n_{CVD}/n_{Non\text{-}CVD}$					
No	146 /2205	42/576	102/947	31/258	44/1258	11/318
Yes	33/430	15/78	15/115	4/23	18/315	11/55
	Odds ratio (95% confidence interval)[a]					
Depression						
No	1 (Ref)	1.1 (0.8 1.6)	1 (Ref)	1.1 (0.73 1.7)	1 (Ref)	1.0 (0.50 2.0)
P values	–	0.5	–	0.5	–	0.10
Yes	1.5 (1.0-2.3)	3.6 (2.0-6.6)	1.8 (1.0-3.4)	2.1 (1.0 6.8)	2.0 (1.1 3.5)	7.0 (3.0 14.0)
P values	0.03	< 0.001	0.05	0.20	0.01	< 0.001

[a]Odds ratio (OR) for Val/Val (G/G) with no depression, Val/Val (G/G) with depression, and Met carriers (A/A plus A/G) with depression, adjusted for age and body mass index. Met carriers (A/A plus A/G) with no depression was the reference group

Table 4 Additive and multiplicative interaction analyses between COMT Val[158]Met and depression for later cardiovascular disease (CVD) ($n = 3525$)

Interaction indices	Estimate (95% CI)
Additive interaction[a]	
RERI	2.06 (− 0.22-4.3)
AP	0.56 (0.24-0.88)
S	4.39 (1.0-18.7)
Multiplicative interaction	Odds ratio (95% CI)
Model 1 - main effects	
Depression (yes)	1.4 (1.0-2.0)
Val/Val	1.3 (1.0-1.8)
Model 2 – main and interaction effects	
Depression (yes)	1.2 (0.70-1.7)
Val/Val	1.1 (0.80-1.6)
Depression x Val[158]Met	2.2 (1.0-4.7)
P-value (Model 2 versus Model 1)	0.10[b]

[a]RERI: the relative excess risk due to interaction
AP the attributable proportion due to interaction
S the synergy index
AP > 0 and S > 1 indicate additive interaction
[b]Log likelihood test (− 2 log likelihood: Model 1 = 1725.6; Model 2 = 1721.2)

partly be due to effects of COMT enzyme activity variation on the metabolism of these transmitters. The influence of depression on the Val/Val-CVD association may in part be through increased inflammation and oxidative stress often seen in the depressed state, [39] which could potentiate a high COMT enzyme activity effect on cardiovascular function. Of the individuals in PART 11% had a non-Swedish origin, among those the vast majority had a Nordic origin. The Swedish population at time of sampling had no strong internal genetic borders [40] and especially the southern/middle parts of Sweden (from where the participants of this study are derived) were more genetically homogeneous [41].

Limitations

Firstly, due to the self-administered sampling at home, the depression cases that participated did likely not represent those most severely depressed. Secondly, only 42% provided DNA samples. Factors associated with public refusal to consent to DNA biobanking in the PART have been reported and reveal that, a lack of personal relevance of DNA contribution and feelings of discomfort related to the DNA being used for purposes other than the respective study were the reasons for low participation [42] The association between depression and risk of later CVD is unlikely influenced by refusal to consent to DNA biobanking. Another limitation of the study is that we did not have individual data on psychotropic drugs medication. Antipsychotic drugs are known to increase risk for CVD [43]. Also, we did not include data from the cause of death register and the outpatient register, hence we might have missed those who died or visited outpatient department due to IHD or stroke without prior hospitalizations.

Conclusion

The risk for later CVD was increased in depressed persons with high activity COMT Val[158]Met genotype (Val/Val), with a synergistic interaction between depression status and *COMT* genotype. This effect on risk for CVD was higher in women and might in part reflect estrogen signaling. The findings warrant further studies.

Abbreviations

CVD: Cardiovascular diseases; HTN: Hypertension; IHD: Ischemic heart Diseases; MDI: Major depression inventory

Funding

Funding for establishing the PART cohort data collection was provided by the Swedish Research Council, the Stockholm County Council and the Karolinska Institutet Faculty Funds (to YF). Funding of this particular study was provided by the regional agreement on medical training and clinical research between Stockholm County Council and Karolinska Institutet (CL), the Swedish research Council (CL) and Karolinska Institutet Foundation funds (JM). The PhD student (AA) was provided support by Faculty Development Award, Aga Khan University Karachi, Pakistan. The funding agencies had no role in the design of the study and collection, analysis, and interpretation of data and in writing the manuscript.

Authors' contributions

The study idea and study design was conceived by AA, YF, JM and CL. AA performed the statistical analyses and wrote the first draft. VM performed genotyping. All authors have been involved in interpretation of the results and made important contributions to the drafting of the manuscript. All authors read and approved the final manuscript.

Competing interests

The authors declare that they have no competing interests.

Author details

[1]Department of Public Health Sciences, Karolinska Institutet, 171 77 Stockholm, Sweden. [2]Department of Medicine, Aga Khan University, Karachi, Pakistan. [3]Department of Molecular Medicine and Surgery, Karolinska Institutet, Stockholm, Sweden. [4]Neurogenetics Unit, Center for Molecular Medicine, Karolinska University Hospital, L8:00, 171 76 Stockholm, Sweden.

References

1. Lohoff FW. Overview of the genetics of major depressive disorder. Curr Psychiatry Rep. 2010;12(6):539–46.
2. Pan A, Sun Q, Okereke OI, Rexrode KM, Hu FB. Depression and risk of stroke morbidity and mortality: a meta-analysis and systematic review. JAMA. 2011; 306(11):1241–9.
3. Di Chiara G, Bassareo V, Fenu S, De Luca MA, Spina L, Cadoni C, et al. Dopamine and drug addiction: the nucleus accumbens shell connection. Neuropharmacology. 2004;47(Suppl 1):227–41.
4. Tunbridge EM, Harrison PJ, Weinberger DR. Catechol-o-methyltransferase, cognition, and psychosis: Val158Met and beyond. Biol Psychiatry. 2006;60(2):141–51.
5. Jose PA, Eisner GM, Felder RA. Regulation of blood pressure by dopamine receptors. Nephron Physiol. 2003;95(2):p19–27.
6. Esler MD. Catecholamines and essential hypertension. Bailliere Clin Endocrinol Metab. 1993;7(2):415–38.
7. Lohmeier TE. The sympathetic nervous system and long-term blood pressure regulation. Am J Hypertens. 2001;14(6 Pt 2):147S–54S.

9. Lachman HM, Papolos DF, Saito T, Yu YM, Szumlanski CL, Weinshilboum RM. Human catechol-O-methyltransferase pharmacogenetics: description of a functional polymorphism and its potential application to neuropsychiatric disorders. Pharmacogenetics. 1996;6(3):243–50.
10. Chen J, Lipska BK, Halim N, Ma QD, Matsumoto M, Melhem S, et al. Functional analysis of genetic variation in catechol-O-methyltransferase (COMT): effects on mRNA, protein, and enzyme activity in postmortem human brain. Am J Hum Genet. 2004;75(5):807–21.
11. Wang M, Ma Y, Yuan W, Su K, Li MD. Meta-Analysis of the COMT Val158Met Polymorphism in Major Depressive Disorder: Effect of Ethnicity. J Neuroimmune Pharmacol. 11(3):434–45.
12. Baekken PM, Skorpen F, Stordal E, Zwart JA, Hagen K. Depression and anxiety in relation to catechol-O-methyltransferase Val158Met genotype in the general population: the Nord-Trondelag health study (HUNT). BMC Psychiatry. 2008;8:48.
13. Voutilainen S, Tuomainen TP, Korhonen M, Mursu J, Virtanen JK, Happonen P, et al. Functional COMT Val158Met polymorphism, risk of acute coronary events and serum homocysteine: the Kuopio ischaemic heart disease risk factor study. PLoS One. 2007;2(1):e181.
14. Annerbrink K, Westberg L, Nilsson S, Rosmond R, Holm G, Eriksson E. Catechol O-methyltransferase val158-met polymorphism is associated with abdominal obesity and blood pressure in men. Metabolism. 2008; 57(5):708–11.
8. Eriksson AL, Skrtic S, Niklason A, Hulten LM, Wiklund O, Hedner T, et al. Association between the low activity genotype of catechol-O-methyltransferase and myocardial infarction in a hypertensive population. Eur Heart J. 2004;25(5):386–91.
15. Aberg E, Fandino-Losada A, Sjoholm LK, Forsell Y, Lavebratt C. The functional Val158Met polymorphism in catechol-O-methyltransferase (COMT) is associated with depression and motivation in men from a Swedish population-based study. J Affect Disord. 2011;129(1–3):158–66.
16. Klein M, Schmoeger M, Kasper S, Schosser A. Meta-analysis of the COMT Val158Met polymorphism in major depressive disorder: the role of gender. World J Biol Psychiatry. 2016;17(2):147–58.
17. Lundberg I, Damstrom Thakker K, Hallstrom T, Forsell Y. Determinants of non-participation, and the effects of non-participation on potential cause-effect relationships, in the PART study on mental disorders. Soc Psychiatry Psychiatr Epidemiol. 2005;40(6):475–83.
18. Bergman P, Ahlberg G, Forsell Y, Lundberg I. Non-participation in the second wave of the PART study on mental disorder and its effects on risk estimates. Int J Soc Psychiatry. 2010;56(2):119–32.
19. Forsberg L RH, Jacobsson A, Nyqvist K, Heurgren M: Kvalitet och innehåll i patientregistret. Utskrivningar från slutenvården 1964–2007 och besök i specialiserad öppenvård (exklusive primärvårdsbesök) 1997–2007. (Quality and content of the Patient Register)(2009–125-15). . ed.^eds E, editor2009.
20. Bech P, Rasmussen NA, Olsen LR, Noerholm V, Abildgaard W. The sensitivity and specificity of the major depression inventory, using the present state examination as the index of diagnostic validity. J Affect Disord. 2001;66(2–3):159–64.
21. Cuijpers P, Dekker J, Noteboom A, Smits N, Peen J. Sensitivity and specificity of the Major Depression Inventory in outpatients. BMC Psychiatry. 2007;7(1).
22. Olsen LR, Jensen DV, Noerholm V, Martiny K, Bech P. The internal and external validity of the Major Depression Inventory in measuring severity of depressive states. Psychol Med. 2003;33(2):351–6.
23. Forsell Y. The major depression inventory versus schedules for clinical assessment in neuropsychiatry in a population sample. Soc Psychiatry Psychiatr Epidemiol. 2005;40(3):209–13.
24. Nilsson AC, Spetz CL, Carsjo K, Nightingale R, Smedby B. [Reliability of the hospital registry. The diagnostic data are better than their reputation]. Lakartidningen. 1994;91(7):598, 603–605.
25. Rothman KJ, Greenland S, Walker AM. Concepts of interaction. Am J Epidemiol. 1980;112(4):467–70.
26. Knol MJ, VanderWeele TJ, Groenwold RH, Klungel OH, Rovers MM, Grobbee DE. Estimating measures of interaction on an additive scale for preventive exposures. Eur J Epidemiol. 2011;26(6):433–8.
27. Padyukov L, Silva C, Stolt P, Alfredsson L, Klareskog L. A gene-environment interaction between smoking and shared epitope genes in HLA-DR provides a high risk of seropositive rheumatoid arthritis. Arthritis Rheum. 2004;50(10):3085–92.
28. Rothman KJ, Greenland S, Lash TL. Modern epidemiology: Lippincott Williams & Wilkins; 2008.
29. Maity A. A Powerful Test for Comparing Multiple Regression Functions. J Nonparametr Stat. 24(3):563–76.
30. Greenland S. Basic problems in interaction assessment. Environ Health Perspect. 1993;101 Suppl 4:59–66.
31. Almas A, Forsell Y, Iqbal R, Janszky I, Moller J. Severity of depression, anxious distress and the risk of cardiovascular disease in a Swedish population-based cohort. PLoS One. 2015;10(10):e0140742.
32. Brunner EJ, Shipley MJ, Britton AR, Stansfeld SA, Heuschmann PU, Rudd AG, et al. Depressive disorder, coronary heart disease, and stroke: dose-response and reverse causation effects in the Whitehall II cohort study. Eur J Prev Cardiol. 2014;21(3):340–6.
33. Van der Kooy K, van Hout H, Marwijk H, Marten H, Stehouwer C, Beekman A. Depression and the risk for cardiovascular diseases: systematic review and meta analysis. Int J Geriatr Psychiatry. 2007;22(7):613–26.
34. Hagen K, Pettersen E, Stovner LJ, Skorpen F, Holmen J, Zwart JA. High systolic blood pressure is associated with Val/Val genotype in the catechol-o-methyltransferase gene. The Nord-Trondelag health study (HUNT). Am J Hypertens. 2007;20(1):21–6.
35. Ge L, Wu HY, Pan SL, Huang L, Sun P, Liang QH, et al. COMT Val158Met polymorphism is associated with blood pressure and lipid levels in general families of Bama longevous area in China. Int J Clin Exp Pathol. 8(11):15055–64.
36. Hsieh YC, Jeng JS, Lin HJ, Hu CJ, Yu CC, Lien LM, et al. Epistasis analysis for estrogen metabolic and signaling pathway genes on young ischemic stroke patients. PLoS One. 2012;7(10):e47773.
37. Jiang H, Xie T, Ramsden DB, Ho SL. Human catechol-O-methyltransferase down-regulation by estradiol. Neuropharmacology. 2003;45(7):1011–8.
38. Xie T, Ho SL, Ramsden D. Characterization and implications of estrogenic down-regulation of human catechol-O-methyltransferase gene transcription. Mol Pharmacol. 1999;56(1):31–8.
39. Dowlati Y, Herrmann N, Swardfager W, Liu H, Sham L, Reim EK, et al. A meta-analysis of cytokines in major depression. Biol Psychiatry. 2010; 67(5):446–57.
40. Lappalainen T, Hannelius U, Salmela E, von Dobeln U, Lindgren CM, Huoponen K, et al. Population structure in contemporary Sweden--a Y-chromosomal and mitochondrial DNA analysis. Ann Hum Genet. 2009; 73(1):61–73.
41. Humphreys K, Grankvist A, Leu M, Hall P, Liu J, Ripatti S, et al. The genetic structure of the Swedish population. PLoS One. 2011;6(8):e22547.
42. Melas PA, Sjoholm LK, Forsner T, Edhborg M, Juth N, Forsell Y, et al. Examining the public refusal to consent to DNA biobanking: empirical data from a Swedish population-based study. J Med Ethics. 2010;36(2):93–8.
43. Kahl KG, Westhoff-Bleck M. Kruger THC. Vascul Pharmacol: Effects of psychopharmacological treatment with antipsychotic drugs on the vascular system; 2017.

10

Identification of *ANKDD1B* variants in an ankylosing spondylitis pedigree and a sporadic patient

Zhiping Tan[1,2*], Hui Zeng[1,2], Zhaofa Xu[3], Qi Tian[3], Xiaoyang Gao[3], Chuanman Zhou[3], Yu Zheng[3], Jian Wang[1,2], Guanghui Ling[4], Bing Wang[5], Yifeng Yang[1,2] and Long Ma[3*]

Abstract

Background: Ankylosing spondylitis (AS) is a debilitating autoimmune disease affecting tens of millions of people in the world. The genetics of AS is unclear. Analysis of rare AS pedigrees might facilitate our understanding of AS pathogenesis.

Methods: We used genome-wide linkage analysis and whole-exome sequencing in combination with variant co-segregation verification and haplotype analysis to study an AS pedigree and a sporadic AS patient.

Results: We identified a missense variant in the ankyrin repeat and death domain containing 1B gene *ANKDD1B* from a Han Chinese pedigree with dominantly inherited AS. This variant (p.L87V) co-segregates with all male patients of the pedigree. In females, the penetrance of the symptoms is incomplete with one identified patient out of 5 carriers, consistent with the reduced frequency of AS in females of the general population. We further identified a distinct missense variant affecting a conserved amino acid (p.R102L) of ANKDD1B in a male from 30 sporadic early onset AS patients. Both variants are absent in 500 normal controls. We determined the haplotypes of four major known AS risk loci, including *HLA-B*27*, *2p15*, *ERAP1* and *IL23R*, and found that only *HLA-B*27* is strongly associated with patients in our cohort.

Conclusions: Together these results suggest that *ANKDD1B* variants might be associated with AS and genetic analyses of more AS patients are warranted to verify this association.

Keywords: Ankylosing spondylitis, Pedigree, *ANKDD1B*, Ankyrin repeat, *HLA-B*27*

Background

Ankylosing spondylitis (AS) is a severe, debilitating and incurable autoimmune disease affecting multi millions of people in the world [1]. AS is the major subtype of spondyloarthritis, a spectrum of inter-related rheumatic diseases that also includes reactive arthritis (ReA), psoriatic arthritis (PsA), juvenile spondyloarthritis (JSpA), enteropathic arthritis (spondylitis/arthritis associated with inflammatory bowel disease), and undifferentiated spondyloarthritis (USpA) (https://www.spondylitis.org) [2, 3].

The symptoms of AS often appear gradually and progress from stiffness and chronic dull pain in the lower back to severe pain felt from the sacroiliac joint. In severe cases, AS can cause a complete fusion (ankylosis) of the spine. Many AS patients suffer severe loss of mobility and as a consequence lose working capabilities.

The average AS prevalence varies among different populations, with 0.24% in Europe, 0.17% in Asia, 0.3% in North America, 0.1% in Latin America and 0.7% in Africa. Based on these ratios, it is estimated that the number of AS cases in Europe and Asia alone could reach 1.30–1.56 million and 4.63–4.98 million, respectively [1].

AS is highly inheritable. The recurrence risks in monozygous twins and first-degree relatives are 63 and 8.2%, respectively [4, 5]. Most AS is presented in sporadic cases, probably reflecting the oligogenic nature of this disease. The human leukocyte antigen B27 (*HLA-B*27*) genotype was found strongly associated with AS [6–8]. Specifically

* Correspondence: zhipingtan@csu.edu.cn; malong@sklmg.edu.cn
[1]Clinical Center for Gene Diagnosis and Therapy, the Second Xiangya Hospital of Central South University, Changsha 410011, China
[3]Center for Medical Genetics, School of Life Sciences, Central South University, Changsha 410081, China
Full list of author information is available at the end of the article

*HLA-B*27* carriers could have a 20-fold increase in the risk of developing spondylarthropathy-related diseases [9], which is exemplified by the fact that most AS patients are *HLA-B*27* positive in the general population. However the presence of *HLA-B*27* genotype is not sufficient for AS pathogenesis, as only 1–5% *HLA-B*27* carriers eventually develop AS [8, 10, 11].

Recently large-scale genome-wide association studies on patients with European ancestry and of the Han Chinese have identified at least 31 non-*HLA-B* genetic loci associated with AS [11–17]. Among these loci, *IL23R*, *2p15*, *ERAP1* exhibit the most significant association [12, 15–17]. Nevertheless these loci, together with *HLA-B*27*, could explain only 24.4% of the heritability of AS [15]. Therefore the major genetic causes of AS remain to be identified. Ideally, AS cases from consanguinity inheritance or large pedigrees could provide a simpler inheritance pattern compared to sporadic cases, which might facilitate the identification of more elusive risk genes of AS.

To further understand the genetics of AS, we employed a combination of genome-wide linkage analysis and next-generation sequencing (NGS) in a three-generation Han Chinese pedigree with five AS patients. The analysis revealed a missense variant affecting a conserved amino acid in the novel gene *ANKDD1B* that segregates with the disease. We further identified a distinct *ANKDD1B* missense variant in a male by surveying a group of sporadic AS patients using exome sequencing. These findings suggest that *ANKDD1B* variants might be related with the pathogenesis of AS.

Methods

Patients and subjects

The study protocol was approved by the Review Board of the Second Xiangya Hospital of the Central South University in China with informed consent from each study participant. The proband (AS9_1) (Fig. 1) was diagnosed with ankylosing spondylitis in 2009 at the Department of Rheumatology of the Second Xiangya Hospital. A follow up of the proband identified a 16-member, three-generation AS9 pedigree (Fig. 2a). The disease history of the five AS9 patients and the sporadic patient sAS_P1 is shown in Additional file 1: Table S1. Medical images of two other patients are also shown in Fig. 1.

DNA extraction

Genomic DNA was extracted from peripheral blood of the family members using a DNeasy Blood & Tissue Kit (Qiagen, Valencia, CA) on the QIAcube automated DNA extraction robot (Qiagen, Hilden, Germany).

Genome-wide linkage analysis

Genomic DNA samples of the AS9 family members were adjusted to a final concentration of 50 ng/μl. The

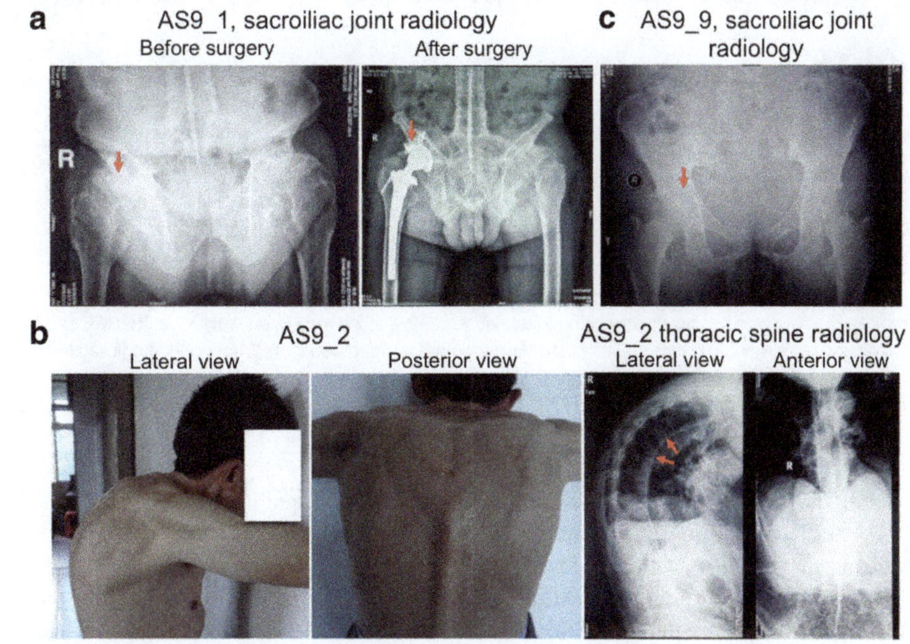

Fig. 1 Medical images of AS9 patients. **a** X-ray pictures of the sacroiliac joints of the proband, AS9_1, before (left) and after (right) joint replacement surgery. Arrows indicate erosion of the right joint before the surgery (left) and the artificial joint after the surgery (right). **b** Medical images of patient AS9_2, showing the deformation of the thoracic spine due to ankylosis (left). X-ray pictures showing the "bamboo"-like spines of AS9_2 (right). Arrows point to the sites of fused vertebrae. **c** Sacroiliitis of patient AS9_9 detected by X-ray photography

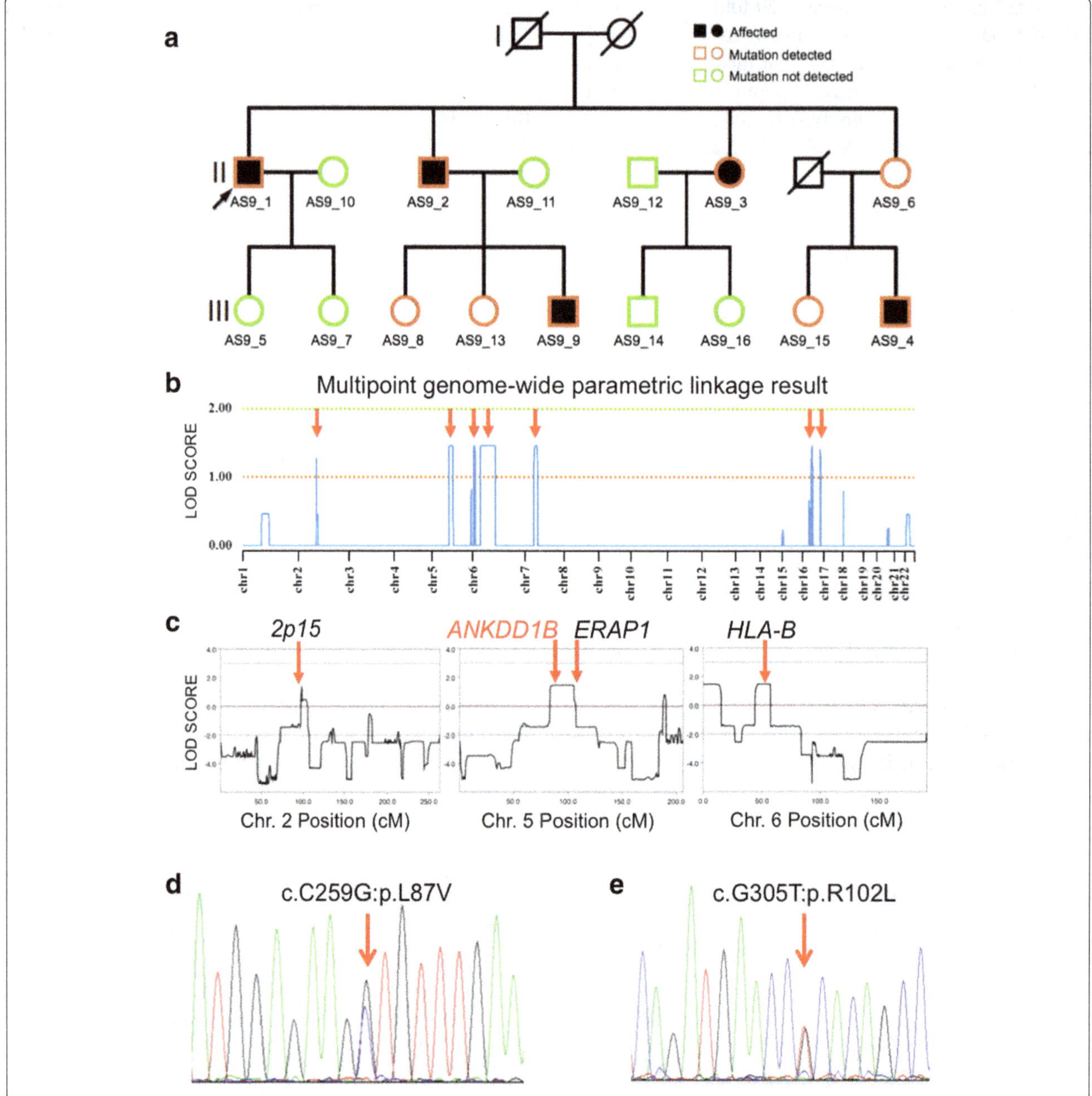

Fig. 2 Whole-genome linkage analysis and exome sequencing identified *ANKDD1B* to be associated with AS. **a** The AS9 pedigree. Generations, non-carriers, non-symptomatic carriers and patients are indicated. Arrow points to the proband. **b** Whole-genome linkage analysis identified seven regions (arrows) on Chr. 2, Chr. 5, Chr. 6, Chr. 7 and Chr. 16 to be significantly linked to disease transmission in the AS9 pedigree. **c** A delineation of the *ANKDD1B* locus and the major known AS risk loci in relation to the linkage regions. **d**, **e** The L87V variant and the R102L variant in *ANKDD1B* as shown in Sanger sequencing chromatograms

Infinium OmniZhongHua-8 v1.3 Beadchip (Illumina Inc., San Diego, USA) and the Illumina BeadScan genotyping system (Beadstation Scanner) were employed to obtain the signal intensities of SNP probes. The Infinium OmniZhongHua-8 v1.3 Beadchip contains 887,270 SNPs that cover common, intermediate and rare variants specific to Chinese populations. The GenomeStudio V1.0 Genotyping Module was used to analyze the genotypes (human genome build 37/Hg19) and evaluate the experimental quality. The call rates of the samples were greater than 99.5%. After no call SNPs, SNPs with minor allele frequency < 0.05, and mismatched SNPs between parents and children were excluded, we chose one SNP per 0.5 cM (7079 SNPs across the genome with an average gap of 379 kb) for multi-point parametric linkage analysis using the merlin (v1.1.2) software based on an autosomal dominant inheritance disease model. Specifically we excluded all females of the third generation from the linkage analysis, since females have a penetrance much lower than males [2]. We treated AS9_6 as patient because she has a symptomatic son.

Whole-exome sequencing

Four members of the AS9 family (AS9_1, AS9_2, AS9_3 and AS9_4) were subjected to whole-exome sequencing analysis. Each individual paired-end Agilent SureSelect library was prepared according to manufacturer's instructions (Agilent) from 1.0 μg genomic DNA sheared with a Covaris S220 sonicator (Covaris, Inc., Woburn, USA). Exome capture was performed with Agilent's SureSelect Human All Exon kit V5, which resulted in ~ 50 Mb DNA sequences of 334,378 exons from 20,965 genes being captured. Paired-end sequencing (150-bp reads) was carried on HiSeq 4000 platform (Illumina). After demultiplexing, paired-end sequences were mapped to the human genome (UCSC hg19) using Burrows-Wheeler Aligner (BWA) [18]. The mean coverage of the target regions obtained for the four samples was 99.9, 99.9, 99.8 and 99.9%, with average sequencing depth of 90.86X, 83.27X, 76.24X and 83.87X for AS9_1, AS9_2, AS9_3 and AS9_4, respectively (Additional file 2: Table S2). Downstream processing was performed using the Genome Analysis Toolkit (GATK), varscan2 and Picard, and variant calls were made with the GATK HaplotypeCaller. Variant annotation was based on Ensembl release 82, and filtering was performed with ANNOVAR Documentation.

127,303, 122,644, 115,062 and 126,720 confidence variants in AS9_1, AS9_2, AS9_3 and AS9_4, respectively, were identified from the exome sequencing (Additional file 3: Table S3). Non-synonymous SNPs or frameshift-causing INDELs with an alternative allele frequency > 0.005 in the NHLBI Exome Sequencing Project Exome Variant Server (ESP6500), dbSNP (build 138) (http://www.ncbi.nlm.nih.gov/projects/SNP/index.html), the 1000 Genomes Browser (released May 2012) (http://www.1000genomes.org/) or the ExAC Browser (http://exac.broadinstitute.org) were excluded prior to analysis. The called SNVs and INDELs were filtered and those predicted by HapMap Genome Browser (release #28) (http://hapmap.ncbi.nlm.nih.gov/), SIFT (http://sift.jcvi.org/), Polyphen2 (http://genetics.bwh.harvard.edu/pph2/) and MutationTaster (http://www.mutationtaster.org/) to be non-deleterious were excluded. By this approach, six candidate variants distributed in five genes were identified in all four patients (Additional file 3: Table S3 and Additional file 4: Table S4), which include *GBP5* (containing two distinct variants), *ANKDD1B*, *TMEM30B*, *CACNA1H* and *RFPL3*.

Variant validation and co-segregation analysis

Sanger sequencing was used to validate the candidate variants found in exome sequencing. Segregation analyses were performed on the family members. The two *ANKDD1B* variants were also examined in the exome sequences of 500 healthy adults of both sexes and different ages, who were recruited by the genome sequencing company Novogene (Beijing) and used as an internal control for genetic variants potentially specific for the Han Chinese. Primer pairs used to amplify fragments encompassing individual variants were designed using an online tool (PrimerQuest, IDT) (http://www.idtdna.com/Primerquest/Home/Index) and the primer sequences for *ANKDD1B* are listed in Additional file 5: Table S5.

Haplotype verification

The genomic sequence for each SNP was obtained from dbSNP database (https://www.ncbi.nlm.nih.gov/projects/SNP/). The genomic DNAs from patients were amplified by PCR using primers listed in Additional file 6: Table S6 and the sequences of the amplified fragments were determined.

Results

The AS9 ankylosing spondylitis pedigree

Using the modified New York criteria for ankylosing spondylitis [19], a diagnosis of AS was made on three individuals (AS9_1, AS9_2, AS9_9) of a three-generation pedigree of the Han Chinese (Fig. 1, Fig. 2a and Additional file 1: Table S1). The family history suggests an autosomal dominant pattern of inheritance, which predominantly affects male members (Fig. 2a). The shared symptoms include: the onset of chronic lower back pain before the age of 20 years, symptomatic sacroiliitis (persistent pain and stiffness lasting > 3 months) and improvement on exercise and worsening with rest. In the proband AS9_1, the symptom was limited to sacroiliitis on both sides, which was verified by radiology (Fig.1a, left). Joint replacement surgery was performed on the right sacroiliac joint of the proband in 2010 (Fig. 1a, right). The proband described that his deceased father also had similar symptoms. For patient AS9_2, the progression of the disease has led to severe deformation of the spine (Fig. 1b, left) and the formation of the "bamboo"-like vertebral joints due to ankylosis (Fig. 1b, right). Patient AS9_9 is the son of patient AS9_2 and began to show mild signs of sacroiliitis before the age of 20 years, which was confirmed by radiology (Fig. 1c).

The other two patients (AS9_3 and AS9_4) were diagnosed based on symptoms that include teenage onset of chronic back pain and symptomatic sacroiliitis (Additional file 1: Table S1). However these symptoms were not verified by radiology due to personal reasons (Additional file 1: Table S1). AS9_3 was not tested for HLA-B*27 positivity as well. We later genotyped rs13202464, a SNP associated with the *HLA-B* locus in the Han Chinese [16] and rs116488202, another verified SNP strongly associated with both Europeans and the Han Chinese [15] (Table 1). We found that AS9_3 shares identical haplotypes at these loci with other HLA-B*27-positive patients of the family, suggesting that AS9_3 is likely HLA-B*27-positive as well.

Genome-wide linkage analysis identified seven risk chromosomal regions in the AS9 pedigree

AS is an oligogenic disease [11] and most AS patients are identified as sporadic cases. The heritability of AS in the AS9 pedigree might provide a rare opportunity for identifying new AS-associated genetic variants.

To identify the potential genetic variants, we performed genome-wide linkage analysis on 10 AS9 family members (six third-generation females were excluded due to the incomplete penetrance of AS in females) based on an autosomal dominant inheritance model (see Methods). Multi-point parametric linkage analysis identified seven regions on five chromosomes with maximum multi-point parametric LOD (logarithm of odds) scores between 1.275 and 1.4608 (Fig. 2b and Table 2). We also identified seven other regions distributed on seven chromosomes, with the maximal LOD scores between 0.2322 and 0.8175 (Fig. 2b).

Whole-exome sequencing identified six candidate variants in the AS9 pedigree

The linkage analysis only provided information concerning the genomic locations of potential genetic variants associated with the AS9 pedigree. To narrow down the genetic variants, we performed exome sequencing on four patients (AS9_1, AS9_2, AS9_3 and AS9_4). In total we obtained on average 4.6 Gbp, 4.2 Gbp, 3.8 Gbp and 4.2 Gbp sequences that covered more than 99% of the exonic regions for AS9_1, AS9_2, AS9_3 and AS9_4, respectively (Additional file 2: Table S2). The sequencing depth for each patient was from 76X for AS9_3 to 90X for AS9_1.

From the exome sequencing (see Methods), we identified six candidate variants distributed in five genes that are shared by all four patients (Additional file 3: Table S3 and Additional file 4: Table S4). These genes include *GBP5* (containing two different variants), *ANKDD1B*, *TMEM30B*, *CACNA1H* and *RFPL3.*

We examined co-segregation of these variants with individuals of the AS9 pedigree and found that the *CACNA1H* variant was absent in the AS9_9 patient, suggesting that *CACNA1H* is probably not a risk locus. MutationTaster (www.mutationtaster.org) prediction indicates that the variants in *GBP5* and *RFPL3* are likely non-disease causing polymorphisms. The variant in *TMEM30B* was reported in the ExAC database (http://exac.broadinsitutute.org) at a frequency of 0.002 and is predicted by the SIFT software (www.sift.jcvi.org) to be a highly tolerated change. We currently could not conclude whether this variant confers any risk for AS. Together these analyses suggest that the genetic variant in *ANKDD1B* is worthy of further consideration.

ANKDD1B variants might be associated with ankylosing spondylitis

We next compared the genomic positions of the five candidate genes (Additional file 4: Table S4) with the

Table 1 Haplotype analysis of major AS risk loci on the study subjects

ID	Phenotype	Sex	ANKDD1B	HLA-B27 rs13202464	HLA-B27 rs116488202	2p15 rs6759298	ERAP1 rs30187	IL23R rs11209026
AS9_1	AS	M	L87 V/+	G/A	C/C	C/G	C/C	G/G
AS9_2	AS	M	L87 V/+	G/A	C/C	C/G	C/C	G/G
AS9_4	AS	M	L87 V/+	G/A	C/C	G/G	T/C	G/G
AS9_9	AS	M	L87 V/+	G/A	C/C	C/G	T/C	G/G
sAS_P1	AS	M	R102L/+	G/A	C/C	G/G	C/C	G/G
AS9_3	AS	F	L87 V/+	G/A	C/C	G/G	T/C	G/G
AS9_6	N	F	L87 V/+	G/A	C/C	G/G	C/C	G/G
AS9_8	N	F	L87 V/+	G/A	C/C	C/G	T/C	G/G
AS9_15	N	F	L87 V/+	G/A	C/C	G/G	T/C	G/G
AS9_13	N	F	L87 V/+	A/A	C/C	C/G	T/C	G/G
AS9_5	N	F	WT	A/A	C/C	G/G	C/C	G/G
AS9_7	N	F	WT	A/A	C/C	G/G	T/C	G/G
AS9_12	N	M	WT	A/A	C/C	C/G	T/C	G/G
AS9_10	N	F	WT	A/A	C/C	C/G	T/C	G/G
AS9_11	N	F	WT	A/A	C/C	C/G	T/C	G/G
AS9_14	N	M	WT	A/A	C/C	G/G	T/C	G/G
AS9_16	N	F	WT	A/A	C/C	C/G	T/C	G/G

Table 2 List of linkage regions with MAX-LOD scores above 1.0

Chr.	Left SNP	Right SNP	MAX-LOD
2	rs17007729	rs17018719	1.275
5	rs3112483	rs13161885	1.4608
6	rs7753332	rs1590328	1.4571
6	rs4710988	rs259686	1.4608
7	rs739749	rs13222756	1.4607
16	rs16947530	rs7184310	1.4598
16	rs17673125	rs16961072	1.4069

whole-genome linkage results (Fig. 2b and c). Interestingly only *ANKDD1B* is contained within one of the seven linkage regions with MAX_LOD score above 1.275 (Table 2), which is between rs3112483 and rs13161885 on Chr. 5 (Fig. 2c and Table 2). This result is consistent with the bioinformatics analysis described above and suggests that *ANKDD1B* is potentially associated with the AS9 pedigree.

We examined the coding exons of *ANKDD1B* in all 16 members of the AS9 family by Sanger sequencing. The L87V variant (Fig. 2d) was verified in the four patients analyzed by exome sequencing and also patient AS9_9 (Fig. 2a), who was not included in our initial exome analysis. The variant was found in AS9_6, who is non-symptomatic but has a symptomatic son. We further detected the L87V variant in three non-symptomatic members of the family (Fig. 2a). Two are daughters of patient AS9_2 and one is the daughter of the non-symptomatic AS9_6. This variant was not detected in seven other non-symptomatic family members (Fig. 2a and Table 1).

ANKDD1B encodes a novel conserved protein with multiple ankyrin repeats and a death domain (Additional file 7: Figure S1). The variant found in the AS9 pedigree changes a conserved leucine to valine at position 87 within the first ankyrin repeat and is predicted to cause a partially deleterious effect on the protein function (www.predictprotein.org).

To further examine the association of *ANKDD1B* with AS, we surveyed the coding exons and splice sites of *ANKDD1B* in 30 sporadic AS patients previously analyzed by whole-exome sequencing (Z. Tan and H. Zeng, unpublished observations). From a 21-year old male patient (sAS_P1, Additional file 1: Table S1), we identified a distinct missense variant that changes a conserved arginine to leucine at position 102 (exon3:c.G305T:p.R102L) within the second ankyrin repeat (Fig. 2e, Table 1 and Additional file 7: Figure S1). This variant is predicted to cause strongly deleterious effect on the protein function (www.predictprotein.org).

The two *ANKDD1B* variants were not found in 500 internal (local) control exomes sequenced. The L87 V variant identified in the pedigree was not identified in NHLBI Exome Sequencing Project Exome Variant Server (ESP6500), the 1000 Genomes Browser as well as the ExAC database. The variant identified in the sporadic male patient (sAS_P1) (c.G305 T:p.R102L) has a SNP number (rs191940699) and is presented in the dbSNP database (www.ncbi.nlm.nih.gov) with a global MAF of 0.0016/8. In addition this SNP is presented in the ExAc database (http://exac.broadinsitutute.org) as a c.G305A:p.R102H variant with an allele frequency of 7.477e-05 (1 out of 13,374 alleles from 6687 individuals in total). In the South Asian population in which this SNP was identified, its allele frequency is 0.0001422 (1 out of 7030 alleles from 3515 individuals). The low values of these frequencies imply a selection against these variants in the general population.

Haplotype analysis of the *ANKDD1B* variant carriers

Besides the linkage region on Chr. 5 that contains *ANKDD1B*, we also identified six other regions (Table 2 and Fig. 2b) with MAX-LOD scores above 1.275. Interestingly, one region on Chr. 6 contains the *HLA-B* locus (Fig. 2c), prompting us to examine the haplotype of *HLA-B*27* in our cohort. We found that the SNP rs13202464 previously reported to tag *HLA-B*27* in Asian populations [16] also predominantly tags the patients (6/6 in patients vs 3/11 in non-AS individuals) (Table 1). However the SNP rs116488202 reported to tag *HLA-B*27* more significantly in both Asian and European populations [15] is presented identically among the patients and normal individuals (Table 1), with the risk minor allele (T) absent in all individuals.

The linkage region on Chr. 2 does not contain the major AS risk locus *2p15* but is at a close distance, with 0.97 Mb between the left outline of this region and the SNP rs6759298 reported to tag *2p15* [15]. We genotyped rs6759298 and found that the risk allele of this SNP does not exhibit an apparent association with AS patients (3/6) vs non-AS individuals (6/11) (Table 1).

The *ERAP1* locus is also significantly associated with AS in the general population [12]. The *ERAP1*-tagging SNP rs30187 [15] is 0.3 Mb apart from the right outline of the linkage region on Chr. 5 (Fig. 2c). 3/6 patients carry the risk allele of rs30187 while 9/11 non-AS individuals are also positive (Table 1), suggesting that the genotype of *ERAP1* might not be associated with AS in our cohort.

No linkage region on Chr. 1 with a MAX-LOD score above 1.0 was identified. However since the AS risk locus *IL23R* is located on Chr. 1, we also genotyped the SNP rs11209026 that tags *IL23R* [15]. We found that all individuals in our cohort are homozygous for the risk allele (Table 1). Therefore we could not evaluate the contribution of the *IL23R* locus to the pathogenesis of our patients.

We compared the other four linkage regions (Table 2, in blue) with all the AS risk loci identified to date [11] and found that none are located within these regions. We postulate that these linkage regions might contain new risk loci for AS or are merely associated with the AS9 family by coincidence.

Discussion

In this study, we combined genome-wide linkage analysis and exome sequencing to identify the *ANKDD1B* gene as a potential locus related ankylosing spondylitis in a Chinese AS pedigree.

AS is an oligogenic disease with over 75% of the heritability unexplained [11]. Of the 32 identified loci associated with AS [11, 15], *HLA-B*27* is the most significant risk factor, followed by *IL23R, 2p15* and *ERAP1* [15]. Among the seven linkage regions we identified in AS9 pedigree (Fig. 2b), one contains the *HLA-B* locus and two others are closely linked to the *2p15* and *ERAP1* loci, respectively (Fig. 2c). This correlation does not appear to be a random coincidence. Instead, it suggests that these linkage regions more or less correspond to the risk loci of AS and could be useful for distinguishing other genetic variants related to AS, e.g., those variants derived from exome sequencing. Indeed, among the six candidate variants that we identified from exome sequencing of the AS9 pedigree, only *ANKDD1B* is contained within a linkage region on Chr. 5 (Fig. 2c). Furthermore, a different *ANKDD1B* variant (R102L) was identified in a sporadic AS patient, emphasizing the potential correlation between *ANKDD1B* variants and AS in the Chinese patients.

The genetic location of *ANKDD1B* is *5q13.3* (www.ensembl.org), which is 0.1 cM away from *5q14.3*, a previously identified risk locus in Asian populations [16]. The significance of *5q14.3* locus was not replicated in the study of European populations [15]. Therefore it is unclear whether *5q14.3* represents an Asian-specific locus or the association of this locus with AS [16] was in fact caused by its closeness with *ANKDD1B*. The linkage region on Chr. 5 identified in this study is also close to but does not contain the risk locus *ERAP1* (Fig. 2c). Whether the haplotype of *ERAP1* affects the identification of this linkage region is unknown. The linkage region that we identified on Chr. 2 is close to another major AS risk locus, *2p15* [15] (Fig. 2c). Currently we could not determine whether the identification of this linkage region is caused by its closeness to *2p15* or it represents a different risk locus for AS. The other linkage regions (Table 2, in blue) do not contain any of the AS risk loci identified so far [11].

ANKDD1B encodes a novel protein containing 10 tandem ankyrin repeats and a death domain and is conserved from zebrafish to human (Additional file 7: Figure S1). Ankyrin repeats are found in proteins involved in inflammatory response, transcription, cell-cycle regulation, cytoskeleton integrity development, cell-cell signaling and protein transport [20]. Death domains are usually regulators of inflammation, innate immune response and cell death through their interactions with TNF (tumor necrosis factor) receptors and Toll-like receptors [21–23].

A protein expression database (www.proteinatlas.org) indicates that the ANKDD1B protein is expressed in muscles, distinct cells of the lymph node and tonsil, a chronic myeloid leukemia cell line (K-562), a multiple myeloma cell line (LP-1) and an ovarian cystadenocarcinoma cell line (EFO-21). In addition the *ANKDD1B* transcript was detected in multiple human tissues including the lymph node and spleen (www.genecards.org). In mouse, the *ANKDD1B* transcript is expressed in higher levels in multiple B- and T-cell lines and in various parts of the nervous system (www.biogps.org). The site of expression and the domain structure of ANKDD1B suggest a function in the immune system.

The complex oligogenic nature of AS hinders the genetic analysis of AS pathogenesis. A previous analysis of AS recurrence in relation to genetic distances estimated that multiplicative interactions involving ~five genetic loci could partially explain the occurrence of AS in the general population [5]. In our pedigree and the sporadic male patient, the presence of the *ANKDD1B* variant and *HLA-B*27* are the most significant factors predicting whether an individual develops AS (Table 1), while the roles of three other GWAS-derived significant loci (*IL23R, 2p15, ERAP1*) could not be evaluated, probably due to the limited size of our cohort.

In the AS9 pedigree, all four male carriers are *HLA-B*27* positive and developed AS (Fig. 2a and Table 1). Four of the five female carriers are *HLA-B*27* positive, while only one developed AS (Fig. 2a and Table 1). This phenomenon is consistent with AS epidemiology in the general population, in which males are three times more frequently affected than females [2].

Besides the AS9 pedigree described in our study, three other Han Chinese AS pedigrees were also described recently [24], in which the *2q36.1-36.3* locus was found to be associated with disease transmission in addition to *HLA-B*27*. This locus has not been associated with AS in other association studies [11]. It is possible that a combination of genome-wide linkage analysis and genome sequencing would narrow down the potential AS-related genetic variants in these pedigrees.

Conclusions

In short, we found that a novel missense variant of the *ANKDD1B* gene might be associated with patients in a rare AS pedigree of the Han Chinese. We also found a different *ANKDD1B* missense variant in a sporadic AS patient. *ANKDD1B* was identified with the combination of genome-wide linkage analysis and exome sequencing and verified to be co-segregated with the patients in a similar manner as the *HLA-B*27* locus, implying that this gene might be related to AS pathogenesis and is worth to be considered for understanding the genetics of AS. Future studies, including verification of this association in more AS patients and analysis of animal models carrying *ANKDD1B* mutations, might provide novel insights into the pathogenesis of AS.

Acknowledgements
We thank the AS9 family members and other individuals for their cooperation. We thank Qiong Fu, Chunyu Liu and Qing Zhou for suggestions.

Funding
The study is supported by a Natural Science Foundation of China grant to ZT (No. 81470445), a MOST grant (2016YFC1201805) and Natural Science Foundation of China grants (No. 31371253 and 31571045) to LM. This study is also partially supported by Key Projects of Changsha Science and Technology (K1306005-31-1). The funding bodies have no roles in the design of the study and collection, analysis, and interpretation of data and in writing the manuscript.

Authors' contributions
ZT and LM secured the funding, instructed the study and wrote the manuscript. HZ, QT and YZ performed the genome-wide linkage and exome sequencing studies and analyzed the data. ZX, XG and CZ performed the haplotype analysis and analyzed the data. JW performed the variant co-segregation analysis and verified the variants. GL, BW and YY diagnosed the patients. All authors have read and approved the manuscript.

Competing interests
The authors declare that they have no competing interests.

Author details
[1]Clinical Center for Gene Diagnosis and Therapy, the Second Xiangya Hospital of Central South University, Changsha 410011, China. [2]Department of Cardiovascular Surgery, the Second Xiangya Hospital of Central South University, Changsha 410011, China. [3]Center for Medical Genetics, School of Life Sciences, Central South University, Changsha 410081, China. [4]Department of Rheumatology, the Second Xiangya Hospital of Cenral South University, Changsha, China. [5]Department of Spine Surgery, the Second Xiangya Hospital Central South University, Changsha 410011, Hunan, China.

References

1. Dean LE, Jones GT, MacDonald AG, Downham C, Sturrock RD, Macfarlane GJ. Global prevalence of ankylosing spondylitis. Rheumatology (Oxford). 2014;53(4):650–7. Epub 2013/12/11. https://doi.org/10.1093/rheumatology/ket387. PubMed PMID: 24324212.
2. Braun J, Sieper J. Ankylosing spondylitis. Lancet. 2007;369(9570):1379–90. Epub 2007/04/24. https://doi.org/10.1016/S0140-6736(07)60635-7. PubMed PMID: 17448825.
3. Stolwijk C, Boonen A, van Tubergen A, Reveille JD. Epidemiology of spondyloarthritis. Rheum Dis Clin N Am 2012;38(3):441–76. Epub 2012/10/23. https://doi.org/10.1016/j.rdc.2012.09.003. PubMed PMID: 23083748; PubMed Central PMCID: PMC4470267.
4. Brown MA, Kennedy LG, MacGregor AJ, Darke C, Duncan E, Shatford JL, et al. Susceptibility to ankylosing spondylitis in twins: the role of genes, HLA, and the environment. Arthritis Rheum 1997;40(10):1823–8. https://doi.org/10.1002/1529-0131(199710)40:10<1823::AID-ART15>3.0.CO;2–1. PubMed PMID: 9336417.
5. Brown MA, Laval SH, Brophy S, Calin A. Recurrence risk modelling of the genetic susceptibility to ankylosing spondylitis. Ann Rheum Dis. 2000;59(11): 883 6. PubMed PMID: 11053066; PubMed Central PMCID: PMCPMC1753017
6. Brewerton DA, Hart FD, Nicholls A, Caffrey M, James DC, Sturrock RD. Ankylosing spondylitis and HL-A 27. Lancet. 1973;1(7809):904–7. Epub 1973/04/28. PubMed PMID: 4123836
7. Schlosstein L, Terasaki PI, Bluestone R, Pearson CM. High association of an HL-A antigen, W27, with ankylosing spondylitis. N Engl J Med. 1973;288(14): 704–6. Epub 1973/04/05. https://doi.org/10.1056/NEJM197304052881403. PubMed PMID: 4688372.
8. Reveille JD. An update on the contribution of the MHC to AS susceptibility. Clin Rheumatol 2014;33(6):749–757. Epub 2014/05/20. doi: https://doi.org/10.1007/s10067-014-2662-7. PubMed PMID: 24838411; PubMed Central PMCID: PMC4488903.
9. Braun J, Bollow M, Remlinger G, Eggens U, Rudwaleit M, Distler A, et al. Prevalence of spondylarthropathies in HLA-B27 positive and negative blood donors. Arthritis Rheum. 1998;41(1):58–67. https://doi.org/10.1002/1529-0131(199801)41:1<58::AID-ART8>3.0.CO;2-G. PubMed PMID: 9433870.
10. Bowness P. Hla-B27. Annu Rev Immunol 2015;33:29–48. Epub 2015/04/12. https://doi.org/10.1146/annurev-immunol-032414-112110. PubMed PMID: 25861975.
11. O'Rielly DD, Uddin M, Rahman P. Ankylosing spondylitis: beyond genome-wide association studies. Curr Opin Rheumatol. 2016;28(4):337–345. https://doi.org/10.1097/BOR.0000000000000297. PubMed PMID: 27224740.
12. Burton PR, Clayton DG, Cardon LR, Craddock N, Deloukas P, Duncanson A, et al. Association scan of 14,500 nonsynonymous SNPs in four diseases identifies autoimmunity variants. Nat Genet 2007;39(11):1329–37. Epub 2007/10/24. https://doi.org/10.1038/ng.2007.17. PubMed PMID: 17952073; PubMed Central PMCID: PMC2680141.
13. Danoy P, Pryce K, Hadler J, Bradbury LA, Farrar C, Pointon J, et al. Association of variants at 1q32 and STAT3 with ankylosing spondylitis suggests genetic overlap with Crohn's disease. PLoS Genet. 2010;6(12): e1001195. Epub 2010/12/15. https://doi.org/10.1371/journal.pgen.1001195. PubMed PMID: 21152001; PubMed Central PMCID: PMC2996314.
14. Evans DM, Spencer CC, Pointon JJ, Su Z, Harvey D, Kochan G, et al. Interaction between ERAP1 and HLA-B27 in ankylosing spondylitis implicates peptide handling in the mechanism for HLA-B27 in disease susceptibility. Nat Genet. 2011;43(8):761–7. Epub 2011/07/12. https://doi.org/10.1038/ng.873. PubMed PMID: 21743469; PubMed Central PMCID: PMC3640413.
15. International Genetics of Ankylosing Spondylitis C, Cortes A, Hadler J, Pointon JP, Robinson PC, Karaderi T, et al. Identification of multiple risk variants for ankylosing spondylitis through high-density genotyping of immune-related loci. Nat Genet. 2013;45(7):730–8. https://doi.org/10.1038/ng.2667. PubMed PMID: 23749187; PubMed Central PMCID: PMCPMC3757343.
16. Lin Z, Bei JX, Shen M, Li Q, Liao Z, Zhang Y, et al. A genome-wide association study in Han Chinese identifies new susceptibility loci for ankylosing spondylitis. Nat Genet 2012;44(1):73–7. Epub 2011/12/06. https://doi.org/10.1038/ng.1005. PubMed PMID: 22138694.
17. Reveille JD, Sims AM, Danoy P, Evans DM, Leo P, Pointon JJ, et al. Genome-wide association study of ankylosing spondylitis identifies non-MHC susceptibility loci. Nat Genet. 2010;42(2):123–7. Epub 2010/01/12. https://doi.org/10.1038/ng.513. PubMed PMID: 20062062; PubMed Central PMCID: PMC3224997.
18. Li H, Durbin R. Fast and accurate short read alignment with Burrows-Wheeler transform. Bioinformatics. 2009;25(14):1754–60. https://doi.org/10.1093/bioinformatics/btp324. PubMed PMID: 19451168; PubMed Central PMCID: PMCPMC2705234.
19. van der Linden S, Valkenburg HA, Cats A. Evaluation of diagnostic criteria for ankylosing spondylitis. A proposal for modification of the New York criteria. Arthritis Rheum. 1984;27(4):361–8. Epub 1984/04/01. PubMed PMID: 6231933
20. Mosavi LK, Cammett TJ, Desrosiers DC, Peng ZY. The ankyrin repeat as molecular architecture for protein recognition. Protein Sci. 2004;13(6):1435–48. Epub 2004/05/21. https://doi.org/10.1110/ps.03554604. PubMed PMID: 15152081; PubMed Central PMCID: PMC2279977.
21. Feinstein E, Kimchi A, Wallach D, Boldin M, Varfolomeev E. The death domain: a module shared by proteins with diverse cellular functions. Trends Biochem Sci. 1995;20(9):342–4. Epub 1995/09/01. PubMed PMID: 7482697
22. O'Neill LA, Dunne A, Edjeback M, Gray P, Jefferies C, Wietek C. Mal and MyD88: adapter proteins involved in signal transduction by toll-like receptors. J Endotoxin Res. 2003;9(1):55–9. Epub 2003/04/15. https://doi.org/10.1179/096805103125001351. PubMed PMID: 12691620.
23. Wajant H. Death receptors. Essays Biochem. 2003;39:53–71. Epub 2003/10/31. PubMed PMID: 14585074

11

Common variant of *BCAS3* is associated with gout risk in Japanese population: the first replication study after gout GWAS in Han Chinese

Masayuki Sakiyama[1,2†], Hirotaka Matsuo[1*†], Hirofumi Nakaoka[3], Yusuke Kawamura[1], Makoto Kawaguchi[1], Toshihide Higashino[1], Akiyoshi Nakayama[1], Airi Akashi[1], Jun Ueyama[4], Takaaki Kondo[4], Kenji Wakai[5], Yutaka Sakurai[6], Ken Yamamoto[7], Hiroshi Ooyama[8] and Nariyoshi Shinomiya[1]

Abstract

Background: Gout is a common disease resulting from hyperuricemia which causes acute arthritis. A recent genome-wide association study (GWAS) of gout identified three new loci for gout in Han Chinese: regulatory factor X3 (*RFX3*), potassium voltage-gated channel subfamily Q member 1 (*KCNQ1*), and breast carcinoma amplified sequence 3 (*BCAS3*). The lack of any replication studies of these three loci using other population groups prompted us to perform a replication study with Japanese clinically defined gout cases and controls.

Methods: We genotyped the variants of *RFX3* (rs12236871), *KCNQ1* (rs179785) and *BCAS3* (rs11653176) in 723 Japanese clinically defined gout cases and 913 controls by TaqMan method. rs179785 of *KCNQ1* is also evaluated by direct sequencing because of difficulties of its genotyping by TaqMan method.

Results: Although the variants of *RFX3* and *BCAS3* were clearly genotyped by TaqMan method, rs179785 of *KCNQ1* was not, because rs179785 (A/G) of *KCNQ1* is located at the last nucleotide ("A") of the 12-bp deletion variant (rs200562977) of *KCNQ1*. Therefore, rs179785 and rs200562977 of *KCNQ1* were genotyped by direct sequencing in all samples. Moreover, by direct sequencing with the same primers, we were able to evaluate the genotypes of rs179784 of *KCNQ1* which shows strong linkage disequilibrium with rs179785 ($D' = 1.0$ and $r^2 = 0.99$). rs11653176, a common variant of *BCAS3*, showed a significant association with gout ($P = 1.66 \times 10^{-3}$; odds ratio [OR] = 0.80); the direction of effect was the same as that seen in the previous Han Chinese GWAS. Two variants of *KCNQ1* (rs179785 and rs179784) had a nominally significant association ($P = 0.043$ and 0.044; OR = 0.85 and 0.86, respectively), but did not pass the significance threshold for multiple hypothesis testing using the Bonferroni correction. On the other hand, rs200562977 of *KCNQ1* and rs12236871 of *RFX3* did not show any significant association with gout.

Conclusion: BCAS3 is a coactivator of estrogen receptor alpha, and the influence of estrogen to serum uric acid level is well known. Our present replication study, as did the previous gout GWAS, demonstrated the common variant of *BCAS3* to be associated with gout susceptibility.

Keywords: Breast carcinoma amplified sequence 3 (BCAS3), Potassium voltage-gated Channel subfamily Q member 1 (KCNQ1), Regulatory factor X3 (RFX3), Single nucleotide polymorphisms (SNP), Urate, Uric acid

* Correspondence: hmatsuo@ndmc.ac.jp
†Masayuki Sakiyama and Hirotaka Matsuo contributed equally to this work.
[1]Department of Integrative Physiology and Bio-Nano Medicine, National Defense Medical College, 3-2 Namiki, Tokorozawa, Saitama 359-8513, Japan
Full list of author information is available at the end of the article

Background

Gout, which can also cause acute arthritis, is a common disease resulting from hyperuricemia. An increasing number of patients nowadays suffer from gout. Although various investigations aiming to elucidate the pathogenesis of this common disease are being conducted worldwide, most of the common genetic causes of gout remain to be clarified. Previous function-based genetic studies [1–3] and genome-wide association studies (GWASs) [4–6] have revealed that gout is associated with several genes, such as ATP-binding cassette transporter, subfamily G, member 2 (*ABCG2/BCRP*) and glucose transporter 9 (*GLUT9/SLC2A9*). Especially, by performing a GWAS of clinically-ascertained gout, our Japanese report identified five gout loci including *MYL2-CUX2* and cornichon family AMPA receptor auxiliary protein 2 (*CNIH-2*) [6]. Subsequent fine mapping analysis of the *MYL2-CUX2* region found that rs671 of aldehyde dehydrogenase 2 (*ALDH2*) is a gout locus which is an Asian specific one [7]. Li et al. recently performed a GWAS of clinically- ascertained gout and identified the following three new loci for gout in Han Chinese: regulatory factor X3 (*RFX3*), potassium voltage-gated channel subfamily Q member 1 (*KCNQ1*) and breast carcinoma amplified sequence 3 (*BCAS3*) [8]. However, there is no replication study of these three loci using other population groups. We therefore performed a replication study using Japanese clinically-defined gout cases and controls.

Methods

Patients and controls

This study was approved by the institutions' Ethical Committees (National Defense Medical College and Nagoya University). All procedures were performed in accordance with the Declaration of Helsinki, with written informed consent obtained from each subject. The cases comprised 723 gout patients assigned from Japanese male outpatients at Ryougoku East Gate Clinic (Tokyo, Japan). All patients were clinically diagnosed with primary gout according to the criteria established by the American College of Rheumatology [9]. Patients with inherited metabolic disorders, including Lesch–Nyhan syndrome and phosphoribosylpyrophosphate synthetase I superactivity, were excluded. Hyperuricemia was defined as the serum uric acid (SUA) level that exceeds 7.0 mg/dl (= 416.36 mol/l) according to the guideline of the Japanese Society of Gout and Nucleic Acid Metabolism [10]. The control group comprised 913 Japanese males without hyperuricemia and gout history, recruited from the participants in the Daiko Study, part of the Japan Multi-Institutional Collaborative Cohort Study (J-MICC Study) [11]. The mean age (± SD) of case and control groups was 45.5 years (± 10.6) and 53.5 years (± 10. 3), respectively, and their mean body mass index was 25. 3 kg/m^2 (± 3.6) and 22.9 kg/m^2 (± 2.9), respectively.

Genotyping

Genomic DNA was extracted from whole peripheral blood cells [12]. Genotyping of the three single nucleotide polymorphisms (SNPs), rs12236871 of *RFX3*, rs179785 of *KCNQ1* and rs11653176 of *BCAS3*, was

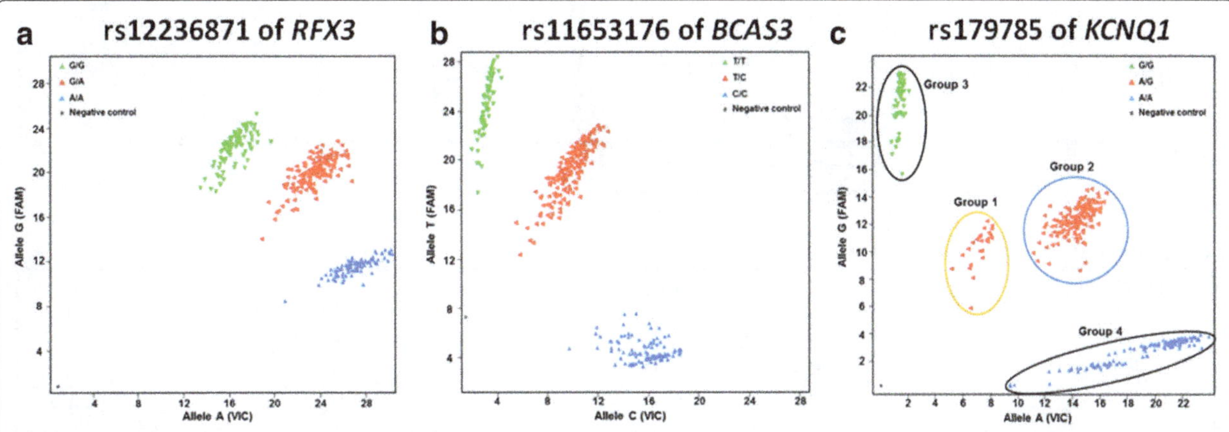

Fig. 1 Allelic discrimination plots of SNPs of *RFX2*, *BCAS3* and *KCNQ1*. **a** Representative plots for rs12236871 of *RFX3*. Well-separated clusters representing each genotype (G/G, G/A and A/A) can be observed. **b** Representative plots of rs11653176 of *BCAS3*. Well-separated clusters are clearly visible, representing each genotype (T/T, T/C and C/C). **c** Representative plots of rs179785 of *KCNQ1*. Computer auto analysis divided these plots into three groups (G/G, A/G and A/A). However, the plots seemed to be clustered into four groups (labeled as Groups 1 to 4). We therefore employed direct sequencing to confirm the genotypes. As a result, a 12-bp deletion variant of *KCNQ1* (rs200562977) was identified in several samples of all of four groups, and rs179785 of *KCNQ1* is located at the last nucleotide of this deletion variant (also see Figs. 2 and 3). Therefore, because it is difficult to genotype rs179785 using the TaqMan method, we performed the subsequent genotyping of rs179785 and rs200562977 by direct sequencing

performed using the TaqMan method (Thermo Fisher Scientific, Waltham, MA, USA) employing a LightCycler 480 (Roche Diagnostics, Mannheim, Germany) [12] with minor modifications. For genotyping *KCNQ1*variants, DNA sequencing analysis was performed with following primers: forward 5'-ACTTCCTGCCTCTGCTTTC-3′ and reverse 5'-TGAAGGAAGTGACCCCTG-3′. Direct sequencing was performed using a 3130xl Genetic Analyzer (Thermo Fisher Scientific) [12].

Data analysis

The software R version 3.1.1 (http://www.r-project.org/) [13] with the GenABEL package was used for all calculations in the statistical analysis. The association analyses were examined using the chi-square test. The pairwise linkage disequilibrium (LD) was calculated using data from the 1000 Genomes phase 3 JPT (Japanese in Tokyo) [14]. All *P* values were two-tailed and *P* values of < 0.05 were regarded as statistically significant.

Results

A representative plots of genotyping results by TaqMan method is shown in Fig. 1. Although allelic discrimination plots of rs12236871 of *RFX3* (Fig. 1a) and rs11653176 of *BCAS3* (Fig. 1b) are clearly divided into three groups for each genotype (major allele homozygote, heterozygote and minor allele homozygote), the plots of rs179785 of *KCNQ1* are clustered into four groups, labeled as Groups 1, 2, 3 and 4 in Fig. 1c. Thus, to confirm the genotypes of samples of Groups 1 and 2, direct sequencing was performed to analyze the DNA sequence around rs179785 of *KCNQ1.* Although the genotypes of almost all the samples in Group 2 shown in Fig. 1c were heterozygous (A/G) for rs179785 (Fig. 2a), the heterozygous 12-bp deletion variant of *KCNQ1*, rs200562977 (Fig. 2b), was frequently found in Group 1 samples in Fig. 1c. Actually, rs179785 (A/G) is located at the last nucleotide ("A") of this 12-bp deletion variant (rs200562977), as shown in Fig. 3. Further direct sequencing analysis revealed that Groups 3 and 4 also include a

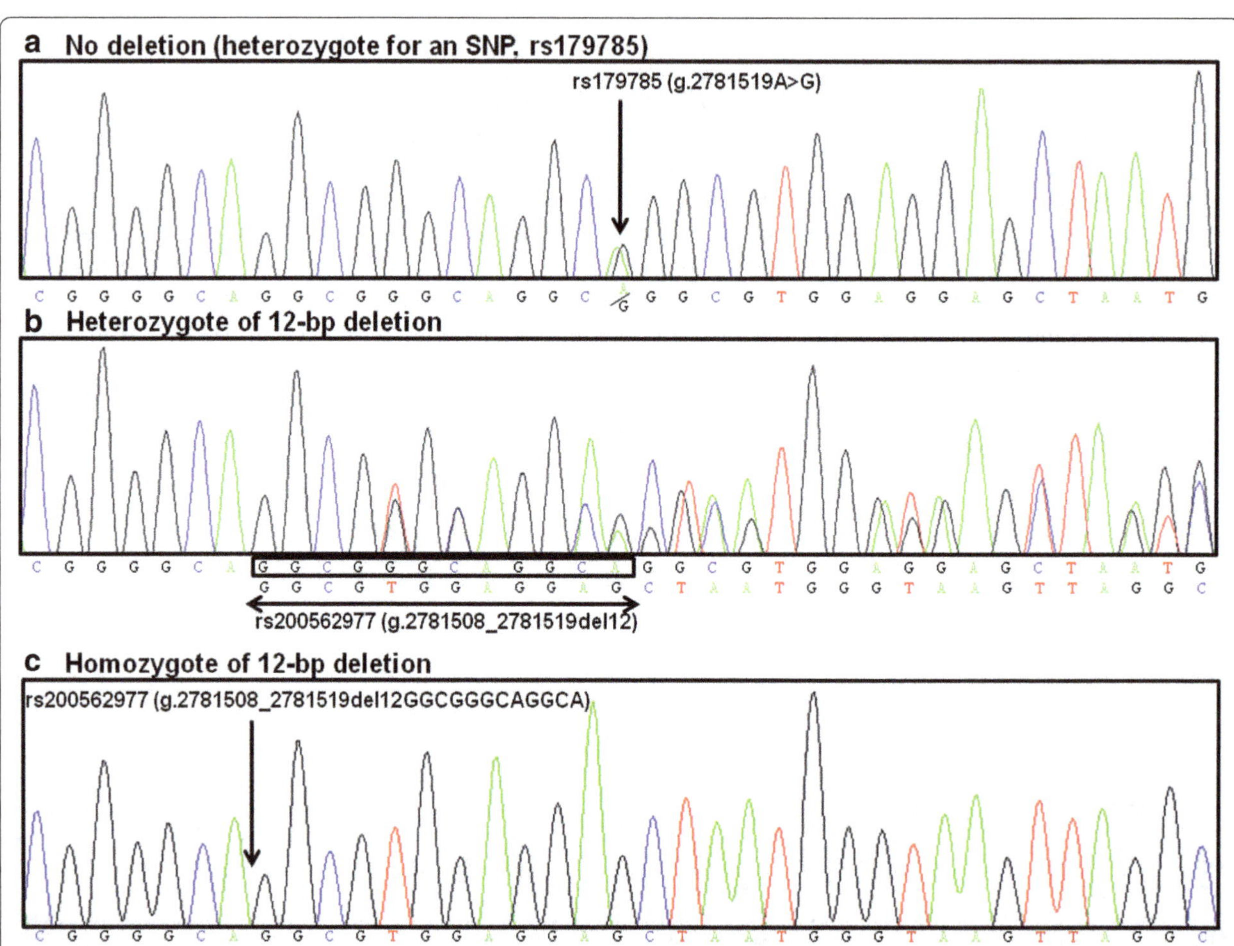

Fig. 2 Common variants of *KCNQ1*, rs179785 and rs200562977, demonstrated by direct sequencing. rs200562977, a 12-bp deletion variant of *KCNQ1*, was identified as a common variant. rs179785 (A/G) is located at the last nucleotide ("A") of 12-bp deletion site for rs200562977. Thus, when there is no deletion (**a**), rs179785 can be properly genotyped. On the other hand, when there is heterozygote (**b**) or homozygote (**c**) of 12-bp deletion, the position of rs179785 disappears

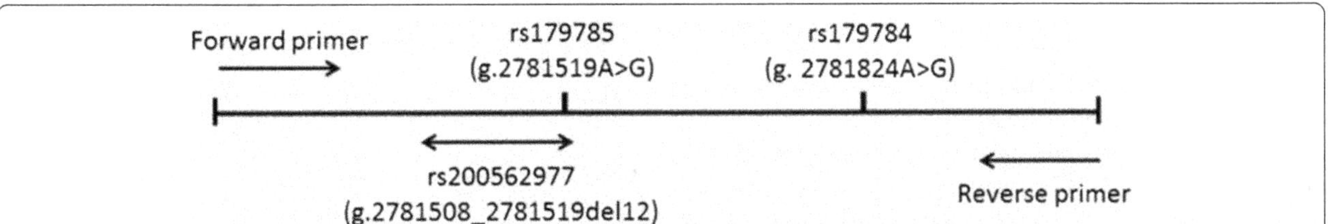

Fig. 3 Location of three variants: rs179785, rs200562977 and rs179784 of *KCNQ1*. rs179785 (A/G) is located at the last nucleotide, "A", of the 12-bp deletion site on rs200562977 (g.2781508_2781519del12GGCGGGCAGGCA). rs179784 is located 305 bp downstream from rs179785 and shows strong linkage disequilibrium with rs179785 (D' = 1.0 and r^2 = 0.99). For direct sequencing of the three variants of *KCNQ1*, the primers were designed as follows: 5′-ACTTCCTGCCTCTGCTTTC-3′ (forward primer) and 5′-TGAAGGAAGTGACCCCTG-3′ (reverse primer), respectively

heterozygous 12-bp deletion variant, and several samples in Groups 2 and 4 exhibit a homozygous 12-bp deletion variant (Fig. 2c). These findings suggest that it is difficult to correctly genotype rs179785 of *KCNQ1* using the TaqMan or DNA micro-array method. Therefore, in subsequent analyses, rs179785 and rs200562977 of *KCNQ1* were genotyped by direct sequencing, not by the TaqMan method, in all samples. Moreover, by direct sequencing with the same primers, we were able to evaluate the genotypes of rs179784 of *KCNQ1*, which is located downstream from rs179785 by 305 bp (Fig. 3), and which shows strong LD with rs179785 (D' = 1.0 and r^2 = 0.99).

All samples were successfully genotyped for the three variants of *KCNQ1* (rs179785, rs200562977 and rs179784) by direct sequencing. The call rates for the two SNPs (rs12236871 and rs11653176) by TaqMan method were more than 97.0%. All the variants were in Hardy-Weinberg equilibrium ($P > 0.05$). Table 1 shows the genotyping results of the three loci (*RFX3, KCNQ1* and *BCAS3*) for 723 clinically-defined gout patients and 913 controls. The common variant of *BCAS3*, rs11653176, showed a significant association with gout ($P = 1.66 \times 10^{-3}$; odds ratio [OR] = 0.80; 95% confidence interval [CI]: 0.70–0.92). The direction of effect was the same as observed in the previous gout GWAS [8]. rs179785 and rs179784 of *KCNQ1* had a nominally significant association (P = 0.043 and 0.044; OR = 0.85 and 0.86; 95% CI: 0.73–0.99 and 0.75–1.00, respectively), but did not pass the significance threshold at P value < 0.017 (= 0.05/3) for multiple hypothesis testing using the Bonferroni correction. On the other hand, rs200562977 of *KCNQ1* and rs12236871 of *RFX3* did not show any significant association with gout.

Discussion

In this study, we were able, for the first time, to replicate the association between rs11653176 of *BCAS3* and gout. rs2079742, another intronic SNP of *BCAS3*, was previously reported to have an association with SUA level at the genome-wide significance level; however, it was not replicated in the same report [5]. BCAS3 is a coactivator of estrogen receptor alpha (ER-α) and is overexpressed in breast cancer cells [15], in which it is associated with tumor grade and proliferation [16]. The influence of sex hormones on SUA level is well known [17]. Especially, estradiol is thought to affect SUA levels through mechanisms modulating renal urate reabsorption and

Table 1 Association analysis of three loci with 723 clinically-defined gout cases and 913 controls

Variant[a]	Gene	Chr.	Position[b]	A1/A2	Genotypes						Alleles frequency model			
					Cases			Controls			Frequency[c]		P value	OR (95% CI)
					A1/A1	A1/A2	A2/A2	A1/A1	A1/A2	A2/A2	Cases	Controls		
rs12236871	*RFX3*	9	3589117	A/G	166	354	172	259	412	239	0.504	0.489	0.390	1.06 (0.92–1.22)
rs179785[d]	*KCNQ1*	11	2781519	A/G	196	277	102	204	379	143	0.418	0.458	0.043	0.85 (0.73–0.99)
rs200562977	*KCNQ1*	11	2781508–2781519	GGCGGGCAGGCA/–	575	142	6	726	173	14	0.107	0.110	0.744	0.96 (0.77–1.20)
rs179784	*KCNQ1*	11	2781824	A/G	288	331	104	304	474	135	0.373	0.407	0.044	0.86 (0.75–1.00)
rs11653176	*BCAS3*	17	59447369	C/T	227	346	148	218	476	219	0.445	0.501	1.66×10^{-3}	0.80 (0.70–0.92)

Chr chromosome, *OR* odds ratio, *CI* confidence interval

[a] dbSNP rs number. The variants of *KCNQ1* were genotyped by direct sequencing because of the presence of common deletion variant (rs200562977), whereas the variants of *RFX3* and *BCAS3* were correctly genotyped by the TaqMan method. In the analysis of rs179785 of *KCNQ1*, 148 cases and 187 controls with a heterozygous or homozygous deletion variant of rs200562977 were excluded because rs179785 is located at the last nucleotide, "A", of rs200562977 (g.2781508_2781519del12GGCGGGCAGGCA). rs179784 of *KCNQ1* shows strong linkage disequilibrium with rs179785 (D' = 1.0 and r^2 = 0.99)

[b] The positions of variants are based on NCBI human genome reference sequence Build 37

[c] 'Frequency' means the frequency of A2

secretion. Increased SUA levels in postmenopausal women could be caused by the loss of estradiol. In addition, SUA levels decrease in postmenopausal patients using postmenopausal hormone compared with patients not using it [18]. Our findings suggest that risk allele (C) of rs11653176 of *BCAS3*, may increase renal urate reabsorption which results in increase of SUA levels and gout risk. Thus, although additional genetic and/or functional analyses will be necessary, the common variant of *BCAS3* might affect gout susceptibility in ways that are attributable to individual differences in responses to the effects of estrogen. Very recently, we have reported further GWAS of clinically-ascertained gout and identified 10 gout loci including *HIST1H2BF-HIST1H4E*, solute carrier family 17 member 1 (*SLC17A1*), solute carrier family 22 member 12 (*SLC22A12*), NIPA like domain containing 1 (*NIPAL1*) and family with sequence similarity 35 member A (*FAM35A*) [19]. Together with these gout loci, *BCAS3*, which is originally identified by the Chinese gout GWAS, will be very important for personalized genome medicine and/or prevention of gout.

Conclusions

In summary, our present replication study demonstrated, as did a previous gout GWAS [8], an association between gout and the common variant of *BCAS3*. These findings suggest that the *BCAS3* locus is likely to have a common pathophysiological risk for gout.

Abbreviations

ABCG2/BCRP: ATP-binding cassette transporter subfamily G member 2/breast cancer resistance protein; BCAS3: Breast carcinoma amplified sequence 3; ER-α: Estrogen receptor alpha; GLUT9/SLC2A9: Glucose transporter 9/solute carrier family 2 member 9; GWAS: Genome-wide association study; J-MICC Study: Japan Multi-Institutional Collaborative Cohort Study; JPT: Japanese in Tokyo; KCNQ1: Potassium voltage-gated channel subfamily Q member 1; LD: Linkage disequilibrium; OR: Odds ratio; RFX3: Regulatory factor X3; SNP: Single nucleotide polymorphisms; SUA: Serum uric acid

Acknowledgements

We would like to thank all the participants for their generous involvement in this study. We are especially indebted to K. Gotanda, Y. Morimoto, M. Miyazawa, S. Shimizu and T. Chiba for genetic analysis. We are indebted to A. Tokumasu, K. Ooyama, H. Tanaka, M. Naito and N. Hamajima for sample collection. We also thank H. Nakashima, T. Nakamura and K. Ichida for helpful discussions.

Funding

This study was supported by grants from the Ministry of Education, Culture, Sports, Science and Technology (MEXT) of Japan, including MEXT KAKENHI (Nos. 25293145, 17 K19863, 17 K19864 and 17H04128), the Ministry of Health, Labour and Welfare of Japan, the Ministry of Defense of Japan, the Kawano Masanori Memorial Foundation for Promotion of Pediatrics, and the Gout Research Foundation of Japan. The study was also supported by a JSPS KAKENHI Grant (No. 16H06277) and Grants-in-Aid for Scientific Research on Priority Areas (No. 17015018) and Innovative Areas (Nos. 221S0001, 221S0002) from the Japanese Ministry of Education, Culture, Sports, Science, and Technology.

Authors' contributions

MS, HM and HN conceived and designed this study. JU, TK, KW and HO collected samples and analyzed clinical data. MS, HM, MK, TH, AN, YK and AA performed genetic analysis. MS and HM performed statistical analyses. YS, KY and NS provided intellectual input and assisted with the preparation of the manuscript. MS and HM wrote the manuscript. MS and HM contributed equally to this work. All authors have read and approved the final version of the manuscript.

Competing interests

The authors declare that they have no competing interests.

Author details

[1]Department of Integrative Physiology and Bio-Nano Medicine, National Defense Medical College, 3-2 Namiki, Tokorozawa, Saitama 359-8513, Japan. [2]Department of Dermatology, National Defense Medical College, Tokorozawa, Japan. [3]Division of Human Genetics, Department of Integrated Genetics, National Institute of Genetics, Mishima, Japan. [4]Program in Radiological and Medical Laboratory Sciences, Pathophysiological Laboratory Sciences, Nagoya University Graduate School of Medicine, Nagoya, Japan. [5]Department of Preventive Medicine, Nagoya University Graduate School of Medicine, Nagoya, Japan. [6]Department of Preventive Medicine and Public Health, National Defense Medical College, Tokorozawa, Japan. [7]Department of Medical Chemistry, Kurume University School of Medicine, Kurume, Japan. [8]Ryougoku East Gate Clinic, Tokyo, Japan.

References

1. Matsuo H, Takada T, Ichida K, Nakayama A, Ikebuchi Y, Ito K, et al. Common defects of ABCG2, a high-capacity urate exporter, cause gout: a function-based genetic analysis in a Japanese population. Sci Transl Med. 2009;1:5ra11.
2. Woodward OM, Köttgen A, Coresh J, Boerwinkle E, Guggino WB, Köttgen M. Identification of a urate transporter, ABCG2, with a common functional polymorphism causing gout. Proc Natl Acad Sci U S A. 2009;106:10338–42.
3. Matsuo H, Ichida K, Takada T, Nakayama A, Nakashima H, Nakamura T, et al. Common dysfunctional variants in ABCG2 are a major cause of early-onset gout. Sci Rep. 2014;2013:3.
4. Sulem P, Gudbjartsson DF, Walters GB, Helgadottir HT, Helgason A, Gudjonsson SA, et al. Identification of low-frequency variants associated with gout and serum uric acid levels. Nat Genet. 2011;43:1127–30.
5. Köttgen A, Albrecht E, Teumer A, Vitart V, Krumsiek J, Hundertmark C, et al. Genome-wide association analyses identify 18 new loci associated with serum urate concentrations. Nat Genet. 2013;45:145–54.
6. Matsuo H, Yamamoto K, Nakaoka H, Nakayama A, Sakiyama M, Chiba T, et al. Genome-wide association study of clinically defined gout identifies multiple risk loci and its association with clinical subtypes. Ann Rheum Dis. 2016;75:652–9. (epub ahead of print, on Feb 2, 2015)
7. Sakiyama M, Matsuo H, Nakaoka H, Yamamoto K, Nakayama A, Nakamura T, et al. Identification of rs671, a common variant of ALDH2, as a gout susceptibility locus. Sci Rep. 2016;6:25360.
8. Li C, Li Z, Liu S, Wang C, Han L, Cui L, et al. Genome-wide association analysis identifies three new risk loci for gout arthritis in Han Chinese. Nat Commun. 2015;6:7041.
9. Wallace SL, Robinson H, Masi AT, Decker JL, McCarty DJ, Yu TF. Preliminary criteria for the classification of the acute arthritis of primary gout. Arthritis Rheum. 1977;20:895–900.
10. The guideline revising committee of Japanese Society of Gout and Nucleic Acid Metabolism in Guideline for the Management of Hyperuricemia and Gout. 2nd ed. Guideline for the Management of Hyperuricemia and Gout. Osaka: Medical Review; 2010.
11. Hamajima N, J-MICC Study Group. The Japan multi-institutional collaborative cohort study (J-MICC study) to detect gene-environment interactions for cancer. Asian Pac J Cancer Prev. 2007;8:317–23.
12. Sakiyama M, Matsuo H, Shimizu S, Chiba T, Nakayama A, Takada Y, et al. Common variant of leucine-rich repeat-containing 16A (LRRC16A) gene is associated with gout susceptibility. Hum Cell. 2014;27:1–4.
13. R Development Core Team, R. Foundation for Statistical Computing, Vienna 2014.

14. 1000 Genomes Project Consortium, Abecasis GR, Altshuler D, Auton A, Brooks LD, Durbin RM, et al. A map of human genome variation from population-scale sequencing. Nature. 2010;467:1061–73.
15. Barlund M, Monni O, Weaver JD, Kauraniemi P, Sauter G, Heiskanen M, et al. Cloning of BCAS3 (17q23) and BCAS4 (20q13) genes that undergo amplification, overexpression, and fusion in breast cancer. Genes Chromosomes Cancer. 2002;35:311–7.
16. Gururaj AE, Singh RR, Rayala SK, Holm C, den Hollander P, Zhang H, et al. MTA1, a transcriptional activator of breast cancer amplified sequence 3. Proc Natl Acad Sci U S A. 2006;103:6670–5.
17. Adamopoulos D, Vlassopoulos C, Seitanides B, Contoyiannis P, Vassilopoulos P. The relationship of sex steroids to uric acid levels in plasma and urine. Acta Endocrinol. 1977;85:198–208.
18. Hak AE, Choi HK. Menopause, postmenopausal hormone use and serum uric acid levels in US women–the third National Health and Nutrition Examination Survey. Arthritis Res Ther. 2008;10:R116.
19. Nakayama A, Nakaoka H, Yamamoto K, Sakiyama M, Shaukat A, Toyoda Y, et al. GWAS of clinically defined gout and subtypes identifies multiple susceptibility loci that include urate transporter genes. Ann Rheum Dis. 2017;76(5):869–77.

12

A variant in *KCNQ1* gene predicts metabolic syndrome among northern urban Han Chinese women

Yafei Liu[1,2†], Chunxia Wang[3†], Yafei Chen[4], Zhongshang Yuan[1], Tao Yu[1], Wenchao Zhang[2], Fang Tang[2], Jianhua Gu[1], Qinqin Xu[1], Xiaotong Chi[5], Lijie Ding[1], Fuzhong Xue[1*] and Chengqi Zhang[2*]

Abstract

Background: Previous studies have reported that the potassium voltage-gated channel subfamily Q member 1 (*KCNQ1*) gene is associated with diabetes in both European and Asian population. This study aims to find a predictable single nucleotide polymorphism (SNP) to predict the risk of metabolic syndrome (MetS) through investigating the association of SNP in *KCNQ1* gene with MetS in Han Chinese women of northern urban area.

Methods: Six SNPs were selected and genotyped in 1381 unrelated women aged 21 and above, who have had physical check-up in Shandong Provincial Qianfoshan Hospital. Cox proportional model was conducted to access the association between SNPs and MetS.

Results: Sixty one women developed MetS between 2010 and 2015 during the 3055 person-year of follow-up. The cumulative incidence density was 19.964/1000 person-year. The SNP rs163182 was associated with MetS both in the additive genetic model (*RR* = 1.658, *95% CI*: 1.144–2.402) and in the recessive genetic model (*RR* = 2.461, *95% CI*: 1.347–4.496). It remained significant after adjustment. This relationship was also observed in MetS components (BMI and SBP).

Conclusion: A novel association between rs163182 and MetS was found in this study, which can predict the occurrence of MetS among northern urban Han Chinese women. More investigations are needed to be done to assess the possible pathway in which *KCNQ1* gene affects MetS.

Keywords: Metabolic syndrome, *KCNQ1*, Single nucleotide polymorphism (SNP), Cohort study

Background

Metabolic Syndrome (MetS) is a complex disorder that is characterized by obesity, hyperglycemia, dyslipidemia, hypertension and insulin resistance [1]. It can increase the risk of type 2 diabetes and cardiovascular disease (CVD) [2]. In recent years, the prevalence of MetS is high (26.8% in females) in urban areas of China, and sex heterogeneity has been found in the relationships between risk factors and MetS [3]. Much research of Genome-Wide Association Studies (GWAS) and candidate gene studies have been conducted in Indian [4], Finnish [5], Chinese [6–9], Taiwanese and Caucasian youth [10]. However, these mechanisms were not consistent among the previous studies, and most of the studies were based on cross-sectional studies. Thus, this study aimed to investigate whether the selected SNPs would be associated with MetS in Chinese women based on a cohort study.

KCNQ1 is a gene that provides instructions for making potassium channels. The gene is expressed in a wild variety of tissues such as cardiac muscle, inner ear, kidney, lung, stomach, and intestine. Cardiac long QT syndrome and congenital deafness are associated with *KCNQ1* gene. However, *KCNQ1* is also expressed in pancreas, and it could influence the insulin secretion [11]. SNPs in *KCNQ1* are significantly associated with lower HOMA-B

* Correspondence: xuefzh@sdu.edu.cn; chengqizhangsd@126.com
†Yafei Liu and Chunxia Wang contributed equally to this work.
[1]Division of Biostatistics, School of Public Health, Shandong University, 44 Wenhua Xilu, Jinan 250010, Shandong, China
[2]Shandong Provincial Qianfoshan Hospital, Shandong University, 16766 Jingshi Rd, Jinan 250014, China
Full list of author information is available at the end of the article

values [12]. Most studies indicated that the *KCNQ1* gene was a diabetes susceptibility gene in different ancestors [13, 14]. Rs231359, rs2237895, rs2237897, rs2237892, and rs231361 polymorphisms were confirmed among Chinese [12, 15, 16]. Type 2 diabetes was the major consequence of MetS [17], and MetS might be an important risk factor for type 2 diabetes [18]. Meanwhile, insulin resistance is a central feature of MetS and the function of the polymorphisms in *KCNQ1* gene for MetS has not been investigated. Previous research had confirmed that both genetic and environmental factors contribute to the pathogenesis of MetS [1, 19]. Some studies only involved few factors such as smoking or drinking.

In this study, we established a cohort study with 1381 females based on the routine health check-up systems in the urban Han Chinese. We aimed to investigate the association among the selected SNPs in the *KCNQ1* gene with MetS in Chinese women after adjusting for potential confounding variables, as well as to provide a genetic basis to establish a prediction model of MetS for the personalized health management for women. Meanwhile, we also explored the relationship between SNP and MetS components.

Methods

Study subjects

This was a cohort study based on the Center for Health Management of Shandong Provincial Qianfoshan Hospital. The health examination database contained persons in Jinan, representing the middle to upper class population of Shandong Province [20, 21]. The participants had two or more records from 2010 to 2015. We selected by a simple random sampling from those who was free of MetS or cardiovascular disease on the first physical examination, and collected their blood samples from April to September 2016. A standardized questionnaire was used to investigate the environmental and dietary risk factors (Additional file 1). Their fasting blood samples were collected and stored in an ultra-low temperature freezer. A total of 1381 women (aged 21 to 81) were included. All individuals were Han Chinese and they were genetically unrelated to each other.

The study was approved by the Ethics Committee of School of Public Health, Shandong University (the number: 20120315). Written informed consent was obtained from all of the participants before the study.

Measurements

The questionnaire, anthropometric and fasting laboratory assay were conducted in each participant. Although there was a general questionnaire in the original cohort [22], the details of lifestyle factors in women were restricted. A detailed questionnaire was applied to these women, including basic demographic information (age, education and occupation), physiological condition (menarche, dysmenorrhea, menopause and reproductive system disease), marriage and pregnancy situation (marriage age, the number of births and abortions), lifestyles (taste preference, sleep, housework, smoking, second-hand smoking and drinking) and family medical history (diabetes, hypertension, obesity, hyperlipidemia and CVDs). Food Frequency Questionnaire (FFQ) was also conducted by asking dietary habits within one month. Some details of the questionnaire are shown in Additional file 2: Table S1.

The anthropometric measurements included weight, height and blood pressure. Weight and height were measured by standardized procedures. Body mass index (BMI) was calculated in accordance with weight/height^2 (kg/m^2). Blood pressure was measured on the right arm by an automated sphygmomanometer after 5-min rest. The biomarkers related to MetS, including systolic blood pressure (SBP), diastolic blood pressure (DBP), fasting plasma glucose (FPG), total cholesterol (TC), triglyceride (TG), low-density lipoprotein-cholesterol (LDL-C) and high-density lipoprotein cholesterol (HDL-C), were measured by the standard clinical and laboratory protocol in the Center for Health Management of Shandong Provincial Qianfoshan Hospital, which was described previously [23, 24].

Diagnosis of MetS

Considering the practical conditions of physical examination management in Shandong Province and the physiological characteristics of our study subjects, the diagnostic criterion adopted in this study is the one that is recommended by Diabetes Society of the Chinese Medical Association (CDS) [25]. MetS was defined as three or more of the following disorders: (1) overweight or obesity (BMI $\geq$ 25.0 kg/M^2); (2) hypertension (SBP $\geq$ 140 mmHg, DBP $\geq$ 90 mmHg or diagnosed before); (3) hyperglycemia (FPG $\geq$ 6.1 mmol/L or 2 h post-meal glucose $\geq$7.8 mmol/L, or diagnosed before); and (4) dyslipidemia (TG $\geq$ 1.7 mmol/L, or HDL $<$ 1.0 mmol/L in female).

SNP selection, genotyping and quality control analysis

We selected six SNPs (rs2237892, rs231361, rs2237895, rs231359, rs2237897 and rs163182) from the *KCNQ1* gene, which were reported to be associated with diabetes [15, 18, 26] . The minor allele frequency (MAF) of the above six SNPs was greater than 0.05 in the Chinese Han population from the NCBI dbSNPs database (http://www.ncbi.nlm.nih.gov/). DNA was extracted from venous blood samples, which were collected in the morning after 8 h of fasting, and then stored in an ultra-low temperature freezer. Genomic DNA extraction and genotyping were accomplished by the company, BioMiao Biological Technology (Beijing) Co., Ltd.

Statistical analyses

Taking missing values of clinical covariates into account, multiple imputations were performed using Amelia II by R3.3.2. All imputation variables had less than 10% missing observations before imputation.

The Hardy-Weinberg Equilibrium (HWE) of six SNPs was performed utilizing the Chi-squared test by R3.3.2. The linkage disequilibrium (LD) was performed by Haploview4.2. Markers of SNP were not included in the analysis, in the conditions that the call rate was less than 95%, and the *P* value from a test of HWE was less than 0.05.

Continuous variables were described with mean (standard deviation) and categorical variables were summarized as percentages. Differences in the baseline between MetS and non-MetS during the follow-up were compared using Student's *t*-test for continuous variables, and Chi-squared test for categorical variables. The Cox proportional hazards model was utilized to discover the association of SNPs in the additive model, dominant model and recessive model after adjusting for potential environmental confounding. The differences between SNPs and metabolic syndrome components were analyzed by the covariance analysis. Aiming to investigate whether SNPs could contribute to the efficiency of the prediction model, we compared the area under receiver operator characteristic curve (AUC) between with and without SNP. A two-tailed *P* value of less than 0.05 was regarded as statistically significant. These statistical analyses were performed using SAS version 9.4.

Results

Basic characteristics

This cohort ($n = 1381$) had a mean age of 39.5 at baseline. During the 3055 person-year of follow-up, 61 women developed MetS between 2010 and 2015. The cumulative incidence density was 19.964/1000 person-year. The baseline characteristics of metabolic syndrome components for participants are shown in Table 1. Cases had significantly higher BMI, SBP, DBP, FPG, TG, TC and LDL-C, but lower HDL-C than controls.

In this study, women rarely smoked or drank. Besides, secondhand smoking showed no statistical significance with MetS. Additional file 2: Table S1 shows the frequency and percentages of environmental variables of the study. Significant differences in marital status, education, sleep, housework time, trip mode, menopausal status, pregnancy information (the number of births and abortions), reproductive system disease, taste preference, intake of fruit and meat between cases and controls were found by simple Cox proportional model (Additional file 2: Table S2).

SNPs in KCNQ1 gene and MetS

Rs231361 was not in genotype quality or Hardy-Weinberg equilibrium ($P < 0.05$) (Additional file 2: Table S3). Hence, it was excluded. The genotype and allele distribution of the five SNPs are shown in Table 2. Only rs163182 showed a difference between MetS and non-MetS both in genotypes ($P = 0.016$) and in allele distribution ($P = 0.010$). We carried out LD mapping in Additional file 3: Figure S1. Rs231359 was isolated compared with the other SNPs ($r^2 = 0$). The r^2 of each pairwise LD among rs2237892, rs163182, rs2237895 and rs2237897 was modest ($0.10 < r^2 < 0.69$).

Table 3 shows the association analyses of the five SNPs with MetS by Cox proportional model. Single SNP analysis revealed that the rs163182 was associated with MetS in the additive genetic model (relative risk (*RR*) =1.658, *95% CI*: 1.144–2.402) and the recessive genetic model (*RR* = 2.461, *95% CI*: 1.347–4.496) (Table 3). Other SNPs suggested no association with MetS. After adjusting for age, the results showed that with the increase of the number of C alleles in rs163182 genotype, *RR* was 1.531 (*95%CI*: 1.064–2.204), and *RR* of CG + CC genotype vs GG was 2.086 (*95%CI*: 1.14–3.816). After adjusting for possible confounding factors (age, marital status, education, sleep, housework, trip mode, menopausal status, the number of births, the number of abortions, reproductive system disease, intake of fruit and fresh meat), the SNP remained significantly associated with MetS in the additive genetic model (*RR* = 1.776, *95% CI*: 1.166–2.704) and the recessive genetic model (*RR* = 2.976, *95% CI*: 1.488–5.951) (Table 3). Other four SNPs in the *KCNQ1* gene had no statistical significance in this study ($P > 0.05$).

Aiming to test and verify the effect of rs136182 on MetS prediction, we compared the performance on two prediction models of MetS using age, menopausal status, the number of births and the intake of fruit, with and without rs163182. The AUC for the prediction model with and without rs163182 was 0.743 (*95% CI*, 0.719–1.766) and 0.756 (*95% CI*, 0.732–0.779) respectively. To a certain extent, the efficiency was improved.

SNP rs163182 and metabolic syndrome components

The association between rs163182 and metabolic components was also explored (Table 4). The difference between SBP and the genotypes (GG, CG and CC) was analyzed under the covariance analysis after adjusting for age ($P = 0.043$). The differences of other biomarkers DBP, FPG, TG and HDL-C were not detected between each three genotypes. The differences between rs163182 genotype and BMI were conducted

Table 1 Baseline clinical characteristics of the women according to the MetS status

	MetS ($n = 61$)	Non-MetS ($n = 1320$)	*T* test	*P*
Age (year)	53.984 ± 12.027	38.812 ± 11.621	−9.950	< 0.001
BMI (kg/m2)	26.588 ± 3.136	22.079 ± 2.923	−11.740	< 0.001
SBP (mmHg)	134.180 ± 15.898	118.698 ± 14.650	−5.690	< 0.001
DBP (mmHg)	79.672 ± 9.916	72.471 ± 9.644	−8.040	< 0.001
FPG (mmol/L)	5.483 ± 0.811	4.997 ± 0.501	−4.640	< 0.001
TG (mmol/L)	1.525 ± 0.852	0.927 ± 0.498	−5.440	< 0.001
TC (mmol/L)	5.149 ± 0.803	4.634 ± 0.846	−4.660	< 0.001
LDL-C (mmol/L)	3.131 ± 0.657	2.633 ± 0.670	−5.680	< 0.001
HDL-C(mmol/L)	1.430 ± 0.292	1.600 ± 0.294	4.430	< 0.001

BMI indicted body mass index, *SBP* systolic blood pressure, *DBP* diastolic blood pressure, *FPG* fasting plasma glucose *TG* triglycerides, *TC* total cholesterol, *LDL-C* low-density lipoprotein-cholesterol, *HDL-C*, high-density lipoprotein-cholesterol

by non-parameters Wilcoxon symbols test, which suggested rs163182 was associated with BMI ($P = 0.032$).

Discussion

In this study, we discovered a novel association between *KCNQ1*-rs163182 and MetS, which suggests that rs163182 is an independent predictor for MetS. Meanwhile, rs163182 was also associated with MetS components (BMI and SBP) in Han Chinese women of northern urban area. Rs163182 may play a role in the biological metabolism.

In the current study, the etiology of MetS refers to environmental confounding factors, genetic susceptibility, as well as their interactions [27, 28]. Identifying genes had the following functions: dramatically improve understanding of the mechanisms of MetS [29], identify people at high risk, and prevent the development of diabetes and CVD. The relationships among SNPs, environmental factors and MetS had received considerable attention. In our study, we reviewed a large amount of literature about SNPs for MetS and its components (obesity, hyperglycemia, dyslipidemia, hypertension and insulin resistance). According to the preliminary study, rs163182, which carried C-allele in the *KCNQ1* gene, was more likely to develop MetS. In addition, it remained statistically significant after adjusting for potential risk factors. That indicates rs163182 in the *KCNQ1* gene is a novel independent predictor for MetS.

It has been confirmed that the *KCNQ1* gene was associated with diabetes in population of both Asian and European descent [13, 14, 30]. Meanwhile, there were few studies about rs163182 [15, 31]. In a genome-wide association study for type 2 diabetes in Han Chinese [15], it validated the association between rs163182 and diabetes ($OR = 1.28$), which was conducted in southern China. However, there was a heterogeneity compared with our study. In our study, the *KCNQ1* rs2237892, rs231361, rs2237895, rs231359, rs2237897, rs163182 and many environmental factors were surveyed. Although we did not find positive results of FPG, we discovered a novel association between rs163182 and MetS. In the study by Chen et al. [32], the *KCNQ1* gene was associated with lipid parameters, TG, HDL-C, and apo A1 in a middle-aged Chinese Han population. A possibility has been mentioned that *KCNQ1* may be a molecule affecting insulin sensitivity [33, 34]. The gene of *KCNQ1* not only plays an important role in blood glucose metabolism but also regulates other metabolic substances. The result that rs163182-C would increase the risk of MetS' occurrence was understood. On the other hand, referring to the causal inference [35], MetS was a risk factor for diabetes and the *KCNQ1* gene was associated with

Table 2 Distribution of genotype and allele of SNPs in the *KCNQ1* gene

SNP	Genotype	number of Genotype		P(G)[a]	Major/minor allele	number of allele		P (A)[b]
	0/1/2	MetS	Non-MetS			MetS	Non-MetS	
rs163182	GG/CG/CC	18/26/14	550/593/156	0.016	G/C	62/54	1693/905	0.010
rs231359	AA/CA/CC	40/18/2	814/445/50	0.782	A/C	98/22	2073/545	0.511
rs2237895	AA/CA/CC	23/32/6	609/570/130	0.361	A/C	78/44	1788/830	0.312
rs2237897	CC/CT/TT	23/29/9	561/592/159	0.685	C/T	75/47	1714/910	0.384
rs2237892	CC/CT/TT	25/32/4	619/564/130	0.308	C/T	82/40	1802/824	0.743

[a]The *P* value of Chi-square test for the genotype between MetS and non-MetS
[b]*P* value of Chi-square test for the allele of SNPs

Table 3 The association analyses of the five SNPs with MetS with Cox proportional model

SNP	*RR (95% CI)*	*P*	Adjusted R^a *(95% CI)*	Adjusted *P*	Adjusted RR^b *(95% CI)*	Adjusted *P*
rs163182						
GG/CG/CC[c]	1.658 (1.144–2.402)	0.008	1.531 (1.064–2.204)	0.022	1.776 (1.166–2.704)	0.007
CG + CC[d]	1.603 (0.919–2.797)	0.096	1.538 (0.881–2.685)	0.130	1.624 (0.878–3.003)	0.122
CC[e]	2.461 (1.347–4.496)	0.003	2.086 (1.14–3.816)	0.017	2.976 (1.488–5.951)	0.002
rs231359						
AA/CA/CC[c]	0.881 (0.553–1.406)	0.596	0.951 (0.596–1.516)	0.832	0.914 (0.551–1.515)	0.727
CA + CC[d]	0.862 (0.504–1.474)	0.586	0.94 (0.549–1.611)	0.823	0.959 (0.538–1.71)	0.887
CC[e]	0.874 (0.213–3.578)	0.851	0.959 (0.234–3.932)	0.954	0.503 (0.068–3.739)	0.502
rs2237895						
AA/CA/CC[c]	1.216 (0.838–1.763)	0.304	1.138 (0.777–1.665)	0.507	1.273 (0.836–1.939)	0.260
CA + CC[d]	1.428 (0.851–2.396)	0.178	1.266 (0.753–2.130)	0.374	1.475 (0.836–2.604)	0.180
CC[e]	0.999 (0.430–2.321)	0.998	0.986 (0.424–2.293)	0.974	1.082 (0.417–2.805)	0.871
rs2237897						
CC/CT/TT[c]	1.188 (0.828–1.705)	0.349	1.187 (0.835–1.687)	0.341	1.296 (0.876–1.915)	0.194
CT + TT[d]	1.267 (0.755–2.126)	0.371	1.341 (0.798–2.253)	0.267	1.383 (0.788–2.43)	0.259
TT[e]	1.235 (0.608–2.506)	0.559	1.123 (0.553–2.280)	0.747	1.46 (0.687–3.101)	0.325
rs2237892						
CC/CT/TT[c]	1.062 (0.728–1.550)	0.754	1.074 (0.739–1.563)	0.707	1.201 (0.792–1.82)	0.389
CT + TT[d]	1.277 (0.766–2.127)	0.348	1.319 (0.791–2.198)	0.289	1.435 (0.821–2.506)	0.205
TT[e]	0.636 (0.231–1.754)	0.382	0.619 (0.225–1.708)	0.355	0.849 (0.295–2.439)	0.761

[a]Adjusted for age
[b]Adjusted for age, marital status, education, sleep, housework, trip mode, menopausal status, the number of births, the number of abortions, reproductive system disease, intake of fruit and fresh meat
[c]Additive model
[d]Dominant model
[e]Recessive model

diabetes. Thus, the *KCNQ1* gene may influence the occurrence of MetS.

We also investigated the role of environmental variables to MetS. Widow or divorce, more housework, peri-menopause or menopause, multiple pregnancies (including birth and abortion), and reproductive system disease would increase the risk of MetS ($RR > 1.0$), while highly-educated people, normal diet (means the taste preference is reasonable), and more fruit or meat would reduce the onset of MetS. That suggested the lifestyle or the information of fertility may influence the MetS, which was consistent with previous studies [36, 37]. We also explored the interactions between rs163182 and these factors, of which the results were negative. That indicates the interactions between rs163182 and environmental factors to MetS are a minor effect.

Table 4 Comparison of metabolic syndrome components between different groups of rs163182 genotypes

	rs163182			P^a	P^b
	GG (*n* = 568)	CG (*n* = 619)	CC (*n* = 170)		
SBP	119.083 ± 14.853	118.877 ± 14.580	122.671 ± 16.859	0.043	0.138
DBP	72.541 ± 9.690	72.673 ± 9.654	74.073 ± 10.500	0.378	0.414
FPG	5.008 ± 0.531	5.003 ± 0.494	5.090 ± 0.602	0.323	0.508
TG	0.927 ± 0.495	0.951 ± 0.526	0.999 ± 0.493	0.433	0.854
HDL-C	1.600 ± 0.297	1.596 ± 0.299	1.564 ± 0.281	0.341	0.753
BMI	22.135 ± 2.871	22.237 ± 3.104	22.899 ± 3.502	0.032[c]	0.020

BMI indicted body mass index, *SBP* systolic blood pressure, *DBP* diastolic blood pressure, *FPG* fasting plasma glucose, *TG* triglycerides, *TC* total cholesterol, *LDL-C* low-density lipoprotein-cholesterol, *HDL-C* high-density lipoprotein-cholesterol
[a]The *P* value of covariance analysis after adjusting for age
[b]The *P* value of the homogeneity test
[c]The *P* value of non-parameters Wilcoxon symbols test for BMI

Aiming to evaluate the prediction effect of rs163182, we calculated AUC with and without rs163182. The result reveals the *KCNQ1* gene may provide a new method for modeling a risk prediction for MetS, which can use rs163182 to achieve the personalized health management in Han Chinese women of northern urban area.

The association between rs163182 and MetS components was also researched. The statistical significance was found among BMI and SBP in rs163182 genotype. The study of Sinha et al. [38] used *KCNQ1* to exhibit both differential methylation and differential gene expression by comparing adipocytes between obese and never-obese women. The *KCNQ1* plays roles in cardiac tissue. Mutations in this gene may impair the function of heart. However, the specific mechanisms need to be further validated.

Considering the survival data in this study, Cox proportional model was applied. To our knowledge, few investigations were conducted by cohort study using Cox proportional model [39] adjusting for other potential variables.

The study also has several limitations. Firstly, the participants comprised only women who came to the Center for Health Management of Shandong Provincial Qianfoshan Hospital, and might not represent the general population. In some way, it could restrict female to avoid gender confounding. Secondly, the time of follow-up in this study was not long enough, that result in the limited number of cases. So this study will be followed up continuously in the future. Thirdly, because of the large population in the Center for Health Management, the subjects were selected simply and randomly based on the database that may be a limitation in some way. In the follow-up study, a more sophisticated strategy could be employed to verify the result, such as a nest case-control study.

Conclusions

It was the first time to discover that rs163182 in *KCNQ1* gene would raise the risk of MetS and elevate the level of BMI and SBP. It partly explains the mechanism of MetS and may provide a new comprehension of molecular mechanism. Of course, further research is needed to evaluate the genetic marker in different populations.

Abbreviations

AUC: Area under receiver operator characteristic curve; BMI: Body mass index; CI: Confidence interval; CVD: Cardiovascular disease; DBP: Diastolic blood pressure; FPG: Fasting plasma glucose; GWAS: Genome Wide Association Study; HDL-C: High-density lipoprotein-cholesterol; HWE: Hardy-Weinberg Equilibrium; KCNQ1: potassium voltage-gated channel subfamily Q member 1; LDL-C: low-density lipoprotein-cholesterol; MAF: Minor allele frequency; MetS: Metabolic syndrome; RR: Relative risk; SBP: Systolic blood pressure; SNP: Single nucleotide polymorphisms; TC: Total cholesterol; TG: Triglycerides

Acknowledgments

The authors wish to acknowledge their colleagues for invaluable work and the participants of the Center for Health Management of Shandong Provincial Qianfoshan Hospital.

Funding

The study was funded by National Natural Science Foundation of China (No.81273082), Taishan industrial expert program (No.tscy20150403) and Project of Priority Research from Department of Science and Technology of Shandong Province (Grant No. 2016GSF201075). The funding agencies were not involved in study design, analysis and interpretation.

Authors' contributions

YL, CW, YC, FX and CZ participated in study conception and design; TY and JG made substaintial contributions to design; YL, CW, YC, TY, JG, XC and LD participated in the collection and cleaning of data; YL, ZY, WZ, FT, QX and XC performed the statistical analyses; YL and CW wrote the manuscript. YC and LD revised the manuscript critically for important intellectual content; FX and CZ contributed to the interpretation of the results and revised the manuscript critically. All authors approved the final version of the manuscript.

Competing interests

The authors declare that they have no competing interests.

Author details

[1]Division of Biostatistics, School of Public Health, Shandong University, 44 Wenhua Xilu, Jinan 250010, Shandong, China. [2]Shandong Provincial Qianfoshan Hospital, Shandong University, 16766 Jingshi Rd, Jinan 250014, China. [3]Jinan Kingmed Center for Clinical Laboratory Co, Ltd., 554 Zhengfeng Rd, Jinan 250010, Shandong, China. [4]Linyi Centre for Adverse Drug Reaction Monitoring, Linyi 276000, Shandong, China. [5]Department of Imaging and Nuclear Medicine, Taishan Medical University, 619 Changcheng Rd, Tai'an 271016, Shandong, China.

References

1. Lusis AJ, Attie AD, Reue K. Metabolic syndrome: from epidemiology to systems biology. Nat Rev Genet. 2008;9(11):819–30. https://doi.org/10.1038/nrg2468.
2. Kaur J. A comprehensive review on metabolic syndrome. Cardiol Res Pract. 2014; https://doi.org/10.1155/2014/943162.
3. Song Q-B, Zhao Y, Liu Y-Q, Zhang J, Xin S-J, Dong G-H. Sex difference in the prevalence of metabolic syndrome and cardiovascular-related risk factors in urban adults from 33 communities of China: the CHPSNE study. Diabetes Vasc Dis Res. 2015;12(3):189–98. https://doi.org/10.1177/1479164114562410.
4. Zabaneh D, Balding DJ. A genome-wide association study of the metabolic syndrome in Indian Asian men. PLoS One. 2010;5(8):1–6. https://doi.org/10.1371/journal.pone.0011961.
5. Kristiansson K, Perola M, Tikkanen E, Kettunen J, Surakka I, Havulinna A, Stancáková A, Barnes C, Widen E, Kajantie E, et al. Genome-wide screen for metabolic syndrome susceptibility loci reveals strong lipid gene contribution but no evidence for common genetic basis for clustering of metabolic syndrome traits. Circ Cardiovasc Genet. 2012;5:242–9. https://doi.org/10.1161/CIRCGENETICS.111.961482.
6. Wang T, Huang Y, Xiao XH, Wang DM, Diao CM, Zhang F, Xu LL, Zhang YB, Li WH, Zhang LL, et al. The association between common genetic variation in the FTO gene and metabolic syndrome in Han Chinese. Chin Med J. 2010;123:1852–8. https://doi.org/10.3760/cma.j.issn.0366-6999.2010.14.005.
7. Yang J, Liu J, Jing L, Li W, Li X, He Y, Ye L. Genetic association study with metabolic syndrome and metabolic-related traits in a cross-sectional sample and a 10-year longitudinal sample of chinese elderly population. PLoS One. 2014;9:e100548.
8. Yan YX, Dong J, Zhang J, Liu F, Wang W, Zhang L, He Y. Polymorphisms in NR3C1 gene associated with risk of metabolic syndrome in a Chinese population. Endocrine. 2014;47:740–8.
9. Ong KL, Jiang CQ, Liu B, Jin Y, Tso A, Tam S, Wong K, Tomlinson B, Cheung B, Lin J. Association of a genetic variant in the apolipoprotein A5 gene with the metabolic syndrome in Chinese. Clin Endocrinol. 2011;74:206–13. https://doi.org/10.1111/j.1365-2265.2010.03899.x

10. Liu PH, Chang YC, Der Jiang Y, Chen W, Chang T, Kuo S, Lee K, Hsiao P, Chiu K, Chuang L. Genetic variants of TCF7L2 are associated with insulin resistance and related metabolic phenotypes in Taiwanese adolescents and Caucasian young adults. J Clin Endocrinol Metab. 2009;94:3575–82. https://doi.org/10.1210/jc.2009-0609.
11. Yamagata K, Senokuchi T, Lu M, Takemoto M, Fazlul Karim M, Go C, Sato Y, Hatta M, Yoshizawa T, Araki E, et al. Voltage-gated K+channel KCNQ1 regulates insulin secretion in MIN6 β-cell line. Biochem Biophys Res Commun. 2011;407:620–5. https://doi.org/10.1016/j.bbrc.2011.03.083.
12. Qi Q, Li H, Loos RJF, Liu C, Wu Y, Hu F, Wu H, Lu L, Yu Z, Lin X. Common variants in KCNQ1 are associated with type 2 diabetes and impaired fasting glucose in a Chinese Han population. Hum Mol Genet. 2009;18:3508–15. https://doi.org/10.1093/hmg/ddp294.
13. Yasuda K, Miyake K, Horikawa Y, Hara K, Osawa H, Furuta H, Hirota Y, Mori H, Jonsson A, Sato Y, et al. Variants in KCNQ1 are associated with susceptibility to type 2 diabetes mellitus. Nat Genet. 2008;40:1092–7. https://doi.org/10.1038/ng.207.
14. Unoki H, Takahashi A, Kawaguchi T, Hara K, Horikoshi M, Andersen G, Ng D, Holmkvist J, Borch-Johnsen K, Jørgensen T, et al. SNPs in KCNQ1 are associated with susceptibility to type 2 diabetes in east Asian and European populations. Nat Genet. 2008;40:1098–102.
15. Li X, Wei D, He H, Zhang J, Wang C, Ma M, Wang B, Yu T, Pan L, Xue F, et al. Association of the adiponectin gene (ADIPOQ) +45 T > G polymorphism with the metabolic syndrome among Han Chinese in Sichuan province of China. Asia Pac J Clin Nutr. 2012;21:296–301.
16. Tsai F, Yang C, Chen C, Chuang L, Lu C, Chang C, Wang T, Chen R, Shiu C, Liu Y, et al. A genome-wide association study identifies susceptibility variants for type 2 diabetes in Han Chinese. PLoS Genet. 2010;6:e1000847. https://doi.org/10.1371/journal.pgen.1000847.
17. Ford ES. Risks for all-cause mortality, cardiovascular disease, and diabetes associated with the metabolic syndrome: a summary of the evidence. Diabetes Care. 2005;28:1769–78. https://doi.org/10.2337/diacare.28.7.1769.
18. Shin JA, Lee JH, Lim SY, Ha HS, Kwon HS, Park YM, Lee WC, Kang MI, Yim HW, Yoon KH, Son HY. Metabolic syndrome as a predictor of type 2 diabetes, and its clinical interpretations and usefulness. J Diabetes Investig. 2013;4:334–43. https://doi.org/10.1111/jdi.12075.
19. Roche HM, Phillips C, Gibney MJ. The metabolic syndrome: the crossroads of diet and genetics. Proc Nutr Soc. 2005;64:371–7. https://doi.org/10.1079/PNS2005445.
20. Zhang W, Chen Q, Yuan Z, Liu J, Du Z, Tang F, Jia H, Xue F, Zhang C. A routine biomarker-based risk prediction model for metabolic syndrome in urban Han Chinese population. BMC Public Health. 2015;15:64. https://doi.org/10.1186/s12889-015-1424-z.
21. Chen Y, Wang C, Liu Y, Yuan Z, Zhang W, Li X, Yang Y, Sun X, Xue F, Zhang C. Incident hypertension and its prediction model in a prospective northern urban Han Chinese cohort study. J Hum Hypertens. 2016:1–7. https://doi.org/10.1038/jhh.2016.23.
22. Ding L, Zhang C, Zhang G, Zhang T, Zhao M, Ji X, Yuan Z, Liu R, Tang F, Xue F. A new insight into the role of plasma fibrinogen in the development of metabolic syndrome from a prospective cohort study in urban Han Chinese population. Diabetol Metab Syndr. 2015;7:110. https://doi.org/10.1186/s13098-015-0103-7.
23. Wu S, Lin H, Zhang C, Zhang Q, Zhang D, Zhang Y, Meng W, Zhu Z, Tang F, Xue F, Liu Y. Association between erythrocyte parameters and metabolic syndrome in urban Han Chinese: a longitudinal cohort study. BMC Public Health. 2013;13:989. https://doi.org/10.1186/1471-2458-13-989.
24. Zhu Z, Liu Y, Zhang C, Yuan Z, Zhang Q, Tang F, Lin H, Zhang Y, Liu L, Xue F. Identification of cardiovascular risk components in urban Chinese with metabolic syndrome and application to coronary heart disease prediction: a longitudinal study. PLoS One. 2013;8:1–10. https://doi.org/10.1371/journal.pone.0084204.
25. Lu YH, Lu JM, Wang SY, Li CL, Liu LS, Zheng RP, Tian H, Wang XL, Yang LJ, Zhang YQ, Pan CY. Comparison of the diagnostic criteria of metabolic syndrome by international diabetes federation and that by Chinese Medical Association diabetes branch. National Medical Journal of China. 2006;86:386–9.
26. Wen W, Zheng W, Okada Y, Takeuchi F, Tabara Y, Hwang J, Dorajoo R, Li H, Tsai F, Yang X, et al. Meta-analysis of genome-wide association studies in east Asian-ancestry populations identifies four new loci for body mass index. Hum Mol Genet. 2014;23:5492–504. https://doi.org/10.1093/hmg/ddu248.
27. Wu Y, Yu Y, Zhao T, Fu Y, Qi Y, Yang G, Yao W, Su Y, Ma Y, Shi J, Jiang J, Kou C. Interactions of environmental factors and APOA1-APOC3-APOA4-APOA5 gene cluster gene polymorphisms with metabolic syndrome. PLoS One. 2016;11(1):e0147946. https://doi.org/10.1371/journal.pone.0147946.
28. Shen J, Arnett DK, Peacock JM, Parnell LD, Kraja A, Hixson JE, Tsai MY, Lai CQ, Kabagambe EK, Straka RJ, Ordovas JM. Interleukin1beta genetic polymorphisms interact with polyunsaturated fatty acids to modulate risk of the metabolic syndrome. J Nutr. 2007;137:1846.
29. Pollex RL, Hegele RA. Genetic determinants of the metabolic syndrome. Nat Clin Pr Cardiovasc Med. 2006;3:482–9. https://doi.org/10.1038/ncpcardio0638
30. Gao K, Wang J, Li L, Zhai Y, Ren Y, You H, Wang B, Wu X, Li J, Liu Z, Li X, Huang Y, Luo XP, Hu D, Ohno K, Wang C. Polymorphisms in four genes (KCNQ1 rs151290, KLF14 rs972283, GCKR rs780094 and MTNR1B rs10830963) and their correlation with type 2 diabetes mellitus in han Chinese in Henan province, China. Int J Environ Res Public Health. 2016;13:1–13. https://doi.org/10.3390/ijerph13030260.
31. Bai H, Liu H, Suyalatu S, Guo X, Chu S, Chen Y, Lan T, Borjigin B, Orlov Y, Posukh O, Yang X, Guilan G, Osipova L, Wu Q, Narisu N. Association analysis of genetic variants with type 2 diabetes in a Mongolian population in China. J Diabetes Res. 2015; https://doi.org/10.1155/2015/613236.
32. Chen Z, Yin Q, Ma G, Qian Q. KCNQ1 gene polymorphisms are associated with lipid parameters in a Chinese Han population. Cardiovasc Diabetol. 2010;9:35. https://doi.org/10.1186/1475-2840-9-35.
33. Boini KM, Graf D, Hennige AM, Koka S, Kempe D, Wang K, Ackermann T, Föller M, Vallon V, Pfeifer K, et al. Enhanced insulin sensitivity of gene-targeted mice lacking functional KCNQ1. Am J Physiol Regul Integr Comp Physiol. 2009;296:R1695–701. https://doi.org/10.1152/ajpregu.90839.2008.
34. Müssig K, Staiger H, Machicao F, Kirchhoff K, Guthoff M, Schäfer S, Kantartzis K, Silbernagel G, Stefan N, Holst J, et al. Association of type 2 diabetes candidate polymorphisms in KCNQ1 with incretin and insulin secretion. Diabetes. 2009;58:1715–20. https://doi.org/10.2337/db08-1589.
35. Pearl J. Causal inference in statistics: an overview. Stat Surv. 2009;3:96–146. https://doi.org/10.1214/09-SS057.
36. Yoo S, Nicklas T, Baranowski T, Zakeri I, Yang S, Srinivasan S, Berenson G. Comparison of dietary intakes associated with metabolic syndrome risk factors in young adults : the Bogalusa heart study. Am J Clin Nutr. 2004;80:841–8.
37. Zuo H, Shi Z, Hu X, Wu M, Guo Z, Hussain A. Prevalence of metabolic syndrome and factors associated with its components in Chinese adults. Metabolism. 2009;58:1102–8. https://doi.org/10.1016/j.metabol.2009.04.008.
38. Arner P, Sinha I, Thorell A, Rydén M, Dahlman-Wright K, Dahlman I. The epigenetic signature of subcutaneous fat cells is linked to altered expression of genes implicated in lipid metabolism in obese women. Clin Epigenetics. 2015;7:1–13. https://doi.org/10.1186/s13148-015-0126-9.
39. Therneau T, Grambsch P. Modeling survival data: extending the cox model. Technometrics. 2002;44:85–6. https://doi.org/10.1198/tech.2002.s656.

13

Genome-wide association study of nocturnal blood pressure dipping in hypertensive patients

Jenni M. Rimpelä[1], Ilkka H. Pörsti[2], Antti Jula[3], Terho Lehtimäki[4], Teemu J. Niiranen[3,5], Lasse Oikarinen[6], Kimmo Porthan[6], Antti Tikkakoski[2], Juha Virolainen[6], Kimmo K. Kontula[1] and Timo P. Hiltunen[1*]

Abstract

Background: Reduced nocturnal fall (non-dipping) of blood pressure (BP) is a predictor of cardiovascular target organ damage. No genome-wide association studies (GWAS) on BP dipping have been previously reported.

Methods: To study genetic variation affecting BP dipping, we conducted a GWAS in Genetics of Drug Responsiveness in Essential Hypertension (GENRES) cohort ($n = 204$) using the mean night-to-day BP ratio from up to four ambulatory BP recordings conducted on placebo. Associations with $P < 1 \times 10^{-5}$ were further tested in two independent cohorts: Haemodynamics in Primary and Secondary Hypertension (DYNAMIC) ($n = 183$) and Dietary, Lifestyle and Genetic determinants of Obesity and Metabolic Syndrome (DILGOM) ($n = 180$). We also tested the genome-wide significant single nucleotide polymorphism (SNP) for association with left ventricular hypertrophy in GENRES.

Results: In GENRES GWAS, rs4905794 near *BCL11B* achieved genome-wide significance ($\beta = -4.8\%$, $P = 9.6 \times 10^{-9}$ for systolic and $\beta = -4.3\%$, $P = 2.2 \times 10^{-6}$ for diastolic night-to-day BP ratio). Seven additional SNPs in five loci had P values $< 1 \times 10^{-5}$. The association of rs4905794 did not significantly replicate, even though in DYNAMIC the effect was in the same direction ($\beta = -0.8\%$, $P = 0.4$ for systolic and $\beta = -1.6\%$, $P = 0.13$ for diastolic night-to-day BP ratio). In GENRES, the associations remained significant even during administration of four different antihypertensive drugs. In separate analysis in GENRES, rs4905794 was associated with echocardiographic left ventricular mass ($\beta = -7.6$ g/m^2, $P = 0.02$).

Conclusions: rs4905794 near *BCL11B* showed evidence for association with nocturnal BP dipping. It also associated with left ventricular mass in GENRES. Combined with earlier data, our results provide support to the idea that *BCL11B* could play a role in cardiovascular pathophysiology.

Keywords: Blood pressure dipping, Genome-wide, Circadian gene, BCL11B, ERAP2, Left ventricular hypertrophy

Background

Blood pressure (BP) follows a diurnal pattern and is generally lower at night than during the day, defined as BP dipping [1]. Attenuated nocturnal BP dipping has been associated with cardiovascular target organ damage and increased risk for cardiovascular events [2, 3]. Recent meta-analysis, examining the prognostic significance of nocturnal systolic BP fall in 17,312 hypertensives from three continents, demonstrated that blunted nighttime BP dipping in untreated hypertensive subjects predicted significantly a variety of cardiovascular end points, including coronary events, strokes, cardiovascular deaths and total deaths [4]. This risk increase was found to be independent of ambulatory 24-h BP levels [4]. In fact, international guidelines for hypertension recommend routine use of 24-h ambulatory BP measurement (ABPM) to assess the nighttime BP and BP dipping [5]. However, the cause of variation in BP dipping is not well established. Better understanding of the phenomenon could help identifying those with increased risk for cardiovascular morbidity and mortality.

Large scale genome-wide association studies (GWAS) have identified several susceptibility loci for elevated BP, which together explain only a few percent of the trait

* Correspondence: timo.hiltunen@hus.fi
[1]Department of Medicine, University of Helsinki and Helsinki University Hospital, 00290 Helsinki, Finland
Full list of author information is available at the end of the article

variance suggesting that many causal loci remain unidentified (for review, see [6]). It is thought that improving accuracy of BP measurements as well as introducing new phenotypic parameters that better correlate to cardiovascular risk could lead to discovery of new genetic loci [6]. Like BP levels, the BP dipping status may be partly inherited; Wang et al. [7] reported that 59% of the heritability in systolic BP (SBP) dipping and 81% of the heritability in diastolic BP (DBP) dipping were due to genetic influence, arousing interest to find the genes that affect BP dipping.

In animal studies, mutation or deletion of core circadian genes operating the internal clock resulted in disruption of the circadian variation of BP [8, 9]. This hypothesis was tested in two candidate gene studies on Taiwanese [10] and Chinese [11] populations that reported suggestive associations between certain circadian gene polymorphisms and BP dipping encouraging further research for their role. A different approach was taken by Wirtwein et al., who recently found that five risk loci for coronary artery disease (CAD), derived from GWASs, were also associated with non-dipping status in patients with CAD [12]. However, no GWASs on BP dipping have been before reported.

We have previously conducted a GWAS on antihypertensive drug responsiveness in the Genetics of Drug Responsiveness in Essential Hypertension (GENRES) study [13], with replication of the data in Finnish participants of the Losartan Intervention for Endpoint Reduction in Hypertension (LIFE) study [14]. A special feature of the GENRES study was the inclusion of four 4-week drug-free placebo periods in its design [15], generating a most useful opportunity to obtain repeated ABPMs and nocturnal BP dipping measurements for every participant. Here we report our GWAS study on BP dipping, mostly based on the GENRES study, but also containing replication data from Finnish patients of two other studies: Haemodynamics in Primary and Secondary Hypertension (DYNAMIC) [16, 17] and Dietary, Lifestyle and Genetic determinants of Obesity and Metabolic Syndrome (DILGOM) [18].

Methods

Discovery cohort – The GENRES platform

Rationale and results of the GENRES study (clinicaltrials.gov NCT03276598, registered retrospectively) have been previously published elsewhere [13–15]. In brief, GENRES is a double-blind, randomized, placebo-controlled cross-over study that was designed to search for genetic variation predicting response to four classes of antihypertensive drugs, conducted at Helsinki University Hospital between years 1999 and 2004 (Additional file 1: Figure S1). Initially, a total of 313 Finnish men (aged 35 to 60 years) with moderate hypertension (DBP ≥ 95 mmHg or previous use of antihypertensive medication) were screened for the study. Secondary hypertension, drug-treated diabetes mellitus, congestive heart failure and CAD were among the exclusion criteria. The study participants underwent 4 different one-month single-drug treatment periods (losartan 50 mg, amlodipine 5 mg, hydrochlorothiazide 25 mg, and bisoprolol 5 mg daily) separated by one-month placebo periods. Twenty-four-hour ABPM was carried out at the end of each drug and placebo period using a device equipped with a position sensor (Diasys Integra; Novacor, Rueil-Malmaison, France). Each subject gave written informed consent and the study was approved by the Ethics Committee of Helsinki University Central Hospital and National Agency of Medicines of Finland.

For the discovery GWAS, we used the ABPMs recorded at the end of each placebo period. BP readings were taken every 15 min when standing and every 30 min when supine. Intense physical activity was not permitted. Daytime was defined as hours between 7 am and 10 pm. Single observations were excluded from the analysis due to low pulse pressure (< 15 mmHg if SBP < 120 mmHg and < 20 mmHg if SBP > 120 mmHg), high heart rates (≥ 110 bpm), lying down during daytime, standing up or being awake at nighttime or high physical activity. For a recording to be accepted, > 15 daytime and > 7 nighttime measurements were required. The mean SBP and DBP dipping of all placebo periods were used as the study variables. A total of 235 unrelated subjects were successfully genotyped and had ABPM data from at least one placebo period. To reduce the effect of day-to-day variation in the dipping phenotype, only the 204 subjects that had ≥3 accepted placebo ABPMs available (173 subjects with four and 31 subjects with three ABPMs) were included in the discovery GWAS.

Replication cohorts

DYNAMIC (clinicaltrials.gov NCT01742702) is an on-going study to investigate hemodynamic changes in primary and secondary hypertension with non-invasive hemodynamic measurement [16, 17]. A total 188 subjects with ABPM dipping available were genotyped. One subject was excluded due to low success rates of genotyping, one subject was excluded due to morbid obesity (body mass index (BMI) > 40) and 3 subjects were excluded due to first degree relativeness; ultimately, 183 subjects were included in this replication cohort. BP was measured with Microlife WatchBP O3 monitor (Microlife AG, Widnau, Switzerland) every 20 min during the day (7 am to 10 pm) and every 30 min during the night (10 pm to 7 am). Single observations were excluded using the same criteria as described for GENRES. Each subject gave written informed consent and the study was approved by the Ethics Committee of Tampere University Hospital.

DILGOM was a population survey conducted in 2007 to assess the effects of environment and genetics on obesity and metabolic syndrome. Four hundred and ninety-four subjects of DILGOM participated in a cardiovascular substudy. In 2014, 290 still living participants of the cardiovascular substudy underwent re-examination including a 24-h ABPM to compare novel and traditional BP measurement methods [18]. Both BP dipping and genetic data were available for 207 unrelated subjects. Four subjects that were morbidly obese (BMI > 40) and 23 subjects that were over the age of 75 were excluded, resulting in 180 subjects to be included in the replication cohort. BP was measured with a Microlife WatchBP O3 monitor (Microlife AG, Widnau, Switzerland) every 20 min during the day (7 am to 10 pm) and every 30 min during the night (10 pm to 7 am). Night-time BP was defined as the mean of all BP values of the actual sleeping period and daytime BP as the mean of all other BP values. Each subject gave written informed consent and the study was approved by the Ethics Committee of the Hospital District of Southwest Finland.

Genotyping methods

The genotyping methods and quality control steps (including exclusions for identity-by-state clustering, gender check, Hardy-Weinberg equilibrium P value $< 1 \times 10^{-5}$ and minor allele frequency < 0.01) for GENRES have been described in detail before [13]. The DNA samples of the GENRES study subjects were genotyped at the Institute for Molecular Medicine Finland (Helsinki, Finland) using the Illumina HumanOmniExpress BeadChip (Illumina, San Diego, CA, USA). After quality control steps a total of 631,844 autosomal SNPs were available for the analysis. Subsequent imputation was performed using IMPUTE2 [19] and the Hapmap2 CEU release 22 reference panel after pre-phasing with ShapeITv2. However, only the genotyped SNPs were used for the GWAS analysis.

The DNA samples of the DYNAMIC study subjects were genotyped at the Institute for Molecular Medicine Finland (Helsinki, Finland) using the Illumina HumanOmniExpress BeadChip (Illumina, San Diego, CA, USA). One subject was excluded due to low success rate (< 95%). The six SNPs used for replication passed the same quality control steps as described for GENRES above.

The genotype data of the DILGOM study subjects was derived from previously conducted GWASs. The DILGOM DNA samples were genotyped with Illumina Cardio-MetaboChip and Illumina 610 K arrays (Illumina, San Diego, CA, USA) at the Wellcome Trust Sanger Institute (Cambridge, UK) and the Institute for Molecular Medicine Finland (Helsinki, Finland). Unobserved SNPs were imputed using 1000 Genomes haplotypes Phase I integrated variant set release (ShapeITv2) in NCBI build 37 version June 2014. If the selected SNP was not genotyped, then the imputed value was used. Info scores for the imputed SNPs used were 0.989 for rs16984571 and 0.998 for rs1230361.

Left ventricular hypertrophy in GENRES

Left ventricular hypertrophy (LVH) was assessed in GENRES from the transthoracic echocardiograms recorded during the first placebo period and from electrocardiograms (ECGs) recorded at the end of each placebo period [20]. Echocardiographically determined left ventricular mass (LVM, in grams) was calculated as $0.8 \times [1.04 \times$ ((interventricular septal thickness + left ventricular end-diastolic diameter + posterior wall thickness)^3 − left ventricular end diastolic diameter^3)] + 0.6 and left ventricle mass index (LVMI) by dividing LVM by body surface area (square meters). LVMI was available for 227 GENRES subjects that were successfully genotyped for rs4905794. The standard resting 12-lead ECG was recorded with Marquette MAC 5000 electrocardiograph (GE Marquette Medical Systems, Milwaukee, Wisconsin, USA) at the end of each placebo period and all measurements were performed blinded to all other data. Sokolow-Lyon voltage (SV1 + RV5 or SV1 + RV6, whichever was greater) and Cornell voltage-duration product [(SV3 + RaVL) × QRS duration] were used as markers of LVH. The indices were calculated from digital ECGs from automatically made ECG measurements with a visual confirmation for all subjects who had completed the whole study. Mean values of all placebo periods were used. A total of 185 subjects, that were successfully genotyped for rs4905794, had these ECG measurements available.

Statistical analysis

Baseline demographics and BP dipping data of all study subjects were analyzed using IBM SPSS Statistics 22.0 (IBM Corp., Armonk, NY, USA). SBP and DBP dipping were analyzed separately as continuous variables, and were calculated as night-to-day BP ratio [3] and expressed as percentage [(mean nighttime BP / mean daytime BP) × 100]. Both variables were adjusted for corresponding daytime BP using linear regression. Lifestyle factors (age, BMI, waist-hip ratio, antihypertensive use before entry to the study, duration of hypertension, smoking, serum creatinine level and daily urinary excretion of sodium after the first placebo period were tested for association with stepwise linear regression and included as covariates if P value for association was < 0.10 for either systolic or diastolic night-to-day BP ratio. The final regression models are presented in Additional file 2: Table S1. These regression variables were approximately normally distributed. The effect of population stratification on night-to-day BP ratio was tested with principal components (PCs) generated with program Smartpca from Eigensoft package [21]. A reduced dataset of 114,487 SNPs with $r^2 < 0.5$ and the long-range linkage disequilibrium (LD) regions excluded [22] was used. Three significant PCs for population stratification with P values < 0.10 were identified with program Twstats from Eigensoft package, but they were not associated with either systolic or diastolic night-to-day BP ratio residuals (all P values > 0.30) and were thus not included in GWAS analysis. The discovery GWAS was done using covariate-adjusted night-to-day BP ratio residuals and linear regression under additive genetic model in PLINK v1.07 [23]. P values $< 5 \times 10^{-8}$ were considered as genome-wide-level significant, while P values $< 1 \times 10^{-5}$ were considered as suggestively significant.

The statistically most significant SNPs from each locus with P value $< 1 \times 10^{-5}$ were selected for replication in two independent Finnish cohorts. For the replication cohorts similar statistical approach was used. Bonferroni corrected P value < 0.004 was regarded as a successful replication [0.05 / (2 studies × 6 SNPs)], considering that systolic and diastolic dipping are highly correlated. P value < 0.05 with the same direction of effect was considered as suggestive replication. We also conducted meta-analyses of the top BP dipping (night-to-day BP ratio) SNPs in all available studies using inverse-variance model with fixed effects in METAL [24]. We defined significant results as P values $< 5 \times 10^{-8}$. P values $< 1 \times 10^{-5}$ were considered to represent a suggestive association.

In addition, we tested association of the genome-wide-significant SNP (rs4905794) with LVMI, Sokolow-Lyon voltage and Cornell voltage-duration product measured in GENRES subjects to further explore the nature of the SNP in relation to target organ damage. We tested for significant covariates and adjusted LVMI with age (standardized $\beta = 3.3$, $P = 0.007$) and Sokolow-Lyon voltage with BMI (standardized $\beta = -0.6$, $P = 0.0003$) using stepwise linear regression (other covariates tested were smoking, waist-hip ratio and previous use of antihypertensive medication). BP levels were not included as covariates (although highly significant) as we presumed the effect of the genotypes to be principally mediated through BP levels. No covariates were significant for Cornell voltage-duration product.

A SNP set-based approach was used to test for association of circadian genes with BP dipping (night-to-day BP ratio). The 24 genes listed in the circadian rhythm pathway in KEGG (Kyoto Encyclopedia of Genes and Genomes) PATHWAY database [25, 26] were selected for testing. All successfully genotyped SNPs located inside the transcript boundaries of each circadian gene were included. Transcript boundaries of the circadian genes were derived from Ensembl Genome Browser (release 87, in NCBI37/hg19) [27, 28]. The set-based tests were conducted in PLINK v1.07 [23]. Using the SBP and DBP dipping (night-to-day BP ratio) residuals calculated as described above, a mean statistic was calculated for each gene based on the single-SNP association results under a linear model. Single SNPs were included in the set if association P value was < 0.05 and r^2 was < 0.5 with other SNPs selected with maximum of five SNPs included for each gene. The dataset was then permuted 10,000 times calculating empirical P value for each gene describing the number of times the permuted set-statistic exceeded the original one for the gene. Bonferroni corrected P value of 0.002 (0.05/24) was used to correct for multiple testing (24 genes).

Finally, we sought to replicate the previously published genetic associations, based on candidate gene studies, with BP dipping. This included five SNPs from Leu et al. [10], two SNPs from Sheng et al. [11] (one of which is shared with Leu et al.) and five SNPs from Wirtwein et al. [12]. Two of these SNPs were not genotyped in GENRES and thus imputed values were used. We considered Bonferroni corrected P value < 0.0045 (0.05/11 SNPs tested) and the same direction of effect as successful replication and P value < 0.05 and the same direction of effect as suggestive replication.

Functional analysis for top associations

We assessed the consequence of the leading SNPs of the loci that achieved P value $< 1 \times 10^{-5}$, using VEP (variant effect predictor) database [29, 30]. To look for putative functional consequences, we annotated each SNP to the closest gene using Ensembl database (release 87) [27, 28] and conducted an expression quantitative trait locus (eQTL) analysis in publicly available Genotype Tissue Expression (GTEx) database [31, 32]. We then used PhenoScanner [33, 34] to find if any of the SNPs had previously reported cardiovascular trait associations at a nominal significance of $P < 0.05$.

The Neale lab has made available basic GWAS results for over 2000 phenotypes from the UK Biobank data of ~ 337,000 unrelated individuals of British ancestry [35]. We looked up our leading SNPs for BP dipping through MR-Base PheWAS database [36] to see if they were associated with SBP or DBP, or with seven sleep traits (sleep duration, getting up in morning, chronotype, nap during day, sleeplessness, snoring, daytime dozing) in the Neale lab data, at a nominal significance of $P < 0.05$.

Results

Genome-wide association study in GENRES

The baseline characteristics of GENRES subjects (the discovery sample) are described in Table 1. Ambulatory BP data used for calculation of the mean BP dipping during placebo administration was derived from four ($n = 173$) or three ($n = 31$) recordings. The Manhattan

Table 1 Clinical characteristics of the discovery cohort (GENRES) and replication cohorts (DYNAMIC and DILGOM)

Variables	GENRES	DYNAMIC	DILGOM
n	204	183	180
Age (years)	50.7 ± 6.3	47.5 ± 11.7	56.3 ± 11.4
Men (%)	100	60	47
Body Mass Index (kg/m^2)	26.4 ± 2.7	27.1 ± 4.2	26.6 ± 4.4
Waist-hip ratio	0.99 ± 0.05	0.91 ± 0.08	0.91 ± 0.09
Current smokers (%)	15.7	15.3	7.8
Blood pressure levels (mmHg)			
Office measurements			
SBP	152 ± 13	145 ± 18	129 ± 18
DBP	100 ± 7	92 ± 12	79 ± 10
Ambulatory recordings			
Daytime			
SBP	144 ± 10	140 ± 13	128 ± 12
DBP	99 ± 6	88 ± 8	78 ± 8
Nighttime			
SBP	118 ± 11	118 ± 13	112 ± 12
DBP	81 ± 6	71 ± 9	65 ± 8
Nocturnal dipping			
Night-to-day BP ratio (%)			
SBP	81.9 ± 5.3	84.2 ± 5.7	87.8 ± 6.2
DBP	81.9 ± 4.8	80.4 ± 6.4	83.7 ± 8.1
Percentage of non-dippers (%)			
	7	16	32

Non-dipper is defined as night-to-day BP ratio > 90% for either systolic or diastolic blood pressure dipping. Values are presented as mean mean ± standard deviation. *Abbreviations*: *SBP* systolic blood pressure, *DBP* diastolic blood pressure, *BP* blood pressure

plots of the GWAS results for BP dipping from the discovery cohort are shown in Fig. 1 and the quantile-quantile plots are depicted in Additional file 3: Figure S2. As detailed in Table 2, one locus (rs4905794 at chromosome 14q32.2 near *BCL11B*) reached genome-wide significance threshold for SBP dipping (systolic night-to-day BP ratio $\beta = -4.8\%$, $P = 9.6 \times 10^{-9}$). The association of rs4905794 was very similar for DBP dipping (diastolic night-to-day BP ratio $\beta = -4.3\%$, $P = 2.2 \times 10^{-6}$). Further five potential loci were identified with suggestive significance ($P < 1 \times 10^{-5}$) (Table 2). Local Manhattan plots of the best loci are presented in Additional file 4: Figure S3A-F. A total of 99 SNPs in 62 loci had P values $< 1 \times 10^{-4}$ for either SBP or DBP dipping.

The GENRES subjects received four different antihypertensive monotherapies in a rotational fashion separated by one-month placebo periods (Additional file 1: Figure S1). We also tested if the associations of the statistically most significant SNPs from the six loci with $P < 1 \times 10^{-5}$ derived from the placebo periods were similar when dipping data during drug administration was analyzed. The results are shown in Additional file 5: Figure S4A-F. The effects of the SNPs were consistently in the same direction as during placebo periods and the associations remained statistically significant.

Replication analysis in DYNAMIC and DILGOM

In the replication step, the lead SNPs (most significantly associated SNP) from the genome-wide significant locus and the five loci with P values $< 1 \times 10^{-5}$ were followed up in two independent Finnish cohorts, DYNAMIC and DILGOM (Table 1). The majority of the DYNAMIC subjects had elevated blood pressure while DILGOM comprised mostly of normotensive individuals (Table 1). The results of the replication analysis are summarized in Table 2. In DYNAMIC, rs4905794 showing genome-wide significance in GENRES had an effect in the same direction, but the association was not statistically significant ($\beta = -0.8\%$, $P = 0.4$ for systolic night-to-day BP ratio and $\beta = -1.6\%$, $P = 0.13$ for diastolic night-to-day BP ratio). The association did not, however, replicate in the population-based DILGOM cohort. Nocturnal BP dipping (night-to-day BP ratio) values according to rs4905794 genotypes in the three study samples are illustrated in Fig. 2. Another SNP, rs16984571 located in *KCNS3* intron, showed effect in the same direction as in GENRES in both replication cohorts, but the associations did not reach statistical significance. In a meta-analysis of all three studies (combined $n = 567$) employing inverse-variance model with fixed effects no SNP showed genome-wide significant P values (Additional file 2: Table S2).

Association of rs4905794 with markers of left ventricular hypertrophy in GENRES

To explore the possible association of the genome-wide-significant SNP (rs4905794) with markers of cardiovascular target organ damage, we tested for the association of this SNP with indices of LVH in GENRES. Using all GENRES subjects with LVMI and rs4905794 genotype data available ($n = 227$, mean LVMI 98.1 ± 18.5 g/m^2), rs4905794 was found to significantly associate with LVMI, with the allele associated with larger dipping also associating with smaller left ventricular mass (G allele $\beta = -7.6$ g/m^2, $P = 0.02$) (Fig. 3a). In the 185 GENRES subjects with ECG recordings and rs4905794 genotype available, the mean Sokolow-Lyon voltage was 25.6 ± 6.7 mm and mean Cornell voltage-duration product was 1444 ± 528 mm × ms. The rs4905794 genotype was associated with Sokolow-Lyon voltage (G allele $\beta = -2.8$ mm, $P = 0.03$) (Fig. 3b). For Cornell voltage-duration product this association had a tendency to the same direction (G allele $\beta = -112$ mm × ms, $P = 0.3$) (Fig. 3c). If BP dipping was included as a covariate in

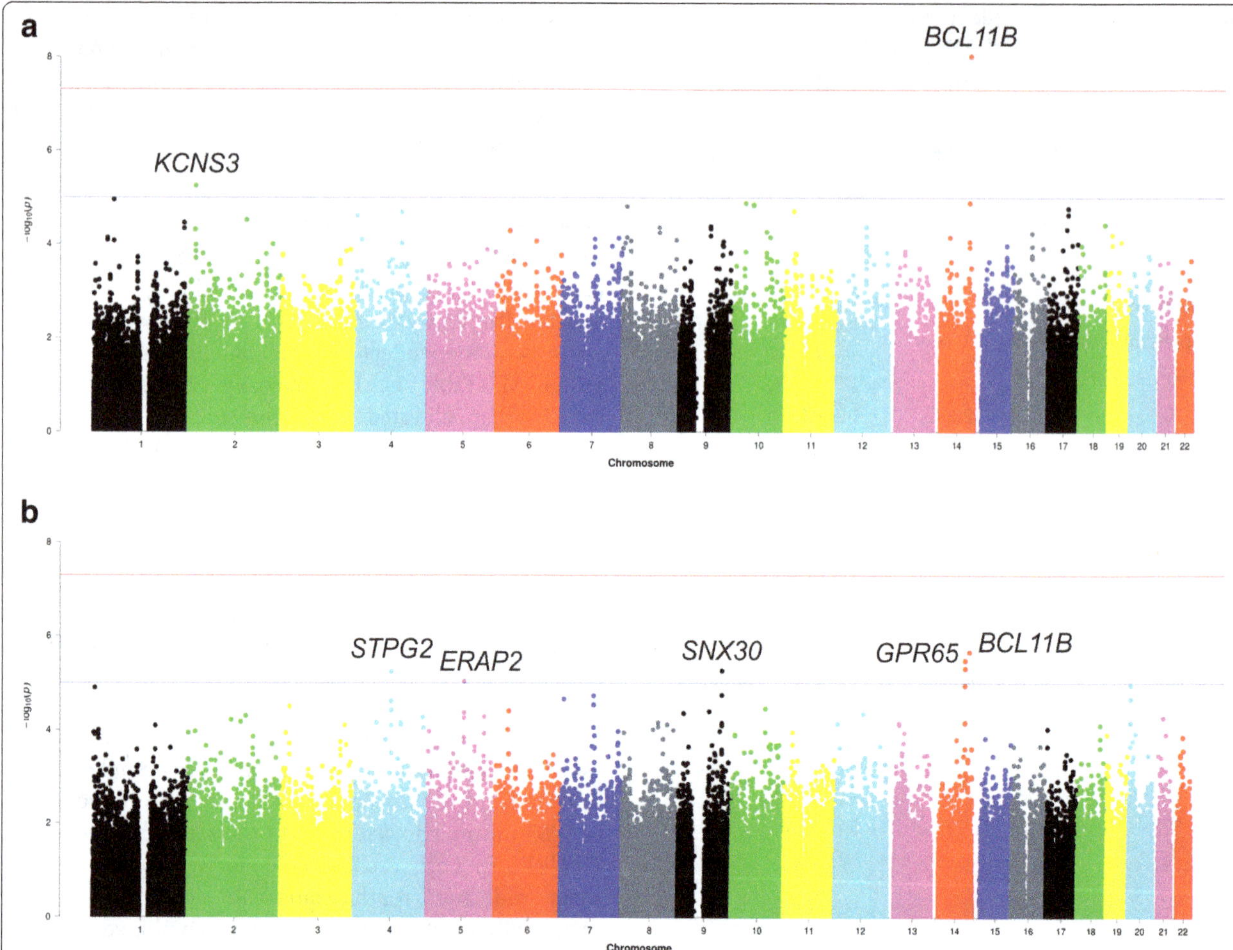

Fig. 1 Manhattan plots of the association *P* values from the discovery GWAS in GENRES. (**a**) SBP dipping (**b**) DBP dipping. The y-axis shows the -$\log_{10}$(*P* values) of each genotyped SNP and the x-axis shows their chromosomal position. The horizontal lines correspond to genome-wide (5×10^{-8}) and suggestive (1×10^{-5}) *P* value thresholds. SNPs above the suggestive threshold are annotated. Abbreviations: GWAS; genome-wide association study; SBP, systolic blood pressure; DBP, diastolic blood pressure; SNP; single nucleotide polymorphism

the analyses, the *P* values for the associations remained the same.

Association of BP dipping with circadian gene polymorphisms

In GENRES GWAS, no SNPs mapping within the transcript boundaries of the selected circadian genes had *P* values $< 1 \times 10^{-4}$ (Additional file 2: Table S3). Using set-based tests to evaluate the combined effect of independent SNPs in each gene, the retinoic acid-related orphan receptor genes (*RORA, RORB, RORC*) had the smallest *P* values (Additional file 2: Table S4). *RORB* had a suggestively significant *P* value 0.03 for association with SBP dipping, but this association did not survive multiple testing. Replication analysis for circadian gene SNPs from two earlier candidate gene studies is summarized in Additional file 2: Table S5. These SNPs did not significantly replicate in our study.

Replication of previously reported associations of CAD SNPs and BP dipping

In our study, rs9818870 was associated with both systolic and diastolic night-to-day BP ratio ($\beta = 1.4\%$, $P = 0.03$ and $\beta = 2.3\%$, $P = 0.002$, respectively) in consistent direction (Additional file 2: Table S5), thus further supporting the association of this SNP with BP dipping. The associations of the other four CAD SNPs found by Wirtwein et al. [12] did not significantly replicate in our study.

Discussion

We report here the first GWAS on nocturnal BP dipping. When using a sample of hypertensive patients subjected to repeated (mostly four times) 24-h ABPMs on placebo, a specific SNP (rs4905794) reached genome-wide significance for association with this phenotype, and five additional loci showed *P* values $< 1 \times 10^{-5}$. It is noteworthy that the associations of all six SNPs remained very

Table 2 Top SNPs associated with blood pressure dipping (night-to-day blood pressure ratio) in GENRES and replication in DYNAMIC and DILGOM

Discovery GWAS in GENRES									Replication in DYNAMIC					Replication in DILGOM				
SNP	Chr	Gene	EA/ OA	SBP/ DBP	EAF	*n*	*β* (%)	*P*	EAF	*n*	*β* (%)	*P*	Direction	EAF	*n*	*β* (%)	*P*	Direction
rs4905794	14	*BCL11B*	G/A	SBP	0.08	204	−4.8	9.6×10^{-9}	0.10	183	−0.8	0.4	same	0.11	180	0.9	0.3	opposite
		eQTL		DBP			−4.3	2.2×10^{-6}			−1.6	0.13	same			1.0	0.4	opposite
rs2119704	14	*GPR65*	A/C	SBP	0.07	204	−2.9	1.7×10^{-3}	0.06	183	1.4	0.2	opposite	0.06	180	0.9	0.5	opposite
		eQTL		DBP			−4.6	3.4×10^{-6}			1.1	0.4	opposite			−0.4	0.8	same
rs10817396	9	*SNX30*	G/A	SBP	0.17	204	1.9	2.4×10^{-3}	0.18	183	0.3	0.7	same	0.20	180	0.3	0.7	same
		intron		DBP			3.1	5.5×10^{-6}			−0.1	0.9	opposite			0.6	0.6	same
rs16984571	2	*KCNS3*	G/A	SBP	0.15	201	−2.7	5.6×10^{-6}	0.14	183	−0.8	0.3	same	0.13	180	−1.2	0.2	same
		intron		DBP			−2.5	1.1×10^{-4}			−0.7	0.4	same			−1.0	0.4	same
rs12509878	4	lncRNA	C/A	SBP	0.34	203	−1.5	9.8×10^{-4}	0.37	183	1.3	0.03	opposite	0.37	180	−1.4	0.03	same
		intron		DBP			−2.2	5.8×10^{-6}			1.1	0.11	opposite			−1.6	0.05	same
rs1230361	5	*ERAP2*	A/C	SBP	0.47	204	1.4	1.1×10^{-3}	0.49	183	0.5	0.4	same	0.45	180	−0.6	0.3	opposite
		intron/eQTL		DBP			2.1	9.3×10^{-6}			0.1	0.9	same			−0.7	0.3	opposite

SNPs with $P < 1 \times 10^{-5}$ for SBP or DBP dipping (covariate-adjusted systolic or diastolic night-to-day BP ratio using additive genetic model) in the discovery GWAS (GENRES) are shown in order of significance. Explanation for selection of related candidate gene is shown under gene name. *Abbreviations*: *GWAS* genome-wide association study, *SNP* single nucleotide polymorphism, *Chr* chromosome, *EA* effect allele, *OA* other allele, *SBP* systolic blood pressure, *DBP* diastolic blood pressure, *EAF* effect allele frequency, *eQTL* expression quantitative trait locus

consistent even when the analyses were conducted during administration of four different antihypertensive drug monotherapies. We sought to replicate the findings in two independent Finnish populations. Compared to GENRES, rs4905794 showed similar, although not statistically significant, association with BP dipping in DYNAMIC, comprising both hyper- and normotensive individuals, but did not replicate in DILGOM, consisting of a population-based sample of individuals. rs4905794 was also associated with LVMI and Sokolow-Lyon voltage in GENRES.

rs4905794 maps to intergenic region on chromosome 14 that is thought to harbor various regulatory features that affect expression of the nearby *BCL11B* gene [37]. In eQTL analysis using publicly available gene expression data sets, rs4905794 was associated with *BCL11B* expression in hippocampus ($n = 111$, $P = 0.001$ in GTEx database [31, 32], Additional file 2: Table S6) and in putamen ($n = 133$, $P = 0.0001$ in Braineac database [38, 39]) with the same direction of effect. rs4905794 has previously been associated with blood lipoprotein(a) level ($P = 7.6 \times 10^{-5}$ in NHLBI Family Heart Study [40] data published in database of genotypes and phenotypes (dbGaP) [41, 42]), a well-defined cardiovascular risk factor [43], that has been shown to closely correlate with nighttime BP level and nocturnal BP dipping [44].

BCL11B codes for a zinc-finger type transcription factor that has an established role in development and maintenance of central nervous system and regulation of T-cell development (for review, see ref. [45]). However, the role of *BCL11B* in regulation BP is not known. A recent GWAS on carotid-femoral pulse-wave velocity, the standard measurement of aortic stiffness, identified SNPs mapping to the same potential 3′ enhancer region near *BCL11B* at genome-wide significance and the top SNP (rs1381289) was also associated with increased risk for CAD events and heart failure [46]. Interestingly, Cherrier et al. have shown that BCL11B has a protective role in cardiomyocytes by repressing P-TEFb-mediated intercellular signaling that otherwise results in hypertrophic cardiomyopathy in mice [47]. In addition, experimental data supports a role for BCL11B in the direct regulation of circadian rhythm. BCL11B was shown to interact with histone deacetylase 1 (HDAC1) [48], and the nucleosome remodeling and histone deacetylase (NuRD) complex [49]. Both HDAC1, as a complex with SIN3 [50], and the NuRD complex [51] are in turn involved in the regulation of rhythmic expression of mammalian circadian clock PER genes in vitro. In summary, *BCL11B* could affect BP regulation and target organ damage through various mechanisms including the regulation of circadian rhythm, supporting the findings from our GWAS.

Available expression and phenotype databases seem to provide support for the role of some of the lead SNPs reported in the present study (Additional file 2: Tables S6 and S7). Three specific SNPs turned out to be eQTLs for nearby genes. Firstly, there was a strong correlation between intergenic SNP rs1230361 genotype and endoplasmic reticulum aminopeptidase 2 (*ERAP2*) expression in all available GTEx datasets (meta-analysis *P* value 1.0×10^{-200}) [31, 32]. In a previous candidate gene study

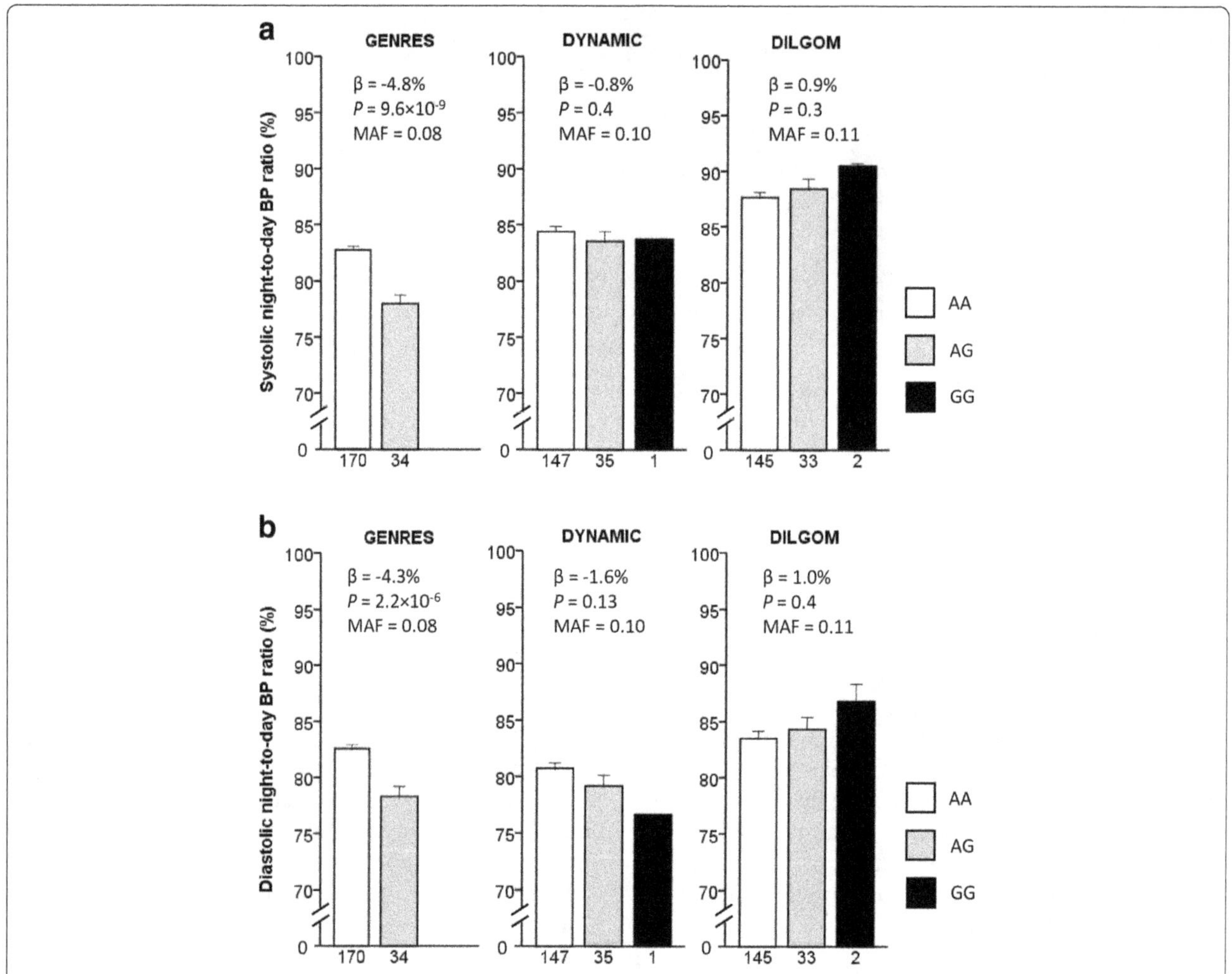

Fig. 2 Mean nocturnal blood pressure dipping according to rs4905794 genotypes in the three study samples. (**a**) SBP dipping (systolic night-to-day blood pressure ratio) (**b**) DBP dipping (diastolic night-to-day blood pressure ratio). Error bars indicate standard error of means. Abbreviations: SBP, systolic blood pressure; DBP, diastolic blood pressure

rs2549782 ($r^2 = 0.40$, $D' = 0.69$ with rs1230361 in GENRES) was shown to be associated with pre-eclampsia [52]. Also, in UK Biobank GWAS data [35, 36], rs1230361 was nominally associated with DBP ($P = 0.002$) supporting the role of this SNP in blood pressure regulation, and with two out of seven available sleep traits (getting up in morning, chronotype). Secondly, rs2119704 was an eQTL for *GPR65* expression (meta-analysis *P* value 2.2×10^{-10}), and rs10817396 for *SNX30* expression (meta-analysis *P* value 4.1×10^{-7}) in selected tissues from the GTEx database [31, 32]. rs10817396 was also associated with both SBP ($P = 0.03$) and DBP ($P = 0.01$) and two out of seven available sleep traits (chronotype, sleeplessness) in UK Biobank GWAS data [35, 36]. It is also noteworthy, that intronic rs16984571 (*KCNS3*), which had an effect in consistent direction in both replication cohorts, also associated with chronotype in UK Biobank GWAS data. *KCNS3* codes for a subunit (Kv9.3) of voltage-gated K^+ channel that regulates the contraction of arterial smooth muscle [53].

Circadian clock genes have been shown to regulate BP in animal studies [8, 9]. In our GWAS of BP dipping, there were no SNPs showing *P* values $< 1 \times 10^{-4}$ and mapping to circadian genes, and in set-based tests no gene showed enrichment of small *P* values. We could not replicate the positive associations of circadian gene polymorphisms with BP dipping reported by Leu et al. [10] and Sheng et al. [11]. However, the carriers of A allele of rs3816358 of *BMAL1* that associated with non-dipping in both Taiwanese (OR = 1.50, $P = 0.03$) [9] and Chinese ($\beta = 3.25\%$, $P = 0.04$) [10] subjects had reduced SBP ($\beta = 0.8\%$, $P = 0.2$) and DBP ($\beta = 1.0\%$, $P = 0.18$) dipping in GENRES. We attempted to replicate the findings of Wirtwein et al. [12] on five CAD risk loci derived from large GWAS studies that were associated with non-dipping status and found that the A allele of rs9818870 in *MRAS* was significantly associated with

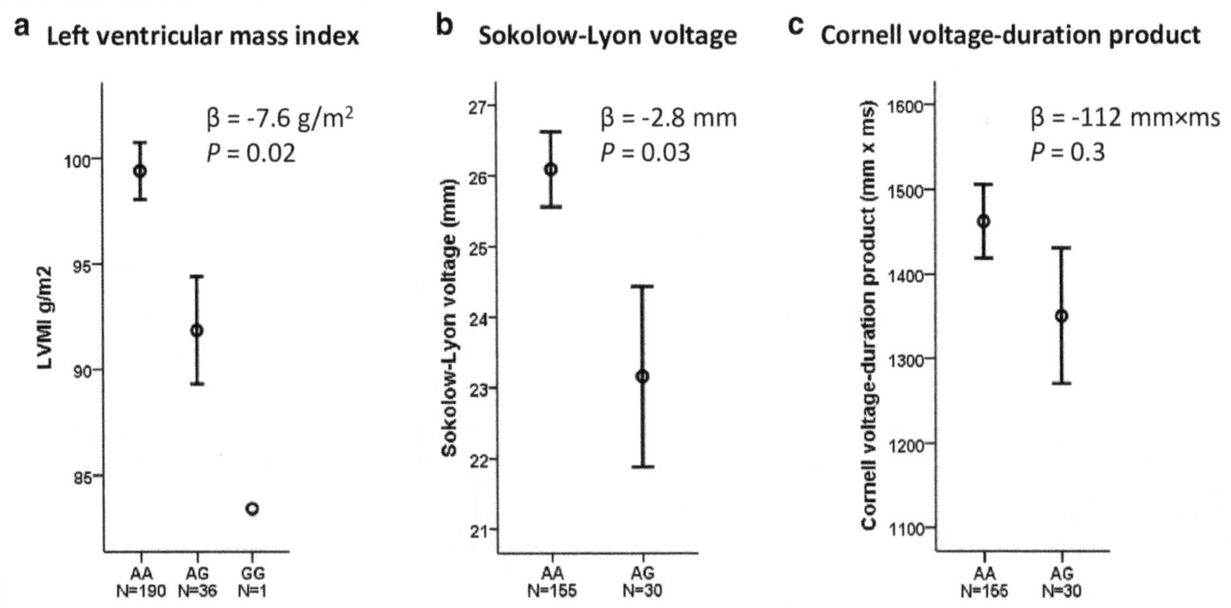

Fig. 3 Markers of LVH according to rs4905794 genotypes in GENRES. (**a**) LVMI ($n = 227$), (**b**) Sokolow-Lyon voltage ($n = 185$) (**c**) Cornell voltage-duration product ($n = 185$). Error bars indicate standard error of means. Abbreviations: LVH, left ventricular hypertrophy; LVMI, left ventricular mass index

reduced SBP and DBP dipping in our hypertensive patients with no evidence of CAD.

The present study has several important limitations. The limited sample size of the discovery cohort (GENRES) and the relatively small sizes of the available replication cohorts constitute an obvious issue. Second, while GENRES and one of the replication samples (DYNAMIC) were dominated by hypertensive individuals, the other (DILGOM) was derived from a population survey. This may have caused a selection bias in GENRES. In addition the definition of awake and sleep period was different in DILGOM compared to GENRES and DYNAMIC. Together, these two issues may have caused smaller effect sizes of the test variable (nocturnal BP dipping), resulting in possible false negative findings in DILGOM. Third, both men and women were included in DYNAMIC and DILGOM, while GENRES consisted of men only. On the other hand, the main strength of our study is the use of repeated (mostly four times) ABPMs during placebo in GENRES. We also believe that acquisition of parallel data under the four different drug monotherapies in GENRES strongly support our data. Even though the results should be interpret with caution due to the small sample size, they encourage further studies using novel well-defined phenotypes to find new genetic associations in human hypertension.

Conclusions

To our knowledge, our study is the first GWAS conducted on BP dipping in human hypertension. Using a carefully controlled pharmacogenetic study platform, we found a genome-wide significant association between BP dipping and rs4905794 near *BCL11B* gene, with similar tendency in another hypertensive patient cohort; however it was not replicated in a population based sample. rs4905794 was also associated with markers of LVH. In addition, we found some support for the association between BP dipping and rs9818870, previously suggested to associate with nondipping pattern in patients with CAD. In contrast, we did not find evidence that polymorphisms of circadian clock genes would play a marked role in determining BP dipping. Together with previous evidence, our results encourage further research into the role of *BCL11B* in pathophysiology of human hypertension.

Additional files

Additional file 1: Figure S1. The GENRES Study design. (DOC 126 kb)

Additional file 2: Table S1. Covariates used for calculation of night-to-day blood pressure ratio residuals in GENRES. **Table S2.** Meta-analysis of blood pressure dipping (night-to-day blood pressure ratio) in all three studies ($n = 567$). **Table S3.** Association of SNPs of circadian genes with blood pressure dipping (night-to-day blood pressure ratio) in GENRES. **Table S4.** Association of circadian genes with blood pressure dipping (night-to-day blood pressure ratio) in GENRES. **Table S5.** Replication of SNPs previously associated with blood pressure dipping in GENRES. **Table S6.** Functional analysis of the lead SNPs associated with blood pressure dipping (night-to-day blood pressure ratio) in GENRES GWAS. **Table S7.** Association of the top blood pressure dipping SNPs with selected UK Biobank GWAS phenotypes. (XLS 167 kb)

Additional file 3: Figure S2. Quantile-quantile plots of the genome-wide association results in the discovery cohort (GENRES). (DOC 80 kb)

Additional file 4: Figure S3A-F. LocusZoom plots of the top loci for blood pressure dipping. (DOC 591 kb)

Additional file 5: Figure S4A-F. Systolic and diastolic blood pressure dipping (night-to-day blood pressure ratio) during placebo and drug treatment periods according to top six SNPs genotypes in GENRES. (DOC 457 kb)

Abbreviations

ABPM: Ambulatory blood pressure measurement; BMI: Body mass index; BP: Blood pressure; CAD: Coronary artery disease; DBP: Diastolic blood pressure; DILGOM: Dietary, lifestyle and genetic determinants of obesity and metabolic syndrome; DYNAMIC: Haemodynamics in primary and secondary hypertension; ECG: Electrocardiogram; eQTL: Expression quantitative trait locus; GENRES: Genetics of drug responsiveness in essential hypertension; GTEx: Genotype tissue expression database; GWAS: Genome-wide association study; LVH: Left ventricular hypertrophy; LVM: Left ventricular mass; LVMI: Left ventricular mass index; PC: Principal component; SBP: Systolic blood pressure; SNP: Single nucleotide polymorphism

Acknowledgements

We thank Ms. Susanna Saarinen for excellent technical help and Reeta Kulmala, RN and Paula Erkkilä, RN for invaluable contribution to the hemodynamic recordings of the DYNAMIC study.

Funding

The GENRES Study was supported by grants from the Sigrid Jusélius Foundation and the Finnish Foundation for Cardiovascular Research. The DYNAMIC study was supported by the Finnish Foundation for Cardiovascular Research, Sigrid Jusélius Foundation, and Päivikki and Sakari Sohlberg Foundation.

Authors' contributions

Design of the work: TPH, KKK. Data Collection: TPH, KKK, IHP, TN, AJ, TL, AT, LO, KP, JV. Data analysis and interpretation: JMR, TPH, KKK. Manuscript preparation: JMR, TPH, KKK. Manuscript revising: IHP, TN, AJ, TL, AT, LO, KP, JV. All authors read and approved the final manuscript.

Competing interests

The authors declare that they have no competing interests.

Author details

[1]Department of Medicine, University of Helsinki and Helsinki University Hospital, 00290 Helsinki, Finland. [2]Faculty of Medicine and Life Sciences, University of Tampere and Tampere University Hospital, Tampere, Finland. [3]National Institute for Health and Welfare (THL), Helsinki, Finland. [4]Department of Clinical Chemistry, Fimlab Laboratories and Finnish Cardiovascular Research Center Tampere, Faculty of Medicine and Life Sciences, University of Tampere, Tampere, Finland. [5]National Heart, Lung, and Blood Institute's and Boston University's Framingham Heart Study, Framingham, MA, USA. [6]Division of Cardiology, Heart and Lung Center, University of Helsinki and Helsinki University Hospital, Helsinki, Finland.

References

1. O'Brien E, Sheridan J, O'Malley K. Dippers and non-dippers. Lancet. 1988;2:397.
2. Verdecchia P, Schillaci G, Guerrieri M, Gatteschi C, Benemio G, Boldrini F, et al. Circadian blood pressure changes and left ventricular hypertrophy in essential hypertension. Circulation. 1990;81:528–36.
3. Fagard RH, Thijs L, Staessen JA, Clement DL, De Buyzere ML, De Bacquer DA. Night-day blood pressure ratio and dipping pattern as predictors of death and cardiovascular events in hypertension. J Hum Hypertens. 2009;23:645–53.
4. Salles GF, Reboldi G, Fagard RH, Cardoso CR, Pierdomenico SD, Verdecchia P, et al. Prognostic effect of the nocturnal blood pressure fall in hypertensive patients: the ambulatory blood pressure collaboration in patients with hypertension (ABC-H) meta-analysis. Hypertension. 2016;67:693–700.
5. ESH/ESC Task Force for the Management of Arterial Hypertension. 2013 practice guidelines for the management of arterial hypertension of the European Society of Hypertension (ESH) and the European Society of Cardiology (ESC): ESH/ESC task force for the Management of Arterial Hypertension. J Hypertens. 2013;31:1925–38.
6. Padmanabhan S, Caulfield M, Dominiczak AF. Genetic and molecular aspects of hypertension. Circ Res. 2015;116:937–59.
7. Wang X, Ding X, Su S, Yan W, Harshfield G, Treiber F, et al. Genetic influences on daytime and night-time blood pressure: similarities and differences. J Hypertens. 2009;27:2358–64.
8. Curtis AM, Cheng Y, Kapoor S, Reilly D, Price TS, Fitzgerald GA. Circadian variation of blood pressure and the vascular response to asynchronous stress. Proc Natl Acad Sci U S A. 2007;104:3450–5.
9. Xie Z, Su W, Liu S, Zhao G, Esser K, Schroder EA, et al. Smooth-muscle BMAL1 participates in blood pressure circadian rhythm regulation. J Clin Invest. 2015;125:324–36.
10. Leu HB, Chung CM, Lin SJ, Chiang KM, Yang HC, Ho HY, et al. Association of circadian genes with diurnal blood pressure changes and non-dipper essential hypertension: a genetic association with young-onset hypertension. Hypertens Res. 2015;38:155–62.
11. Sheng CS, Cheng YB, Wei FF, Yang WY, Guo OH, Li FK, et al. Diurnal blood pressure rhythmicity in relation to environmental and genetic cues in untreated referred patients. Hypertension. 2017;69:128–35.
12. Wirtwein M, Melander O, Sjogren M, Hoffman M, Narkiewicz K, Gruchala M, et al. The relationship between gene polymorphisms and dipping profile in patients with coronary heart disease. Am J Hypertens. 2016;29:1094–102.
13. Hiltunen TP, Donner KM, Sarin AP, Saarela J, Ripatti S, Chapman AB, et al. Pharmacogenomics of hypertension: a genome-wide, placebo-controlled cross-over study, using four classes of antihypertensive drugs. J Am Heart Assoc. 2015;4:e001521.
14. Rimpela JM, Kontula KK, Fyhrquist F, Donner KM, Tuiskula AM, Sarin AP, et al. Replicated evidence for aminoacylase 3 and nephrin gene variations to predict antihypertensive drug responses. Pharmacogenomics. 2017;18:445–58.
15. Hiltunen TP, Suonsyrja T, Hannila-Handelberg T, Paavonen KJ, Miettinen HE, Strandberg T, et al. Predictors of antihypertensive drug responses: initial data from a placebo-controlled, randomized, cross-over study with four antihypertensive drugs (the GENRES study). Am J Hypertens. 2007;20:311–8.
16. Tikkakoski AJ, Tahvanainen AM, Leskinen MH, Koskela JK, Haring A, Viitala J, et al. Hemodynamic alterations in hypertensive patients at rest and during passive head-up tilt. J Hypertens. 2013;31:906–15.
17. Kangas P, Tahvanainen A, Tikkakoski A, Koskela J, Uitto M, Viik J, et al. Increased cardiac workload in the upright posture in men: noninvasive hemodynamics in men versus women. J Am Heart Assoc. 2016;5:10. 1161
18. Lindroos AS, Johansson JK, Puukka PJ, Kantola I, Salomaa V, Juhanoja EP, et al. The association between home vs. ambulatory night-time blood pressure and end-organ damage in the general population. J Hypertens. 2016;34:1730–7.
19. Howie BN, Donnelly P, Marchini J. A flexible and accurate genotype imputation method for the next generation of genome-wide association studies. PLoS Genet. 2009;5:e1000529.
20. Porthan K, Virolainen J, Hiltunen TP, Viitasalo M, Väänänen H, Dabek J, et al. Relationship of electrocardiographic repolarization measures to echocardiographic left ventricular mass in men with hypertension. J Hypertens. 2007;25:1951–7.
21. Patterson N, Price AL, Reich D. Population structure and eigenanalysis. PLoS Genet. 2006;2:e190.
22. Price AL, Weale ME, Patterson N, Myers SR, Need AC, Shianna KV, et al. Long-range LD can confound genome scans in admixed populations. Am J Hum Genet. 2008;83:132–5.
23. Purcell S, Neale B, Todd-Brown K, Thomas L, Ferreira MA, Bender D, et al. PLINK: a tool set for whole-genome association and population-based linkage analyses. Am J Hum Genet. 2007;81:559–75.
24. Willer CJ, Li Y, Abecasis GR. METAL: fast and efficient meta-analysis of genomewide association scans. Bioinformatics. 2010;26:2190–1.
25. Kanehisa M, Furumichi M, Tanabe M, Sato Y, Morishima KKEGG. New perspectives on genomes, pathways, diseases and drugs. Nucleic Acids Res. 2017;45:D353–61.
26. KEGG PATHWAY Database. Kanehisa laboratories, Kyoto, Japan. 2017. http://www.genome.jp/kegg/pathway.html. Accessed 7 Apr 2017.
27. Aken BL, Ayling S, Barrell D, Clarke L, Curwen V, Fairley S, et al. The Ensembl gene annotation system. Database (Oxford). 2016;2016:baw093.
28. Ensembl Genome Browser. The European bioinformatics institute (EMBL-EBI), Hinxton, Cambridgeshire, UK. 2017. http://ensembl.org. Accessed 7 Apr 2017.
29. McLaren W, Gil L, Hunt SE, Riat HS, Ritchie GR, Thormann A, et al. The Ensembl variant effect predictor. Genome Biol. 2016;17:122-016-0974-4.
30. Variant Effect Predictor VEP. The European bioinformatics institute (EMBL-EBI), Hinxton, Cambridgeshire, UK. 2017. http://www.ensembl.org/info/docs/tools/vep/index.html. Accessed 7 Apr 2017.

31. The GTEx Consortium. Genetic effects on gene expression across human tissues. Nature. 2017;550:204–13.
32. The Genotype-Tissue Expression (GTEx) Portal. The broad institute of MIT and Harvard, Cambridge, MA. 2017. http://www.gtexportal.org. Accessed 24 Oct 2017.
33. Staley JR, Blackshaw J, Kamat MA, Ellis S, Surendran P, Sun BB, et al. PhenoScanner: a database of human genotype-phenotype associations. Bioinformatics. 2016;32:3207–9.
34. Phenoscanner (v1.1) – A database of human genotype-phenotype associations. University of Cambridge, UK. 2017. http://www.phenoscanner.medschl.cam.ac.uk/phenoscanner. Accessed 7 Apr 2017.
35. UK Biobank GWAS Results. The Neale lab, analytical and translational genetic unit (ATGU), Massachusetts General Hospital, Boston, MA. 2017 http://www.nealelab.is. Accessed 16 May 2018.
36. MR-Base PheWAS database. University of Bristol, Bristol, UK. 2018. http://phewas.mrbase.org/. Accessed 16 May 2018.
37. Nagel S, Scherr M, Kel A, Hornischer K, Crawford GE, Kaufmann M, et al. Activation of TLX3 and NKX2-5 in t(5;14)(q35;q32) T-cell acute lymphoblastic leukemia by remote 3'-BCL11B enhancers and coregulation by PU.1 and HMGA1. Cancer Res. 2007;67:1461–71.
38. Ramasamy A, Trabzuni D, Guelfi S, Varghese V, Smith C, Walker R, et al. Genetic variability in the regulation of gene expression in ten regions of the human brain. Nat Neurosci. 2014;17:1418–28.
39. Braineac - the brain eQTL almanac. The UK Brain Expression Consortium (UKBEC). http://www.braineac.org. Accessed 7 Apr 2017.
40. Higgins M, Province M, Heiss G, Eckfeldt J, Ellison RC, Folsom AR, et al. NHLBI family heart study: objectives and design. Am J Epidemiol. 1996;143:1219–28.
41. Tryka KA, Hao L, Sturcke A, Jin Y, Wang ZY, Ziyabari L, et al. NCBI's database of genotypes and phenotypes: dbGaP. Nucleic Acids Res. 2014;42:D975–9.
42. dbGaP database of genotypes and phenotypes. National center for biotechnology information, National Library of medicine (NCBI/NLM). 2017. https://www.ncbi.nlm.nih.gov/projects/gap/cgi-bin/study.cgi?study_id=phs000221.v1.p1. Accessed 7 Apr 2017.
43. Nordestgaard BG, Langsted A. Lipoprotein (a) as a cause of cardiovascular disease: insights from epidemiology, genetics, and biology. J Lipid Res. 2016;57:1953–75.
44. Antonicelli R, Testa R, Bonfigli AR, Sirolla C, Pieri C, Marra M, et al. Relationship between lipoprotein(a) levels, oxidative stress, and blood pressure levels in patients with essential hypertension. Clin Exp Med. 2001;1:145–50.
45. Lennon MJ, Jones SP, Lovelace MD, Guillemin GJ, Brew BJ. Bcl11b-a critical neurodevelopmental transcription factor-roles in health and disease. Front Cell Neurosci. 2017;11:89.
46. Mitchell GF, Verwoert GC, Tarasov KV, Isaacs A, Smith AV, Yasmin, et al. Common genetic variation in the 3'-BCL11B gene desert is associated with carotid-femoral pulse wave velocity and excess cardiovascular disease risk: the AortaGen consortium. Circ Cardiovasc Genet. 2012;5:81–90.
47. Cherrier T, Le Douce V, Eilebrecht S, Riclet R, Marban C, Dequiedt F, et al. CTIP2 is a negative regulator of P-TEFb. Proc Natl Acad Sci U S A. 2013;110:12655–60.
48. Fu W, Yi S, Qiu L, Sun J, Tu P, Wang Y. BCL11B-mediated epigenetic repression is a crucial target for histone deacetylase inhibitors in cutaneous T-cell lymphoma. J Invest Dermatol. 2017;137:1523–32.
49. Cismasiu VB, Adamo K, Gecewicz J, Duque J, Lin Q, Avram D. BCL11B functionally associates with the NuRD complex in T lymphocytes to repress targeted promoter. Oncogene. 2005;24:6753–64.
50. Duong HA, Robles MS, Knutti D, Weitz CJ. A molecular mechanism for circadian clock negative feedback. Science. 2011;332:1436–9.
51. Kim JY, Kwak PB, Weitz CJ. Specificity in circadian clock feedback from targeted reconstitution of the NuRD corepressor. Mol Cell. 2014;56:738–48.
52. Johnson MP, Roten LT, Dyer TD, East CE, Forsmo S, Blangero J, et al. The ERAP2 gene is associated with preeclampsia in Australian and Norwegian populations. Hum Genet. 2009;126:655–66.
53. Cox RH, Fromme S. Comparison of voltage gated K^+ currents in arterial myocytes with heterologously expressed K_v subunits. Cell Biochem Biophys. 2016;74:499–511.

14

Exome sequencing identifies novel dysferlin mutation in a family with pauci-symptomatic heterozygous carriers

Mahjoubeh Jalali-Sefid-Dashti[1], Melissa Nel[2], Jeannine M. Heckmann[3†] and Junaid Gamieldien[4*†]

Abstract

Background: We investigated a South African family of admixed ancestry in which the first generation (G1) developed insidious progressive distal to proximal weakness in their twenties, while their offspring (G2) experienced severe unexpected symptoms of myalgia and cramps since adolescence. Our aim was to identify deleterious mutations that segregate with the affected individuals in this family.

Methods: Exome sequencing was performed on five cases, which included three affected G1 siblings and two pauci-symptomatic G2 offspring. As controls we included an unaffected G1 sibling and a spouse of one of the G1 affected individuals. Homozygous or potentially compound heterozygous variants that were predicted to be functional and segregated with the affected G1 siblings, were further evaluated. Additionally, we considered variants in all genes segregating exclusively with the affected (G1) and pauci-symptomatic (G2) individuals to address the possibility of a pseudo-autosomal dominant inheritance pattern in this family.

Results: All affected G1 individuals were homozygous for a novel truncating p.Tyr1433Ter *DYSF* (dysferlin) mutation, with their asymptomatic sibling and both pauci-symptomatic G2 offspring carrying only a single mutant allele. Sanger sequencing confirmed segregation of the variant. No additional potentially contributing variant was found in the *DYSF* or any other relevant gene in the pauci-symptomatic carriers.

Conclusion: Our finding of a truncating dysferlin mutation confirmed dysferlinopathy in this family and we propose that the single mutant allele is the primary contributor to the neuromuscular symptoms seen in the second-generation pauci-symptomatic carriers.

Keywords: Exome, Dysferlinopathy, Myalgia, Cramps, Pauci-symptomatic carriers

Background

Dysferlinopathies are a group of autosomal recessive muscular dystrophies caused by mutations in the dysferlin gene, *DYSF* [1, 2], and is typified by markedly reduced or absent dysferlin protein on immunohistochemical staining in muscle [3]. It most frequently presents as a distal myopathy affecting first the posterior distal leg compartment (Miyoshi muscle dystrophy), limb-girdle muscle dystrophy (LMGD2B) and a combination of the aforementioned, "proximodistal" myopathy [4, 5]. Clinical manifestations can be significantly varied even between individuals in a family bearing the same mutation, which indicates a possible role for genetic modifiers [6–8].

A definitive diagnosis of dysferlinopathy can only be made when pathogenic mutations are identified in the large (>233Kbp, 58 exons, >6Kbp coding sequence) dysferlin (*DYSF*) gene [9], which lacks mutation hotspots. It was recently demonstrated that next generation sequencing (NGS) targeting the coding regions of the *DYSF* gene enables efficient and accurate genetic diagnosis of dysferlinopathy [10]. Whole exome sequencing (WES), however, may provide additional advantages as an unbiased diagnostic strategy in families requesting a definitive diagnosis and genetic counselling [11], particularly in atypical

* Correspondence: junaid@sanbi.ac.za

†Jeannine M. Heckmann and Junaid Gamieldien contributed equally to this work.

[4]South African National Bioinformatics Institute, University of the Western Cape, Private Bag X17, Bellville 7535, South Africa

Full list of author information is available at the end of the article

disease presentations and/or when unexpected phenotypes are suspected.

We present an exome sequencing study in a non-consanguineous family actively seeking a diagnosis for the neuromuscular symptoms experienced by themselves and their children over a period of 25 years. The first generation (G1) presented with a predominant distal 'posterior calf' myopathy starting in early adulthood. This was suggestive of classical autosomal recessive Miyoshi myopathy caused by compound heterozygous or homozygous dysferlin gene mutation(s), since neither of their parents had been diagnosed with muscular dystrophy. However, at least five of the second generation (G2) offspring had been attending neurological services with mainly exercise-induced muscle cramps over a number of years starting in adolescence.

Methods

Patients and clinical evaluations

The study and subject consent forms were approved by the University of Cape Town Health Sciences faculty human ethics research committee (REF 552/2013) and the study carried out in accordance with the approved guidelines and regulations. We studied two generations of a South African family of mixed genetic ancestry that likely includes ancestors from Africa, Europe as well as Madagascar and Java as previously described [12]. Family members of G1 and G2 had been attending the adult and paediatric neurology clinics attached to the University of Cape Town for 25 years. After signed informed consent, blood was obtained for WES from G1 individuals, three affected (I-2, I-4 and I-5), one unaffected sibling (I-1) and one unrelated unaffected family member (I-3) as controls, and two members from G2 with neuromuscular symptoms and areflexia, II-2 and II-5. Structured folder reviews were performed to obtain previous examination details, laboratory data including those of muscle biopsies and clinical electrophysiological studies.

Whole exome capture, sequencing and variant calling

Paired-end exome sequencing was performed at 50× coverage by CLIA accredited Otogenetics Corporation, Norcross, GA, USA using the Agilent SureSelect Human V5 + UTR capture kit and the Illumina HiSeq2000/2500 platform. After quality control, reads for each patient were aligned to the hg19 human reference genome using NOVOALIGN [13], PCR duplicates were removed using Picard [14], followed by indel realignment and base quality score recalibration, variant calling and quality evaluation using the Genome Analysis ToolKit [15] version 3.6 to produce a high-confidence set of variants for each sample.

Identification of likely function-impacting candidate variants

Variants were annotated using ANNOVAR [16] and were filtered based on both autosomal recessive and dominant inheritance models. For the recessive model, we identified variants that were homozygous in the three affected G1 siblings, wild-type in their unaffected sibling, and wild-type or heterozygous in the unrelated unaffected family member and the G2 offspring. For the autosomal dominant model, we identified variants that were heterozygous in all the affected/pauci-symptomatic family members, and where both related and unrelated controls were wild-type. For initial filtering, variants with a minor allele frequency > 1% in public databases, namely the 1000 Genomes Project [17], the NHLBI-ESP 6500 Exome Sequencing Project [18] and the Exome Aggregation Consortium [19] databases were filtered out, as were those present in the currently unreleased Southern African Human Genome Program [20] variant dataset. Nonsense, frameshift and splicing variants were automatically selected as preliminary candidates, while missense variants were further evaluated if they passed the recommended deleteriousness score thresholds for any one of FATHMM [21] or the MetaSVM and MetaLR ensemble prediction methods [22].

Results

Clinical findings

Three affected individuals from G1 had developed progressive muscle weakness in their twenties, two of whom also had prominent exercise-induced myalgia, and five individuals from the second generation developed neuromuscular symptoms in adolescence (Fig. 1). Two individuals from G1 (I-4 and I-5) presented with the distal Miyoshi muscle dystrophy phenotype and one (I-2) with a "proximodistal" phenotype. Two cases from G2 had areflexia and marginally raised CK (II-2 and II-5), and three (II-1, II-6, II-7 and II-8) had normal reflexes. Individuals I-1, II-3, and II-4 had no neuromuscular symptoms or signs. The offspring of 1–1 were asymptomatic adults, and those of I-4 had not reached adolescence and were not examined.

The index case (I-4), first examined at age 26, complained of two years of progressive thinning of the distal legs and quadriceps, an inability to stand on his toes, and myalgia in his legs aggravated by exercise. Later, he noticed weakness in the hands. The clinical presentation was a distal, posterior compartment muscular dystrophy with markedly raised creatine kinase (CK) levels (> 47× upper limit of normal (ULN)). However, the tendon reflexes were either absent (legs) or reduced (arms), and four years later all the reflexes were absent. Electrophysiology showed normal nerve conductions, and myopathic features on needle electromyography (EMG). Electrocardiography was normal. A deltoid muscle biopsy

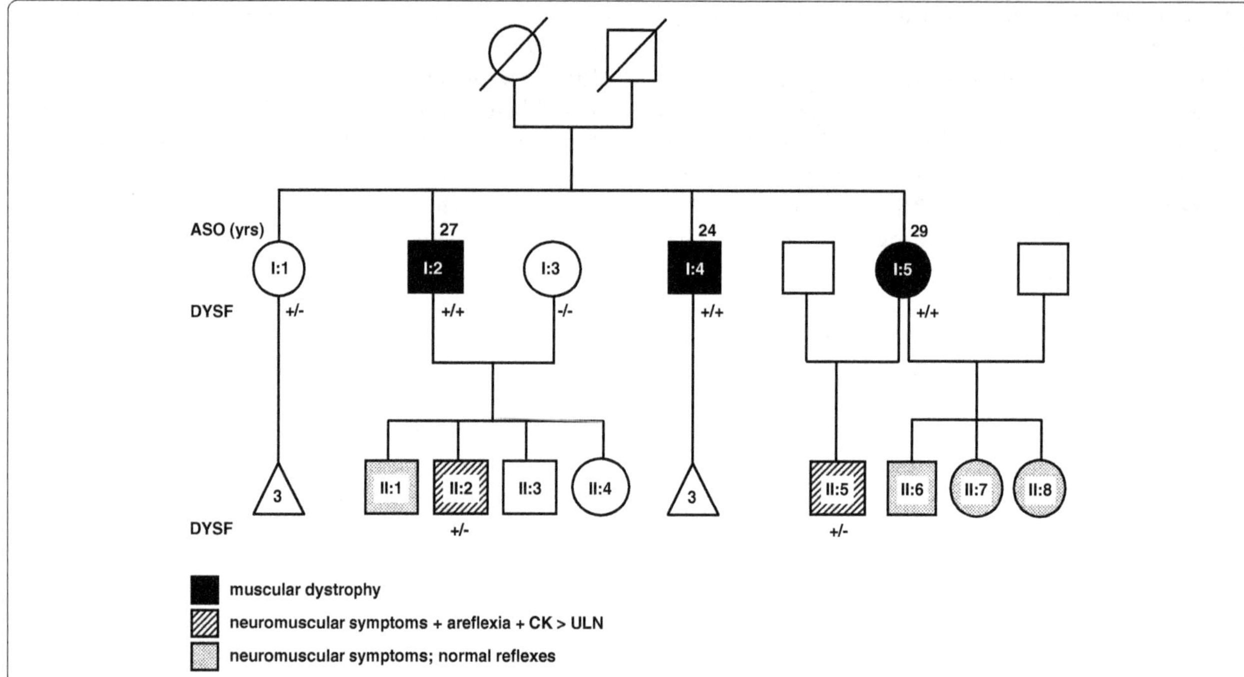

Fig. 1 Family pedigree and validated genotypes for the novel DYSF stop gain variants. Circles represent females and squares represent males. White figures (excluding triangles) symbolize unaffected members; solid symbolize disease cases, striped represent cases with neuromuscular symptoms, areflexia and elevated creatine kinase (CK) levels above the upper limit of normal (ULN); and speckled symbolize cases with neuromuscular symptoms but normal deep tendon reflexes. Individuals denoted by triangles were of uncertain clinical status and "/" indicate deceased individuals. ASO refers to age at symptom onset in years (yrs). Generation 1 (G1) refers to I:1 to I:5 and G2 refers to II:1 to II:8. DYSF refers to the dysferlin gene. '+' refers to the presence of the DYSF mutation, '-'to wild-type DYSF, +/− refers to heterozygous individuals and +/+ to homozygous individuals

confirmed a dystrophic process without inflammatory infiltrates; no special staining was available. At that time, his two asymptomatic sisters (one was Case I-5, aged 21, see below) and mother were noted to have normal CK levels (CK ≈ 61 IU/L; $N = 26–140$ IU/L), although his father, aged 51, complained of muscle cramps and had a slightly raised CK level (249 IU/L) which was 1.5× above the upper level of normal expected for age and sex. Approximately 15 years after symptom onset, I-4 required bilateral crutches to mobilize, and 10 years later became wheelchair bound. The pattern of weakness had progressed to severe limb girdle and distal weakness. Although sensation was previously recorded as intact, the last examination at age 49 showed evidence of a mild sensory stocking neuropathy.

Case I-2 presented at age 29 with a history of progressive leg weakness since mid-twenties, noting difficulty climbing stairs, getting up from chairs and exercise-induced muscle cramps, especially in his calves. His examination showed wasting of the biceps and distal legs, mild proximo-distal posterior leg weakness, and reduced/absent reflexes. Later he exhibited a waddling gait. The CK level was 20× ULN. A muscle biopsy at age 40 showed features of muscle dystrophy and immunohistochemistry showed absence of dysferlin in the presence of positive merosin, emerin, caveolin, dystrophin and sarcoglycan staining. Fifteen years later he required crutches to mobilize.

Case I-5 presented at age 34 with increasing difficulty in walking, climbing stairs, rising from a seated position, and general muscle fatigue since her late twenties. The arms showed tapering distally and the posterior compartment of the legs, marked wasting. Her tendon reflexes were globally depressed and there was marked weakness of the posterior compartment leg muscles. Her CK level was > 30× ULN. A muscle biopsy of the left biceps showed similar results to her brother except that dysferlin staining was initially present and dystrophin was absent, but the positive control (spectrin) showed partial staining. Her disability increased substantially and at age 45 years she was largely confined to a wheelchair. A repeat biopsy of the right biceps showed absent dysferlin staining.

II-2 was examined at age 18 years. He had normal early motor development but was noted to fall more than usual as a child whilst running. Muscle cramps and stiffness, especially with physical activity, was noted during early adolescence. At age 15 he had increasing difficulty with riding his bicycle, climbing stairs as well as gait instability and stopped playing sport. He fell frequently. The neurological examination showed mild wasting of the biceps despite well-developed muscles elsewhere. His tendon jerks were absent. Power testing was normal, but he had a mild waddling gait. Sensation and coordination testing were normal. Clinical electrophysiology was refused. The CK level was at the upper the limit of normal (ULN) for his age (218 IU/L).

II-5 had experienced muscle pain, and episodes of cramp and stiffness lasting several hours to 1–2 days since the age of 12–13 years. These symptoms were, and still are, aggravated by physical activity. Since his early twenties he has also noticed increasing clumsy ankles and occasional give-in weakness of the legs. Examination at age 25 showed floppy ankles but no obvious wasting in his hands or feet. His tendon reflexes were globally absent and he had mild weakness of toe flexors but not of the plantar flexors. The remaining motor, sensory (all modalities) and coordination systems were normal. The CK level was slightly elevated (193 IU/L; 1.1× ULN for age and sex). Nerve conduction studies were normal. EMG of the medial head of gastrocnemius showed no spontaneous activity and normal motor units.

Cases II-1, II-6, II-7 and II-8 had been experiencing neuromuscular symptoms since the ages of 12 to 13 years, mainly myalgia, stiffness and/or muscle cramps. These symptoms occurred either in the hands or legs and were frequently provoked by mild physical activity including writing with a pen or walking upstairs, respectively.

Exome sequencing and filtering for candidate deleterious variants

WES was performed on I-2, I-4 and I-5 from G1, one unaffected sibling (I-1) and one unrelated unaffected family member (I-3) as controls, and on two members from G2 with neuromuscular symptoms and areflexia, II-2 and II-5. Approximately 50,000 variants were identified for each individual. Six variants segregated with all three symptomatic G1 individuals using the recessive model, of which three were in exonic regions, and one each in a 3′-untranslated region (UTR), intronic and intergenic regions, respectively. A novel nonsense $C > G$ mutation located at position 4299 in exon 39 (NCBI RefSeq: NM_003494) of the dysferlin gene (*DYSF*) was identified as responsible for the family's muscular dystrophy after filtering out common variants and those not predicted to impact protein function. Sanger sequencing confirmed the mutation to be homozygous in affected individuals of G1, and carrier status in I-1, II-2 and II-5. The p.Tyr1433Ter (NP_003485.1) mutation results in the loss of the sixth (C2E) and seventh (C2F) domains of the dysferlin protein (Fig. 2).

No other potentially deleterious dysferlin variant was found in the exomes of the two pauci-symptomatic G2 *DYSF*-mutant carriers. As they also presented with neuromuscular symptoms and areflexia in absence of distinct myopathy, we further filtered for rare or novel variants predicted to impact protein function that segregated exclusively with symptomatic individuals in both G1 and G2. Only two novel heterozygous missense mutations were identified in the *LRP2* (low density lipoprotein-related protein 2) and *GXYLT1* (glucoside xylosyltransferase 1) genes, which have no known roles in neuromuscular disease.

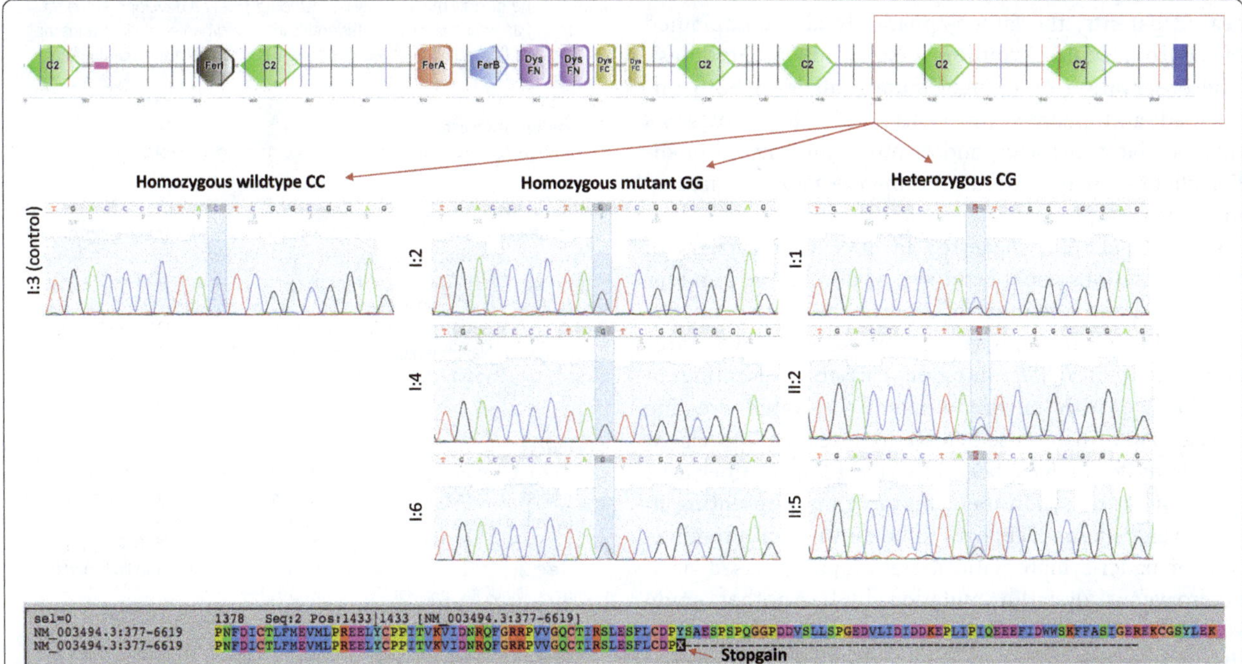

Fig. 2 Protein level consequence of the identified novel stop-gain dysferlin gene (*DYSF*) mutation. The diagram illustrates the loss of two C2 domains in *DYSF* gene due to the identified novel stop-gain. The chromatogram illustrates the Sanger sequencing validation for mutant and wild-type alleles in the affected and unaffected family members. The protein alignment illustrates the nonsense mutation and protein truncation

Discussion

The G1 symptomatic individuals developed mainly distal posterior compartment myopathy in their legs during their early twenties with extremely high CK levels at the time of diagnosis. The first generation's symptoms were indicative of Miyoshi myopathy/dysferlinopathy, since neither of their parents was diagnosed with myopathy even after age 60. Using WES, we confirmed autosomal recessive dysferlinopathy in this South African family, caused by a novel truncating p.Tyr1433Ter mutation in the *DYSF* gene, which accounts for the muscle dystrophy in the first generation. An asymptomatic G1 sibling also carried one copy of the *DYSF* mutation.

Several of their offspring experienced neuromuscular symptoms starting in adolescence to the extent that they had been followed at the pediatric neurology service for several years. The current study found that all the G2 cases with neuromuscular symptoms have only one copy of the novel nonsense *DYSF* mutation and no other potentially disease-causing variants in the gene. Although we postulated that co-occurrence of another mutation in a second gene could potentially be causing or contributing to the neuromuscular symptoms observed in G2, we only found two novel heterozygous missense mutations in the *LRP2* and *GXYLT1* genes, neither of which are reasonable candidates based on their known cellular functions and disease associations. We therefore suggest that the single mutated *DYSF* allele could be responsible for the less severe neuromuscular symptoms in G2. Interestingly, of the two inferred heterozygous deceased parents, the father apparently also complained of neuromuscular symptoms (see Clinical Findings). The observation of a single mutant allele in both unaffected and pauci-symptomatic individuals suggests that variable penetrance, and/or other unidentified modifier allele(s), may underlie the manifestation of neuromuscular symptoms.

Fanin et al. [23] suggested in 2006 that carriers of *DYSF* mutations could be at risk of developing a milder phenotype and a number of reports have since contributed evidence to support this hypothesis. Two unrelated cases of *DYSF* mutation carriers presenting in middle age with muscle weakness, elevated creatine kinase, abnormal muscle MRI and reduced levels of muscle dysferlin, have been reported [24]. Another case of a bent spine syndrome/camptocormia, presenting in the seventh decade, appears to be an unusual presentation of pauci-symptomatic dysferlinopathy based on a heterozygous dysferlin mutation [25]. Another study was able to support a diagnosis of primary dysferlinopathy in symptomatic carriers with findings of abnormal dysferlin gene expression in skeletal muscle and monocytes [26]. Of note is that the two patients studied were unrelated but carried the same mutated allele, which suggests that certain mutations may have a higher likelihood than others of producing symptoms in carriers.

Conclusion

We confirm dysferlinopathy in this family due to a novel truncating p.Tyr1433Ter *DYSF* mutation. Our report highlights the importance of considering variable penetrance of heterozygous dysferlin mutations in the context of pauci-symptomatic younger offspring.

Abbreviations

ASO: Age of symptom onset; CK: Creatine kinase; CLIA: Clinical Laboratory Improvement Amendments; *DYSF*: Dysferlin; EMG: Electromyography; G1: First generation; G2: Second generation; *GXYLT1*: Glucoside xylosyltransferase 1; IUL: International Units Per Litre; LMGD2B: Limb-girdle muscular dystrophy; *LRP2*: Low density lipoprotein-related protein 2; MRI: Magnetic resonance imaging; NGS: Next generation sequencing; PCR: Polymerase chain reaction; ULN: Upper limit of normal; UTR: Untranslated region; WES: Whole exome sequencing

Acknowledgements

We gratefully acknowledge the participation of all the participants.

Funding

The South African National Research Foundation (NRF) supported (i) MJSD with a postdoctoral scholarship and associated research costs. JG was partly funded by a South African Medical Research Council grant (SHIP-NCD-003). The funding agencies had no involvement in the design of the study and the collection, analysis, and interpretation of data, or the drafting and editing of the manuscript.

Authors' contributions

MJSD performed the exome data processing/analysis, functional variant identification and causative variant prioritization, and drafted the manuscript. MN contributed to clinical genetics, sample collection/prep and Sanger verification. JH ran the clinical, clinical genetics and patient consent components, and had a role in manuscript drafting and editing. JG oversaw the bioinformatics analyses including pipeline development, data processing and candidate variant identification, and had a role in manuscript drafting and final editing. All authors agreed to the submission of the final manuscript.

Competing interests

The authors declare that they have no competing interests.

Author details

[1]South African Medical Research Council Bioinformatics Unit, South African National Bioinformatics Institute, University of the Western Cape, Bellville 7535, South Africa. [2]Division of Neurology, Department of Medicine, University of Cape Town, Observatory 7925, South Africa. [3]E8-74, Neurology, New Groote Schuur Hospital Observatory, Cape Town 7925, South Africa. [4]South African National Bioinformatics Institute, University of the Western Cape, Private Bag X17, Bellville 7535, South Africa.

References

1. Bashir R, Britton S, Strachan T, Keers S, Vafiadaki E, Lako M, et al. A gene related to Caenorhabditis elegans spermatogenesis factor fer-1 is mutated in limb-girdle muscular dystrophy type 2B. Nat Genet. 1998;20:37–42.
2. Liu J, Aoki M, Illa I, Wu C, Fardeau M, Angelini C, et al. Dysferlin, a novel skeletal muscle gene, is mutated in Miyoshi myopathy and limb girdle muscular dystrophy. Nat Genet. 1998;20:31–6.
3. Klinge L, Aboumousa A, Eagle M, Hudson J, Sarkozy A, Vita G, et al. New aspects on patients affected by dysferlin deficient muscular dystrophy. J Neurol Neurosurg Psychiatry. 2010;81:946–53.
4. Laval SH, Bushby KMD. Limb-girdle muscular dystrophies–from genetics to molecular pathology. Neuropathol Appl Neurobiol. 2004;30:91–105.
5. Nguyen K, Bassez G, Krahn M, Bernard R, Laforêt P, Labelle V, et al. Phenotypic study in 40 patients with dysferlin gene mutations: high frequency of atypical phenotypes. Arch Neurol. 2007;64:1176–82.

6. Weiler T, Bashir R, Anderson LV, Davison K, Moss JA, Britton S, et al. Identical mutation in patients with limb girdle muscular dystrophy type 2B or Miyoshi myopathy suggests a role for modifier gene(s). Hum Mol Genet. 1999;8:871–7.
7. Illarioshkin SN, Ivanova-Smolenskaya IA, Greenberg CR, Nylen E, Sukhorukov VS, Poleshchuk VV, et al. Identical dysferlin mutation in limb-girdle muscular dystrophy type 2B and distal myopathy. Neurology. 2000;55:1931–3.
8. Ueyama H, Kumamoto T, Nagao S, Masuda T, Horinouchi H, Fujimoto S, et al. A new dysferlin gene mutation in two Japanese families with limb-girdle muscular dystrophy 2B and Miyoshi myopathy. Neuromuscul Disord. 2001;11:139–45.
9. Tagawa K, Ogawa M, Kawabe K, Yamanaka G, Matsumura T, Goto K, et al. Protein and gene analyses of dysferlinopathy in a large group of Japanese muscular dystrophy patients. J Neurol Sci. 2003;211:23–8.
10. Shin HY, Jang H, Han JH, Park HJ, Lee JH, Kim SW, et al. Targeted next-generation sequencing for the genetic diagnosis of dysferlinopathy. Neuromuscul Disord. 2015;25:502–10.
11. Rehm HL. Disease-targeted sequencing: a cornerstone in the clinic. Nat Rev Genet. 2013;14:295–300.
12. Heckmann JM, Owen EP, Little F. Myasthenia gravis in south Africans: racial differences in clinical manifestations. Neuromuscul Disord. 2007;17:929–34.
13. Hansen NF. Variant calling from next generation sequence data. Methods Mol Biol. 2016;1418:209–24.
14. BroadInstitute. Picard Tools - By Broad Institute [Internet]. 2016 [cited 2016 Jun 9]. Available from: http://broadinstitute.github.io/picard/
15. McKenna A, Hanna M, Banks E, Sivachenko A, Cibulskis K, Kernytsky A, et al. The genome analysis Toolkit: a MapReduce framework for analyzing next-generation DNA sequencing data. Genome Res. 2010;20:1297–303.
16. Wang K, Li M, Hakonarson H. ANNOVAR: functional annotation of genetic variants from high-throughput sequencing data. Nucleic Acids Res. 2010;38:e164.
17. 1000 Genomes Project Consortium {fname}, Abecasis GR, Auton A, Brooks LD, MA DP, Durbin RM, et al. An integrated map of genetic variation from 1,092 human genomes. Nature. 2012:491, 56–65.
18. Fu W, O'Connor TD, Jun G, Kang HM, Abecasis G, Leal SM, et al. Analysis of 6,515 exomes reveals the recent origin of most human protein-coding variants. Nature. 2013;493:216–20.
19. Lek M, Karczewski KJ, Minikel EV, Samocha KE, Banks E, Fennell T, et al. Analysis of protein-coding genetic variation in 60,706 humans. Nature Nature Publishing Group. 2016;536:285–91.
20. Pepper MS. Launch of the southern African human genome Programme. South African Med J. 2011;101:287–8.
21. Shihab HA, Rogers MF, Gough J, Mort M, Cooper DN, Day INM, et al. An integrative approach to predicting the functional effects of non-coding and coding sequence variation. Bioinformatics. 2015;31:1536–43.
22. Dong C, Wei P, Jian X, Gibbs R, Boerwinkle E, Wang K, et al. Comparison and integration of deleteriousness prediction methods for nonsynonymous SNVs in whole exome sequencing studies. Hum Mol Genet. 2015;24:2125–37.
23. Fanin M, Nascimbeni AC, Angelini C. Muscle protein analysis in the detection of heterozygotes for recessive limb girdle muscular dystrophy type 2B and 2E. Neuromuscul Disord. 2006;16:792–9.
24. Illa I, De Luna N, Dominguez-Perles R, Rojas-Garcia R, Paradas C, Palmer J, et al. Symptomatic dysferlin gene mutation carriers: characterization of two cases. Neurology. 2007;68:1284–9.
25. Gáti I, Danielsson O, Gunnarsson C, Vrethem M, Häggqvist B, Fredriksson B-A, et al. Bent spine syndrome: a phenotype of dysferlinopathy or a symptomatic DYSF gene mutation carrier. Eur Neurol. 2012;67:300–2.
26. Meznaric M, Gonzalez-Quereda L, Gallardo E, de Luna N, Gallano P, Fanin M, et al. Abnormal expression of dysferlin in skeletal muscle and monocytes supports primary dysferlinopathy in patients with one mutated allele. Eur J Neurol. 2011;18:1021–3.

15

Identification of deletion-duplication in *HEXA* gene in five children with Tay-Sachs disease from India

Jayesh Sheth[1*], Mehul Mistri[1], Lakshmi Mahadevan[2], Sanjeev Mehta[3], Dhaval Solanki[4], Mahesh Kamate[5] and Frenny Sheth[1]

Abstract

Background: Tay-Sachs disease (TSD) is a sphingolipid storage disorder caused by mutations in the *HEXA* gene. To date, nearly 170 mutations of *HEXA* have been described, including only one 7.6 kb large deletion.

Methods: Multiplex Ligation-dependent Probe Amplification (MLPA) study was carried out in 5 unrelated patients for copy number changes where heterozygous and/or homozygous disease causing mutation/s could not be identified in the coding region by sequencing of *HEXA* gene.

Results: The study has identified the presence of a homozygous deletion of exon-2 and exon-3 in two patients, two patient showed compound heterozygosity with exon 1 deletion combined with missense mutation p.E462V and one patient was identified with duplication of exon-1 with novel variants c.1527-2A > T as a second allele.

Conclusion: This is the first report of deletion/duplication in *HEXA* gene providing a new insight into the molecular basis of TSD and use of MLPA assay for detecting large copy number changes in the *HEXA* gene.

Keywords: Tay-Sachs disease, ß-hexosaminidase-A, *HEXA* gene; MLPA

Background

Tay-Sachs disease (TSD) [MIM* 606869] is one of the common sphingolipid storage disorder in India [1]. It is a rare neurodegenerative lysosomal storage disorder (LSD) caused by a deficiency of ß-hexosaminidase-A (Hex-A) (HEXA; EC: 3.2.1.52) enzyme. It occurs due to the inability of Hex-A enzyme to cleave the terminal N-acetyl hexosamine residues from GM2 ganglioside due to a mutation in *HEXA* gene. As a result, GM2 ganglioside is accumulated in various tissues especially in neuronal cells instead of further metabolizing into GM3 gangliosides [2, 3]. The clinical phenotype varies widely with an acute infantile form of early onset leading to rapid neuroregression and early death to a progressive later onset form compatible with a longer survival [2].

The human *HEXA* gene is mapped on chromosomes 15q23-q24 with 35.56 kb spans, containing 14 exons [4]. As per HGMD (Human Gene Mutation Database), nearly 170 mutations have been reported so far in the gene that causes TSD; that include 130 single base substitutions, 29 small deletions, 6 small insertions, 2 indels and 1 large deletion of 7.6 kb (http://www.hgmd.cf.ac.uk/). Of these only 7.6 kb deletion is reported as a largest one in *HEXA* gene which covers 70% of infantile TSD cases in French Canadians [5].

Our earlier studies on Indian patients affected with TSD revealed various novel and known missense, nonsense, splice site mutation and frameshift mutations [6, 7]. In the present study, Multiplex Ligation-dependent Probe Amplification (MLPA) - based approach (MRC-Holland, P199-B) was used to investigate for the potential occurrence of large *HEXA* deletions/duplications in addition to common mutation(s) screening and bidirectional sequencing of *HEXA* gene.

* Correspondence: jshethad1@gmail.com
[1]Biochemical and Molecular Genetics, FRIGE's Institute of Human Genetics, FRIGE House, Satellite, Ahmedabad, Gujarat 380 015, India
Full list of author information is available at the end of the article

Methods

The present study was carried out as a part of National Taskforce multicentric project of Indian Council of

Table 1 Clinical, biochemical and molecular details of the Indian patients with Tay–Sachs disease

Patient ID	Age at diagnosis (Months/ Sex	Native State	Cosan-guinity	Hex-A activity (MUGS) (nmol/ hr./mg) = (x)	Total Hex activity (MUG) = (y)	[a] Hex A % = (x/y) X 100	Genotypes		Phenotypes
							Nucleotide level (Allele from Father/ Allele from Mother)	Protein level (Allele from Father/ Allele from Mother)	
1	18/M	Gujarat	No	0.9	1292.1	0.07	Exon-2-3del/ Exon-2-3del	Not	Regression of milestone, cherry red spot, abnormal muscle tone, hyperacusis, seizures, abnormal MRI,
2	14/M	Gujarat	No	1.05	Not done	–	Exon-2-3del/ Exon-2-3del	Not applicable	Regression of milestone, cherry red spot, poor vision, abnormal muscle tone, hyperacusis, seizures, abnormal MRI, abnormal EEG
3	12/F	Gujarat	No	3.8	2185.7	0.17	c.1385A > T/Exon-1 deletion	p.E462V/ Not applicable	Regression of milestone, cherry red spot, abnormal muscle tone, seizures, hyperacusis, hearing impairment
4	13/F	Gujarat	No	2.5	1635	0.15	c.1385A > T/Exon-1 deletion	p.E462V/ Not applicable	Regression of milestone, hypotonia, hyperacusis, cherry red spot, abnormal MRI
5	13/ M	Karnataka	Yes	1.78	2198.2	0.08	c.1527-2 A > T/Exon-1 duplication	Not applicable	Regression of milestone, cherry red spot, hypotonia

Normal total-Hexosaminidase values using MUG substrate in our controls – 723 to 2700 nmol/hr./mg protein and normal Hex-A activity using MUGS substrate- 80 to 410 nmol/hr./mg

[a]The MUG/MUGS ratio for Hex A is 3.7:1 [10]

Medical Research (ICMR) and Department of Health Research (DHR), Government of India. The present study has been approved by the institutional ethics committee in accordance with the Helsinki declaration. A written informed consent was obtained from the parents before enrollment.

Patients

MLPA study was carried out in 5 enzymatically confirmed TSD patients for deletion/duplication analysis where disease causing mutation was not identified in the coding region of the gene and/or single disease causing allele was identified by common mutations screening and bi-directional sequencing of *HEXA* gene.

Multiplex ligation-dependent probe amplification (MLPA) analysis of *HEXA* gene

The genomic DNA was isolated from whole blood using salting out method [8]. MLPA analysis was carried out using P199-B2 HEXA P probe mix (MRC-Holland, Amsterdam, The Netherlands) in cases where Sanger sequencing failed to identify any pathological variant. The procedure was carried out according to the manufacturer's recommendations using100 ng of genomic DNA. It was denatured at 98 °C for 5 min and hybridized overnight at 60 °C with the SALSA probe mix P199-B2 (*HEXA* gene, exons 1-14). Samples were then treated for ligation for 15 min at 54 °C. The reaction was stopped by incubation at 98 °C for 5 min. Finally, PCR amplification was carried out with the specific SALSA FAM PCR primers. Amplification products were run on an ABI PRISM 3100 Genetic Analyzer (Applied Biosystems, USA). Copy number differences of various exons between test and control DNA samples were detected by analyzing the MLPA peak patterns.

Results

Molecular analysis was carried out in 75 TSD cases with deficiency of Hex-A and normal Total-Hex enzyme activity. Of these, 70 TSD patients have been identified with both coding mutations in *HEXA* gene while in 3 patients only one coding mutation was detected and in 2 patients no coding mutation was identified. Hence, MLPA study was carried out in these 5 unrelated patients to rule out copy number changes where heterozygous and/or homozygous disease causing variant could not be identified in the coding region by sequencing *HEXA* gene.

Consanguinity was present in 1/5 (20%) families. The mean age at presentation was 13.8 months (±2.48). All the cases were classified as infantile as they were presented with seizures, cherry red spot on the fundus, exaggerated startle, hypotonia, brisk deep tendon reflexes and regression of learned skill. The CT/MRI study of the brain was available in 3/5 cases and showed characteristic findings of a decrease in thalami and decreased attenuation of basal ganglia isodense with white matter, and one case had dysmyelination. A significant deficiency of Hex A activity was observed in the leukocytes of all five patients. The geographic/ethnic background, age at onset, age at last observation, enzyme activities and the genotypes identified are shown in Table 1.

The MLPA analysis of *HEXA* gene showed the presence of homozygous deletion of exon-2 and exon-3 in two patients, two patients showed compound heterozygosity for exon 1 deletion and missense mutation p.E462V as a second allele and one patient was identified with duplication of exon-1 with novel splice site variant c.1527-2A > T as a second allele (Table 2 and Fig. 1). In Silico analysis of the novel variant was identified as disease causing by Mutation taster and NNsplice site 0.9 algorithm.

Discussion

The clinical appearance and neuroimaging features of infantile TSD seen in our patients were consistent with the defined phenotype. All patients presented with the severe infantile form of the disease irrespective of the genotype. The results of enzyme activity measurements (Hex-A expressed as a percentage of Total-Hex activity)

Table 2 MPLA analysis for deletion/duplication study of *HEXA* gene

Patient ID	Deletions/ Duplications	No of Exons Deleted/ Duplicated	[c] MLPA probe ratio (Dosage quotient)	Clinical relevance
1	Homozygous deletions	2 (Exon 2 and 3)	0.0	Yes
2	Homozygous deletions	2 (Exon 2 and 3)	0.0	Yes
3[a]	Heterozygous deletion	1 (Exon 1)	0.5	Yes
4[a]	Heterozygous deletion	1 (Exon 1)	0.5	Yes
5[b]	Heterozygous duplication	1 (Exon 1)	1.3	Yes

[a]Compound heterozygous with p.E462V as a second allele
[b]Compound heterozygous with c.1527-2A > T as a second allele
[c]>MLPA ratios (dosage quotient) of below 0.7 or above 1.3 are indicative of a deletion (copy number change from two to one) or duplication (copy number change from two to three), respectively. A dosage quotient of 0.0 indicates a homozygous deletion, 0.35 to 0.65 indicates heterozygous deletion, 1.3 to 1.55 indicates heterozygous duplication and 1.7 to 2.2 indicates homozygous duplication

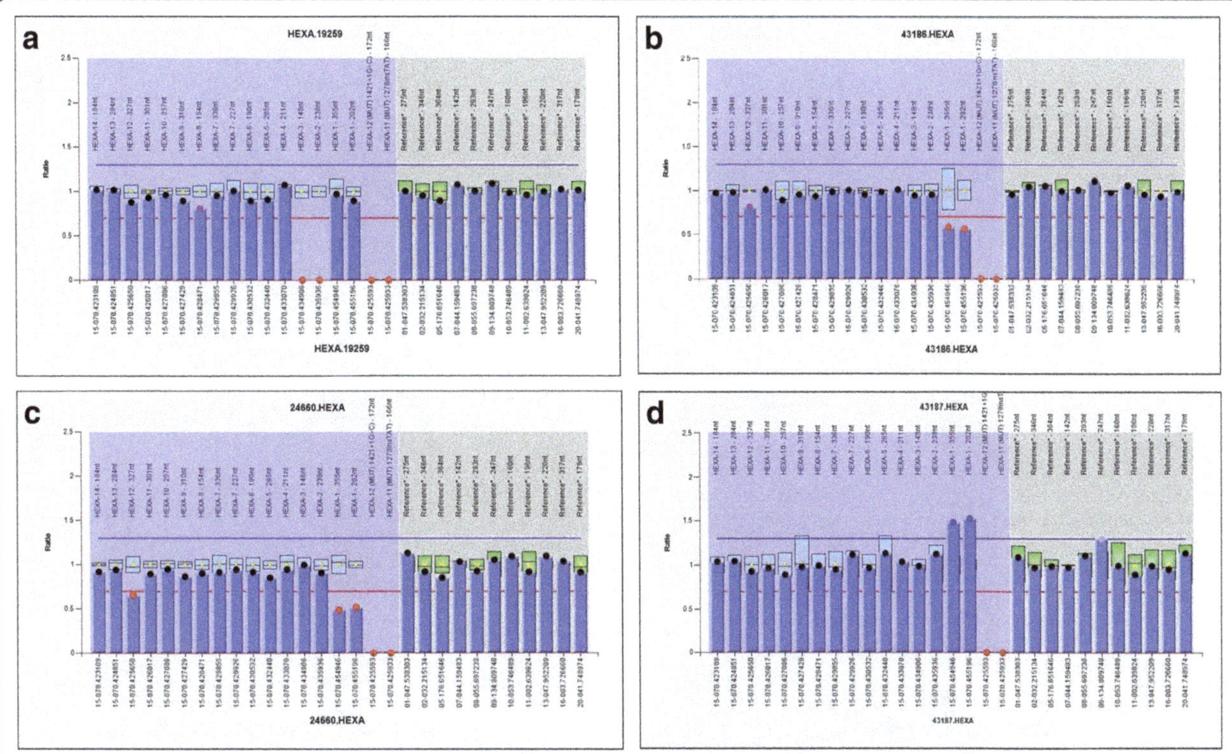

Fig. 1 MLPA analysis of *HEXA* gene (**a**): homozygous deletion of exon 2 & 3; (**b**) & (**c**): heterozygous deletion of exon 1; (**d**): heterozygous duplication of exon 1

varied from 0 to 0.2%. This is consistent with previous observations that infantile TSD patients have values ranging from 0 to 2% [9, 10].

During the course of the analysis we could not identify the second disease-causing allele in three patients and no variant was identified in two patients after sequencing the entire coding region of *HEXA* gene. Among the possible underlying reason for these findings, we suspected the presence of a deletion or duplication in the gene. Therefore using MLPA specific for *HEXA* gene we could identify two large deletions and one large duplication in an Indian TSD patients for the first time that include homozygous deletion of exon 2 & 3 in two cases, compound heterozygous deletion of exon-1 with second founder mutation p.E462V in two cases [6] and compound heterozygous duplication of exon-1 with second novel splice site variant c.1527-2A > T (Table 1). The carrier frequency of p.E462V mutation is ~ 1/500 which was earlier reported by Mistri et al. in 2012 [6]. In addition to this, recently the said variant was also reported only in one South Asian sample (http://gnomad.broadinstitute.org/variant/15-72638612-T-A). As has been known, the 7.6 kb deletion is the major mutation causing TSD in the French Canadian population; it removes part of intron-1, all of exon-1 and extends 2 kb upstream, encompassing the putative promoter region [4]. Although, this deletionwas never identified in our large cohort of Indian patient with TSD. Nonetheless, large deletion encompassing one or two exons or duplication of one exon are never reported and identified as a first disease causing variation in *HEXA* gene so far. Severity of phenotype in all five patients could be explained by the truncation of normal protein structure due to exon deletion/duplication in the gene.

This experimental approach of determination towards quantitative copy number variation in identifying large deletion and/or duplication is novel and reported here for the first time. The present study and earlier publications from our group [6, 7] also demonstrates that Indian TSD patients mainly portray infantile onset with severe phenotype irrespective of the genotype. None of our patients showed juvenile or late onset presentation. Though, it is highly likely that they are missed due to lack of awareness and failure of clinical identification as well. However, there are few mutations that have been identified in the late-onset phenotypes [11].

Conclusion

The present study demonstrates that large deletion and/or duplication in *HEXA* gene needs to be considered as the second tier approach in thegenomic sites where no variants are observed by conventional Sanger sequencing.

Abbreviations

Hex-A: β-hexosaminidase-A; LSDs: Lysosomal storage disorders; MLPA: Multiplex Ligation-dependent Probe Amplification; TSD: Tay-Sachs disease

Acknowledgements

We are grateful to the patients and their families who kindly agreed to participate in this study.

Funding

This work is supported by the Department of Health Research/Indian Council of Medical Research [grant no. BMS-54/2009], Government of India. Funding agency was not involved in the study design, specimen collection, analysis, interpretation of the data and preparation of the manuscript.

Authors' contributions

MM, JS were involved in the designing of the study, standardization of technical procedure, preparation of manuscript. MM was also involved in processing of sample for enzymes study and molecular analysis. JS will also act as a guarantor. MM, LM was involved in processing of samples for MLPA study. SM, MK, DS were involved in clinical information of all cases. FS has critically evaluated the manuscript. All the authors read and approved the manuscript.

Competing interests

The authors declare that they have no competing interests.

Author details

[1]Biochemical and Molecular Genetics, FRIGE's Institute of Human Genetics, FRIGE House, Satellite, Ahmedabad, Gujarat 380 015, India. [2]Medgenome Labs Pvt Ltd, Bangalore, India. [3]Usha Deep Hospital, Ahmedabad, Gujarat, India. [4]Mantra Child Neurology & Epilepsy Clinic, Bhavnagar, Gujarat, India. [5]Department of Pediatric Neurology, KLES Prabhakar Kore Hospital, Belgaum, Karnataka, India.

References

1. Sheth J, Mistri M, Sheth F, Shah R, Bavdekar A, Godbole K, et al. Burden of lysosomal storage disorders in India: experience of 387 affected children from a single diagnostic facility. JIMD Rep. 2014;12:51–63.
2. Gravel RA, Kaback MM, Proia RL, Sandhoff K, Suzuki K. The GM2 gangliosidosis. In: Scriver CR, Beaudet AL, Sly WS, Valle D, editors. The metabolic and molecular bases of inherited disease. New York: McGraw-Hill; 1995. p. 3827–76.
3. Sonnino S, Chigorno V. Ganglioside molecular species containing C18- and C20-sphingosine in mammalian nervous tissues and neuronal cell cultures. Biochim Biophys Acta. 2000;1469:63–77.
4. Proia L, Neufeld EF. Synthesis of beta-hexosaminidase in cell-free translation and in intact fibroblasts: an insoluble precursor alpha chain in a rare form of Tay-Sachs disease. Proc Nat Acad Sci. 1982;79:6360–4.
5. Myerowitz R, Hogikyan ND. Different mutations in Ashkenazi Jewish and non-Jewish French Canadians with Tay-Sachs disease. Science. 1986; 232(4758):1646–8.
6. Mistri M, Tamhankar P, Sheth F, Sanghavi D, Kondurkar P, Patil S, et al. Identification of novel mutations in *HEXA* gene in children affected with Tay Sachs disease from India. PLoS One. 2012;7(6):e39122.
7. Sheth J, Mistri M, Datar C, Kalane U, Patil S, Kamate M, et al. Expanding the spectrum of HEXA mutations in Indian patients with Tay-Sachs disease. Mol Genet Metab Rep. 2014;1:425–30.
8. Miller SA, Dykes DD. Polesky HF. A simple salting out procedure for extracting DNA from human nucleated cells. Nucleic Acids Res. 1988; 16(3):1215.
9. Kaback M, Desnick R. Pagon R, Bird T, Dolan C, Stephens K, editors. Hexosaminidase A Deficiency. Available from: http://www.ncbi.nlm.nih.gov/bookshelf/br.fcgi?book=gene&part=tay-sachs (Accessed 17 Sept 2017)
10. Hou Y, Tse R, Mahuran DJ. The direct determination of the substrate specificity of the α-active site in heterodimeric β-hexosaminidase a. Biochemistry. 1996;35:3963–9.
11. Mahuran DJ. Biochemical consequences of mutations causing the GM2 gangliosidosis. Biochem Biophys Acta. 1999;1455:105–38.

Clinical characteristics and spectrum of *NF1* mutations in 12 unrelated Chinese families with neurofibromatosis type 1

Bin Mao[1], Siyu Chen[1], Xin Chen[1], Xiumei Yu[2], Xiaojia Zhai[1], Tao Yang[1], Lulu Li[1], Zheng Wang[1], Xiuli Zhao[1*] and Xue Zhang[1*]

Abstract

Background: Neurofibromatosis type 1 (NF1) is a common autosomal dominant disorder caused by a heterozygous germline mutation in the tumor suppressor gene *NF1*. Because of the existence of highly homologous pseudogenes, the large size of the gene, and the heterogeneity of mutation types and positions, the detection of variations in NF1 is more difficult than that for an ordinary gene.

Methods: In this study, we collected samples from 23 patients among 46 study participants from 12 unrelated Chinese families with NF1. We used a combination of Sanger sequencing, targeted next-generation sequencing, and multiplex ligation-dependent probe amplification to identify potential mutations of different types.

Results: Seven recurrent mutations and four novel mutations were identified with the aforementioned methods, which were subsequently confirmed by either restriction fragment length polymorphism analysis or Sanger sequencing. Truncating mutations accounted for 73% (8/11) of all mutations identified. We also exhaustively investigated the clinical manifestations of NF1 in patients via acquired pathography, photographs and follow-up. However, no clear genotype–phenotype correlation has been found to date.

Conclusion: In conclusion, the novel mutations identified broaden the spectrum of *NF1* mutations in Chinese; however, obvious correlations between genotype and phenotype were not observed in this study.

Keywords: Neurofibromatosis type 1, The *NF1* gene, Clinical manifestations, Chinese

Background

Neurofibromatosis type 1 (NF1; MIM: 162200) is one of the most common autosomal dominant inherited diseases with an incidence of 1 in 2500–3000 individuals [1]. Caused by a germline heterozygous mutation in the tumor suppressor gene neurofibromin 1 (*NF1*; MIM: 613113) located on chromosome 17q11.2, NF1 is characterized by typical café-au-lait spots and cutaneous neurofibromas [2]. Individuals with NF1 are predisposed to plexiform neurofibromas, axillary and inguinal freckling, Lisch nodules of the iris, benign and malignant tumors, and renal artery stenosis, among a list of other abnormalities [3]. Although NF1 is a classical monogenic disease with complete penetrance by adulthood, clinical symptoms may vary in patients who come from the same family, or even for the same patient at different life stages. Complex though the clinical manifestations of patients may be, individuals in this study were diagnosed as NF1 only when they met two or more of the National Institutes of Health Diagnostic Criteria for NF1 [4].

NF1 is one of the largest known genes with a genomic size of 282 kb, consisting of 57 constitutive exons and three alternatively spliced exons [5]. Owing to its extremely frequent incidence of mutation (circa 1 in 10,000 gametes per generation) without obvious mutational hot spots, over 2600 *NF1* mutations have hitherto been reported in the Human Gene Mutation Database (HGMD). Single nucleotide substitutions and small deletions (20 bp or less) account for 71% of currently known mutations.

* Correspondence: xiulizhao@ibms.pumc.edu.cn; xuezhang@pumc.edu.cn
[1]Department of Medical Genetics, Institute of Basic Medical Sciences, Chinese Academy of Medical Sciences & School of Basic Medicine, Peking Union Medical College, Beijing 100005, China
Full list of author information is available at the end of the article

Moreover, approximately half of all NF1 cases are de novo mutations [6]. In addition, the large size of the *NF1* gene, the existence of homologous pseudogenes dispersed on other chromosomes [7], the diversity of mutation types and positions, and the great variety of lesions make traditional mutation detection in patients with NF1 a complicated, time-consuming and laborious process [8]. With the superiority of being high throughput and its rapidity, the next-generation sequencing can make up for any deficiency in the single Sanger sequencing method to some extent. In addition, multiplex ligation-dependent probe amplification (MLPA) for the detection of copy number was incorporated in our methods. Hence, we adopted various approaches such as Sanger sequencing, targeted next-generation sequencing, and MLPA so as to overcome challenges in the detection of *NF1* mutations in patients.

Despite several reports with regard to genotype–phenotype correlations in patients [9–11], the underlying causes of sophisticated clinical manifestations among patients have not yet been elucidated [12]. Nevertheless, the causes of polymorphisms in genotype–phenotype correlations may be assigned to modifier genes, gender, loss of heterozygosity (based on the two-hit hypothesis) [13], tumor microenvironment, and heterogeneity in the regulation of signaling pathways [3]. Consequently, it is of great significance to identify the causative mutation and assess the prognosis of NF1 patients, if genotype–phenotype correlations can be clarified, before the onset of symptoms.

In brief, we examined 12 non-consanguineous Chinese families from which patients were diagnosed with NF1. A molecular diagnosis and clinical characterization of NF1 patients were undertaken to identify causative mutations and evaluate any correlations between genotype and phenotype.

Methods

Patients

We studied 12 unrelated families with NF1 from different regions in China that included seven cases with positive family histories (Families 1–5 and 11–12; Fig. 1) and five sporadic cases (Families 6–10; Additional file 1: Figure S1), including 23 patients and 23 unaffected individuals. Peripheral blood samples of all 46 participants, as well as clinical data and photographs of patients, were obtained after written informed consent from all participants and from parents or legal guardians of children under the age of 18. Long-term follow-up was also performed with several contactable patients to evaluate progression of the disease. Age of patients was recorded at their last visit in this study. This study was approved by the Institutional Review Board (IRB) of the Institute of Basic Medical Sciences, Chinese Academy of Medical Sciences, Beijing, China (015–2015).

Sanger sequencing

For earlier probands in Families 1–8 and other study participants in Families 4–12, the identification and verification of mutations were carried out with conventional Sanger sequencing. Genomic DNA was extracted by a traditional proteinase K and phenol/chloroform method. Genomic DNA and cDNA reference sequences of *NF1* (hg19; NM_000267.3) were downloaded from

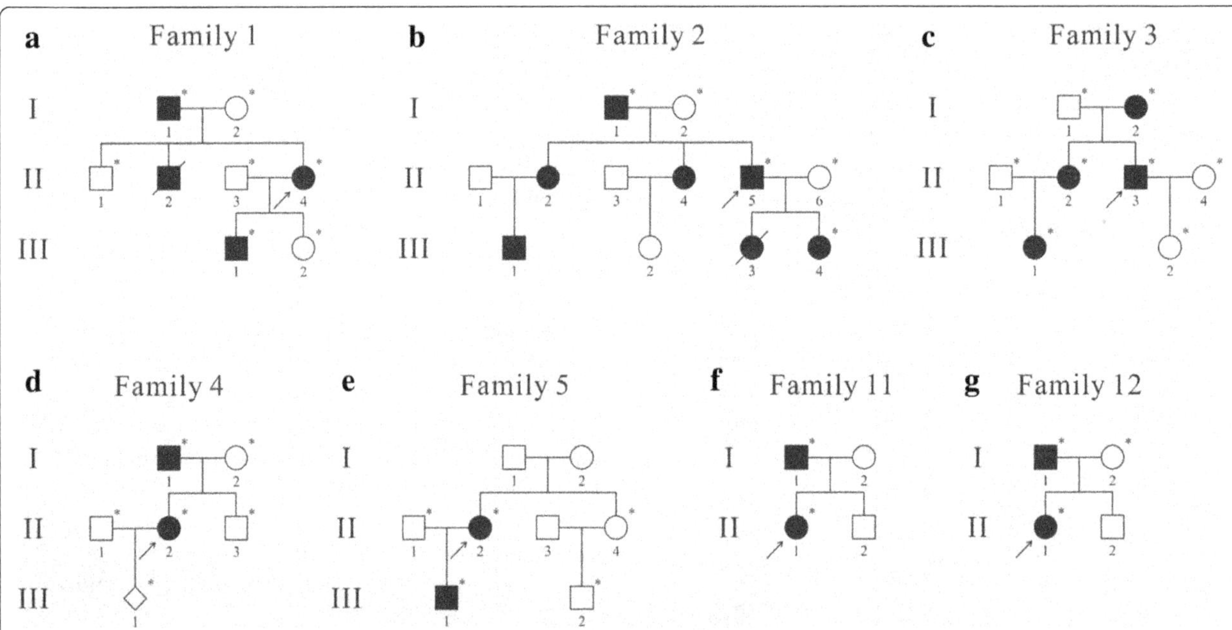

Fig. 1 Pedigrees of families with positive family histories. The arrows indicate the probands in each family. The asterisks denote that peripheral blood samples of individuals had been acquired. **a-g**: Pedigrees of Families 1-5 and 11–12

the University of California, Santa Cruz (UCSC) Genome Browser. Primers were designed via Primer Premier 5 (version 5.00; PREMIER Biosoft, Palo Alto, CA, USA) to amplify and sequence exons and flanking intronic regions of *NF1* (Additional file 1: Table S1). The specificity of the primers was checked using the UCSC Genome Browser BLAT and *In-Silico* PCR online tools. Sequencing data was analyzed using CodonCode Aligner (version 6.0.2.6; CodonCode, Centerville, MA, USA).

Targeted next-generation sequencing

The mutation identification of later probands in Families 9–12 was performed through targeted next-generation sequencing. A NimbleGen capture panel (Roche, Basel, Switzerland) was designed and assessed to detect potential variants in the probands. The capture panel comprised 10,308 bp that covered all exons together with flanking intronic regions (± 15 bp) of the *NF1* and *NF2* genes.

Genomic DNA was extracted using a QIAamp DNA Blood Midi Kit (QIAGEN, Hilden, Germany) in accordance with the manufacturer's instructions. Genomic DNA was then fragmented for the paired-end library (200–250 bp) using an ultrasonicator LE220 (Covaris, Woburn, MA, USA). The library was enriched through array hybridization at 47 °C for 64–72 h, with elution and post-capture amplification afterwards. The library was then inspected using a 2100 Bioanalyzer (Agilent, Santa Clara, CA, USA) and ABI StepOne (Thermo Fisher Scientific, Waltham, MA, USA) to estimate the size, concentration, and magnitude of the enrichment of the reads.

After the assessment of read quality, captured library sequencing was implemented on a HiSeq2500 System high-throughput sequencing system (Illumina, San Diego, CA, USA) for 90 cycles per read following the manufacturer's instructions. Image analysis, error estimation and base calling were performed with Pipeline software (version 1.3.4; Illumina) to generate raw data.

MLPA

For the proband in whom a causative mutation was not identified by Sanger sequencing or targeted next-generation sequencing, P081 (version C1) and P082 (version C1) MLPA probemixes (MRC-Holland, Amsterdam, the Netherlands) were applied to detect copy number variation in conformity with the manufacturer's instructions. Capillary electrophoresis results of MLPA samples were analyzed by Coffalyser.Net software (version 140,721.1958; MRC-Holland).

Bioinformatics analysis

The raw data from targeted next-generation sequencing was screened by filtering criteria to remove low-quality and contaminated reads [14]. Reads were then aligned to the human genome reference (hg19) by a Burrows Wheeler Aligner–backtrack software package [15]. The sequencing coverage and depth of the target region, single nucleotide variant (SNV) and indel calling, were analyzed after alignment. Software Short Oligonucleotide Analysis Package–snp (version 1.03; Beijing Genomics Institute, Beijing, China) [16] and Sequence Alignment/Map tools (version 1.4) [17] were used to detect SNVs and indels, respectively. After acquisition of the allele frequency from the UCSC Genome and ExAC Browsers database to eliminate the possibility of single nucleotide polymorphism (SNP), we consulted the HGMD and other references to study relevant reports about screened variants in all probands.

For missense variants, the online tools Polymorphism Phenotyping v2 (PolyPhen-2) [18], Scale-Invariant Feature Transform (SIFT) [19], and Mutation Taster [20] were utilized to predict the pathogenicity of each variant. Multiple sequence alignment and conservative analysis were performed by ClustalX software (version 2.1; Conway Institute, University College Dublin, Dublin, Republic of Ireland). The amino acid sequences of human neurofibromin (NP_000258.1) and that of 11 different vertebrates were obtained from the National Center for Biotechnology Information (NCBI) protein database (FASTA format). For frame shift variants (small deletions and single nucleotide duplication), DNAMAN (version 5.2.2; Lynnon Biosoft, San Ramon, CA, USA) was used to predict how the reading frame was interrupted and to calculate the number of nucleotides before a premature stop codon.

Restriction fragment length polymorphism

Restriction fragment length polymorphism (RFLP) was used, together with nested PCR and restriction endonuclease, to discriminate between genotypes of patients and that of unaffected individuals in Families 1–3 with larger pedigrees. In addition to the primers used for Sanger sequencing, nested PCR primers were designed to enhance the specificity of small DNA fragments or to introduce a mismatch nucleotide to create a new restriction site (Additional file 1: Table S1). Sequence differences between wild-type and mutant alleles resulted in the gain or loss of a restriction site that led to size differences between amplicons of different alleles after the restriction endonuclease reaction. The restriction endonucleases (New England Biolabs, Ipswich, MA, USA) *Taq*$^{\alpha}$ I (restriction site: T|CGA), *Alu* I (restriction site: AG|CT), and *Sac* II (restriction site: CCGC|GG) were applied to Families 1, 2, and 3, respectively. Polyacrylamide gel electrophoresis (PAGE) using an 8% neutral polyacrylamide gel was then performed to separate DNA fragments of different sizes. Electrophoresis conditions included 1 × TBE as electrophoresis buffer and a constant voltage of

Table 1 Available clinical symptoms of NF1 patients

Family number	Family history	Patient number	Pedigree number	Age	Gender	Number of café-au-lait spots	Largest diameter of café-au-lait spots	Number of NFs	Largest Diameter of NFs	Plexiform NFs	Axillary/Inguinal Freckling	Location of Skin Lesions
1	Yes	1	II-4	35–39	Female	7	5.5 cm	300–400	3.5 cm	Yes	Yes	Trunk, Neck, Chin, Forehead
		2	III-1	15–19	Male	N/A						
		3	I-1	75–79	Male	5	4 cm	200–300	2 cm	Yes	Yes	Trunk, Neck, Chin, Cheek
2	Yes	4	II-5	25–29	Male	13	5.5 cm	10–20	1.5 cm	No	Yes	Trunk
		5	III-4	0–4	Female	3	2.5 cm	0	–	No	No	Trunk, Lower Limbs
		6	I-1	55–59	Male	N/A						
3	Yes	7	II-3	50–54	Male	9	6 cm	300–400	2 cm	Yes	Yes	Trunk, Limbs, Neck, Chin
		8	II-2	40–44	Female	N/A						
		9	III-1	10–14	Female	N/A						
		10	I-2	65–69	Female	3	5 cm	1000–2000	3 cm	Yes	Yes	Trunk, Limbs
4	Yes	11	II-2	25–29	Female	13	4.5 cm	10–20	2 cm	No	Yes	Trunk, Lower Limbs
		12	I-1	45–49	Male	14	5 cm	20–30	2 cm	No	Yes	Trunk, Limbs
5	Yes	13	II-2	45–49	Female	12	4 cm	50–100	1.5 cm	No	Yes	Trunk, Lower Limbs, Neck
		14	III-1	10–14	Male	N/A						
6	No	15	II-1	15–19	Female	28	7 cm	0	–	No	Yes	Trunk, Upper Limbs
7	No	16	II-1	40–44	Female	14	4.5 cm	50–100	1.5 cm	Yes	Yes	Trunk, Limbs
8	No	17	II-1	15–19	Female	34	5 cm	0	–	No	Yes	Trunk, Limbs
9	No	18	II-1	30–34	Female	9	7.5 cm	200–300	2.5 cm	Yes	Yes	Trunk
10	No	19	II-1	30–34	Female	7	3.5 cm	0	–	No	Yes	Trunk, Neck
11	Yes	20	II-1	25–29	Female	16	4 cm	100–200	1.5 cm	No	Yes	Trunk, Neck
		21	I-1	45–49	Male	N/A						
12	Yes	22	II-1	25–29	Female	8	6.5 cm	100–200	1 cm	No	Yes	Trunk, Limbs, Neck, Forehead
		23	I-1	55–59	Male	6	3 cm	200–300	1.5 cm	No	Yes	Trunk, Upper Limbs

NFs neurofibromas, *N/A* not available

350 V for 3–5 h. Silver staining was used for the final step of the chromogenic reaction.

Results

Clinical manifestations

A general description of the clinical manifestations of 23 NF1 patients are listed in Table 1, with typical symptoms shown in Fig. 2. It is regrettable that on account of advanced age, geographical distances, or for personal reasons, the detailed clinical data and photographs of six patients (Patients 2, 6, 8, 9, 14 and 21) were not available except for their peripheral blood samples. Of the readily obtained clinical symptoms of the remaining 17 patients, café-au-lait spots were observed in all 17 patients and were found spotted in one or more skin regions immediately after birth in Patients 1, 5, 7, 11, 15, 16, 17, 19, 20 and 22. Axillary or inguinal freckling was the second most common phenotype that accounted for 94% (16/17) of cases. Additionally, 13 (76%) patients suffered from cutaneous neurofibromas, six (35%) of which were also found to have plexiform neurofibromas. In terms of the location of skin lesions, these were present on the trunk in all 17 (100%) patients, followed by limbs (upper and lower limbs) in 11 (65%), neck in seven (41%) and face (chin, forehead and cheek) in four (24%).

NF1 mutation Spectrum

We identified 11 different germline mutations in probands from the 12 families mentioned above; these were located in different exons across the gene (Fig. 3 and Table 2). In other words, a mutational hot spot was not detected according to our findings. Remarkably, the proportion of truncating mutations approached 73% (8/11), and was composed of four (36%) nonsense mutations (c.1246C>T, p.R416*; c.2062G>T, p.E688*; c.3826C>T, p.R1276*; c.6102C>A, p.C2034*), three (27%) small deletions (c.4802delT, p.L1601Cfs*2; c.5428delT, p.W1810Gfs*32; c.1754_1757delTAAC, p.T586Vfs*18), and one (9%) single nucleotide duplication (c.6791dupA, p.Y2264*). In addition, the remaining three (27%) variants were all missense mutations (c.5791T>C, p.W1931R; c.4469T>C, p.L1490P; c.1885G>A, p.G629R). For the proband in Family 12 (Patient 22) in whom a causative mutation was not identified by targeted next-generation sequencing, an

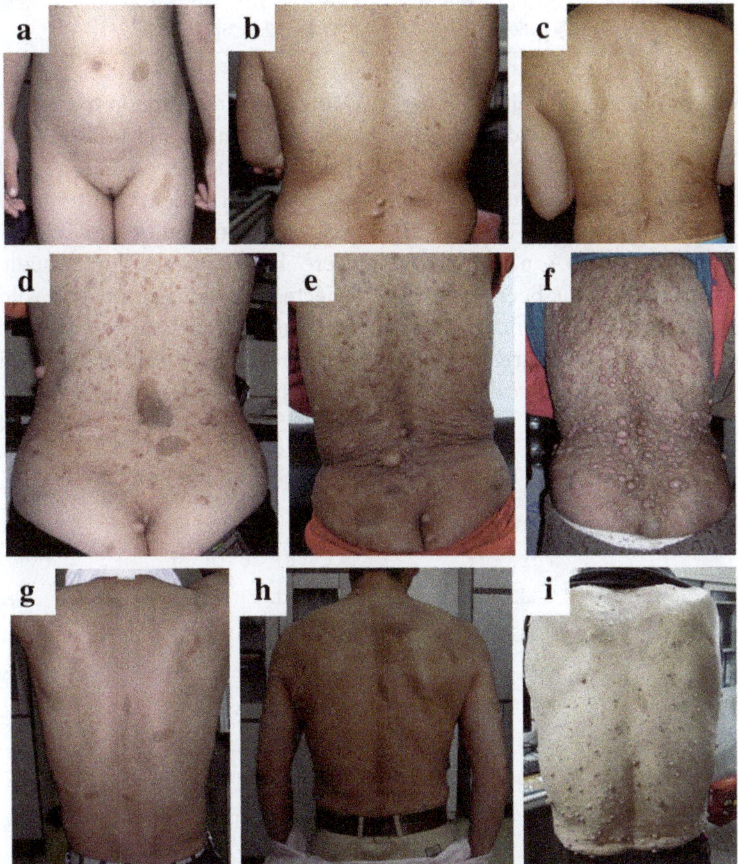

Fig. 2 Clinical signs of NF1 in several patients. **a**: Café-au-lait spots on the abdomen and left leg of prepubertal female Patient 17; **b**–**i**: Café-au-lait spots and neurofibromas on the back of postpubertal females without (Patients 11 and 20) or with (Patients 18, 1, and 10) histories of pregnancy, and postpubertal males (Patients 4, and 7 in 2007 and 2017, respectively)

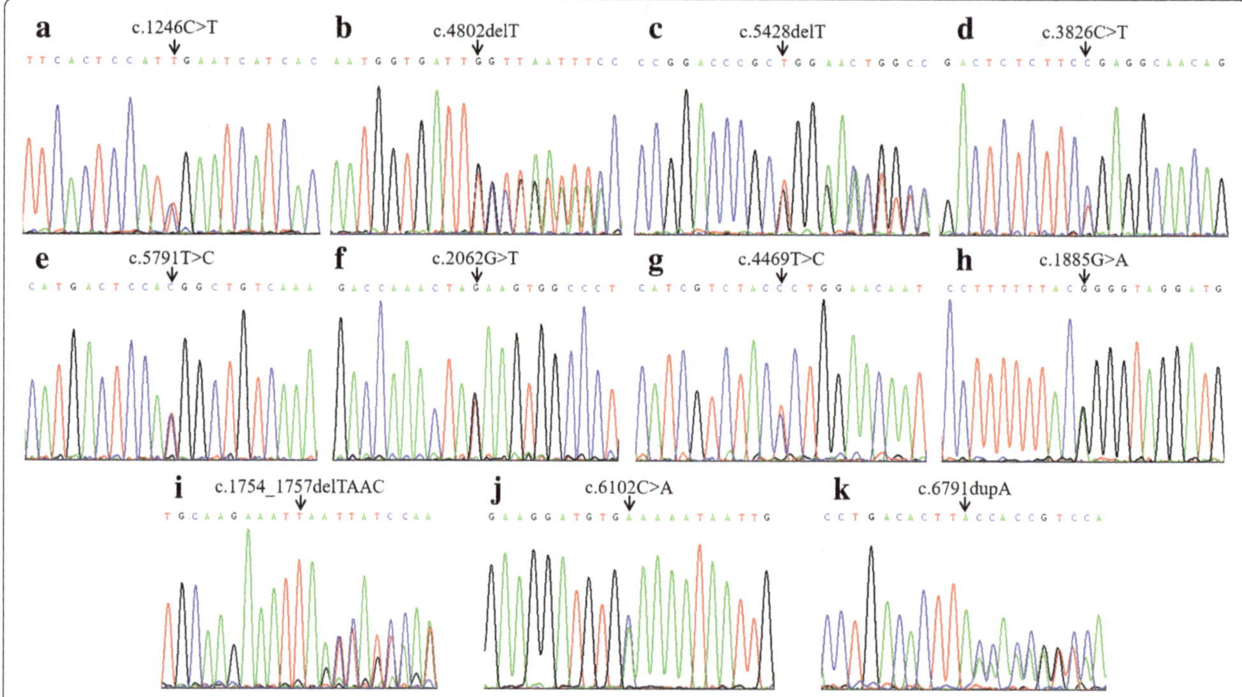

Fig. 3 Mutations identified in the probands of Families 1–11. Mutations detected by Sanger sequencing: **a**: Patient 1, c.1246C>T; **b**: Patient 4, c.4802delT; **c**: Patient 7, c.5428delT; **d**: Patient 11, c.3826C>T; **e**: Patient 13, c.5791T>C; **f**: Patient 15, c.2062G>T; **g**: Patient 16, c.4469T>C; **h**: Patient 17 c.1885G>A; **i**: Patient 18, c.1754_1757delTAAC; **j**: Patient 19, c.6102C>A; **k**: Patient 20, c.6791dupA

abnormal copy number was not detected in either Patient 22 or her father (Patient 23) using MLPA (Additional file 1: Figure S2).

Furthermore, the mutations we identified in Families 2 (c.4802delT, p.L1601Cfs*2), 3 (c.5428delT, p.W1810Gfs*32), 6 (c.2062G>T, p.E688*), and 10 (c.6102C>A, p.C2034*), respectively, as far as we know, have not been reported previously. It is noteworthy that the four novel mutations are all truncating mutations that are generally considered to introduce a premature stop codon in the reading frame.

Mutation verification in the families

For individuals in Families 1–3, a nested PCR–restriction endonuclease reaction–neutral PAGE method was adopted. All patients in the three families were found to carry the same mutation as that of the probands, and were heterozygotes for mutant alleles, while all unaffected individuals only had wild-type alleles (Fig. 4).

Sanger sequencing was performed to verify mutations in individuals of Families 4–11. It turned out that other patients in the families all carried mutations identical to that of the probands, while unaffected individuals were

Table 2 NF1 mutations identified in this study

Family Number	Mutation Position	Nucleotide Change	Amino Acid Change	Mutation Type	References
1	Exon 11	c.1246C>T	p.R416*	Nonsense	Reported[a]
2	Exon 36	c.4802delT	p.L1601Cfs*2	Deletion	Novel
3	Exon 37	c.5428delT	p.W1810Gfs*32	Deletion	Novel
4	Exon 28	c.3826C>T	p.R1276*	Nonsense	Reported
5	Exon 39	c.5791T>C	p.W1931R	Missense	Reported
6	Exon 18	c.2062G>T	p.E688*	Nonsense	Novel
7	Exon 33	c.4469T>C	p.L1490P	Missense	Reported
8	Exon 17	c.1885G>A	p.G629R	Missense	Reported
9	Exon 16	c.1754_1757delTAAC	p.T586Vfs*18	Deletion	Reported
10	Exon 41	c.6102C>A	p.C2034*	Nonsense	Novel
11	Exon 45	c.6791dupA	p.Y2264*	Duplication	Reported

[a]The mutation has been reported in the Human Gene Mutation Database (HGMD; Professional 2016.4)

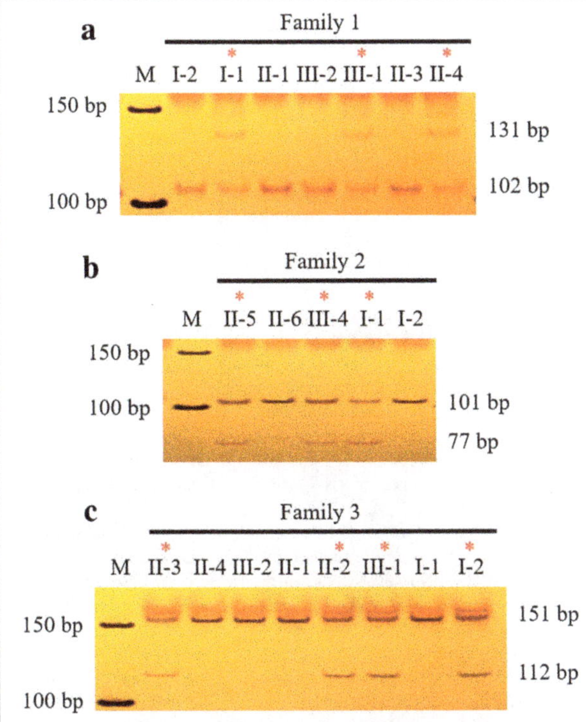

Fig. 4 Neutral polyacrylamide gel electrophoresis (PAGE) of DNA samples from all study participants in Families 1–3. A 50-bp DNA Ladder was used as a marker (lane M). Red asterisks denote affected individuals. The numbers on the left and right of the figures represent the size of markers and DNA fragments, respectively. **a**: Neutral PAGE of DNA samples from participants in Family 1. The wild-type allele had a *Taq*$^{\alpha}$ I restriction site, and was therefore digested into 29-bp (not shown) and 102-bp fragments; **b**: Neutral PAGE of DNA samples from participants in Family 2. The mutation c.4802delT resulted in a gain of the *Alu* I restriction site after the forward primer (*NF1*-family 2F; Additional file 1: Table S1) introduced a mismatch nucleotide in its 3′ end, and the mutant allele was subsequently digested into 24-bp (not shown) and 77-bp fragments; **c**: Neutral PAGE of DNA samples from participants in Family 3. The mutant allele was digested into 39-bp (not shown) and 112-bp fragments by *Sac* II since the deletion of thymidylate produced a new restriction site

all homozygotes for wild-type alleles (data available on request).

Genotype–phenotype correlations

Patients who had rather serious clinical manifestations (from Families 1, 3 and 9) were all heterozygotes for the truncating mutation. However, other patients with milder symptoms carried similar truncating or missense mutations. Furthermore, patients who carried the same mutation within the one family exhibited diverse clinical symptoms. For example, Patient III-3 in Family 2 (samples not available), whose father (II-5; Patient 4) merely manifested moderate symptoms, died of acute infantile spasm 10.5 months after birth as a complication of NF1, while her affected sister (III-4; Patient 5) fortunately survived. Moreover, the phenotype of Patient 1 was slightly more severe than that of her father (Patient 3).

Discussion

In this study, we utilized a synthetic method of Sanger sequencing, targeted next-generation sequencing, and MLPA to detect potential mutations in patients. We also investigated the clinical presentations of each patient with NF1 to elucidate the factors associated with the severity of the disease phenotype.

As a consequence, 11 different mutations scattered in different exons of *NF1* were identified in 12 unrelated Chinese families with NF1, suggesting a positive detection rate of 92% (11/12). Though no mutational hot spot was discovered, our attention was drawn to the observation that about three quarters of the mutations identified were truncating mutations. Consequently, a truncated neurofibromin with a partial or absolute functional loss may be produced, or the protein may become degraded as a result of its abnormal termination, resulting in the inactivation of the negative regulatory protein. Therefore, the pathogenicity of the four novel truncating mutations that we identified is proverbially acknowledged because of a prematurely disrupted reading frame. Furthermore, we detected three different missense mutations that had been previously reported [21–26]. Nonetheless, multiple sequence alignment and in silico analysis were still performed to authenticate their pathogenicity (Additional file 1: Figure S3 and Table S2). Moreover, for Family 12 in whom a causative mutation was not found by either targeted next-generation sequencing or MLPA, we conjectured the existence of a deep intronic mutation.

Maruoka et al. [27] described a c.6853_6854insA (hg19; NM_001042492.2) *NF1* mutation that was identical to the mutation we found in Family 11 (Table 2). However, we thought a description of c.6791dupA (hg19; NM_000267.3) rather than c.6790_6791insA may be more appropriate in keeping with the standard human sequence variant nomenclature of the Human Genome Sequence Variation Society (HGVS) [28] and Mutalyzer website (version 2.0.23; Leiden University Medical Center, Leiden, the Netherlands) [29]. Likewise, the amino acid change in the c.1754_1757delTAAC mutation in Family 9 (Table 2) should be depicted as p.T586Vfs*18 [30], instead of p.L585fs*18 [31].

According to our observations, clinical manifestations in patients who had the same mutation within a family, and the same patient at different stages of their life, may be highly discrepant. Additionally, with regard to the polymorphisms in genotype–phenotype correlations, possible causes may be modifier genes, gender, or heterogeneity in the regulation of signaling pathways, to name a few.

Alterable though the phenotype of NF1 may be, the progression of NF1 was ascribed to age and pregnancy according to a long-term follow-up of several contactable patients. In general, it was older patients who usually manifested severer symptoms, while prepubertal patients displayed a comparatively mild phenotype with only café-au-lait spots. For example, Patient 7's symptoms gradually worsened in the form of an increase in the number and size of cutaneous neurofibromas during a 10-year observation period (from 2007 to 2017; Fig. 2). Patients 1, 7, 16, 20 and 22 recalled that cutaneous neurofibromas appeared and symptoms became worse in their adolescence. Furthermore, some females with NF1 (Patients 1, 8, 10 and 18) complained of a marked exacerbation of disease after pregnancy (Fig. 2), as also described by Griffiths et al. [32]. These observations indicated that a patient's physical condition, particularly their hormone levels, played a vital role in the development of NF1.

Conclusions

Our research, via an integrated methodology, extends the *NF1* mutation spectrum in the Chinese population. Although a comprehensive investigation of the clinical profiles of patients was undertaken, we rarely found correlations between genotype and phenotype in NF1. Nevertheless, we noticed during follow-up observation that age and hormone levels were associated with the severity of disease.

Abbreviations

HGMD: Human Gene Mutation Database; *HGVS*: Human Genome Sequence Variation Society; *IRB*: Institutional Review Board; *MLPA*: multiplex ligation-dependent probe amplification; *NCBI*: National Center for Biotechnology Information; *NF1*: neurofibromatosis type 1; *PAGE*: polyacrylamide gel electrophoresis; *PolyPhen-2*: Polymorphism Phenotyping v2; *RFLP*: restriction fragment length polymorphism; *SIFT*: Scale-Invariant Feature Transform; *SNP*: single nucleotide polymorphism; *SNV*: single nucleotide variant; *UCSC*: University of California, Santa Cruz

Acknowledgments

We thank all patients and their families for their participation in this study.

Funding

This work was supported by the National Key Research and Development Program of China (2016YFC0905100) to Xue Zhang and Xiuli Zhao.

Authors' contributions

BM, SYC, XC and XJZ performed the experiments; BM, SYC, XC, XJZ, TY, LLL and ZW analyzed the data; XLZ and XMY studied the patients and collected the clinical samples; BM drafted and wrote the manuscript; XZ and XLZ designed the study. All authors read and approved the final manuscript.

Competing interests

The authors declare that they have no competing interests.

Author details

[1]Department of Medical Genetics, Institute of Basic Medical Sciences, Chinese Academy of Medical Sciences & School of Basic Medicine, Peking Union Medical College, Beijing 100005, China. [2]Department of Obstetrics and Gynecology, the First Affiliated Hospital of Hebei North University, Zhangjiakou 075061, China.

References

1. Williams VC, Lucas J, Babcock MA, Gutmann DH, Korf B, Maria BL. Neurofibromatosis type 1 revisited. Pediatrics. 2009;123(1):124–33.
2. Lin X, Chen H, Zhu W, Lian S. A novel frameshift mutation of the NF1 gene in a Chinese pedigree with neurofibromatosis type 1. Indian J Dermatol Venereol Leprol. 2017;83(2):231–3.
3. Monroe CL, Dahiya S, Gutmann DH. Dissecting clinical heterogeneity in Neurofibromatosis type 1. Annu Rev Pathol. 2017;12:53–74.
4. Neurofibromatosis. Conference statement. National Institutes of Health consensus development conference. Arch Neurol. 1988;45(5):575–8.
5. Hinman MN, Sharma A, Luo G, Lou H. Neurofibromatosis type 1 alternative splicing is a key regulator of Ras signaling in neurons. Mol Cell Biol. 2014; 34(12):2188–97.
6. Valero MC, Pascual-Castroviejo I, Velasco E, Moreno F, Hernandez-Chico C. Identification of de novo deletions at the NF1 gene: no preferential paternal origin and phenotypic analysis of patients. Hum Genet. 1997;99(6):720–6.
7. Luijten M, Redeker S, Minoshima S, Shimizu N, Westerveld A, Hulsebos TJ. Duplication and transposition of the NF1 pseudogene regions on chromosomes 2, 14, and 22. Hum Genet. 2001;109(1):109–16.
8. Cunha KS, Oliveira NS, Fausto AK, de Souza CC, Gros A, Bandres T, Idrissi Y, Merlio JP, de Moura Neto RS, Silva R, et al. Hybridization capture-based next-generation sequencing to evaluate coding sequence and deep Intronic mutations in the NF1 gene. Genes. 2016;7(12):133.
9. Alkindy A, Chuzhanova N, Kini U, Cooper DN, Upadhyaya M. Genotype-phenotype associations in neurofibromatosis type 1 (NF1): an increased risk of tumor complications in patients with NF1 splice-site mutations? Hum Genomics. 2012;6:12.
10. Upadhyaya M, Ruggieri M, Maynard J, Osborn M, Hartog C, Mudd S, Penttinen M, Cordeiro I, Ponder M, Ponder BA, et al. Gross deletions of the neurofibromatosis type 1 (NF1) gene are predominantly of maternal origin and commonly associated with a learning disability, dysmorphic features and developmental delay. Hum Genet. 1998;102(5):591–7.
11. Upadhyaya M, Huson SM, Davies M, Thomas N, Chuzhanova N, Giovannini S, Evans DG, Howard E, Kerr B, Griffiths S, et al. An absence of cutaneous neurofibromas associated with a 3-bp inframe deletion in exon 17 of the NF1 gene (c.2970-2972 delAAT): evidence of a clinically significant NF1 genotype-phenotype correlation. Am J Hum Genet. 2007;80(1):140–51.
12. Faden DL, Asthana S, Tihan T, DeRisi J, Kliot M. Whole exome sequencing of growing and non-growing cutaneous Neurofibromas from a single patient with Neurofibromatosis type 1. PLoS One. 2017;12(1):e0170348.
13. Emmerich D, Zemojtel T, Hecht J, Krawitz P, Spielmann M, Kuhnisch J, Kobus K, Osswald M, Heinrich V, Berlien P, et al. Somatic neurofibromatosis type 1 (NF1) inactivation events in cutaneous neurofibromas of a single NF1 patient. Eur J Hum Genet. 2015;23(6):870–3.
14. Wei X, Ju X, Yi X, Zhu Q, Qu N, Liu T, Chen Y, Jiang H, Yang G, Zhen R, et al. Identification of sequence variants in genetic disease-causing genes using targeted next-generation sequencing. PLoS One. 2011;6(12):e29500.
15. Li H, Durbin R. Fast and accurate short read alignment with burrows-wheeler transform. Bioinformatics (Oxford, England). 2009;25(14):1754–60.
16. Li R, Li Y, Fang X, Yang H, Wang J, Kristiansen K, Wang J. SNP detection for massively parallel whole-genome resequencing. Genome Res. 2009;19(6): 1124–32.
17. Li H, Handsaker B, Wysoker A, Fennell T, Ruan J, Homer N, Marth G, Abecasis G, Durbin R. Genome project data processing S: the sequence alignment/map format and SAMtools. Bioinformatics (Oxford, England). 2009;25(16):2078–9.

18. Adzhubei IA, Schmidt S, Peshkin L, Ramensky VE, Gerasimova A, Bork P, Kondrashov AS, Sunyaev SR. A method and server for predicting damaging missense mutations. Nat Methods. 2010;7(4):248–9.
19. Ng PC, Henikoff S. Predicting deleterious amino acid substitutions. Genome Res. 2001;11(5):863–74.
20. Schwarz JM, Cooper DN, Schuelke M, Seelow D. MutationTaster2: mutation prediction for the deep-sequencing age. Nat Methods. 2014;11(4):361–2.
21. Hudson J, Wu CL, Tassabehji M, Summers EM, Simon S, Super M, Donnai D, Thakker N. Novel and recurrent mutations in the neurofibromatosis type 1 (NF1) gene. Hum Mutat. 1997;9(4):366–7.
22. van Minkelen R, van Bever Y, Kromosoeto JN, Withagen-Hermans CJ, Nieuwlaat A, Halley DJ, van den Ouweland AM. A clinical and genetic overview of 18 years neurofibromatosis type 1 molecular diagnostics in the Netherlands. Clin Genet. 2014;85(4):318–27.
23. Duat Rodriguez A, Martos Moreno GA, Martin Santo-Domingo Y, Hernandez Martin A, Espejo-Saavedra Roca JM, Ruiz-Falco Rojas ML, Argente J: Phenotypic and genetic features in neurofibromatosis type 1 in children. Anales de pediatria (Barcelona, Spain : 2003) 2015, 83(3):173–182.
24. Gasparini P, D'Agruma L, Pio de Cillis G, Balestrazzi P, Mingarelli R, Zelante L. Scanning the first part of the neurofibromatosis type 1 gene by RNA-SSCP: identification of three novel mutations and of two new polymorphisms. Hum Genet. 1996;97(4):492–5.
25. Kiel C, Serrano L. Structure-energy-based predictions and network modelling of RASopathy and cancer missense mutations. Mol Syst Biol. 2014;10:727.
26. Kim MJ, Cheon CK. Neurofibromatosis type 1: a single center's experience in Korea. Korean J Pediatr. 2014;57(9):410–5.
27. Maruoka R, Takenouchi T, Torii C, Shimizu A, Misu K, Higasa K, Matsuda F, Ota A, Tanito K, Kuramochi A, et al. The use of next-generation sequencing in molecular diagnosis of neurofibromatosis type 1: a validation study. Genet Test Mol Biomarkers. 2014;18(11):722–35.
28. den Dunnen JT, Dalgleish R, Maglott DR, Hart RK, Greenblatt MS, McGowan-Jordan J, Roux AF, Smith T, Antonarakis SE, Taschner PE. HGVS recommendations for the description of sequence variants: 2016 update. Hum Mutat. 2016;37(6):564–9.
29. Wildeman M, van Ophuizen E, den Dunnen JT, Taschner PE. Improving sequence variant descriptions in mutation databases and literature using the Mutalyzer sequence variation nomenclature checker. Hum Mutat. 2008; 29(1):6–13.
30. Hutter S, Piro RM, Waszak SM, Kehrer-Sawatzki H, Friedrich RE, Lassaletta A, Witt O, Korbel JO, Lichter P, Schuhmann MU, et al. No correlation between NF1 mutation position and risk of optic pathway glioma in 77 unrelated NF1 patients. Hum Genet. 2016;135(5):469–75.
31. Upadhyaya M, Spurlock G, Majounie E, Griffiths S, Forrester N, Baser M, Huson SM, Gareth Evans D, Ferner R. The heterogeneous nature of germline mutations in NF1 patients with malignant peripheral serve sheath tumours (MPNSTs). Hum Mutat. 2006;27(7):716.
32. Griffiths S, Thompson P, Frayling I, Upadhyaya M. Molecular diagnosis of neurofibromatosis type 1: 2 years experience. Familial Cancer. 2007; 6(1):21–34.

17

Heterozygous versus homozygous phenotype caused by the same *MC4R* mutation: novel mutation affecting a large consanguineous kindred

Max Drabkin[1], Ohad S. Birk[1,2*] and Ruth Birk[3*]

Abstract

Background: The hypothalamic G-protein-coupled-receptor melanocortin-4 receptor (MC4R) is a key player in the central circuit regulating energy expenditure and appetite. Heterozygous loss-of-function *MC4R* mutations are the most common known genetic cause of monogenic human obesity, with more than 200 mutations described to date, affecting 2–3% of the population in various cohorts tested. Homozygous or compound heterozygous *MC4R* mutations are much less frequent, and only few families have been described in which heterozygotes and homozygotes of the same mutation are found.

Methods: We performed exome sequencing in a consanguineous Bedouin family with morbid obesity to identify the genetic cause of the disease. Clinical examination and biochemical assays were done to delineate the phenotype.

Results: We report the frequency of *MC4R* mutations in the large inbred Bedouin Israeli population. Furthermore, we describe consanguineous inbred Bedouin kindred with multiple individuals that are either homozygous or heterozygous carries of the same novel *MC4R* mutation (c.124G > T, p.E42*). All family members with the homozygous mutation exhibited morbid early-onset obesity, while heterozygote individuals had either a milder overweight phenotype or no discernable phenotype compared to wild type family members. While elder individuals homozygous or heterozygous for the *MC4R* mutation had abnormally high triglycerides, cholesterol, glucose and HbA1C levels, most did not.

Conclusions: *MC4R* mutation homozygotes exhibited morbid early-onset obesity, while heterozygotes had a significantly milder overweight phenotype. Whereas obesity due to *MC4R* mutations is evident as of early age – most notably in homozygotes, the metabolic consequences emerge only later in life.

Keywords: MC4R, Obesity, Mutation, Homozygous, Heterozygous

Background

Obesity, affecting more than 30% of adults and children worldwide [1], is a complex trait affected by diet in conjunction with environmental and genetic factors [2]. The melanocortin-4 receptor (MC4R) is a key player in the leptin-regulated melanocortin circuit, essential for central energy regulation [3]. Predominantly expressed in the hypothalamus, the G-protein-coupled-receptor MC4R acts in signaling satiety, consequently decreasing food intake: upon binding of its endogenous ligand, the neuropeptide melanocyte stimulating hormone (α-MSH), MC4R activates adenylate cyclase, enhancing cAMP synthesis and levels, thereby generating a satiety signal. In line with the role of MC4R in satiety signaling and regulation of food intake, MC4R null mutant (MC4R $^{-/-}$) mice develop severe obesity, while heterozygous (MC4R $^{+/-}$) mice present a mildly obese intermediate phenotype [4].

Mutations in members of the leptin-regulated melanocortin circuit have been shown to result in human obesity. Most notably, human obesity has been associated with

* Correspondence: obirk@bgu.ac.il; ruthb@ariel.ac.il
[1]The Morris Kahn Laboratory of Human Genetics at the National Institute of Biotechnology in the Negev, Ben-Gurion University of the Negev, Beer-Sheva, Israel
[3]Department of Nutrition, Faculty of Health Sciences, Ariel University, Ariel, Israel
Full list of author information is available at the end of the article

mutations in leptin (LEP) [5], leptin receptor (LEPR) [6], prohormone convertase 1 (PC1) [7], proopiomelanocortin (POMC) [8] and melanocortin-4 receptor (MC4R) [9–15]. In fact, heterozygous loss-of-function *MC4R* mutations have been shown to be the most common known genetic cause of human obesity. Initial studies by Farooqi et al. [16] estimated that about 6% of early onset morbidly obese patients harbor *MC4R* mutations. Consequently, other large cohort studies, mostly in Caucasian European and American populations, demonstrated lower calculated prevalence of about < 2% [17–21]. The prevalence of *MC4R* mutations in severely obese populations in other ethnicities, such as Asians, was found to be low or not relevant [16].

Homozygous or compound heterozygous carriers of *MC4R* mutations are rare [15, 16, 22, 23]. Previous studies suggest that the obesity in these rare cases develops earlier in life, and is more severe than for heterozygous carriers; notably, these homozygous individuals do not display any discernible additional unrelated phenotypes [16]. Only few families have been described to date in which multiple heterozygotes and homozygotes of the same mutation are found [16]. We now describe large consanguineous inbred kindred with individuals that are either homozygous or heterozygous carries of the same novel *MC4R* mutation, and review the literature of such families described to date.

Methods

Subjects and clinical phenotyping

Sixteen affected and unaffected individuals of consanguineous Bedouin kindred were studied (Fig. 1a). DNA samples were obtained following informed consent and approval of the Soroka Medical Center Internal Review Board (0316–14-SOR) according to Helsinki ethical guidelines. Clinical phenotyping was determined by an experienced team of pediatrics specialists and clinical geneticists for all affected individuals, their parents and siblings. Blood samples, as well as measurements of weight and height, were taken from all participants on the same day.

Whole exome sequencing

Genomic DNA was isolated from peripheral blood using The E.Z.N.A. SQ Blood DNA Kit (Omega Bio-tek, Norcross,GA, USA). Whole exome sequencing (HiSeq2000, Illumina, San Diego, CA, USA) of two affected individuals (III:5 & IV:1, Fig. 1a) was performed using paired-end (2 × 100) protocol at a mean coverage of 100-fold (85–90% of all exonic nucleotides were covered by > 100 reads), as previously described [24]. For exome enrichment, we used NimbleGen SeqCap EZ Human Exome Library v2.0 (Roche NimbleGen, Madison, WI, USA) targeting 44.1 Mb regions. Sequencing read alignment, variant calling and annotation were performed by DNAnexus (DNAnexus Inc., Mountain View, CA, USA; dnanexus.com).

Data were analyzed using QIAGEN's Ingenuity® Variant Analysis™ software (www.qiagen.com/ingenuity) from QIAGEN Redwood City. Using their filtering cascade, we excluded common variants which demonstrated an allele frequency higher than 0.5% in AFC (Allele Frequency Community - including ExAC and CGI), in the 1000 genomes project and in NHLBI ESP exomes (National Heart, Lung, and Blood Institute Exome Sequencing Project). In addition, we excluded variants which appeared in a homozygous state or that presented an allele frequency of higher than 2% in our in-house whole exome sequencing database of 120 Bedouin control samples. Furthermore, we kept variants which were predicted to have a deleterious effect upon protein coding sequences (e.g. Frameshift, in-frame indel, stop codon change, missense or predicted to disrupt splicing by MaxEnt Scan) and variants which were experimentally observed to be associated with a phenotype: pathogenic, possibly pathogenic or disease-associated, according to the Human Gene Mutation Database (HGMD). Following the above filtering, of the remaining variants we selected only homozygous variants that were shared between both affected individuals sequenced.

Mutation screening

Validation of the *MC4R* variant in all affected family members was performed by Sanger sequencing. Primers used for PCR: Forward 5'-ATCAATTCAGGGGG ACACTG; Reverse 5'-AACGCTCACCAGCATATCAG. Annealing temperature used was 60 °C and the extension time was set for 30 s. Segregation analysis within the entire kindred was performed by restriction analysis using the primers mentioned above for PCR, based on an NheI restriction site generated through the *MC4R* c.124 G > T mutation. PCR products (207 bp amplicon) were incubated for 3 h with the enzyme NheI (New England Biolabs) which cuts selectively only the mutant allele (163 and 44 bp fragments), and subsequently loaded onto a 2% agarose gel for electrophoresis.

Results

Molecular genetic studies

In search for the molecular basis of the familial obesity, whole-exome sequencing analysis was done for two remotely related affected individuals of the kindred, namely III:5 & IV:1 (Fig. 1a). Data were filtered for normal variants as described in the materials and methods section. Following the above filtering, only a single homozygous variant was found that was shared between the two individuals: g.chr18: 58039459C < A, c.124 G > T, p.E42* in *MC4R*. No other variants (heterozygous or homozygous) in *MC4R* or in any other obesity-related gene were identified in any of the two subjects tested through whole

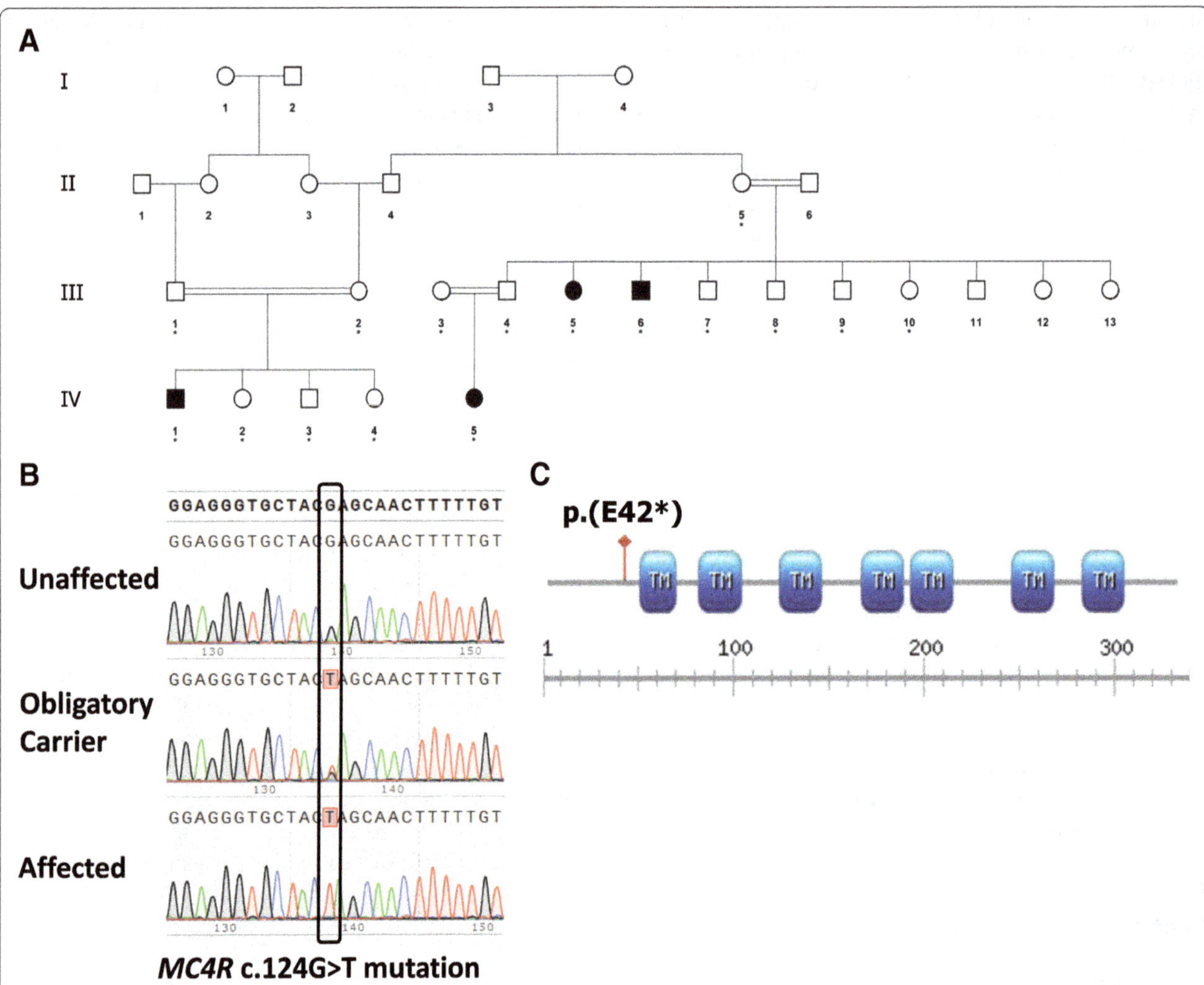

Fig. 1 Pedigree of the studied kindred and the *MC4R* mutation. **a** Pedigree of a consanguineous Bedouin family presenting with a phenotype of autosomal recessive early-onset obesity (individuals with phenotypic morbid obesity are marked as affected; asterisk marks individuals whose DNA was available for analysis). **b** The c.124 G > T, p.(E42*) *MC4R* mutation: Sanger sequencing of an unaffected individual (III:7), an obligatory carrier (II:5) and a morbidly-obese affected individual (IV:1). **c** Schematic representation of the p.(E42*) mutation in *MC4R* predicted to truncate almost 90% of the protein (TM, Transmembrane domain)

exome sequencing. The *MC4R* mutation, validated by Sanger sequencing (Fig. 1b), was found to segregate within the family as expected for autosomal recessive heredity (data not shown). There is no evidence of the reported mutation being present in the Genome Aggregation Database (gnomAD, http://gnomad.broadinstitute.org/), a database of 123,136 exome sequences and 15,496 whole-genome sequences from unrelated individuals sequenced as part of various disease-specific and population genetic studies. The mutation truncates the 332-amino acid MC4R protein at amino acid 42, eliminating all its 7 transmembrane domains, hence practically all its functional domains (Fig. 1c). The mutation was not found in 120 whole exome sequences of local Bedouin controls in our in-house database.

As delineated in Table 1, of those 120 Bedouin control non-related individuals, one carried a heterozygous c.606C > A p.F202 L *MC4R* mutation previously associated with obesity, and two individuals carried heterozygous synonymous variants (c.594C > T, c.690C > T) previously described as possibly associated with obesity, though likely non-pathogenic [25–27]. Clinical obesity-related information regarding those individuals is not available. Interestingly, 4 of the 120 Bedouin controls were heterozygous for the c.307G > A p.V103I *MC4R* variant previously associated with protection from obesity [28] (ExAC frequency for this variant is 0.01743).

Clinical characterization

Sixteen individuals of a consanguineous Bedouin kindred were studied (ages 1–58 years, 21.7 ± 14.7 SD), of which 4 were homozygous for the *MC4R* mutation, 7 were heterozygous for the mutation and 5 were homozygous for the wild type sequence. As shown in Table 2, height,

Table 1 *MC4R* variants identified in 120 ethnically matched controls, excluding sequenced members of the studied kindred

Mutation Type	Transcript Variant	Protein Variant	No. of subjects with genotype (All heterozygous)	dbSNP ID	ExAC Frequency
Synonymous	c.594C > T	p.I198I	1	61,741,819	0.003676
Synonymous	c.690C > T	p.P230P	1	148,026,669	2.472e-05
Missense	c.606C > A	p.F202 L	1	138,281,308	0.0008488
Missense	c.307G > A	p.V103I	4	2,229,616	0.01743
Stop gain	c.124G > T	p.E42	0	–	–

weight and body mass index (BMI) were measured for all, and fasting blood values of cholesterol, triglycerides, LDL, HDL, glucose and HbA1C were available for most. In cases where more than one measurement was available, the average of the measurements was calculated and is presented.

Homozygotes for the p.E42* *MC4R* mutation exhibited average BMI of 44.83 (44.83 ± 9.7 SD), indicative of extreme obesity (obesity class III) and significantly higher than the BMI of both heterozygous and wild type family members ($p < 0.005$). Individuals heterozygous for the mutation had an average BMI of 29.22 (29.22 ± 10.2 SD), within the upper limits of BMI values defined as overweight. Average BMI of family members homozygous for the wild type *MC4R* allele was 24.46 (24.46 ± 8.98 SD), within BMI normal values.

Fasting blood triglycerides, cholesterol, LDL, HDL, glucose and HbA1C levels were measured for most individuals studied. As seen in Table 2, only the eldest of the 4 homozygous individuals (III:5, Fig. 1a, age 30–35 years) had extremely high levels of cholesterol, triglycerides, LDL, glucose and HbA1C, while the other 3 (ages 5–10 and 25–30 years) had normal values. Similarly, of the 7 heterozygotes, high levels of triglycerides, glucose and HbA1C were found only in the eldest individual (age range 55–60 years, versus age ranges 5–10, 20–25, 25–30, 25–30, 25–30, 30–35 of heterozygotes with normal levels).

Discussion

MC4R mutations are the most common known genetic cause of obesity, affecting 2–3% of the population in various cohorts tested [16, 29]. To date, about 200 *MC4R* genetic variants have been identified, including at least 122 missense mutations, 2 in-frame deletion mutations, 7 nonsense mutations and dozens of frameshift mutations [3, 30], altogether affecting more than 30% of the receptor coding sequence. While it has been suggested that obesity due to *MC4R* mutations can be caused by either haplo-insufficiency or dominant negative activity exerted by the mutant receptor, co-transfection studies show that the extreme majority of

Table 2 Phenotypic delineation of the 16 family members studied

ID	Sex	Genotype	Age (years)	BMI	Cholesterol (mg/dl)	LDL (mg%)	HDL (mg/dl)	TG (mg/dl)	Glucose (mg/dl)	HbA1C (%)
III:5	F	Hom	25–30	48	358	N/A	63	444	413	16
III:6	M	Hom	25–30	57	156	107	36	66	86	6.2
IV:1	M	Hom	5–10	36 (3.1)	153	93	28	162	73	5.5
IV:5	F	Hom	5–10	37 (3.1)	150	80	37	165	88	5.7
II:5	F	Het	55–60	35	172	70	45	284	363	12.1
III:4	M	Het	30–35	22	148	83	52	66	89	N/A
III:1	M	Het	25–30	26	209	132	41	180	217	7.4
III:3	F	Het	25–30	48	184	127	45	61	80	N/A
III:2	F	Het	25–30	32	193	119	41	164	90	5.6
III:9	M	Het	20–25	24	157	87	48	111	89	N/A
IV:2	F	Het	5–10	17 (1.0)	N/A	N/A	N/A	N/A	116	N/A
III:8	M	WT	25–30	33	244	169	35	202	82	N/A
III:10	F	WT	20–25	20	N/A	N/A	N/A	N/A	74	N/A
III:7	M	WT	20–25	35	179	114	49	82	94	N/A
IV:3	M	WT	1–5	17	N/A	N/A	N/A	N/A	94	N/A
IV:4	F	WT	1–5	18	N/A	N/A	N/A	N/A	81	N/A

Hom homozygous, *Het* heterozygous, *WT* wild type, *F* female, *M* Male. Age adjusted Z scores of BMI values for Het / Hom children (compared to WHO norms) given in parenthesis. N/A not available. Ages (years) given in ranges to obscure patient identity

mutations analyzed do not have dominant negative activity [3, 15, 31, 32]. Therefore, it is suggested that haplo-insufficiency is the main route through which these mutations exert their effect. While loss-of-function mutations in *MC4R* cause familial forms of obesity, two rare gain-of-function *MC4R* polymorphisms have been identified that are associated with protection against obesity [19]. In fact, we show that in our cohort of 120 control Bedouin whole exome sequences, 4 individuals are heterozygous for one of these variants, namely c.307G > A, p.V103I. Meta analysis of previously published data showed that this gain-of function mutation has a modest negative association with obesity [19]. It is of interest that the prevalence of the p.V103I variant in the Israeli Bedouin community seems to be higher than worldwide (ExAC frequency 0.01743). Notably, another gain-of-function c.751A > C p.I251L *MC4R* variant, that is more clearly negatively associated with obesity worldwide [19], was not found in our Bedouin cohort. Obviously, larger cohorts within this large inbred Bedouin community [33] should be tested to validate statistical significance of these observations.

In families with *MC4R*-associated obesity, obesity tends to have an autosomal dominant mode of transmission, but the penetrance of the disease can be incomplete and the clinical expression variable (moderate to severe obesity), underscoring the role of the environment and other possible modulating genetic factors [34, 35]. As heterozygous *MC4R* mutation carriers are obese, yet present with partial penetrance of the mutations, O'Rahilly and colleagues concluded that the mode of inheritance in MC4R deficiency is codominance with modulation of expressivity and penetrance of the phenotype [36]. It has been suggested that the varying onset and severity of obesity in heterozygous *MC4R* mutation carriers are related to the severity of the functional effects of the mutations. In fact, with many human *MC4R* mutations identified, several research groups (Tao et al. [3], MacKenzie [29], Vaisse et al. [14], Farooqi et al. [15]) classified the *MC4R* mutations based on possible functional consequences: mutations that cause intracellular-retaining of the receptor, defective expression, defective binding, defects in both basal and ligand-induced signaling, etc. However, as only a minority of the variants underwent in-depth functional analysis, validity of such classifications in the context of clinical phenotypic association awaits further studies.

Homozygous or compound heterozygous carriers of *MC4R* mutations are rare [15, 22, 23]. Only few families have been described to date in which multiple heterozygotes and homozygotes of the same mutation are found. We now identified a novel *MC4R* truncation mutation, putatively abolishing all 7 transmembrane domains of the molecule (Fig. 1c). Previous studies reported phenotypic variation in consequences of heterozygous *MC4R* deletion mutations [19, 20]. As the cohort we studied is small, while the average BMI in heterozygous individuals was higher than in wild type family members (29.22 versus 24.24.46, respectively), this difference was not statistically significant, neither in adults nor in children.

Unique to our study, we delineated the mutation-related phenotype in large consanguineous kindred with 4 homozygous and 7 heterozygous individuals, as well as 5 wild type family members. This unique kindred, of few identified thus far, allows insights as to phenotypic effects in heterozygotes versus homozygotes of the same mutation. As evident in Table 2, although the cohort is too small to establish statistical significance, the data clearly point to early-onset obesity in individuals homozygous for the *MC4R* mutation: of the children (ages 1–7 years) within the kindred, the two homozygotes were morbidly obese (BMI 37 and 37; Z scores 3.12, 3.08) as compared to the two wild type individuals (BMI 18 and 17) and the heterozygous individual (BMI 17) that were within normal BMI values (85th BMI-per age percentile). In fact, in spite of the fact that a single kindred is described, the clear morbid obesity (average BMI 44.83) in homozygous individuals is statistically significant compared to the overweight (average BMI 29.22) in heterozygous individuals and the higher end of normal weight (average BMI 24.46) seen in wild type family members. This is in line with previous reports, showing a dramatically more consistent and severe obesity phenotype in homozygotes for *MC4R* mutations than in heterozygotes [16]. Furthermore, the obesity in the homozygotes is of early onset, with BMI Z scores ~ 3 in individuals ages 5–10 years. While previous studies of *MC4R* heterozygotes have shown age-dependent differences in expressivity and a stronger effect in females [16, 18–21, 34], the cohort in the present study is too small to reach conclusions in this regard. Interestingly, although all affected individuals share the same mutation and reside in the same environment (practically the same household), there is variability in phenotypic expression, in the heterozygous individuals in particular, suggesting possible effects of modifier genes. In fact, future studies of such kindreds might be conducive to elucidation of such modifiers.

Previous reports of homozygotes vs heterozygotes of the same *MC4R* mutations did not systematically describe related blood biochemistry values. Fasting blood triglycerides, cholesterol, LDL, HDL, glucose and HbA1C levels were measured for most individuals in our studied kindred. As seen in Table 2, only the eldest of the 4 homozygous individuals (III:5, Fig. 1a, age 30–35 years) had extremely high levels of cholesterol, triglycerides, LDL, glucose and HbA1C, while the other 3 (ages 5–10 and 25–30 years) had normal values. Similarly, of the 7 heterozygotes, high levels of triglycerides, glucose and HbA1C were found only in the eldest individual (age range 55–60 years vs age ranges 5–10, 20–25, 25–30, 25–30, 25–30, 30–35).

Conclusions

Through studies of a large inbred kindred we demonstrate a novel *MC4R* mutation, practically eliminating all functional domains of the encoded protein. We show that the phenotype in homozygotes for the mutation is significantly more severe than that of heterozygous carriers of the same mutation. While obesity, as delineated through BMI measurements, is evident in homozygotes (yet not necessarily in heterozygotes) at early ages, the metabolic consequences of *MC4R*-related obesity appear in both heterozygotes and homozygotes only at later ages.

Abbreviations

BMI: Body mass index; LEP: Leptin; LEPR: Leptin receptor; MC4R: Melanocortin-4 receptor; PC1: Prohormone convertase 1; PCR: Polymerase chain reaction; POMC: Proopiomelanocortin

Acknowledgements

We thank the kindred participating in the study.

Funding

Funding for this research was provided by the Legacy Heritage Bio-Medical Program of the Israel Science Foundation (grant no. 1520/09) awarded to Prof. Ruth Birk and Prof. Ohad Birk.

Authors' contributions

MD did the experiments, interpreted data and contributed to writing the manuscript. OSB interpreted data and contributed to writing the manuscript. RB initiated the study, interpreted data and wrote the manuscript. All authors have read and approved the manuscript.

Competing interests

Prof. Ohad Birk is an associate editor of BMC Medical Genetics. The authors declare that they have no competing interests.

Author details

[1]The Morris Kahn Laboratory of Human Genetics at the National Institute of Biotechnology in the Negev, Ben-Gurion University of the Negev, Beer-Sheva, Israel. [2]Genetics Institute, Soroka University Medical Center, Faculty of Health Sciences, Ben-Gurion University of the Negev, Beer-Sheva, Israel. [3]Department of Nutrition, Faculty of Health Sciences, Ariel University, Ariel, Israel.

References

1. Spiegelman BM, Flier JS. Adipogenesis and obesity: rounding out the big picture. Cell. 1996;87:377–89.
2. Braunschweig, G. & Fantuzzi, C. *Adipose Tissue and Adipokines in Health and Disease*. (Springer, 2014). doi:https://doi.org/10.1007/978-1-62703-770-9
3. Tao Y-X, Segaloff DL. Functional characterization of melanocortin-4 receptor mutations associated with childhood obesity. Endocrinology. 2003;144: 4544–51.
4. Dubern B. MC4R and MC3R Mutations. In Frelut ML, editor. The ECOG's eBook on Child and Adolescent Obesity. 2015. Retrieved from ebook.ecog-obesity.eu
5. Montague CT, et al. Congenital leptin deficiency is associated with severe early-onset obesity in humans. Nature. 1997;387:903–8.
6. Clement K, et al. A mutation in the human leptin receptor gene causes obesity and pituitary dysfunction. Nature. 1998;392:398–401.
7. Jackson RS, et al. Obesity and impaired prohormone processing associated with mutations in the human prohormone convertase 1 gene. Nat Genet. 1997;16:303–6.
8. Krude H, Biebermann H, Luck W, Horn R, Brabant G, Grüters A. Severe Early-Onset Obesity, Adrenal Insufficiency and Red Hair Pigmentation Caused by POMC Mutations in Humans. Nat. Genet. 1999;**19**:155–7.
9. Yeo GSH, et al. A frameshift mutation in MC4R associated with dominantly inherited human obesity. Nat Genet. 1998;20:111–2.
10. Vaisse C, Clement K, Guy-Grand B, Froguel P. A frameshift mutation in human MC4R is associated with a dominant form of obesity. Nat Genet. 1998;20:113–4.
11. Gu W, et al. Identification and functional analysis of novel human melanocortin-4 receptor variants. Diabetes. 1999;48:635–9.
12. Hinney A, et al. Several mutations in the melanocortin-4 receptor gene including a nonsense and a frameshift mutation associated with dominantly inherited obesity in humans. J Clin Endocrinol Metab. 1999;84:1483–6.
13. Sina M, et al. Phenotypes in three pedigrees with autosomal dominant obesity caused by haploinsufficiency mutations in the melanocortin-4 receptor gene. Am J Hum Genet. 1999;65:1501–7.
14. Vaisse C, et al. Melanocortin-4 receptor mutations are a frequent and heterogeneous cause of morbid obesity. J Clin Invest. 2000;106:253–62.
15. Farooqi IS, et al. Dominant and recessive inheritance of morbid obesity associated with melanocortin 4 receptor deficiency. J Clin Invest. 2000;106: 271–9.
16. Farooqi IS, Keogh JM, Yeo GSH, Lank EJ, Cheetham T, O'Rahilly S. Clinical spectrum of obesity and mutations in the melanocortin 4 receptor gene. N Engl J Med. 2003;348:1085–95.
17. Hinney A, et al. Melanocortin-4 receptor gene: case-control study and transmission disequilibrium test confirm that functionally relevant mutations are compatible with a major gene effect for extreme obesity. J Clin Endocrinol Metab. 2003;88:4258–67.
18. Valli-Jaakola K, et al. Identification and characterization of melanocortin-4 receptor gene mutations in morbidly obese finnish children and adults. J Clin Endocrinol Metab. 2004;89:940–5.
19. Stutzmann F, et al. Prevalence of melanocortin-4 receptor deficiency in europeans and their age-dependent penetrance in multigenerational pedigrees. Diabetes. 2008;57:2511–8.
20. Roth CL, et al. A novel melanocortin-4 receptor gene mutation in a female patient with severe childhood obesity. Endocrine. 2009;36:52–9.
21. Calton MA, et al. Association of functionally significant Melanocortin-4 but not Melanocortin-3 receptor mutations with severe adult obesity in a large north American case-control study. Hum Mol Genet. 2009;18:1140–7.
22. Lubrano-Berthelier C, Le Stunff C, Bougnères P, Vaisse C. A homozygous null mutation delineates the role of the Melanocortin-4 receptor in humans. J Clin Endocrinol Metab. 2004;89:2028–32.
23. Dubern B, et al. Homozygous null mutation of the Melanocortin-4 receptor and severe early-onset obesity. J Pediatr. 2007;150:613–8.
24. Perez Y, et al. *UNC80* mutation causes a syndrome of hypotonia, severe intellectual disability, dyskinesia and dysmorphism, similar to that caused by mutations in its interacting cation channel *NALCN*. *J. Med. Genet.* jmedgenet-2015-103352. 2015; https://doi.org/10.1136/jmedgenet-2015-103352.
25. Rettenbacher E, et al. A novel non-synonymous mutation in the melanocortin-4 receptor gene (MC4R) in a 2-year-old Austrian girl with extreme obesity. Exp Clin Endocrinol Diabetes. 2007;115:7–12.
26. Logan M, et al. Allelic variants of the Melanocortin 4 receptor (*MC4R*) gene in a south African study group. Mol Genet Genomic Med. 2016;4:68–76.
27. van den Berg L, et al. Melanocortin-4 receptor gene mutations in a Dutch cohort of obese children. Obesity. 2011;19:604–11.
28. Young EH, et al. The V103I polymorphism of the MC4R gene and obesity: population based studies and meta-analysis of 29 563 individuals. Int J Obes (Lond). 2007;31:1437–41.
29. MacKenzie RG. Obesity-associated mutations in the human melanocortin-4 receptor gene. Peptides. 2006;27:395–403.
30. Loos RJF, et al. Melanocortin-4 receptor gene and physical activity in the Québec family study. Int J Obes. 2005;29:420–8.
31. Yeo GSH, et al. Mutations in the human melanocortin-4 receptor gene associated with severe familial obesity disrupts receptor function through multiple molecular mechanisms. Hum Mol Genet. 2003;12:561–74.
32. Ho G, MacKenzie RG. Functional characterization of mutations in melanocortin-4 receptor associated with human obesity. J Biol Chem. 1999; 274:35816–22.
33. Markus B, Alshafee I, Birk OS. Deciphering the fine-structure of tribal admixture in the Bedouin population using genomic data. Heredity (Edinb). 2013;112:182–9.

34. Lubrano-Berthelier C, et al. Melanocortin 4 receptor mutations in a large cohort of severely obese adults: prevalence, functional classification, genotype-phenotype relationship, and lack of association with binge eating. J Clin Endocrinol Metab. 2006;91:1811–8.
35. Hinney A, et al. Prevalence, spectrum, and functional characterization of melanocortin-4 receptor gene mutations in a representative population-based sample and obese adults from Germany. J Clin Endocrinol Metab. 2006;91:1761–9.
36. O'Rahilly S, Sadaf Farooqi I, Yeo GSH, Challis BG. Minireview: human obesity - lessons from monogenic disorders. Endocrinology. 2003;144:3757–64.

18

An African perspective on the genetic risk of chronic kidney disease

Cindy George[1*], Yandiswa Y Yako[2], Ikechi G Okpechi[3,4], Tandi E Matsha[5], Francois J. Kaze Folefack[6,7] and Andre P Kengne[1]

Abstract

Background: Individuals of African ethnicity are disproportionately burdened with chronic kidney disease (CKD). However, despite the genetic link, genetic association studies of CKD in African populations are lacking.

Methods: We conducted a systematic review to critically evaluate the existing studies on CKD genetic risk inferred by polymorphism(s) amongst African populations in Africa. The study followed the HuGE handbook and PRISMA protocol. We included studies reporting on the association of polymorphism(s) with prevalent CKD, end-stage renaldisease (ESRD) or CKD-associated traits. Given the very few studies investigating the effects of the same single nucleotide polymorphisms (SNPs) on CKD risk, a narrative synthesis of the evidence was conducted.

Results: A total of 30 polymorphisms in 11 genes were investigated for their association with CKD, ESRD or related traits, all using the candidate-gene approach. Of all the included genes, *MYH9, AT1R* and *MTHFR* genes failed to predict CKD or related traits, while variants in the *APOL1, apoE, eNOS, XPD, XRCC1, renalase, ADIPOQ,* and *CCR2* genes were associated with CKD or other related traits. Two SNPs (rs73885319, rs60910145) and haplotypes (G-A-G; G1; G2) of the apolipoprotein L1 (*APOL1*) gene were studied in more than one population group, with similar association with prevalent CKD observed. The remaining polymorphisms were investigated in single studies.

Conclusion: According to this systematic review, there is currently insufficient evidence of the specific polymorphisms that poses African populations at an increased risk of CKD. Large-scale genetic studies are warranted to better understand susceptibility polymorphisms, specific to African populations.

Keywords: Chronic kidney disease, End-stage renal disease, Genetics, Africa

Background

Chronic kidney disease (CKD) is fast becoming a leading public health issue in Africa, with an estimated prevalence of 14.3% in the general population, and 36.1% in high-risk populations [1]. Due in part to increasing rates of type 2 diabetes, hypertension and obesity, the prevalence of CKD continues to rise [2]. However, marked variability in the incidence of CKD between population groups, suggests additional factors contributing to CKD aetiology [3]. Indeed, prevalent end-stage renal disease (ESRD), which is the terminal stage of CKD, is 4-fold higher among African ethnicity as compared to European ethnicity [4, 5] and individuals of African ethnicity progress faster from moderately decreased kidney function to ESRD [6]; thus highlighting African ethnicity as a contributing risk factor for CKD [4, 5].

Over the past decade, through the use of genome-wide association studies (GWAS), researchers have identified various genomic regions with common genetic variants associated with CKD traits [7]. However, a limitation of the majority of GWAS's conducted to date is the paucity of studies conducted in individuals of African ancestry and even less in Africans living in Africa [7–10]. Despite, Africa being one of the most ethnically and genetically diverse regions of the world [11], these populations are understudied, with most of the common loci associated with CKD in non-African populations not being replicated in African populations. Though African migrants living in Europe and America are genetically linked with African ancestry [12, 13], these

* Correspondence: cindy.george@mrc.ac.za
[1]Non-Communicable Diseases Research Unit, South African Medical Research Council, Parow Valley, PO Box 19070, Cape Town, South Africa
Full list of author information is available at the end of the article

genetic variants cannot be extrapolated to Africans residing in Africa. This is mainly due to genetic admixture of American and European populations, as well as differences in environment, cultural and lifestyles [11]. Accordingly, identification of genetic loci for CKD in African populations will help to advance our understanding of the underpinnings of CKD in individuals of African descent.

There is currently no systematic review evaluating the CKD-associated genes found in African populations residing in Africa. The main purpose of this review is thus to critically evaluate the existing studies on CKD genetic risk inferred by polymorphisms amongst African populations in Africa, and explore the specific effect these genetic loci have on CKD development in the African population.

Methods

Protocol and registration

The review was conducted using the Preferred Reporting Items for Systematic Reviews and Meta-Analysis PRISMA framework [14] and HuGENET™ HuGE Review handbook [15]. The methods of the analysis and inclusion criteria were specified in advance and documented in a protocol in the PROSPERO database (registration number: CRD42017058440).

Selection of eligible studies, types of studies and sources of information

Relevant studies published until August 2017 were identified through a comprehensive electronic search of major databases such as MEDLINE (via PubMed), EBSCOhost, Scopus, and Web of Science, using an African search filter [16] and without any starting date or language restrictions. Medical Subject Headings (MeSH) terms and Boolean operators, such as AND/OR/NOT, were used to string terms together (refer to Additional files 1, 2, 3 and 4: Tables S1–S4). Publication bibliographies were searched to further enhance the search strategy.

Data collection

Two authors (CG and YYY) independently conducted the database searches and sequentially (titles, abstracts and then full texts) screened them for inclusion (Fig. 1). In situations of disagreements between the two authors, a third author (APK) arbitrated for eligibility. The inclusion criteria was that a study had to be an original study

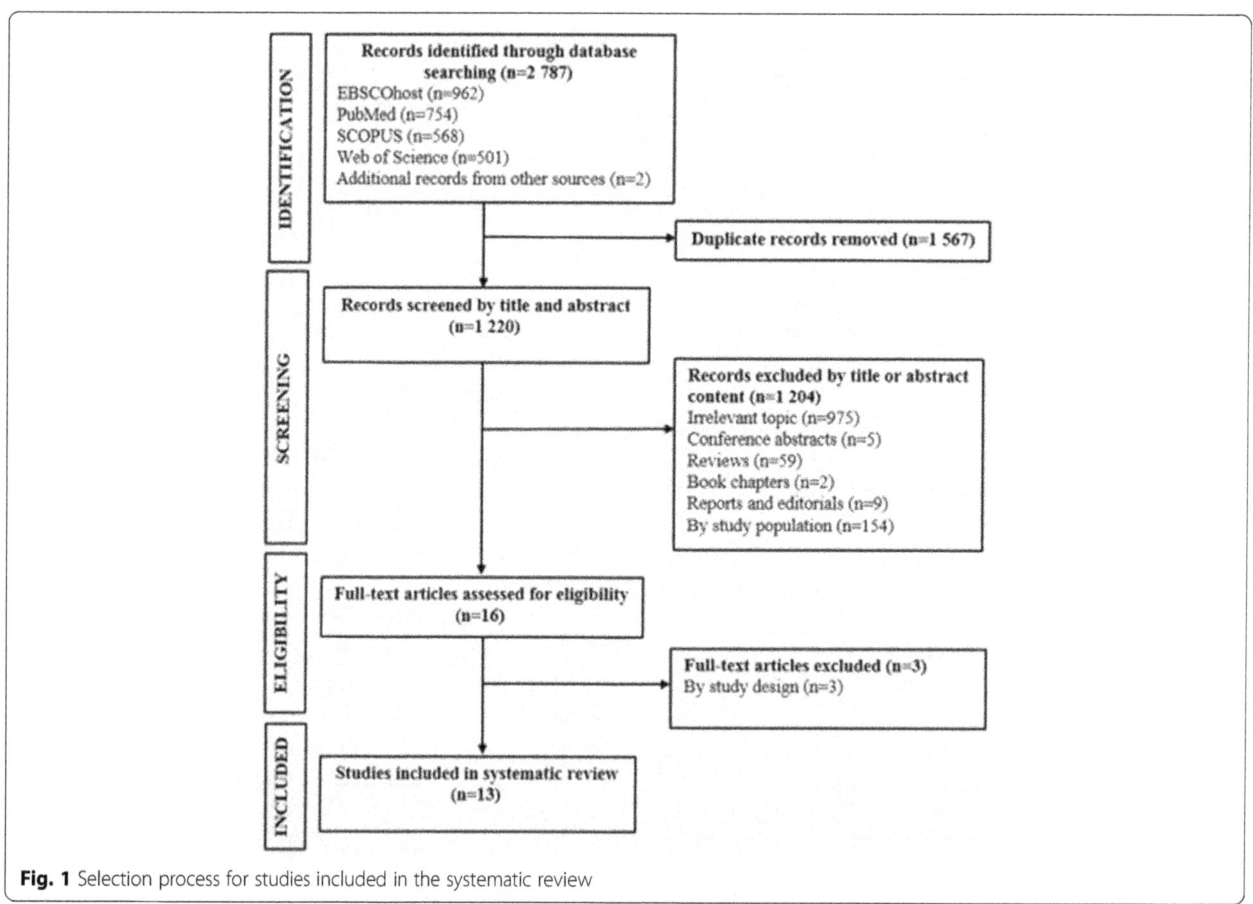

Fig. 1 Selection process for studies included in the systematic review

containing independent data that were obtained from case-control or cohort studies, which specifically conducted genetic association analyses on African populations residing in Africa. These studies had to report on study population characteristics, methods, CKD or renal traits (such as serum creatinine, estimated glomerular filtration rate (eGFR), urinary albumin excretion), genes and polymorphisms, genotyping technique(s), statistical analyses, and report on allele and genotype frequencies. Studies were excluded if, [1] the conducted analyses were exclusively on migrant African populations, [2] the entire cohort consisted of only high-risk individuals (a population of only type 2 diabetic or hypertensive patients), [3] the study did not report the estimate effects and/or *p*-values, allele and genotype frequencies, and if [4] the study was a meta-analysis, review or any other form of publication that do not have primary data. Full articles were obtained for all abstracts and titles that met inclusion criteria as well as those that certainty of inclusion was unclear. The two authors (CG and YYY) screened the full-text articles, and selected full manuscripts according to the inclusion criteria. Disagreements were resolved through discussion or if consensus were not met, reviewed by a third author (APK). The reasons for excluding studies were also recorded.

Data extraction, assessment and synthesis

The data extracted from selected articles included the name of the first author and year of publication, study setting and design, population characteristics, genetic models used for measures of association, adjustment (if any) for confounding variables, allele and genotype frequencies, and the study outcome. Data extraction was done by one author (CG), and another author (YYY) verified the accuracy and validity of extracted data. As recommended by Sagoo et al. [17], we assessed the existence of bias considering the following: case definition, population stratification, reporting of methods used (sample size of a study population, genotyping method and its reliability/accuracy, validation of results, statistical analyses). Given the very few studies investigating the effects of the same SNPs on CKD risk across different settings/countries, attempting to pool studies were deemed meaningless, thus, we opted to conduct a narrative synthesis of the evidence instead of a meta-analysis.

Results

Study selection

We retrieved 2787 citations (962 from EBSCOhost; 754 from MEDLINE; 568 from SCOPUS; 501 from Web of Science; 2 from publication bibliography) from our searches. Of these, 2771 citations were not eligible for inclusion for the following reasons: duplicate ($n = 1567$) or irrelevant to this review based on the title or abstract ($n = 1204$). Consequently, 16 full-text articles were reviewed and of those, three citations were excluded, based on not meeting the inclusion criteria of this review, resulting in 13 eligible articles retained for the systematic review (Fig. 1).

Characteristics of included studies

Table 1 describes the characteristics of the genetic studies included in this review. All the studies were conducted between 2009 and 2016 with the vast majority conducted in Egypt ($n = 7$), followed by Nigeria and South Africa ($n = 2$, each), and Morocco and Tunisia each with only one reported study on CKD genetic association. Overall, nine studies (69.2%) were from three north-African countries [18–26] and the rest from sub-Saharan African countries [27–30]. The study population ranged from 87 to 859 participants per study, with the mean age ranging from 8.7 to 58.9 years and a male predominance in all except the two South African studies, where only 22–23% were male [27, 28]. Of the thirteen studies included, kidney dysfunction was characterized mainly by an estimated glomerular filtration rate (eGFR) equal to or less than 60 ml/min/ 1.73m^2 [18, 23, 25, 27, 28]. The remaining studies used other surrogate measures to determine kidney dysfunction, which included ESRD (undergoing haemodialysis) [19, 21, 22, 24, 26], elevated serum creatinine levels [20] and a combination of serum creatinine levels greater or equal to 170 μmol/l and dipstick proteinuria greater or equal to 2 [30] or serum creatinine above 1.4 mg/dl (men) and 1.2 mg/dl (women) and urinary albumin to creatinine ratio (ACR) above 30 mg/g [29]. The CKD patients included in these studies were of different aetiologies, reflective of the diversity in nephropathy present in Africa.

Table 2 summarizes the polymorphisms investigated in the included studies. Thirty different polymorphisms (including SNP, indels and repeats) in 11 genes have been studied in various population groups in Africa. Of the polymorphisms investigated by selected studies, only three SNPs of the *APOL1* gene (rs73885319, rs60910145, rs71785313) were studied in more than one population group, which included the Yoruba [29] and Igbo [30] tribes of Nigeria and the South African mixed-race population group [27]. The remaining 27 polymorphisms of the *MYH9, apoE, AT1R, eNOS, MTHFR, XPD, XRCC1, renalase, ADIPOQ* and *CCR2* genes were each studied in only one ethnic group. Eight of the included genetic association studies assessed the distribution of allele frequency by formally testing for Hardy-Weinberg equilibrium (HWE), and one study assumed HWE without formal testing [21]. Of those formally tested, only one polymorphism showed a departure from HWE (*MYH9* rs4821480), and was

Table 1 Characteristics of genetic studies conducted in Africa

Authors	Study design	Country	Population	Sample size (case/control)	Mean age (years±SD)	Male (%) (case/control)	Measure of kidney dysfunction	Type of nephropathy
Tayo et al. [29]	Case-control	Nigeria	Yoruba tribe	87/79	42.1 ± 16.9 (case) 35.2 ± 8.2 (control)	53/51	*Serum creatinine* (> 1.4 mg/dl, men; > 1.2 mg/dl, women) *Spot urine* (ACR > 30 mg/g)	Hypertension-associated (50.5%) HIV-associated (9.2%) Proteinuric (40.2%)
Ulasi et al. [30]	Case-control	Nigeria	Igbo tribe	44/43	46.6 ± 17.8 (case) 42.7 ± 10.9 (control)	57/63	Serum creatinine (≥170 µmol/l or proteinuria ≥2+)	HIV-associated (18.2%) NS (81.8%)
Matsha et al. [28]	Cross-sectional	South Africa	Mixed-race	*By MDRD* 68/648 *By CKD-EPI* 67/649	53.6 ± 14.9 (total)	22.1 (total)	eGFR (< 60 ml/min/1.73m^2 based on MDRD and CKD-EPI equations)	NS
Matsha et al. [27]	Cross-sectional	South Africa	Mixed-race	*By MDRD* 79/780 *By CKD-EPI* 73/786	53.1 ± 14.1 (total)	22.7 (total)	eGFR (< 60 ml/min/1.73m^2 based on MDRD and CKD-EPI equations)	NS
Lahrach et al. [21]	Case-control	Morocco	NS	109/97	44.9 ± 14.4 (case) 46.8 ± 11.8 (control)	NS	ESRD undergoing haemodialysis	NS
Hanna et al. [19]	Case-control	Egypt	NS	50/44	37.9 ± 14.3 (case) NS (control)	64/NS	ESRD undergoing haemodialysis	Diabetic nephropathy (26%) Hypertensive nephrosclerosis (22%) Systemic lupus erythematosus (8%) Polycystic kidney disease (10%) Idiopathic (34%)
Kerkeni et al. [20]	Case-control	Tunisia	NS	100/120	51.0 ± 15.0 (case) 54.0 ± 10.0 (control)	55/73	Serum creatinine (thresholds NS; groups included MRF, SRF and ESRD)	Non-diabetes CKD with the following aetiologies: Chronic glomerular nephritis (41%) Chronic tubulointerstitial nephropathy (30%) Vascular nephropathy (23%) Idiopathic (6%)
Elshamaa et al. [18]	Case-control	Egypt	NS	78/30	9.14 ± 7.59 (CT); 10.62 ± 3.49 (MHD) (case) 8.7 ± 4.51 (control)	51/67	eGFR (according to K/DOQ1 guidelines): *Undergoing CT* GFR (range, 15–29 ml/min/1.73m^2) *Undergoing MHD* GFR (range, 5–15 ml/min/1.73m^2)	Advanced CKD with the following aetiology: Renal hypoplasia/dysplasia (20.5%) Obstructive uropathies (17.9%) Neurogenic bladder (7.7%) Metabolic (2.6%) Hereditary nephropathies (21.8%) Glomerulopathy (2.6%) Idiopathic (26.9%)
Radwan et al. [22]	Case-control	Egypt	NS	98/102	47.8 ± 14.2 (total)	50/56	ESRD undergoing hemodialysis	Hypertension-associated (44.9%) Diabetes-associated (11.2%) Preeclampsia (4%) Drug-induced (3%) Glomerulonephritis (6.1%) Obstructive uropathy (5.1%) Atrophic kidney (3%)

Table 1 Characteristics of genetic studies conducted in Africa *(Continued)*

Authors	Study design	Country	Population	Sample size (case/control)	Mean age (years±SD)	Male (%) (case/control)	Measure of kidney dysfunction	Type of nephropathy
								Systemic lupus erythematosus (5.1%) Polycystic kidney (2%) Combined polycystic kidney and hypertension (1%) Combined DM and hypertension (6.1%) Amyloidosis and hypertension (1%) Idiopathic (7.1%)
Rezk et al. [23]	Case-control	Egypt	NS	178 (83 NT; 95 HT)/ 178	47.4 ± 9.3 (case) NS (control)	NS	eGFR (according to K/DOQ1 guidelines)	Hypertension-associated (53.4%) NS (46.6%)
Abdallah et al. [26]	Case-control	Egypt	NS	139/50	NS	48.2/NS	ESRD undergoing hemodialysis	NS
Elshamaa et al. [25]	Case-control	Egypt	NS	78/70	9.14 ± 7.59 (CT); 10.62 ± 3.49 (MHT) (case) 10.7 ± 4.51 (control)	51/57	eGFR (according to K/DOQ1 guidelines): *Undergoing CT* GFR (range, 15–29 ml/min/1.73m^2) *Undergoing MHD* GFR (range, 5–15 ml/min/1.73m^2)	Advanced CKD with the following aetiology: Renal hypoplasia/dysplasia (20.5%) Obstructive uropathies (17.9%) Neurogenic bladder (7.7%) Metabolic (2.6%) Hereditary nephropathies (21.8%) Glomerulopathy (2.6%) Idiopathic (26.9%)
Elhelbawy et al. [24]	Case-control	Egypt	NS	70/30	60.2 ± 9.4 (case) 58.9 ± 10.7 (control)	61.4/63.3	ESRD undergoing hemodialysis	NS

ACR albumin/creatinine ratio, *CKD* chronic kidney disease, *CKD-EPI* Chronic Kidney Disease Epidemiology Collaboration, *CT* conservative treatment, *DM* diabetes mellitus, *eGFR* estimated glomerular filtration rate, *ESRD* end-stage renal disease, *HT* hypertensive, *K/DOQI* NKF Kidney Disease Outcomes Quality Initiative, *MDRD* Modification of Diet in Renal Disease, *MHD* maintenance hemodialysis, *MRF* moderate renal failure, *NS* not specified, *NT* normotensive, *PCR* polymerase chain reaction, *RFLP* restriction fragment length polymorphism, *SRF* severe renal failure, *SSA* sub-Saharan Africa

Table 2 Polymorphisms investigated in African studies

Author	Gene (chromosome region)	Polymorphism	Minor allele frequency: case/control (%)	Genotyping method	HWE	Adjustment	Effect estimate OR/HR (95% CI)	Outcome
Tayo et al. [29]	*APOL1* (22q12.3)	rs9622363	A: 25.86/29.75	Custom Fluidigm ™ 96.96 array platform; TaqMan genotyping assay	0.788	Age Gender	OR (additive): 0.76 (0.45 to1.31); $p = 0.875$ OR (dominant): 0.88 (0.47 to 1.66); $p = 0.999$ OR (recessive): 0.24 (0.05 to 1.29); $p = 0.377$	CKD
		rs73885319	A: 44.19/26.58		1.00		OR (additive): 2.29 (1.39 to 3.77); $p = 0.005$ OR (dominant): 2.59 (1.34 to 5.00); $p = 0.025$ OR (recessive): 3.85 (1.31 to 11.36); $p = 0.038$	
		rs60910145	G: 50.00/30.13		0.114		OR (additive): 2.04 (1.32 to 3.17); $p = 0.006$ OR (dominant): 2.54 (1.31 to 4.92); $p = 0.034$ OR (recessive): 3.12 (1.35 to 7.20); $p = 0.015$	
		G2: rs71785313	D: 8.62/12.66		1.00		OR (additive): 0.61 (0.29 to 1.31); $p = 0.701$ OR (dominant): 0.64 (0.29 to 1.40); $p = 0.816$ OR (recessive): NS	
		G1: rs73885319 and rs60910145	44.19/26.92 (A-G haplotype)				OR (additive): 2.25 (1.36 to 3.71); $p = 0.005$ OR (dominant): 2.52 (1.30 to 4.88); $p = 0.051$ OR (recessive): 3.80 (1.29 to 11.22); $p = 0.026$	
			50.00/69.87 (G-T haplotype)				OR (additive): 0.49 (0.32 to 0.76); p = 0.005 OR (dominant): 0.32 (0.14 to 0.73); $p = 0.018$ OR (recessive): 0.40 (0.21 to 0.77); $p = 0.031$	
	MYH9 (22q12.3)	rs11912763	A: 38.51/27.22		1.00		OR (additive): 1.68 (1.02 to 2.76); $p = 0.197$ OR (dominant): 2.03 (1.06 to 3.87); $p = 0.183$ OR (recessive): 1.70 (0.58 to 4.94); $p = 0.872$	
		rs2032487	T: 18.39/26.28		0.770		OR (additive): 0.68 (0.40 to 1.16); $p = 0.580$ OR (dominant): 0.64 (0.33 to 1.23); $p = 0.645$ OR (recessive): 0.55 (0.14 to 2.22); $p = 0.934$	
		rs4821481	T: 18.39/26.58		0.777		OR (additive): 0.66 (0.39 to 1.13); $p = 0.532$ OR (dominant): 0.61 (0.32 to 1.18); $p = 0.583$	

Table 2 Polymorphisms investigated in African studies *(Continued)*

Author	Gene (chromosome region)	Polymorphism	Minor allele frequency: case/control (%)	Genotyping method	HWE	Adjustment	Effect estimate OR/ HR (95% CI)	Outcome
							OR (recessive): 0.55 (0.14 to 2.24); $p = 0.940$	
		rs5750248	C: 25.86/36.08		1.00		OR (additive): 0.61 (0.37 to 0.99); $p = 0.225$ OR (dominant): 0.56 (0.29 to 1.05); $p = 0.354$ OR (recessive): 0.46 (0.15 to 1.41); $p = 0.627$	
		rs5750250	A: 26.16/37.97		0.635		OR (additive): 0.56 (0.34 to 0.94); $p = 0.141$ OR (dominant): 0.51 (0.27 to 0.97); $p = 0.208$ OR (recessive): 0.44 (0.14 to 1.38); $p = 0.576$	
Ulasi et al. [30]	*APOL1* (22q12.3)	G1: rs73885319 and rs60910145 G2: rs71785313	59/30 20/23	PCR-sequencing; PCR-RFLP	NS	Age Gender BMI HIV	OR: 4.8 (1.6 to 14.9); p = 5.1E-03	CKD
Matsha et al. [28]	*MYH9* (22q12.3)	rs5756152	G: 12.4 (overall)	PCR-sequencing; TaqMan genotyping assay	> 0.999	Age Gender Diabetes ACR	OR (additive): − 2.3 (− 5.6 to 0.9); $p = 0.16$ OR (additive): 1.91 (− 1.32 to 5.15); $p = 0.25$ OR (additive): 1.83 (− 1.23 to 4.89); $p = 0.24$ OR (additive): − 1.6 (− 18.9 to 15.6); $p = 0.85$	Serum creatinine eGFR(MDRD) eGFR (CKD-EPI) ACR
		rs4821480	T: 30.3 (overall)		0.053		NS	
		rs12107	A: 22.2 (overall)		0.908		OR (additive): 0.4 (− 2.2 to 2.9); $p = 0.78$ OR (additive): − 0.07 (− 2.61 to 2.46); $p = 0.95$ OR (additive): 0.13 (− 2.27 to 2.54); $p = 0.91$ OR (additive): 1.0 (− 12.6 to 14.5); $p = 0.90$	Serum creatinine eGFR(MDRD) eGFR (CKD-EPI) ACR
Matsha et al. [27]	*APOL1* (22q12.3)	rs73885319	G: 3.6 (overall)	PCR-sequencing; TaqMan genotyping assay	0.150	Age Gender Diabetes Hypertension	OR (additive): -0.018 (-0.069 to 0.0034); p=0.503 OR (dominant): -0.026 (-0.080 to 0.028); p=0.341 OR (recessive): 0.191 (-0.094 to 0.478); p=0.189	Serum creatinine
							OR (additive): 0.99 (-4.42 to 6.40); p=0.720 OR (dominant): 1.75 (-9.93 to 7.44); p=0.546 OR (recessive): -18.54 (-48.59 to 11.51); p=0.227	eGFR(MDRD)
							OR (additive): 2.07 (-2.40 to 6.55); p=0.364	eGFR (CKD-EPI)

Table 2 Polymorphisms investigated in African studies *(Continued)*

Author	Gene (chromosome region)	Polymorphism	Minor allele frequency: case/control (%)	Genotyping method	HWE	Adjustment	Effect estimate OR/ HR (95% CI)	Outcome
							OR (dominant): 2.96 (-1.74 to 7.66); p=0.217 OR (recessive): -18.90 (-43.76 to 5.96); p=0.136	
							OR (additive): 0.76 (0.27 to 2.16); p=0.601 OR (dominant): 0.56 (0.18 to 1.79); p=0.307 OR (recessive): 23.47 (0.92 to 599.29); p=0.074	CKD (MDRD)
							OR (additive): 1.08 (0.38 to 3.03); p=0.887 OR (dominant): 0.81 (0.26 to 2.54); p=0.720 OR (recessive): 42.72 (1.22 to ∞); p=0.047	CKD (CKD-EPI)
							OR (additive): -0.126 (-0.446 to 0.195); p=0.442 OR (dominant): -0.096 (-0.436 to 0.245); p=0.583 OR (recessive): -1.02 (-2.62 to 0.57); p=0.210	ACR
		rs60919145	G: 3.4 (overall)		0.127		OR (additive): -0.020 (-0.072 to 0.033); p=0.466 OR (dominant): -0.029 (-0.084 to 0.026); p=0.307 OR (recessive): 0.192 (-0.094 to 0.478); p=0.289	Serum creatinine
							OR (additive): 1.26 (-4.27 to 6.79); p=0.656 OR (dominant): 2.09 (-3.73 to 7.91); p=0.482 OR (recessive): -18.54 (-48.59 to 11.51); p=0.227	eGFR(MDRD)
							OR (additive): 2.28 (-2.29 to 6.86); p=0.328 OR (dominant): 3.24 (-1.57 to 8.06); p=0.187 OR (recessive): -18.90 (-43.76 to 5.96); p=0.136	eGFR (CKD-EPI)
							OR (additive): 0.80 (0.28 to 2.27); p=0.665 OR (dominant): 0.59 (0.18 to 1.89); p=0.350 OR (recessive): 23.47 (0.92 to 599.29); p=0.074	CKD (MDRD)
							OR (additive): 1.12 (0.39 to 3.16); p=0.836 OR (dominant): 0.84 (0.27 to 2.65); p=0.767 OR (recessive): 42.72 (1.22	CKD (CKD-EPI)

Table 2 Polymorphisms investigated in African studies *(Continued)*

Author	Gene (chromosome region)	Polymorphism	Minor allele frequency: case/control (%)	Genotyping method	HWE	Adjustment	Effect estimate OR/ HR (95% CI)	Outcome
							to ∞); p=0.047	
							OR (additive): -0.178 (-0.504 to 0.147); p=0.283 OR (dominant): -0.154 (-0.502 to 0.193); p=0.384 OR (recessive): -1.02 (-2.62 to 0.57); p=0.210	ACR
		rs71785313	Del: 5.8 (overall)		0.420		OR (additive): 0.019 (-0.022 to 0.060); p=0.367 OR (dominant): -0.020 (-0.024 to 0.064); p=0.382 OR (recessive): 0.038 (-0.144 to 0.219); p=0.684	Serum creatinine
							OR (additive): -2.38 (-6.68 to 1.93); p=0.323 OR (dominant): -2.35 (-6.99 to 2.30); p=0.323 OR (recessive): -7.16 (-26.19 to 11.87); p=0.461	eGFR(MDRD)
							OR (additive): -2.91 (-6.46 to 0.65); p=0.110 OR (dominant): -3.03 (-6.88 to 0.81); p=0.123 OR (recessive): -5.99 (-21.74 to 9.76); p=0.456	eGFR (CKD-EPI)
							OR (additive): 0.86 (0.39 to 1.93); p=0.712 OR (dominant): 0.91 (0.38 to 2.14); p=0.823 OR (recessive): 0.0	CKD (MDRD)
							OR (additive): 1.00 (0.42 to 2.34); p=0.993 OR (dominant): 1.07 (0.43 to 2.66); p=0.890 OR (recessive): 0.0	CKD (CKD-EPI)
							OR (additive): 0.035 (-0.207 to 0.277); p=0.777 OR (dominant): 0.050 (-0.214 to 0.314); p=0.710 OR (recessive): -1.123 (-1.134 to 0.888); p=0.811	ACR
Lahrach et al. [21]	*apoE* (19q13.32)	e2 (rs7412-T, rs429358-T)	3.0/6.0	PCR-sequencing; gelelectrophoresis	NS	None	OR (NS): 0.473 (0.181 to 1.235); p=0.093	ESRD
		e3 (rs7412-C, rs429358-T	73.0/82.0 (Reference)				Reference group	
		e4 (rs7412-C, rs429358-C)	24.0/12.0				OR (NS): 0.491 (0.277 to 0.870); p=0.009 (UA)	
Hanna et al. [19]	*AT1R* (3q24)	A1166C	C: 86.0/83.0	PCR-RFLP	NS	Age Gender	HR (NS): 1.254 (0.658 to 2.389); p=0.491	ESRD

Table 2 Polymorphisms investigated in African studies *(Continued)*

Author	Gene (chromosome region)	Polymorphism	Minor allele frequency: case/control (%)	Genotyping method	HWE	Adjustment	Effect estimate OR/ HR (95% CI)	Outcome
Kerkeni et al. [20]	*eNOS* (7q36.1)	G894T (exon7)	T: 27.0/22.1	PCR-RFLP	Satisfied HWE (p-value NS)	Age Gender Smoking Hypertension Dyslipidaemia Cholesterol Homocysteine MTHFR C677T eNOS G894T	EE not reported; p=0.028 (difference in allele frequency)	CKD
Elshamaa et al. [18]	*eNOS* (7q36.1)	4a (intron4)	CT and MHD/controls: 32.8 and 33.7/22.7 CT and MHD/controls: 67.2 and 66.3/78.3	PCR-sequencing; gelelectrophoresis	Satisfied HWE (p-value NE)	Age Hypertension SBP DBP Serum NO	EE not reported; p<0.05 (patient groups vs control)	Advanced CKD (ESRD)
Radwan et al. [22]	*XPD* (9)	Asp312Asn	Asn: 35.0/36.0	PCR-RFLP	Satisfied HWE (p-value NE)	NS	OR (NS): 0.93 (0.53 to 1.64); p=0.93	ESRD
		Lys751Gln	Gln: 37.0/37.0				OR (NS): 0.98 (0.55 to 1.74); p=0.94	
	XRCC1 (NS)	Arg399Gln	Gln: 34.0/19.0				OR (NS): 2.48 (1.36 to 4.52); p=0.002	
Rezk et al. [23]	*Renalase* (10q23.21)	rs2296545	C: 28.7/16.3 C: 29.4/16.3 (hypertensive CKD/controls)	PCR-RFLP	Satisfied HWE (p-value NE)	NS	OR: 2.14 (1.07 to 4.26); p=0.04 OR: 2.10 (1.07 to 4.26); p=0.041 (hypertensive CKD/controls)	CKD Hypertensive CKD
Abdallah et al. [26]	*Renalase* (10q23.21)	rs2576178	G: 56/16	PCR-sequencing; gelelectrophoresis	NS	NS	OR: 7.188 (3.5 to 14.7); p<0.05	ESRD
		rs10887800	G: 26/12				OR: 12.3 (5.6 to 27.1); p<0.05	
Elshamaa et al. [25]	*ADIPOQ* (3q27.3)	rs1501299G>T;	T: 18.6/10.7 T (CT/MHD): 15.6/20.7	PCR-sequencing; gelelectrophoresis	Satisfied HWE (p-value NE)	NS	p=0.04 (TT genotype distribution between cases and controls)	Advanced CKD (ESRD)
		rs2241766T>G	G: 0.0/0.0 G (CT/MHD): 0.0/0.0					
Elhelbawy et al. [24]	*CCR2* (3q21.31)	G190A	G: 75.7/90.0 A: 24.3/10.0	PCR-RFLP	NS	NS	OR: 2.8 (1.40 to 5.51); p<0.05 OR: 4.1 (1.27 to 13.03); p<0.05 OR: 2.9 (1.14 to 7.3); p<0.05	CKD

ACR albumin/creatinine ratio, *BMI* body mass index, *CKD* chronic kidney disease, *CKD-EPI* Chronic Kidney Disease Epidemiology Collaboration, *CRF* chronic renal failure, *CT* conservative treatment, *DBP* diastolic blood pressure, *EE* effect estimate, *eGFR* estimated glomerular filtration rate, *ESRD* end-stage renal disease, *HIV* human immunodeficiency virus, *HR* hazard ratio, *HWE* Hardy–Weinberg equilibrium, *MAF* minor allele frequency, *MDRD* Modification of Diet in Renal Disease, *MHD* maintenance hemodialysis, *NO* nitric oxide, *NS* not specified, *OR* odds ratio, *SBP* systolic blood pressure, *UA* unadjusted

subsequently removed from further association analysis in that study [28]. Adjustment for confounders was not consistent across studies, with six studies not providing information on the degree of adjustment or variables accounted for [21–26]. The remaining seven studies all adjusted for at least age and gender [18–20, 27–30]. In all studies, the genomic DNA was extracted from whole blood samples and genotyped by methods including TaqMan genotyping assays, polymerase chain reaction restriction fragment length polymorphism (PCR-RFLP) and gel-electrophoresis and confirmed by PCR-sequencing.

Association of genetic markers with CKD and related traits

According to the studies included in this review, some SNP's investigated in the *MYH9* [28], *AT1R* [19], and *MTHFR* [20] genes failed to predict prevalent CKD, ESRD or related traits (serum creatinine, eGFR and ACR), while variants in the *APOL1* [27, 29, 30], *apoE* [21], *eNOS* [18, 20], *XPD* [22], *XRCC1* [22], *renalase* [23, 26], *ADIPOQ* [31] and *CCR2* [24] genes were associated with either prevalent CKD or progression of CKD, ESRD, or other surrogate measures of renal function.

The majority of CKD-associated polymorphisms were conducted in single studies. In a Moroccan population, the e4 allele and the E3E4 genotype of the *apoE* gene demonstrated a significant association with ESRD (OR = 0.491; $p = 0.009$ and OR = 0.316, $p < 0.001$, e4 and E3E4, respectively) [21]. However, this association was unadjusted for any potential confounder effects. Both Kerkeni et al. [20] and Elshamaa et al. [18] conducted genetic association studies on SNPs in the *eNOS* gene, adjusting for potential confounders, albeit different population groups and different SNPs. According to Kerkeni et al. [20], the *eNOS* SNP found in exon 7 (G894 T) was an independent risk factor of severity of CKD ($p = 0.01$) in Tunisian adults. Similarly, Elshamaa et al. [18] found the a-allele in the *eNOS* (intron 4) gene to predict ESRD in Egyptian children ($p < 0.05$) [18]. Radwan et al. [22] investigated three polymorphisms in the DNA repair genes (*XPD* and *XRCC1*) and found that patients with *XRCC1–399 Arg/Gln* genotype had a significantly higher risk of developing ESRD (OR: 2.48; 95% CI: 1.36–4.52). Furthermore, the haplotypes containing *XRCC1–399 Arg/Gln* and *XPD-312 Asp/Asn* as well as *XRCC1–399 Arg/Gln* and *XPD-751 Lys/Gln* were significantly associated with the development of ESRD (OR: 8.35, 95%CI: 1.94–35.85, $p = 0.004$ and OR: 9.22, 95%CI: 2.14–39.71, $p = 0.003$, respectively). Two studies, both in Egyptian populations, investigated polymorphisms of the renalase gene [23, 26]. Rezk et al. [23] found that patients with the CC genotype and carriers of C allele of the rs2296545 renalase gene were significantly more likely to have prevalent CKD (CC genotype; OR: 4.84, 95%CI: 1.28–18.2, $p = 0.02$ and C-carrier; OR: 2.14, 95%CI: 1.07–4.26, $p = 0.04$). Abdallah et al. [26], conversely found that carriers of the G allele of the rs2576178 and rs10887800 *renalase* gene were associated with increased risk of developing ESRD (OR: 7.188, 95%CI: 3.5–14.7, $p < 0.05$ and OR: 12.3, 95%CI: 5.6–27.1; $p < 0.05$). However, in both studies no adjustments were made for potential confounders. ADIPOQ+276G > T was also investigated for association with ESRD in Egyptian children [31]. This study suggested that the +276G > T allele may indirectly contribute to CKD susceptibility by increasing adiponectin levels (p = 0.04). Elhelbawy et al. [24] found a significant association between *CCR2*–641 and chronic renal failure, particularly the AG genotype (OR = 2.8, 95% CI = 1.40–5.51), combined AG and GG genotypes (OR = 4.1, 95% CI = 1.27–13.03) and A allele (OR = 2.9, 95% CI = 1.14–7.3).

As seen in Table 2, only polymorphisms in the *APOL1* gene were investigated in more than one ethnic group, with the observed association similar in at least two population groups. Indeed, according to the study conducted in the Yoruba tribe of Nigeria [29], two single *APOL1* SNPs (rs73885319 and rs60910145) were significantly associated with CKD under all genetic models, with the largest effect under the recessive model (OR: 3.85 and 3.12 for rs73885319, and rs60910145, respectively). Furthermore, due to the linkage disequilibrium (D-prime = 1.00, $r^2 = 0.82$) between the two SNPs, adjusting for either SNP resulted in no association for the other SNP. Similarly, albeit a different population (mixed-race South Africans), Matsha et al. [27] found the same two single SNPs (rs73885319 and rs60910145) to be associated with prevalent CKD, however only under the recessive model ($p = 0.047$) (as measured by the CKD-EPI eGFR equation), even after adjusting for multiple confounders. The study did not observe an association between these single *APOL1* SNPs and any of the other surrogate measures of kidney function. Tayo et al. [29] also investigated the adjusted association of *APOL1* haplotypes, namely the G-A-G haplotype (rs9622363–rs73885319–rs60910145) and the G1 haplotype (rs73885319 and rs60910145) and found both to be significantly associated with CKD under all models of genetic association (G-A-G, ORs: 2.26; $p = 0.005$, OR: 2.54; $p = 0.023$ and OR: 3.79; $p = 0.041$ for the additive, dominant and recessive modes; G1, OR: 2.25; $p = 0.006$, OR: 2.52; $p = 0.025$ and OR: 3.80; p = 0.041 for the additive, dominant and recessive modes). Ulasi et al. [30] also conducted a study on the *APOL1* G1 haplotype (rs73885319 and rs60910145) and G2 (rs71785313) (Wt:G1 or Wt:G2; G1:G1 or G1:G2 or G2:G2) in the Igbo tribe of Nigeria. This study found no significant effect of the Wt:G1 or Wt:G2 one-copy, but observed a high association between *APOL1* two-risk alleles (G1:G1 or G1:G2 or G2:G2) and CKD (OR: 4.8; $p = 5.1E\text{-}03$), even after adjusting for various confounders.

Discussion

To the best of our knowledge, this is the first comprehensive report of the current evidence on genetic polymorphisms associated with renal disease amongst populations in Africa. This review highlights the lack of genetic association studies conducted within the borders of Africa, despite the known genetic link to CKD and the genetic diversity in Africa.

All the studies included in this review used the candidate gene approach, and amongst these, only *MYH9* polymorphisms has been previously investigated by GWAS and showed directional association with CKD in populations elsewhere [10]. Indeed, multiple *MYH9* SNPs have been identified as powerful predictors of non-diabetic kidney disease in African Americans [32], Hispanic-Americans [33], and individuals of European ancestry [34]. However, from this review we found no evidence for the associative role of *MYH9* polymorphisms in non-diabetic CKD patients in Africa, as all eight SNPs investigated in populations from Nigeria and South Africa failed to predict prevalent CKD or any other surrogate measure of kidney function [28, 29]. Differences in linkage disequilibrium structure might however explain the lack of genetic association in studies conducted in these African populations. Indeed, previous studies have shown that the G1 and G2 risk variants of the *APOL1* gene are in strong linkage disequilibrium with variants in *MYH9*. Indeed, most of the association previously attributed to *MYH9* variants or haplotypes with CKD could be explained by their genetic linkage with *APOL1* polymorphisms in populations of African ancestry residing outside the African continent [35, 36]. In contrast, the studies included in this review instead observed independent association between four SNPs of the *APOL1* gene and with either prevalent CKD, serum creatinine, eGFR or ACR in the included studies [27, 29, 30]. This strong association between *APOL1* polymorphisms and non-diabetic kidney disease found in studies in this review have been replicated in several studies [37–45] since the initial findings reported in African Americans [35, 36]. In addition, as reported in all the above mentioned studies, the risk is mostly conferred by the presence of two copies of the risk alleles, that is, homozygous or compound heterozygous compared to no or one *APOL1* risk variant [35, 36]. It would therefore be of great interest if larger population studies are conducted to ascertain the kidney disease-*APOL1* association across African population groups.

Currently, the role of the polymorphisms in the *apoE* [21], *eNOS* [18, 20], *XPD* [22], *XRCC1* [22], *renalase* [23, 26], *ADIPOQ* [31] and *CCR2* [24] genes in the aetiology of CKD remains controversial and further larger studies should be conducted to confirm these results in population groups within Africa. Certainly, various polymorphisms have been associated, both directly and indirectly, with increased CKD risk in certain populations and decreased CKD risk in others or alternatively have no convincing association. This is true for the polymorphisms investigated in the current review. For example, Lahrach et al. [21] showed that the e4 allele and the E3E4 genotype of the *apoE* gene demonstrated a strong association with ESRD, similar to a study conducted in a Swedish population [46]. However, a study conducted in African Americans and European Americans showed an opposite effect, with the e4 allele being associated with decreased risk of ESRD progression and decreased risk of prevalent ESRD [47], with no association found between the e4 allele and CKD in Asian populations [48]. The genetic link between *eNOS* (4a; intron4) and ESRD [18] and CKD severity (G894 T; exon7) [20] have also been studied in two African populations, and in both studies, as in various other studies [49–51], the polymorphisms under investigation were found to be significantly associated with kidney disease. However, this association between polymorphisms of *eNOS* and kidney disease is not fully elucidated, as the direction and magnitude have been found to differ by population and even within the same population. For example, Bellini et al. [52] demonstrated a strong association between *eNOS* 4a polymorphism and ESRD risk in a Brazilian population, while Marson et al. [53] found no significant correlation between *eNOS* 4a polymorphism and ESRD risk in a similar Brazilian population group. The association between DNA repair genes (XPD and XRCC1) and kidney disease is not commonly investigated, and with the exception of the study reviewed in this publication [22], has only been investigated previously in a Turkish population [54]. Both studies showed an association between DNA repair gene polymorphisms and ESRD development. However, the effect estimates amongst the African population were higher than that reported in the Turkish population. From the included studies, it is evident that investigating regional differences in the relationship between genes and CKD risk within Africa has relevance, considering the genetic diversity among ethnic population groups in the continent [55].

Our study has some limitations, which include the small number of existing studies, which precluded statistical analysis by means of meta-analysis. Furthermore, as a result of existing genetic association studies not always reporting on key methodological information that includes testing the HWE, the sample size/power calculations, clear description of controls, consideration and correction for population stratification, as well as the levels of adjustment, it is difficult to draw definitive inferences from these studies. In addition, the sample size of the included studies was much smaller than other studies conducted outside of Africa, thus as a result it is possible that with larger sample sizes, additional previously proposed candidate genes may have reached statistical significance. Indeed, with the largest included study comprising 859 participants [27], it is highly likely that most existing studies on the genetics of kidney disease in Africa have been underpowered to replicate existing loci or estimate effects with precision. Furthermore, the majority of included studies were conducted in Egyptian populations, thus not covering all the scope of genetic variations that exist on the African continent. The age range, which varied from approximately 9–60 years, and the range of covariates included in adjustment of the estimates of association also differed substantially across studies and could possibly affect between-studies comparisons. In addition, since we had no access to individual participant data, refined analyses and accounting for potential confounders and other types of bias, could not be executed. However, despite the shortcomings of this review, the strength resides in the fact that, according to our knowledge, this is the first study to systematically and comprehensively review the existing data on genetic association studies of CKD in the context of Africa.

Conclusion

The putative genetic risk factors that have emerged from current data represent the most promising kidney disease susceptibility genes described to date in populations within Africa. However, larger-scale genetic association studies are needed to further expand our knowledge of the underlying genetic mechanisms of kidney disease among populations within Africa.

Abbreviations

ACR: Albumin to creatinine ratio; *ADIPOQ*: Gene encoding adiponectin; *apoE*: Gene encoding apolipoprotein E; *APOL1*: Apolipoprotein L1; *AT1R*: Gene encoding angiotensin II receptor type 1; BMI: Body mass index; *CCR2*: Gene encoding C-C chemokine receptor type 2; CKD: Chronic kidney disease; CKD-EPI: Chronic Kidney Disease Epidemiology Collaboration; CRF: Chronic renal failure; CT: Conservative treatment; DBP: Diastolic blood pressure; DM: Diabetes mellitus; EE: Effect estimate; eGFR: Estimated glomerular filtration rate; *eNOS*: Gene encoding endothelial nitric oxide synthase; ESRD: End-stage renal disease; GWAS: Genome-wide association studies; HIV: Human immunodeficiency virus; HR: Hazard ratio; HT: Hypertensive; HWE: Hardy-Weinberg equilibrium; K/DOQI: NKF Kidney Disease Outcomes Quality Initiative; MAF: Minor allele frequency; MDRD: Modification of Diet in Renal Disease; MeSH: Medical Subject Headings; MHD: Maintenance hemodialysis; MRF: Moderate renal failure; *MTHFR*: Gene encoding Methylene tetrahydrofolate reductase; *MYH9*: Gene encoding myosin, heavy chain 9; NO: Nitric oxide; NS: Not specified; NT: Normotensive; OR: Odds ratio; PCR-RFLP: Polymerase chain reaction restriction fragment length polymorphism; SAMRC: South African Medical Research Council; SBP: Systolic blood pressure; SNP: Single nucleotide polymorphisms; SRF: Severe renal failure; SSA: Sub-Saharan Africa; UA: Unadjusted; *XPD*: Gene encoding xeroderma pigmentosum group D; *XRCC1*: Gene encoding X-ray repair cross-complementing protein 1

Funding

Financial support, through means of infrastructure, was provided by the South African Medical Research Council (SAMRC). The SAMRC as an organization was not directly involved in the design of the study and collection, analysis, interpretation of data or in writing the manuscript.

Authors' contributions

CG, YYY and APK contributed to the conception, the design of the study and drafting the manuscript. CG, YYY, IGO, TEM, FJKF and APK critically revised the manuscript for important intellectual content and all co-authors (CG, YYY, IGO, TEM, FJKF, APK) approved the final version of the manuscript.

Competing interests

The authors declare that they have no competing interests.

Author details

[1]Non-Communicable Diseases Research Unit, South African Medical Research Council, Parow Valley, PO Box 19070, Cape Town, South Africa. [2]Department of Human Biology, Faculty of Health Sciences, Walter Sisulu University, Mthatha, South Africa. [3]Department of Medicine, Division of Nephrology and Hypertension, University of Cape Town, Cape Town, South Africa. [4]Kidney and Hypertension Research Unit, University of Cape Town, Cape Town, South Africa. [5]Department of Biomedical Sciences, Faculty of Health and Wellness Science, Cape Peninsula University of Technology, Bellville, Cape Town, South Africa. [6]Faculty of Medicine and Biomedical Sciences, University of Yaounde I, Yaounde, Cameroon. [7]Medicine Unit, Yaounde University Teaching Hospital, Yaounde, Cameroon.

References

1. Ene-Iordache B, Perico N, Bikbov B, Carminati S, Remuzzi A, Perna A, et al. Chronic kidney disease and cardiovascular risk in six regions of the world (ISN-KDDC): a cross-sectional study. Lancet Glob Health. 2016;4(5):e307–19.
2. Ayodele OE, Alebiosu CO. Burden of chronic kidney disease: an international perspective. Adv Chronic Kidney Dis. 2010;17(3):215–24.
3. Jha V, Garcia-Garcia G, Iseki K, Li Z, Naicker S, Plattner B, et al. Chronic kidney disease: global dimension and perspectives. Lancet. 2013; 382(9888):260–72.
4. Kiberd BA, Clase CM. Cumulative risk for developing end-stage renal disease in the US population. J Am Soc Nephrol. 2002;13(6):1635–44.
5. Peralta CA, Risch N, Lin F, Shlipak MG, Reiner A, Ziv E, et al. The Association of African Ancestry and Elevated Creatinine in the coronary artery risk development in young adults (CARDIA) study. Am J Nephrol. 2010;31(3): 202–8.
6. Hsu CY, Lin F, Vittinghoff E, Shlipak MG. Racial differences in the progression from chronic renal insufficiency to end-stage renal disease in the United States. J Am Soc Nephrol. 2003;14(11):2902–7.
7. Wuttke M, Kottgen A. Insights into kidney diseases from genome-wide association studies. Nat Rev Nephrol. 2016;12(9):549–62.
8. Kottgen A, Glazer NL, Dehghan A, Hwang SJ, Katz R, Li M, et al. Multiple loci associated with indices of renal function and chronic kidney disease. Nat Genet. 2009;41(6):712–7.
9. Kottgen A, Pattaro C, Boger CA, Fuchsberger C, Olden M, Glazer NL, et al. New loci associated with kidney function and chronic kidney disease. Nat Genet. 2010;42(5):376–84.
10. O'Seaghdha CM, Fox CS. Genome-wide association studies of chronic kidney disease: what have we learned? Nat Rev Nephrol. 2012;8(2):89–99.
11. Tishkoff SA, Williams SM. Genetic analysis of African populations: human evolution and complex disease. Nat Rev Genet. 2002;3(8):611–21.
12. Bryc K, Velez C, Karafet T, Moreno-Estrada A, Reynolds A, Auton A, et al. Colloquium paper: genome-wide patterns of population structure and admixture among Hispanic/Latino populations. Proc Natl Acad Sci U S A. 2010;107(Suppl 2):8954–61.
13. Tishkoff SA, Reed FA, Friedlaender FR, Ehret C, Ranciaro A, Froment A, et al. The genetic structure and history of Africans and African Americans. Science. 2009;324(5930):1035–44.
14. Moher D, Liberati A, Tetzlaff J, Altman DG. Preferred reporting items for systematic reviews and meta-analyses: the PRISMA statement. PLoS Med. 2009;6(7):e1000097.
15. Bray M, Higgins J, Ioannidis J, Khoury M, Little J, Manolio T, et al. The HuGENet™ HuGE Review Handbook, version 1.0. In: Little J, Higgins JPT, editors. The HuGENetTM HuGE review handbook. Version 1.0. 2006. Available at: http://www.med.uottawa.ca/public-health-genomics/web/assets/documents/hug_review_handbook_v1_o.pdf. Accessed 23 Jan 2017.
16. Pienaar E, Grobler L, Busgeeth K, Eisinga A, Siegfried N. Developing a geographic search filter to identify randomised controlled trials in Africa: finding the optimal balance between sensitivity and precision. Health Inf Libr J. 2011;28(3):210–5.

17. Sagoo GS, Little J, Higgins JP. Systematic reviews of genetic association studies. Human Genome Epidemiol Network PLoS Med. 2009;6(3):e28.
18. Elshamaa MF, Sabry S, Badr A, El-Ahmady M, Elghoroury EA, Thabet EH, et al. Endothelial nitric oxide synthase gene intron4 VNTR polymorphism in patients with chronic kidney disease. Blood Coagul Fibrinolysis. 2011;22(6):487–92.
19. Hanna MOF, Shahin RMH, Meshaal SS, Kostandi IF. Susceptibility and progression of end stage renal disease are not associated with angiotensin II type 1 receptor gene polymorphism. J Rec Signal Transd. 2015;35(5):381–5.
20. Kerkeni M, Letaief A, Achour A, Miled A, Trivin F, Maaroufi K. Endothelial nitric oxide synthetase, methylenetetrahydrofolate reductase polymorphisms, and cardiovascular complications in Tunisian patients with nondiabetic renal disease. Clin Biochem. 2009;42(10–11):958–64.
21. Lahrach H, Essiarab F, Timinouni M, Hatim B, El Khayat S, Er-Rachdi L, et al. Association of apolipoprotein E gene polymorphism with end-stage renal disease and hyperlipidemia in patients on long-term hemodialysis. Ren Fail. 2014;36(10):1504–9.
22. Radwan WM, Elbarbary HS, Alsheikh NM. DNA repair genes XPD and XRCC1 polymorphisms and risk of end-stage renal disease in Egyptian population. Ren Fail. 2015;37(1):122–8.
23. Rezk NA, Zidan HE, Elnaggar YA, Ghorab A. Renalase gene polymorphism and epinephrine level in chronic kidney disease. Appl Biochem Biotechnol. 2015;175(4):2309–17.
24. Elhelbawy NG, Elzorkany KM, Abdelatty AF. Chemokine receptor 2 (CCR2) G190A polymorphism in chronic renal failure patients requiring hemodialysis. Egypt Soc Biochem Mol Biol. 2016;34(1/2):67–76.
25. Elshamaa MF, Sabry SM, El-Sonbaty MM, Elghoroury EA, Emara N, Raafat M, et al. Adiponectin: an adipocyte-derived hormone, and its gene encoding in children with chronic kidney disease. BMC Res Notes. 2012;5:174.
26. Abdallah ES, Sabry D. Renalase gene polymorphisms in end-stage renal disease patients: an Egyptian study. J Amer Sci. 2013;9(1):346–9.
27. Matsha TE, Kengne AP, Masconi KL, Yako YY, Erasmus RT. APOL1 genetic variants, chronic kidney diseases and hypertension in mixed ancestry south Africans. BMC Genet. 2015;16:69.
28. Matsha TE, Masconi K, Yako YY, Hassan MS, Macharia M, Erasmus RT, et al. Polymorphisms in the non-muscle myosin heavy chain gene (MYH9) are associated with lower glomerular filtration rate in mixed ancestry diabetic subjects from South Africa. PLoS One. 2012;7(12):e52529.
29. Tayo BO, Kramer H, Salako BL, Gottesman O, McKenzie CA, Ogunniyi A, et al. Genetic variation in APOL1 and MYH9 genes is associated with chronic kidney disease among Nigerians. Int Urol Nephrol. 2013;45(2): 485–94.
30. Ulasi II, Tzur S, Wasser WG, Shemer R, Kruzel E, Feigin E, et al. High population frequencies of APOL1 risk variants are associated with increased prevalence of non-diabetic chronic kidney disease in the Igbo people from South-Eastern Nigeria. Nephron Clin Pract. 2013;123(1–2):123–8.
31. El-Shal AS, Zidan HE, Rashad NM. Adiponectin gene polymorphisms in Egyptian type 2 diabetes mellitus patients with and without diabetic nephropathy. Mol Biol Rep. 2014;41(4):2287–98.
32. Kao WH, Klag MJ, Meoni LA, Reich D, Berthier-Schaad Y, Li M, et al. MYH9 is associated with nondiabetic end-stage renal disease in African Americans. Nat Genet. 2008;40(10):1185–92.
33. Behar DM, Rosset S, Tzur S, Selig S, Yudkovsky G, Bercovici S, et al. African ancestry allelic variation at the MYH9 gene contributes to increased susceptibility to non-diabetic end-stage kidney disease in Hispanic Americans. Hum Mol Genet. 2010;19(9):1816–27.
34. O'Seaghdha CM, Parekh RS, Hwang SJ, Li M, ttgen AK, Coresh J, et al. The MYH9/APOL1 region and chronic kidney disease in European-Americans. Hum Mol Genet. 2011;20(12):2450–6.
35. Genovese G, Friedman DJ, Ross MD, Lecordier L, Uzureau P, Freedman BI, et al. Association of trypanolytic ApoL1 variants with kidney disease in African Americans. Science. 2010;329(5993):841–5.
36. Tzur S, Rosset S, Shemer R, Yudkovsky G, Selig S, Tarekegn A, et al. Missense mutations in the APOL1 gene are highly associated with end stage kidney disease risk previously attributed to the MYH9 gene. Hum Genet. 2010; 128(3):345–50.
37. Genovese G, Friedman DJ, Pollak MR. APOL1 variants and kidney disease in people of recent African ancestry. Nat Rev Nephrol. 2013;9(4): 240–4.
38. Wasser WG, Tzur S, Wolday D, Adu D, Baumstein D, Rosset S, et al. Population genetics of chronic kidney disease: the evolving story of APOL1. J Nephrol. 2012;25(5):603–18.
39. Behar DM, Kedem E, Rosset S, Haileselassie Y, Tzur S, Kra-Oz Z, et al. Absence of APOL1 risk variants protects against HIV-associated nephropathy in the Ethiopian population. Am J Nephrol. 2011;34(5):452–9.
40. Buckley R. Apolipoprotein G1 and G2 variants may partially explain a higher prevalence of lupus-nephritis ESRD in African Americans. MD Conf Express. 2012:10.
41. Cohen DL, Townsend RR. Is it variants in the apolipoprotein I1 gene, or blood pressure control, that predicts progression of nondiabetic hypertensive nephropathy in african americans? J Clin Hypertens. 2013;15(7): 445–6.
42. Colares VS, Titan SMDO, Pereira ADC, Malafronte P, Cardena MM, Santos S, et al. MYH9 and APOL1 gene polymorphisms and the risk of CKD in patients with lupus nephritis from an admixture population. PLoS One. 2014;9(3).
43. Estrella MM, Li M, Tin A, Abraham AG, Shlipak MG, Penugonda S, et al. The association between APOL1 risk alleles and longitudinal kidney function differs by HIV viral suppression status. Clin Infect Dis. 2015; 60(4):646–52.
44. Fine DM, Wasser WG, Estrella MM, Atta MG, Kuperman M, Shemer R, et al. APOL1 risk variants predict histopathology and progression to ESRD in HIV-related kidney disease. J Am Soc Nephrol. 2012;23(2):343–50.
45. Foster MC, Coresh J, Fornage M, Astor BC, Grams M, Franceschini N, et al. APOL1 variants associate with increased risk of CKD among African Americans. J Am Soc Nephrol. 2013;24(9):1484–91.
46. Roussos L, Flor n C, Carlson J, Svensson PJ, Wallmark A, Ekberg H. Increased prevalence of apolipoprotein E3/E4 genotype among Swedish renal transplant recipients. Nephron. 1999;83(1):25–30.
47. Hsu CC, Kao WH, Coresh J, Pankow JS, Marsh-Manzi J, Boerwinkle E, et al. Apolipoprotein E and progression of chronic kidney disease. JAMA. 2005; 293(23):2892–9.
48. Choi SW, Kweon SS, Choi JS, Rhee JA, Lee YH, Nam HS, et al. Association between apolipoprotein E polymorphism and chronic kidney disease in the Korean general population: dong-gu study. Kor J Fam Med. 2014;35(6):276–82.
49. Nagase S, Suzuki H, Wang Y, Kikuchi S, Hirayama A, Ueda A, et al. Association of ecNOS gene polymorphisms with end stage renal diseases. Mol Cell Biochem. 2003;244(1–2):113–8.
50. Noiri E, Satoh H, Taguchi J, Brodsky SV, Nakao A, Ogawa Y, et al. Association of eNOS Glu298Asp polymorphism with end-stage renal disease. Hypertension. 2002;40(4):535–40.
51. Wang Y, Kikuchi S, Suzuki H, Nagase S, Koyama A. Endothelial nitric oxide synthase gene polymorphism in intron 4 affects the progression of renal failure in non-diabetic renal diseases. Nephrol Dial Transplant. 1999;14(12): 2898–902.
52. Bellini MH, Figueira MN, Piccoli MF, Marumo JT, Cendoroglo MS, Neto MC, et al. Association of endothelial nitric oxide synthase gene intron 4 polymorphism with end-stage renal disease. Nephrology (Carlton). 2007; 12(3):289–93.
53. Marson BP, Dickel S, Ishizawa MH, Metzger IF, Izidoro-Toledo T, da Costa BE, et al. Endothelial nitric oxide genotypes and haplotypes are not associated with end-stage renal disease. DNA Cell Biol. 2011;30(1):55–9.
54. Trabulus S, Guven GS, Altiparmak MR, Batar B, Tun O, Yalin AS, et al. DNA repair XRCC1 Arg399Gln polymorphism is associated with the risk of development of end-stage renal disease. Mol Biol Rep. 2012;39(6): 6995–7001.
55. Sanchez-Quinto F, Botigue LR, Civit S, Arenas C, Avila-Arcos MC, Bustamante CD, et al. North African populations carry the signature of admixture with Neandertals. PLoS One. 2012;7(10):e47765.

Factor XIII polymorphism and risk of aneurysmal subarachnoid haemorrhage in a south Indian population

Arati Suvatha[1], M. K. Sibin[2], Dhananjaya I. Bhat[3], K. V. L. Narasingarao[3], Vikas Vazhayil[3] and G. K. Chetan[1*]

Abstract

Background: The rupture of a brain aneurysm causes bleeding in the subarachnoid space and is known as aneurysmal subarachnoid haemorrhage (aSAH). In our study, we evaluated the association of *factor XIII* polymorphism and the risk of Aneurysmal subarachnoid haemorrhage (aSAH) in South Indian population.

Methods: The study was performed in 200 subjects with aSAH and 205 healthy control subjects. Genotyping of rs5985(c.103G > T (p.Val35Leu)) and rs5982(c.1694C > T (p.Pro564Leu)) polymorphism was performed by Taqman® allelic discrimination assay.

Results: In our study, Val/Leu genotype frequency was higher in control subjects (18%) compared to aSAH patients (9%).The Val/Leu genotype was associated with lower risk of aSAH (OR = 0.48, 95%CI = 0.26–0.88, p = 0.02). When compared with Val allele, Leu allele was significantly associated with lower risk of aSAH (OR = 0.55, 95%CI = 0.32–0.95, p = 0.03). In subtyping, we found a significant association of Leu/Leu genotype with the Basilar top aneurysm (OR = 3.59, 95%CI = 1.11–11.64, p = 0.03). In c.1694C > T (p.Pro565Leu) variant, Pro/Pro Vs Pro/Leu genotype (OR = 2.06, 95%CI = 1.10–3.85, p = 0.02) was significantly associated with higher risk of aSAH. The 564Leu allelic frequency in aSAH patients (36%) was higher when compared with that in healthy controls (30%) in our study. When allele frequency (Pro Vs Leu) was compared, 564Leu allele was found to be significantly associated with higher aSAH risk (OR = 1.36, 95%CI = 1.01–1.83, p = 0.04). (OR = 1.36, 95%CI = 1.01–1.83, p = 0.04). Regarding rs5985 and rs5982, significant association was found in the log-additive model (OR = 0.57, 95%CI = 0.33–0.97, p = 0.034; OR = 1.32, 95%CI = 1.00–1.72, p = 0.043).

Conclusion: These results suggest that 34Leu allele was a protective factor for lower risk of aSAH whereas 564Leu allele was associated with higher risk of aSAH in South Indian population.

Keywords: Aneurysmal subarachnoid haemorrhage, Factor XIII, Polymorphism, Basilar top aneurysm

Background

Subarachnoid hemorrhage (SAH) caused by rupture of a cerebral aneurysm is the reason for approximately 85% of cases with spontaneous SAH [1]. It accounts for 5% of all stroke cases and is associated with high rate of mortality and morbidity [2]. Rebleeding and delayed cerebral ischemia are the two major complications that are associated with poor prognosis and high mortality rate in SAH [3]. The first-degree relatives of patients with SAH have a three-fold increased risk for the rupture of an aneurysm when compared with general population [4]. But the role of genetic factors which contribute to the risk of SAH is poorly defined. Most candidate gene studies have considered proteins associated with connective tissue organization [5–7]. The reason for SAH occurrence was not only due to weakened vessel wall structure but also due to rupture of vessel wall [8]. A few studies have investigated the role of fibrinolytic system and coagulation factors association with the risk of aSAH [9–11].

Coagulation factor XIII belongs to transglutaminase family which circulates as a heterotetramer, composed of two A subunits and two B subunits [12]. During coagulation,

* Correspondence: drchetangk@gmail.com
[1]Department of Human Genetics, National Institute of Mental Health and Neuro Sciences, Bangalore, Karnataka 560029, India
Full list of author information is available at the end of the article

thrombin activates the catalytic factor XIII A subunit and crosslinks the fibrin molecules to increase the clot stability [13]. During fibrinolysis, factor XIII A activates anti plasmin which inhibits the plasmin from degrading the crosslinked fibrin structure [14]. Thus, factor XIII A subunit plays a significant role both in coagulation and fibrinolysis. Also, it plays a key role in extracellular remodelling, angiogenesis, atherosclerosis, wound healing and tissue repair [15].

In humans, the Coagulation factor XIII A chain (*F13A*) gene is located on chromosome 6p 24–25 [16]. The factor XIII A is 83 kDa protein, which consists of 732 amino acids [17]. *F13A* gene consists of 15 exons and 14 introns [18]. The nine polymorphisms in *F13A* genes are c.103G > T(p.Val35Leu), c.614A > T(p.Tyr204Phe), c.996A > C (p.Pro 332Pro), c.1652C > T(p.Thr550Ile), c.1694C > T (p.Pro564-Leu), c.1704A > G (p.Glu567Glu), c.1696 T > A (p.Leu588 Gl), c.1951G > A (p.Val650Ile) and c.1954G > C (p.Glu652 Gln) [19]. Among them, the common *F13A* polymorphisms are c.103G > T (p.Val35Leu)and c.1694C > T (p.Pro564Leu).

In the Asian and Caucasian population, the allele frequency of 34Leu allele is 0.13 and 0.25 [20]. In Han Chinese population, the c.103G > T (p.Val35Leu) polymorphism was associated with the risk of ischemic cardiovascular and cerebrovascular diseases [21].In Caucasian population, c.103G > T (p.Val35Leu) polymorphism was associated with the risk of intracerebral hemorrhage and brain infarction [22, 23].In the Asian and Caucasian population, the allele frequency of 564Leu allele is 0.29 and 0.21 [17]. The c.1694C > T(p.Pro564Leu) polymorphism was associated with decreased factor XIII plasma levels with increased factor XIII activity [24]. When stratified by gender c.1694C > T (p.Pro564Leu) polymorphism was associated with risk of haemorrhagic stroke in women aged < 45 years in Caucasian population [10]. The aim of the present study is to investigate the association of c.103G > T (p.Val35Leu) and c.1694C > T (p.Pro564Leu) polymorphisms with the risk of aSAH in a South Indian population.

Methods

Study population

A total of 200 patients with aneurysmal subarachnoid haemorrhage and 205, age and sex- matched healthy controls were selected randomly from general population during the period of 2015–2017. The healthy controls were unrelated to patients but were of the same ethnicity. Also, patients were unrelated to each other. The patients were recruited from the Department of Neurosurgery, NIMHNAS, Bangalore, India and their demographic and clinical details were collected from the medical records department of the hospital. The neurological grade was classified based on World Federation of neurological surgeons (WFNS) scale and all grades were included in this study. The inclusion criteria for selecting patients with aSAH was the presence of symptoms suggestive of aSAH combined with the finding of subarachnoid blood on CT and a proven aneurysm on conventional angiography. Exclusion criteria for selecting patients were 1.the presence of neuropsychiatric conditions like dementia, Parkinson's disease, epilepsy, psychoses 2. SAH resulted from a mycotic aneurysm, arterio-venous malformation, or head trauma. The inclusion criteria for healthy controls were 1. the absence of clinical symptoms of aSAH 2. similar demographic characteristics of patients such as adult group over 18 years old, gender, ethnicity and dietary habits, 3. no medical history of haemorrhage and no family history of aSAH in first degree relatives. The study protocol was approved by the Institute of ethics committee for human studies, NIMHANS, Bangalore. Written informed consent was obtained from all the participants included in the study.

DNA extraction and genotyping

Five milliliter blood sample was collected from all the participants and genomic DNA was isolated from blood using commercially available Machery-Nagel (MN) kit according to manufacturer's protocol. DNA with a purity of 1.75–1.85 was used for genotyping analysis. Purity and quantity of DNA was analysed by Nanodrop ND2000c spectrophotometer. Genotyping of c.103G > T (p.Val35-Leu) (rs5985) and c.1694C > T (p.Pro564Leu) (rs5982) was performed using Taqman® allelic discrimination assay (Applied Biosystems, Foster City, CA) with a commercially available primer probe set (assay ID C_1639938_20, C_8786720_10). Experiments were performed in duplicates in Applied Biosystem7500 Fast real-time machine.

Statistical analysis

R.3.0.11 statistical software was used to statistically analyse the data. The continuous variables were expressed as mean ± SD and categorical variables were expressed as absolute values and percentages. The difference in genotype and allele frequencies between groups were analysed by $\chi 2$ test. Association between *F13A* genotypes or alleles and aSAH risk were expressed as odds ratio (OR) with 95% confidence intervals (CI), adjusted for the confounding effects of smoking, hypertension, drinking and diabetes mellitus using the logistic regression model. p-value < 0.05 was considered significant. The Hardy-Weinberg equilibrium calculation and additive effect of SNPs was calculated using the online tool SNPStats, https://www.snpstats.net/start.html [25]. Prediction of functional effect of two SNPs mapped in genetic variants of *F13A* gene was done using SIFT (http://sift.jcvi.org/) and PolyPhen-2 (http://genetics.bwh.harvard.edu/pph/data/index.html) [26].The linkage disequilibrium (LD) and haplotype frequency were estimated using Haploview software (version 4.2). The meta-analysis study was performed for fixed and random effect model using Review manager5.2. The test for heterogeneity was estimated by I^2 statistics. p-value < 0.10 was considered as significant for heterogeneity among the studies. Fixed effect model was used to find out the OR with 95%CI when there was no heterogeneity; otherwise, random effect model was applied [27]. Val/Val and Pro/Pro genotypes were the wild- type homozygote genotype for *F13A* gene, while Leu/Leu genotype was the rare homozygous genotype. The dominant and recessive models for this study were Val/Val Vs Val/Leu + Leu/Leu, Pro/Pro Vs Pro/Leu + Leu/Leu, Val/Val + Val/Leu Vs Leu/Leu and Pro/Pro+ Pro/Leu Vs Leu/Leu.

Results

Characteristics of study population

Demographic characteristics of aSAH patients and controls were already published previously (DOI: https://doi.org/10.1186/s11658-017-0059-8). There were no significant differences in gender and mean age between aSAH patients and healthy controls.

Factor XIII polymorphism and risk of aSAH

The distribution of *factor XIII* genotype and allele frequencies is shown in Table 1.The distribution of genotype frequencies of controls are in Hardy–Weinberg equilibrium (rs5985; $p = 0.99$, rs5982; $p = 0.79$). In our study, for c.103G > T(p.Val35Leu) and c.1694C > T (p.Pro564Leu) variants there was no significant difference in genotypes ($\chi^2 = 5.81$; df = 2; $p = 0.05$); ($\chi^2 = 5.41$; df = 2; $p = 0.06$) between cases and controls. However, in allele frequencies ($\chi^2 = 4.12$; df = 1; $p = 0.04$); ($\chi^2 = 3.89$; df = 1; $p = 0.04$) there was a significant difference for c.103G > T (p.Val35Leu) and c.1694C > T (p.Pro564Leu) variants between cases and controls.

The result of logistic regression analyses is shown in Table 2 and Additional file 1: Table S1. In c.103G > T (p.Val35Leu) variant, the Val/Leu genotype frequency was higher in control subjects (18%) when compared with that in aSAH patients (9%).The presence of one copy of 34Leu allele was associated with lower risk of aSAH (Val/Val Vs Val/Leu; OR = 0.45, 95%CI = 0.24–0.84; p = 0.013). In the dominant model of inheritance, there was a significant association between c.103G > T (p.Val35Leu) polymorphism and risk of aSAH (Val/Val Vs Val/Leu + Leu/Leu; OR = 0.48, 95%CI = 0.26–0.84; $p = 0.013$). However, the presence of two copies of 34Leu allele was not significantly associated with aSAH risk (Val/Val Vs Leu/Leu; OR = 1.19, 95%CI = 0.16–8.65; $p = 0.858$).Likewise, the recessive model of c.103G > T (p.Val35Leu) polymorphism did not have any statistical significance. A significant association was found in the log-additive model for rs5985 (c.103G > T (p.Val35Leu)) with an OR of 0.57 (95% CI = 0.33–0.97; $p = 0.034$). In our study, the 34Leu allelic frequency in healthy controls subjects (10%) was higher than that in aSAH patients (6%). When allele frequency (Val Vs Leu) was compared, 34Leu allele was significantly associated with lower aSAH risk (OR = 0.55, 95%CI = 0.32–0.95; $p = 0.030$).

In c.1694C > T (p.Pro564Leu) variant, the Leu/Leu genotype was higher in aSAH patients (17%) when compared with that in healthy controls (9.5%). The presence of two copies of the 564Leu allele was significantly associated with higher risk of aSAH (Pro/Pro Vs Leu/Leu; OR = 2.00, 95%CI = 1.15–3.76; $p = 0.034$).Also, in the recessive model of inheritance, there was a significant association between c.1694C > T (p.Pro564Leu) polymorphism and risk of aSAH (Pro/Pro+ Pro/Leu Vs Leu/Leu; OR = 1.94, 95%CI = 1.05–3.58; $p = 0.034$). Similarly, a significant association was found in the log-additive

Table 2 Logistic Regression Analysis of association between *F13A* SNPs and aSAH risk

Genotype & Allele	Adjusted OR[a] (95%CI)	p-value
c.103G > T (p.Val35Leu) Model		
Dominant	0.48(0.26–0.89)	**0.020**
Recessive	1.30(0.18–9.41)	0.791
Log-Additive model	0.57 (0.33–0.97)	**0.034**
c.1694C > T (p.Pro564Leu) Model		
Dominant	1.25(0.83–1.86)	0.275
Recessive	1.94(1.05–3.58)	**0.034**
Log-Additive model	1.32 (1.00–1.72)	**0.043**

OR Odds Ratio
[a]Adjusted for smoking, alcohol consumption, hypertension and diabetes
p-values < 0.05 are given in bold

Table 1 Genotypes and allele frequency of *F13A* polymorphisms in aSAH Cases and Controls

	Alleles		Genotypes		
	n(%)	*n*(%)	*n*(%)	*n*(%)	*n*(%)
c.103G > T (p.Val35Leu)	Val	Leu	Val/Val	Val/Leu	Leu/Leu
Control subjects (205)	371(93)	39(10)	168(84)	35(17.5)	2(1)
aSAH patients (200)	378(95)	22(6)	180(90)	18(9)	2(1)
c.1694C > T (p.Pro564Leu)	Pro	Leu	Pro/Pro	Pro/Leu	Leu/Leu
Control subjects (205)	292(73)	118 (30)	106(53)	80(40)	19(9.5)
aSAH patients (200)	258(65)	142(36)	92(46)	74(37)	34(17)

model for rs5982 (c.1694C > T (p.Pro564Leu)) with an OR of 1.32 (95% CI = 1.00–1.72; $p = 0.043$). Our studies showed that 564Leu allelic frequency in aSAH patients (36%) was higher than that in healthy controls (30%). When allele frequency (Pro Vs Leu) was compared, 564Leu allele was significantly associated with higher aSAH risk (OR = 1.36, 95%CI = 1.01–1.83; $p = 0.040$). However, there was no significant association in heterozygous genotype and dominant model of inheritance with the risk of aSAH.

When aneurysm was classified according to the location, size and WFNS grade, only the Leu/Leu genotype in c.103G > T (p.Val35Leu) variant was statistically significant with basilar top aneurysm (OR = 3.59, 95%CI = 1.11–11.64; $p = 0.030$). Classification of aneurysm according to c.103G > T (p.Val35Leu) and c.1694C > T (p.Pro564Leu) variants is shown in Table 3. Multiple comparisons were performed between male versus female, hypertensive versus non-hypertensive, diabetic versus non- diabetic patients with different c.103G > T (p.Val35Leu) and c.1694C > T (p.Pro564Leu) genotypic model and allele frequencies. None of the comparison showed statistical significance with c.103G > T (p.Val35-Leu) and c.1694C > T (p.Pro564Leu) variants.

Prediction of the functional effect of studied SNPs was done with two annotation programs, namely SIFT (Sorting Intolerant from Tolerant) and PolyPhen-2 (Polymorphism Phenotyping). Using SIFT algorithm, the normalized probability score for rs5985 and rs5982 was > 0.05 (1 and 0.14) and predicted to be tolerated. Using PolyPhen-2 algorithm, the normalized probability score for rs5985 and rs5982 was < 0.2 (0 and 0.003) and predicted as benign. According to the sequence and structural homology-based approach, the studied nsSNPs has tolerated/benign functional prediction score (Additional file 2: Table S2).

Linkage disequilibrium (LD) and haplotype analysis of *factor XIII* and aSAH

Haploview software was used to estimate the LD between the two-studied polymorphism. There was no significant LD (D' = 0.17) observed among the polymorphism (Fig. 1), which suggest the strongest evidence of recombination.

Table 3 c.103G > T (p.Val35Leu) and c.1694C > T (p.Pro564Leu) Variants in aSAH subtypes

Variable	Case	Val/Val (p)	Val/Leu (p)	Leu/Leu (p)	Val	Leu	Val Vs Leu (p)	Pro/Pro (p)	Pro/Leu (p)	Leu/Leu (p)	Pro	Leu	Pro Vs Leu (p)
Total	200	180	18	2	378	22		92	74	34	258	142	
Site of Aneurysm													
ACOM	86	75(0.86)	11(0.38)	0(0.62)	161	11	0.67	42 (0.79)	26 (0.44)	18(0.51)	110	62	0.90
PCOM	12	11(0.96)	1(0.94)	0(0.45)	23	1	0.78	4 (0.58)	7(0.35)	1(0.50)	15	9	0.84
ICA	36	32(0.96)	3(0.90)	1(0.40)	67	5	0.62	16(0.91)	16(0.57)	4(0.44)	48	24	0.72
MCA	37	36(0.76)	1(0.24)	0(0.96)	73	1	0.16	14 (0.56)	17(0.50)	6(0.92)	45	29	0.54
Multiple	22	20(0.97)	2(0.98)	0(0.71)	42	2	0.79	13 (0.50)	6(0.52)	3(0.73)	32	12	0.27
Basilar top	7	6(0.93)	0(0.82)	1(**0.03**)	12	2	0.18	3 (0.91)	2(0.75)	2(0.52)	8	6	0.57
Size of aneurysm													
Small(< 15 mm)	159	141(0.92)	17(0.62)	1(0.70)	299	19	0.78	76(0.83)	55(0.74)	28(0.89)	207	111	0.86
Large(15-25 mm)	37	36(0.76)	0	1(0.42)	72	2	0.32	15(0.70)	17(0.50)	5(0.65)	47	27	0.87
Giant(> 25 mm)	4	3(0.81)	1(0.37)	0	7	1	0.41	1(0.58)	2 (0.73)	1(0.73)	4	4	0.40
WFNS Grade													
Grade I	91	82(0.99)	8(0.95)	1(0.93)	172	10	0.99	38(0.67)	31(0.73)	22(0.24)	107	75	0.18
Grade II	42	36(0.84)	5(0.59)	1(0.48)	77	7	0.32	21(0.77)	17(0.77)	4(0.29)	59	25	0.31
Grade III	51	47(0.91)	4(0.81)	0	98	4	0.52	26(0.71)	20(0.40)	5(0.27)	72	30	
Grade IV	16	15(0.91)	1(0.73)	0	31	1	0.57	7(0.91)	6(0.97)	3(0.88)	20	12	0.82
Male	77	73(0.78)	4(0.33)	0	150	4	0.15	39(0.68)	26(0.72)	12(0.81)	104	50	0.50
Female	123	107(0.14)	14(0.53)	2(0.62)	228	18	0.35	53(0.75)	48(0.80)	22(0.86)	154	92	0.62
Hypertension (+)	37	32(0.33)	5(0.44)	0	69	5	0.66	14(0.56)	18(0.38)	5(0.65)	46	28	0.70
Diabetes mellitus (+)	71	65(0.93)	5(0.63)	1(0.78)	136	7	0.78	34(0.86)	25(0.85)	12(0.98)	93	49	0.83
Alcohol (+)	57	53(0.88)	4(0.66)	0	110	4	0.39	29(0.69)	18(0.60)	10(0.93)	76	38	0.66
Smoking (+)	58	54(0.87)	4(0.64)	0	112	4	0.37	31(0.55)	19(0.68)	8(0.61)	81	35	0.28

p-value < 0.05 are given in bold

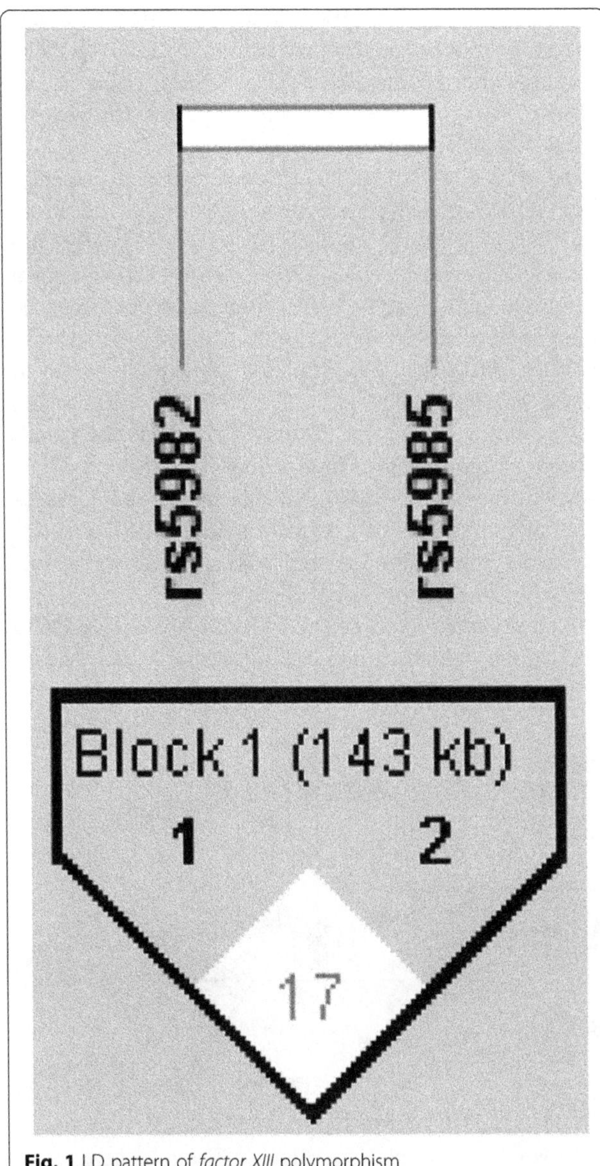

Fig. 1 LD pattern of *factor XIII* polymorphism

The haplotype frequency estimation among patients and controls is shown in Table 4. The frequency of Leu:Val haplotype (c.1694C > T (p.Pro564Leu): c.103G > T (p.Val35Leu)) was significantly higher in controls than in aSAH patients ($p = 0.01$). Whereas the frequency of Pro:Leu (c.1694C > T (p.Pro564Leu): c.103G > T (p.Val35Leu)) haplotype was significantly higher in aSAH patients than in controls ($p = 0.03$).Pro:Val (c.1694C > T (p.Pro564Leu): c.103G > T (p.Val35Leu)) was the most frequent haplotype and was observed in more than 60% in both aSAH patients and controls.

Meta-analysis of *factor XIII* polymorphism with risk of aSAH

We performed the meta-analysis with previously reported studies along with our present study to verify the association between *F13A* gene polymorphism and risk of aSAH. The meta -analysis of c.103G > T (p.Val35Leu) variant could not predict any significant association with aSAH risk in fixed effect and random effect models. There was significant heterogeneity in Val Vs Leu ($p = 0.02$) and in dominant model ($p = 0.03$). However, in c.1694C > T (p.Pro564Leu) variant there was significant association in Pro Vs Leu allele, Pro/Pro Vs Leu/Leu genotype and in dominant model of inheritance (Pro Vs Leu, OR = 1.36, 95%CI =1.12–1.66; $p = 0.002$; Pro/Pro Vs Leu/Leu, OR = 2.49, 95%CI =1.53–4.06; $p = 0.0002$; Pro/Pro Vs Pro/Leu + Leu/Leu, OR = 2.19, 95%CI = 1.37–3.50; $p = 0.001$) (Fig. 2).

Discussion

Spontaneous subarachnoid hemorrhage (non-traumatic) remains as one of the considerable neurosurgical problems that affect 25,000 to 28,000 people yearly [28]. In cerebrovascular disorders, the role of multifactorial and multigene have been studied progressively. The difference in phenotype in persons carrying same genetic mutation suggests the role of multiple factors in the pathogenesis of the disease [29]. This study was carried out to analyse whether *F13A* polymorphism was associated with the risk of aSAH.

Extracellular matrix remodelling dysfunction, atherosclerosis and fibrinolytic dysfunction were considered as important pathogenic mechanisms in the formation and rupture of a cerebral aneurysm [30–32]. Coagulation factor XIII A chain plays a significant role in extracellular matrix (ECM) remodelling and tissue repair [33]. Cross-linking of collagen and fibronectin to each other by F13A during extracellular matrix formation and wound healing was an important physiological event in stabilizing the ECM [34]. F13A in the cellular form plays a significant role in triggering atherosclerosis [18]. F13A helps in angiotensin I receptor dimerization which activates the monocyte adhesion to endothelium cells and this was considered as one of the pathogenic mechanism in the progression of atherosclerosis [33]. In the fibrinolytic system, the primary mechanism to prolong fibrinolysis is crosslinking of α_2 -anti plasmin and fibrin by F13A [35]. It has been shown that properties of F13A were affected by its gene variants [19] and it was suggested that *F13A* variants play a key role in the pathogenesis of a cerebral aneurysm by affecting the vessel wall stability, triggering atherosclerosis and decreasing clot stability [20].

F13A polymorphism was associated with the severity of outcome in atherothrombotic ischemic stroke [36], primary intracerebral hemorrhage [37] brain infarction [38] and deep vein thrombosis [39]. Many case-control studies reported the association of *F13A* polymorphism and risk of aSAH. Ladenvall et al. reported that 34Leu and 564Leu carriers had an increased risk of aSAH in

Table 4 Haplotype frequency distribution among patients and controls

Haplotypes	Frequencies in controls (%)	Frequencies in patients (%)	χ2	*p*
Pro:Val	60.6	64.1	1.08	0.29
Leu:Val	33.9	26.1	5.86	0.01
Pro:Leu	3.9	7.3	4.47	0.03
Leu:Leu	1.6	2.4	0.71	0.40

Order of SNPs in *F13A* haplotypes: c.1694C > T (p.Pro564Leu), c.103G > T (p.Val35Leu); χ2: Chi-square test; *p*: probability value

the Swedish population [9], but there was no association between c.103G > T (p.Val35Leu) variant and nonfatal haemorrhagic stroke in young white women in U.S population [10]. Another study done by Rugriok et al. reported that c.103G > T (p.Val35Leu) and c.1694C > T (p.Pro564Leu) polymorphisms did not have any association with the risk for aSAH in Caucasian population [11]. In Spanish population, the prevalence of 34 Leu allele was higher in aSAH than in primary intracerebral hemorrhage group [40]. The meta-analysis of four studies including the present study suggested that there was no significant association with c.103G > T (p.Val35-Leu) polymorphism and risk of aSAH, whereas the c.1694C > T (p.Pro564Leu) polymorphism showed significant association with risk of aSAH.

The c.103G > T (p.Val35Leu) polymorphism present at exon 2 of *F13A* gene increases the activation rate of coagulation and affects the fibrin structure [41]. The fibrin clot which is crosslinked by 34Leu variants has thinner fibres, smaller pore and altered permeation characteristics when compared with fibrin clot crosslinked by Val34 variant [19]. Also, the clot formation time was shorter for 34Leu variant samples [42]. The c.1694C > T (p.Pro564-Leu) polymorphism present at exon 12 affects the specific activity of the enzyme. Also, c.1694C > T (p.Pro564Leu) variant causes lower plasma F13A levels and increases F13A activity [43]. In the present study, 34Leu allele was associated with lower risk and 564Leu allele was associated with the higher risk for aSAH.

The protective effect of the *F13A* c.103G > T (p.Val35-Leu) polymorphism is not well understood and needs to

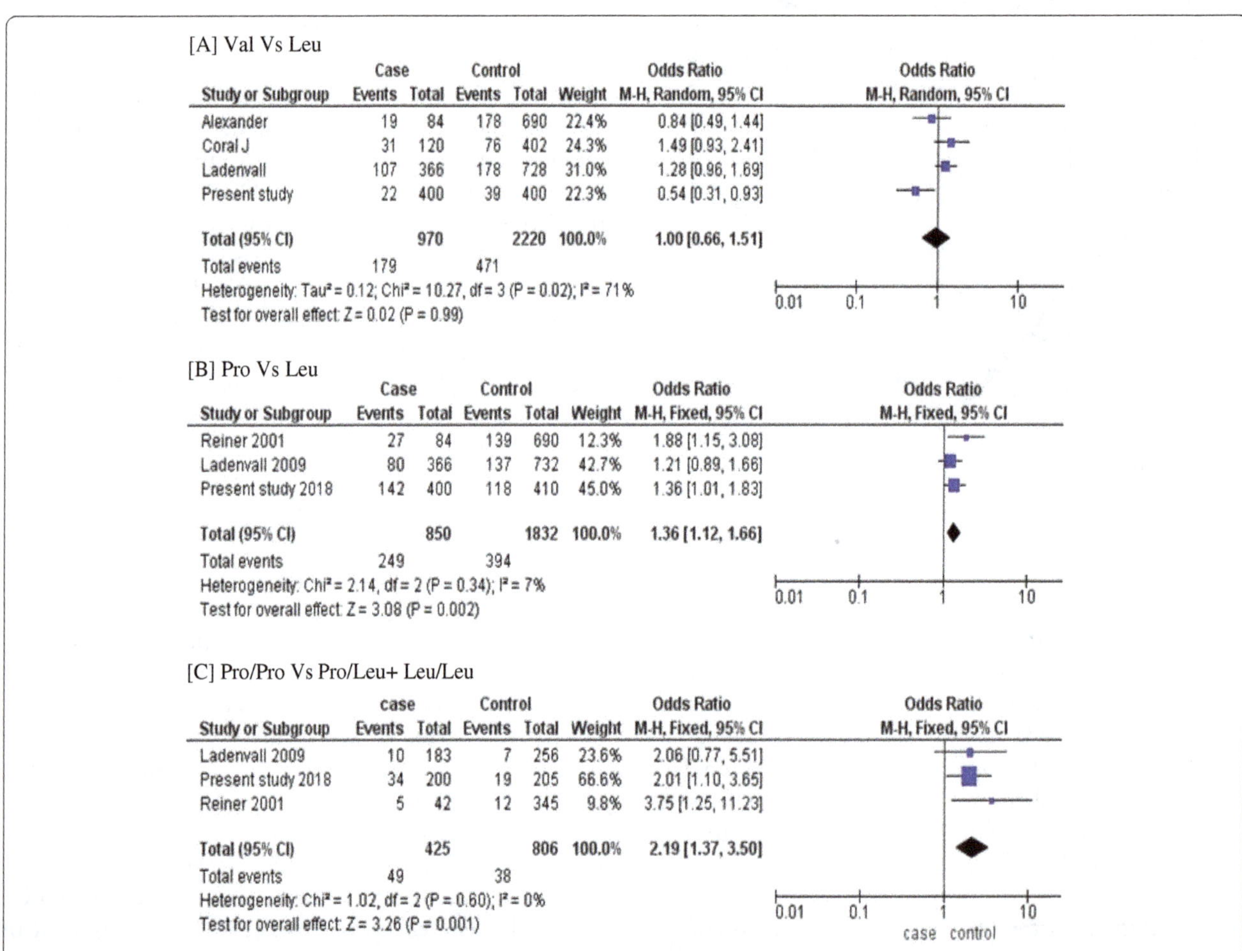

Fig. 2 Metanalysis of *factor XIII* gene variants. **a** c.103G > T (p.Val35Leu) (Val Vs Leu) (**b**) c.1694C > T (p.Pro564Leu) (Pro Vs Leu) (**c**) c.1694C > T (p.Pro564Leu) (Pro/Pro Vs Pro/Leu + Leu/Leu)

be elucidated. The protective effect c.103G > T (p.Val35-Leu) polymorphism was reported in few studies on myocardial infraction and venous thrombosis [44–47]. .An increased F13A activity was reported in 34Leu carriers, higher activity in Leu homozygotes and intermediate activity in Leu heterozygote [43]. This was because of proximity of polymorphism to the thrombin activation site. Kohler et al. reported that the higher F13A activation results in ineffective cross linking [48]. Van Wersch et al. reported that in pregnant women, F13A levels were higher in smokers than in non -smokers [49]. In our study number of smokers in patients were higher than that in controls. Elbaz et al. reported that the ORs associated with smoking were lower in 34Leu carriers than in noncarriers. This suggests that the protective effect of polymorphism was more significant than effect of smoking in 34Leu carriers [22]. The investigation of F13A activity in healthy controls while taking the effect of smoking and c.103G > T (p.Val35Leu) polymorphism in to account will be helpful for better understanding.

Basilar top aneurysm is the most common aneurysm seen in the posterior fossa circulation. It was characterised with higher bleeding tendency and worst clinical outcome after rupture [50]. In this study, 42.8% of patients with basilar top aneurysm had WFNS grade 1 and 71.4% of patients had WFNS grade 2 and 3. Therefore, most of the patients with basilar top aneurysm had the worst clinical outcome in this study.34Leu variant affects clot stability and thereby associated with the bleeding tendency [51]. Basilar top aneurysm was characterised by bleeding tendency and this explains the reason for the association between Leu/Leu genotype and basilar top aneurysm in this study.

The SIFT algorithm predicts the 'damaging' and 'non--damaging' (tolerated) SNPs based on the sequence homology and physical properties of sequence submitted [52]. The PolyPhen-2 algorithm predicts the nsSNPs in three distinct categories: 'probably damaging', 'possibly damaging' and 'benign' SNPs based on the structural homology-based approach using functional point of view [53]. The SNPs predicted as damaging /deleterious in both sequence and structural homology-based approach are considered as 'high-confidence' nsSNP, since they have higher impact on the function of protein [52, 54]. The rs5985 and rs5982 SNPs do not have any direct structural-functional effect on factor XIII A protein according to SIFT and PolyPhen-2 annotation programs. But the studied SNPs might have effect on factor XIII A protein through other indirect pathway.

There are previous reports of linkage disequilibrium (LD) between the variants of *F13A* gene [9, 10]. LD is the non-random association of alleles in two or more loci [55]. LD block (haplotype) is clinically important for the identification of disease causing genes and the origin of mutations [56]. Haplotypes occurs when SNPs are situated near to each other in the chromosome and are inherited in blocks [57]. In both the haplotypes, we found a significant association with the risk of aSAH. Haplotypes are more powerful than individual polymorphism for detecting susceptibility alleles associated with diseases [56, 57].

Conclusion

Our study established that 34Leu carriers are associated with a lower risk and 564Leu carriers are association with a higher risk of aSAH in South Indian population. To the best of our knowledge, this is the first case-control study that has reported the association of *F13A* polymorphism with the risk of aSAH in South Indian population. Larger studies are required from other ethnic populations to determine the association of *factor XIII* polymorphism with the risk of aSAH, especially in the subtypes.

Abbreviations

ACOM: Anterior communicating artery; aSAH: aneurysmal subarachnoid haemorrhage; CI: Confidence interval; F13A: Factor XIII A subunit; ICA: Internal carotid artery; MCA: Middle cerebral artery; OR: Odds ratio; PCOM: Posterior communicating artery; WFNS: World Federation of Neurological Surgeons

Acknowledgements

Arati S acknowledges Department of Science and Technology (DST) [SR/WOS A/LS-1040/2014], Government of India for providing Women Scientist fellowship.

Funding

The study is funded by Department of Science and Technology (DST) [SR/WOS A/LS-1040/2014].

Authors' contributions

AS performed sample collection, DNA extraction, genotyping, participated in its design, acquired data, interpreted the results, and drafted and revised the manuscript. SMK participated in the design of the study, helped in the interpretation of results, performed statistical analyses and contributed in the writing of the manuscript. DIB, KVLN and VV made theoretical contributions and approved the version of the manuscript to be published. CGK co-conceived the study, helped in the study design, contributed to the review of manuscript and gave the final approval to publish. All authors read and approved the final manuscript.

Competing interests

The authors have declared that no competing interests exist on the materials or methods used in this study and findings specified in this paper.

Author details

[1]Department of Human Genetics, National Institute of Mental Health and Neuro Sciences, Bangalore, Karnataka 560029, India. [2]Department of Biochemistry, Armed Forces Medical College, Pune 411040, India. [3]Department of Neurosurgery, National Institute of Mental Health and Neuro Sciences, Bangalore 560029, India.

References

1. Marder CP, Narla V, Fink JR, Tozer Fink KR. Subarachnoid hemorrhage: beyond aneurysms. Am J Roentgenol. 2014;202:25–37.
2. Maddahi A, Povlsen G, Edvinsson L. Regulation of enhanced cerebrovascular expression of proinflammatory mediators in experimental subarachnoid

hemorrhage via the mitogen-activated protein kinase kinase/extracellular signal-regulated kinase pathway. J Neuroinflammation. 2012;9:274.

3. Sehba FA, Hou J, Pluta RM, Zhang JH. The importance of early brain injury after subarachnoid hemorrhage. Prog Neurobiol. 2012;97:14–37.
4. Bor AS, Rinkel GJE, Adami J, Koffijberg H, Ekbom A, Buskens E, Blomqvist P, Granath F. Risk of subarachnoid haemorrhage according to number of affected relatives: a population based case–control study. Brain. 2008;131:2662–5.
5. Song MK, Kim MK, Kim TS, Joo SP, Park MS, Kim BC, Cho KH. Endothelial nitric oxide gene T-786C polymorphism and subarachnoid hemorrhage in Korean population. J Korean Med Sci. 2006;21:922–6.
6. Hofer A, Hermans M, Kubassek N, Sitzer M, Funke H, Stögbauer F, Ivaskevicius V, Oldenburg J, Burtscher J, Knopp U, Schoch B. Elastin polymorphism haplotype and intracranial aneurysms are not associated in Central Europe. Stroke. 2003;34:1207–11.
7. Van den Berg JSP, Pals G, Arwert F, Hennekam RCM, Albrecht KW, Westerveld A, Limburg M. Type III Collagen deficiency in saccular intracranial aneurysms. Stroke. 1999;30:1628–31.
8. Cui V, Kouliev T, Wood J. A case of cerebral aneurysm rupture and subarachnoid hemorrhage associated with air travel. Open Access Emerg Med. 2014;6:23.
9. Ladenvall C, Csajbok L, Nylén K, Jood K, Nellgård B, Jern C. Association between factor XIII single nucleotide polymorphisms and aneurysmal subarachnoid hemorrhage. J Neurosurg. 2009;110:475–81.
10. Reiner AP, Schwartz SM, Frank MB, Longstreth WT, Hindorff LA, Teramura G, Rosendaal FR, Gaur LK, Psaty BM, Siscovick DS. Polymorphisms of coagulation factor XIII subunit a and risk of nonfatal hemorrhagic stroke in young white women. Stroke. 2001;1:2580–7.
11. Ruigrok YM, Slooter AJ, Rinkel GJ, Wijmenga C, Rosendaal FR. Genes influencing coagulation and the risk of aneurysmal subarachnoid hemorrhage, and subsequent complications of secondary cerebral ischemia and rebleeding. Acta Neurochir. 2010;152:257–62.
12. Richardson VR, Cordell P, Standeven KF, Carter AM. Substrates of factor XIII-A: roles in thrombosis and wound healing. Clin Sci. 2013;124:123–37.
13. Komaromi I, Bagoly Z, Muszbek L. Factor XIII: novel structural and functional aspects. J Thromb Haemost. 2011;9:9–20.
14. Bakker EN, Pistea A, VanBavel E. Transglutaminases in vascular biology: relevance for vascular remodeling and atherosclerosis. J Vasc Res. 2008;45:271–8.
15. Schröder V, Kohler HP. New developments in the area of factor XIII. J Thromb Haemost. 2013;11:234–44.
16. Heng CK, Lal S, Saha N, Low PS, Kamboh MI. The impact of factor XIIIa V34L polymorphism on plasma factor XIII activity in the Chinese and Asian Indians from Singapore. Hum Genet. 2004;114:186–91.
17. Muszbek L, Bereczky Z, Bagoly Z, Komáromi I, Katona É. Factor XIII: a coagulation factor with multiple plasmatic and cellular functions. Physiol Rev. 2011;91:931–72.
18. Muszbek L, Bereczky Z, Bagoly Z, Shemirani AH, Katona E. Factor XIII and atherothrombotic diseases. Semin Thromb Hemost. 2010;31:018–33.
19. Ariëns RA, Lai TS, Weisel JW, Greenberg CS, Grant PJ. Role of factor XIII in fibrin clot formation and effects of genetic polymorphisms. Blood. 2002;100:743–54.
20. Ariëns RAS, Kohler HP, Mansfield MW, Grant PJ. Subunit antigen and activity levels of blood coagulation factor XIII in healthy individuals. Arterioscler Thromb Vasc Biol. 1999;19:2012–6.
21. Tu CQ, Wu JZ, Xie CY, Pan CY, Li JH, Huang MQ, Zhang X. Association between polymorphism of coagulation factor XIII Val34Leu and ischemic arterial thrombotic diseases in Han population. Chin J Clin Rehabil. 2005;9:70–1.
22. Ma J, Li H, You C, Liu Y, Ma L, Huang S. Blood coagulation factor XIII-A subunit Val34Leu polymorphisms and intracerebral hemorrhage risk: a meta-analysis of case-control studies. Br J Neurosurg. 2015;29:672–7.
23. Elbaz A, Poirier O, Canaple S, Chédru F, Cambien F, Amarenco P. The association between the Val34Leu polymorphism in the factor XIII gene and brain infarction. Blood. 2000;95:586–91.
24. Gallivan L, Markham AF, Anwar R. The Leu564 factor XIIIA variant results in significantly lower plasma factor XIII levels than the Pro564 variant. Thromb Haemost. 1999;81:1368–70.
25. Sole X, Guino E, Valls J, Iniesta R, Moreno V. SNPStats: Aweb tool for the analysis of association studies. Bioinformatics. 2006;22:1928–9.
26. Lee PH, Shatkay H. F-SNP: computationally predicted functional SNPs for disease association studies. Nucleic Acids Res. 2007;36:820–4.
27. DerSimonian R, Laird N. Meta-analysis in clinical trials. Control Clin Trials. 1986;7:177–88.
28. Carpenter CR, Hussain AM, Ward MJ, Zipfel GJ, Fowler S, Pines JM, Sivilotti ML. Spontaneous subarachnoid hemorrhage: a systematic review and Meta-analysis describing the diagnostic accuracy of history, physical examination, imaging, and lumbar puncture with an exploration of test thresholds. Acad Emerg Med. 2016;23:963–1003.
29. Shawky RM. Reduced penetrance in human inherited disease. Egypt J Med Hum Genet. 2014;15:103–11.
30. Steucke KE, Tracy PV, Hald ES, Hall JL, Alford PW. Vascular smooth muscle cell functional contractility depends on extracellular mechanical properties. J biomechan. 2015;4812:3044–51.
31. Tang BH, McKenna PJ, Rovit RL. Primary fibrinolytic syndrome associated with subarachnoid hemorrhage: a case report. Angiology. 1973;4:627–34.
32. Chalouhi N, Ali MS, Jabbour PM, Tjoumakaris SI, Gonzalez LF, Rosenwasser RH, Koch WJ, Dumont AS. Biology of intracranial aneurysms: role of inflammation. J Cereb Blood Flow Metab. 2012;32:1659–76.
33. Nina P, Schisano G, Chiappetta F, Papa ML, Maddaloni E, Brunori A, Capasso F, Corpetti MG, Demurtas F. A study of blood coagulation and fibrinolytic system in spontaneous subarachnoid hemorrhage: Correlation with Hunt-Hess grade and outcome. Surg Neurol. 2001;55:197–203.
34. Mosher DF, Schad PE, Vann JM. Cross-linking of collagen and fibronectin by factor XIIIa. Localization of participating glutaminyl residues to a tryptic fragment of fibronectin. J Biol Chem. 1980;255:1181–8.
35. Rijken DC, Abdul S, Malfliet JJMC, Leebeek FWG, Uitte de Willige S. Compaction of fibrin clots reveals the antifibrinolytic effect of factor XIII. J Thromb Haemost. 2016;14:1453–61.
36. Shemirani AH, Antalfi B, Pongrácz E, Mezei ZA, Bereczky Z, Csiki Z. Factor XIII-A subunit Val34Leu polymorphism in fatal atherothrombotic ischemic stroke. Blood Coagul Fibrinolysis. 2014;25:364–8.
37. Gemmati D, Serino ML, Ongaro A, Tognazzo S, Moratelli S, Resca R, Morett M, Scapoli GL. A common mutation in the gene for coagulation factor XIII-A (VAL34Leu): a risk factor for primary intracerebral hemorrhage is protective against atherothrombotic diseases. Am J Hematol. 2001;67:183–8.
38. Akar N, Dönmez B, Deda G. FXIII gene Val34Leu polymorphism in Turkish children with cerebral infarct. J Child Neurol. 2007;22:222–4.
39. Margaglione M, Bossone A, Brancaccio V, Ciampa A, Di Minno G. Factor XIII Val34Leu polymorphism and risk of deep vein thrombosis. Thromb Haemost. 2000;84:1118–9.
40. Corral J, Iniesta JA, González-Conejero R, Villalón M, Vicente V. Polymorphisms of clotting factors modify the risk for primary intracranial hemorrhage. Blood. 2001;97:2979–82.
41. Dickneite G, Herwald H, Korte W, Allanore Y, Denton CP, Cerinic MM. Coagulation factor XIII: a multifunctional transglutaminase with clinical potential in a range of conditions. Thromb Haemost. 2015;114:686–97.
42. Wartiovaara U, Mikkola H, Szoke G, Haramura G, Karpati L, Balogh I, Lassila R, Muszbek L, Palotie A. Effect of Val34Leu polymorphism on the activation of the coagulation factor XIII-A. Thromb Haemost. 2000;84:595–600.
43. Anwar R, Gallivan L, Edmonds SD, Markham AF. Genotype/phenotype correlations for coagulation factor XIII: specific normal polymorphisms are associated with high or low factor XIII specific activity. Blood. 1999;93:897–905.
44. Kohler HP, Stickland MH, Ossei-Gerning N, Carter A, Mikkola H, Grant PJ. Association of a common polymorphism in the factor XIII gene with myocardial infarction. Thromb Haemost. 1998;80:8–13.
45. Catto AJ, Kohler HP, Coore J, Mansfield MW, Stickland MH, Grant PJ. Association of a common polymorphism in the factor XIII gene with venous thrombosis. Blood. 1999;93:906–8.
46. Wartiovaara U, Perola M, Mikkola H, Tötterman K, Savolainen V, Penttilä A, Grant PJ, Tikkanen MJ, Vartiainen E, Karhunen PJ, Peltonen L. Association of FXIII Val34Leu with decreased risk of myocardial infarction in Finnish males. Atherosclerosis. 1999;142:295–300.
47. Franco RF, Reitsma PH, Lourenco D, Maffei FH, Morelli V, Tavella MH, Araujo AG, Piccinato CE, Zago MA. Factor XIII Val34Leu is a genetic factor involved in the aetiology of venous thrombosis. Thromb Haemost. 1999;81:676–9.
48. Kohler HP, Ariëns RAS, Whitaker P, Grant PJ. A common coding polymorphism in the FXIII A-subunit gene (FXIIIVal34Leu) affects cross-linking activity. Thromb Haemost. 1998;80:704.
49. Van Wersch JWJ, Vooijs MEEC, Ubachs JMH. Coagulation factor XIII in pregnant smokers and non-smokers. Int J Clin Lab Res. 1997;27:68–71.
50. Sekhar LN, Tariq F, Morton RP, Ghodke B, Hallam DK, Barber J, Kim LJ. Basilar tip aneurysms: a microsurgical and endovascular contemporary series of 100 patients. Neurosurgery. 2012;72:284–99.
51. Korte W. Catridecacog: a breakthrough in the treatment of congenital factor XIII A-subunit deficiency? J Blood Med. 2014;5:107.
52. Dobson RJ, Munroe PB, Caulfield MJ, Saqi MA. Predicting deleterious nsSNPs: an analysis of sequence and structural attributes. BMC Bioinformatics. 2006;7:217.

20

Novel mutations in *ALDH1A3* associated with autosomal recessive anophthalmia/ microphthalmia, and review of the literature

Siying Lin[1], Gaurav V. Harlalka[1], Abdul Hameed[2], Hadia Moattar Reham[3], Muhammad Yasin[3], Noor Muhammad[3], Saadullah Khan[3], Emma L. Baple[1], Andrew H. Crosby[1] and Shamim Saleha[3*]

Abstract

Background: Autosomal recessive anophthalmia and microphthalmia are rare developmental eye defects occurring during early fetal development. Syndromic and non-syndromic forms of anophthalmia and microphthalmia demonstrate extensive genetic and allelic heterogeneity. To date, disease mutations have been identified in 29 causative genes associated with anophthalmia and microphthalmia, with autosomal dominant, autosomal recessive and X-linked inheritance patterns described. Biallelic *ALDH1A3* gene variants are the leading genetic causes of autosomal recessive anophthalmia and microphthalmia in countries with frequent parental consanguinity.

Methods: This study describes genetic investigations in two consanguineous Pakistani families with a total of seven affected individuals with bilateral non-syndromic clinical anophthalmia.

Results: Using whole exome and Sanger sequencing, we identified two novel homozygous *ALDH1A3* sequence variants as likely responsible for the condition in each family; missense mutation [NM_000693.3:c.1240G > C, p. Gly414Arg; Chr15:101447332G > C (GRCh37)] in exon 11 (family 1), and, a frameshift mutation [NM_000693.3:c. 172dup, p.Glu58Glyfs*5; Chr15:101425544dup (GRCh37)] in exon 2 predicted to result in protein truncation (family 2).

Conclusions: This study expands the molecular spectrum of pathogenic *ALDH1A3* variants associated with anophthalmia and microphthalmia, and provides further insight of the key role of the *ALDH1A3* in human eye development.

Keywords: Autosomal recessive anophthalmia and microphthalmia, *ALDH1A3* gene, Mutations, Variants, Exome sequencing, Consanguineous families

Background

Anophthalmia and microphthalmia are severe congenital developmental defects of the eye. In the clinical context, anophthalmia refers to complete absence of the globe in the orbit, whilst microphthalmia refers to the presence of a small globe within the orbit. Both anophthalmia and microphthalmia are more commonly bilateral, although they can also present unilaterally. These are relatively rare defects, occurring with an estimated combined incidence of 1 in 10,000 live births [1]. Anophthalmia and microphthalmia can occur as isolated malformations, or as part of a syndrome. Both syndromic and non-syndromic forms of anophthalmia and microphthalmia have been associated with autosomal recessive, autosomal dominant and X-linked patterns of inheritance, and display extensive genetic heterogeneity [2]. Mutations in numerous genes including *RAX, PAX6, SOX2, OTX2, VSX2, RARB, BMP7, BCOR, BMP4, FOXE3, STRA6, SMOC1, SHH, SNX3,*

* Correspondence: shamimsaleha@yahoo.com
[3]Department of Biotechnology and Genetic Engineering, Kohat University of Science and Technology (KUST), Kohat, Khyber Pakhtunkhwa 26000, Pakistan
Full list of author information is available at the end of the article

MFRP, PRSS56, GDF3, GDF6, TENM3, C12orf57, YAP1, *ABCB6, ATOH7, VAX1, NDP, ALDH1A3* and *SMARCA4* have all been described in association with microphthalmia, and some, including *RAX, PAX6, SOX2, OTX2, RARB, BMP7, BCOR, BMP4, FOXE3, STRA6, SMOC1, GDF6* and *ALDH1A3* have also been described in association with anophthalmia [3–5]. *SOX2* mutations are the major single-gene cause of anophthalmia and microphthalmia, accounting for ~ 10–15% of all cases [6]. Mutations in other genes have been shown to account for another ~ 25% of cases of anophthalmia and microphthalmia [7]. In up to 50–60% of cases however, the underlying genetic cause remains undetermined [2, 8].

Mutations in the aldehyde dehydrogenase 1 family, member A3 (*ALDH1A3*) gene have been found in association with autosomal recessive anophthalmia and microphthalmia in individuals of different ethnicities. Notably, mutations of this gene appear to be the major cause of these conditions in consanguineous families of Pakistani origin [3, 6]. The *ALDH1A3* gene encodes a NAD-dependent aldehyde dehydrogenase, which is among one of three retinaldehyde dehydrogenases (the others being *ALDH1A1* and *ALDH1A2*) that play a key role in the biosynthesis of retinoic acid from retinaldehyde. Retinoic acid functions as a ligand for DNA-binding retinoid receptors that directly regulate transcription of specific target genes in the retinoic-acid signaling pathway in vertebrates [9], and promotes neuronal differentiation in the embryonic nervous system [10]. It also has an important function in the normal early embryonic development of ocular and nasal regions [11].

In this study, we identified homozygous novel missense and frameshift sequence alterations in *ALDH1A3* that segregate with the disease phenotype in consanguineous Pakistani families with isolated anophthalmia, and discuss our findings alongside existing literature in this area.

Methods

Ascertainment of family

This study was approved by the ethical committee, Kohat University of Science and Technology (KUST; Pakistan), and families were subsequently recruited. Informed written consent was obtained from parents, and consent was obtained on behalf of their children. A consanguineous family, extending over four generations and comprising of 4 living affected and 12 unaffected members, was recruited from the Khyber Pakhtunkhwa region of Pakistan. All the affected individuals were in the fourth generation. Another consanguineous family, extending over two generations with three affected and five unaffected members, was also recruited from same region of Pakistan. Blood samples were collected from affected and unaffected individuals, and all affected individuals were clinically evaluated by an ophthalmologist for obtaining medical and family histories and clinical assessment.

Genetic studies

Following informed consent, genomic DNA from the blood samples was extracted using the ReliaPrep™ kit (Blood gDNA Miniprep System, Promega) according to the manufacturer's protocol. To identify the causative gene, whole-exome sequencing was performed on a single affected individual in each family (subject IV: 7 in family 1 and II: 1 in family 2, Fig. 1) to develop a profile of variants not present in publicly available databases and rare sequence variants. Coding regions were captured by HiSeq2000 using paired-end (2 × 100) protocol at a mean coverage depth of 30X at the Otogenetics Corporation (Norcross, GA, USA). The Agilent SureSelect Human All ExonV4 (51 Mb) enrichment kit was used for exome enrichment. The sequence reads were aligned to the human genome reference sequence [hg19] and read alignment, variant calling, and annotation were performed by DNAnexus (DNAnexus Inc., Mountain View, CA; https://dnanexus.com).

Allele-specific primers were designed using Primer3 web software (primer sequences are available upon request) to evaluate segregation of variants via dideoxy sequencing. Polymerase chain reaction (PCR) was undertaken for all recruited family members using allele-specific primers following standard conditions, with products sequenced by Source BioScience LifeSciences (https://www.sourcebioscience.com/). Pathogenicity of the identified missense sequence variation in the *ALDH1A3* gene was also analyzed using PolyPhen-2 (http://genetics.bwh.harvard.edu/pph2/), PROVEAN (http://provean.jcvi.org/index.php) and SIFT (http://provean.jcvi.org/index.php) specialized prediction software. To compare and correlate the *ALDH1A3* gene variants with the phenotype, all reported variants were retrieved from HGMD (http://www.hgmd.cf.ac.uk/ac/search.php), OMIM (https://www.ncbi.nlm.nih.gov/omim/) and PubMed (https://www.ncbi.nlm.nih.gov/pubmed/) databases.

Results

Subjects

Pedigree analysis of recruited consanguineous Pakistani families suggested an autosomal recessive inheritance of the disease in these families (Fig. 1). In total, seven living affected individuals with normal intelligence as well as 13 healthy individuals including parents and siblings from both families were investigated. The four affected individuals IV:3, IV:5, IV:7 and IV:8 were 13, 18, 14 and 12 years of age in first family, while three affected individuals II:1, II:4 and II:8 were 19, 10, 4 years of age in second family respectively at the time of examination. On the basis of basic clinical ophthalmic assessment, bilateral isolated anophthalmia was the major finding in all affected members

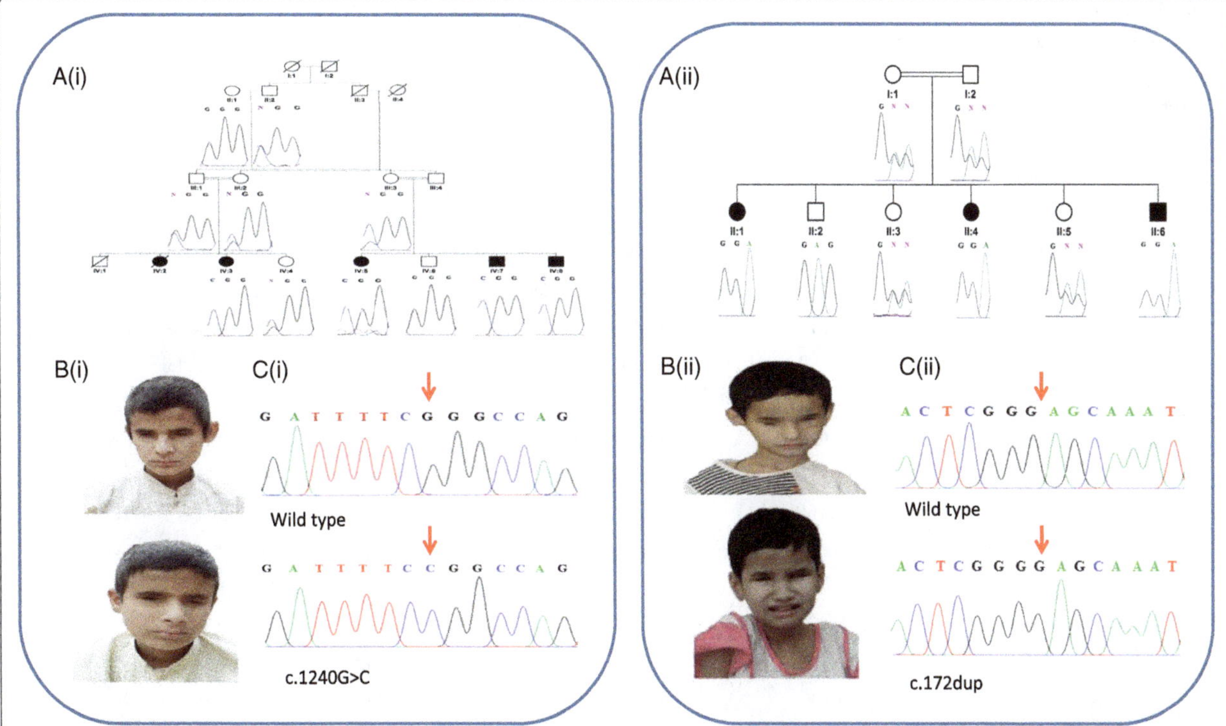

Fig. 1 **A** Pedigrees of the Pakistani families investigated, and genetic findings. **A(i)** and **A(ii).** Family 1 (Ai) and family 2 (Aii) pedigrees showing segregation of the variants identified in each case. **B(i)** and **B(ii).** Photographs of two affected individuals in both families with non-syndromic clinical anophthalmia **C(i)** and **C(ii).** Sequence chromatograms showing wild-type alongside *ALDH1A3* [NM_000693.3:c.1240G > C, p.Gly414Arg; Chr15:101447332G > C (GRCh37)] in exon 11 (family 1), and, a frameshift mutation [NM_000693.3:c.172dup, p.Glu58Glyfs*5; Chr15:101425544dup (GRCh37)] variants

of the investigated families. No other neurological and behavioral features were observed in affected individuals.

Genetic findings

The exome data was first inspected to exclude previously described variants in genes known to cause ocular disease. Variants were then assessed and filtered for rare, non-synonymous exonic or splice variants, with a population frequency of < 0.01 in control databases (including the Genome Aggregation Database; gnomAD, the Exome Aggregation Consortium; ExAC, and the 1000 Genomes Project). A single candidate novel homozygous missense variant [NM_000693.3:c.1240G > C; Chr15:101447332G > C (GRCh37)] was identified in exon 11 of *ALDH1A3* (Fig. 1) in first family. This variant leads to a substitution of glycine with arginine and at the evolutionary conserved position 414 (p.Gly414Arg) according to the UCSC Human Genome (GRCh37/ hg19) and Ensemble databases (Additional file 1 A). The p.Gly414Arg variant is not listed in the Genome Aggregation Database (gnomAD). In silico analysis of p.Gly414Arg using PolyPhen-2, PROVEAN and SIFT predicted it to be damaging or deleterious with a score of 1.000, – 7.559 and 3.25 respectively (Additional file 1 B). In family 2, a novel variant [NM_000693.3:c.172dup; Chr15:101425544dup (GRCh37)] was identified in exon 2 of the *ALDH1A3* gene (Fig. 1). This single base pair duplication is predicted to result in a frameshift followed by a premature stop codon (p. Glu58Glyfs*5). The variants in families 1 and 2 segregate as expected for an autosomal recessive condition in each family, and both variants are summarized in Table 1 alongside all other reported disease-associated *ALDH1A3* variants; a schematic representation of each mutation in *ALDH1A3* is also shown in Fig. 2.

Discussion

The *ALDH1A3* (NG_012254.1) gene comprises 13 exons spanning ~ 36 kb on chromosome 15 (15q26.3), encoding a 512-amino acid NAD-dependent aldehyde dehydrogenase localized in the cytoplasm, nucleus, endoplasmic reticulum and mitochondria [12]. Structural analysis reveals that *ALDH1A3* shares high structural homology with other types of aldehyde dehydrogenases. ALDH1A3 assembles as a tetramer, however, each of its monomeric units is independently able to oxidize retinaldehyde into retinoic acid using NAD as a cofactor. Each monomeric unit folds into 13 α-helices, 19 β-sheets and the connecting loops, arranged into three functional domains: the NAD-binding domains (L20-D149 and I171–G282), the catalytic domain (G283–M482), and the C-terminal oligomerization domains (K150–P170 and S483–L507), [11].

Table 1 Summary of all reported *ALDH1A3* variants associated with anophthalmia and microphthalmia

Type of mutation	Mutations	Variants	Ethnicity	Patients #	Clinical diagnosis	Literature
Missense	c.211G > A	p. Val71Met	Israeli	9	AM	Mory et al. [15]
	c.265C > T	p. Arg89Cys	Pakistani	2	AM	Fares-Taie et al. [6]
	c.287G > A	p.Arg96His	Chinese	1	A	Liu et al. [21]
	c.434C > T	p. Ala145Val	Saudi Arabian	2	M	Aldahmesh et al. [14]
	c.521G > A	p.Cys174Tyr	Lebanese	3	AM	Roos et al. [16]
	c.709G > A	p.Gly237Arg	Chinese & Iranian	3	A	Liu et al. [21]; Dehghani et al. [19]
	c.845G > C	p.Gly282Ala	Arabic	2	M	Alabdullatif et al. [20]
	c.964G > A	p.Val322Met	Indian	1	A	Ullah et al. [3]
	c.1064C > G	p.Pro355Arg	Egyptian	1	A	Abouzeid et al. [17].
	c.1105A > T	p. Ile369Pro	Saudi Arabian	3	M	Aldahmesh et al. [14]
	c.1144G > A	p.Gly382Arg	Egyptian	4	A	Abouzeid et al. [17]
	c.1231G > A	p.Glu411Lys	Sri Lankan	1	M	Abouzeid et al. [17]
	c.1398C > A	p.Asn466Lys	Turkish	2	AM	Semerci et al. [18]
	c.1477G > C	p. Ala493Pro	Turkish	1	AM	Fares-Taie et al. [6]
	c. 1240G > C	p.Gly414Arg	Pakistani	4	A	Present study
Nonsense	c.568A > T	p.Lys190	Egyptian	2	AM	Yahyavi et al. [5]
	c.898G > T	p.Glu300	Spanish	1	M	Abouzeid et al. [17]
	c.1165A > T	p.Lys389	Hispanic	1	AM	Yahyavi et al. [5]
Splicing	c.204 + 1G > A Alteration of the WT donor site	affecting splicing	Egyptian	2	AM	Abouzeid et al. [17]
	c.475 + 1G > T Skipping of exon 5	p. Asp159-Pro179 del	Moroccan	1	AM	Fares-Taie et al. [6]
	c.666G > A Skipping of exon 6	p.Trp180_Glu222del	Turkish	7	AM	Semerci et al. [18] Plaisancié et al. [13]
	c.1391 + 1G > T Alteration of the WT donor site	affecting splicing	Egyptian	1	A	Abouzeid et al. [17]
Frameshift	c.1310_1311delAT	p.Tyr437Trpfs*44	Pakistani	4	A	Ullah et al. [3]
	c.172dup	p. Glu58Glyfs*5	Pakistani	3	A	Present study

WT wild type, *AM* anophthalmia and microphthalmia, *A* anophthalmia, *M* microphthalmia

The first evidence of involvement of *ALDH1A3* variants in autosomal recessive anophthalmia and microphthalmia in humans was provided by Fares-Taie et al. in 2013 [6]. Since then, mutations of *ALDH1A3* have been identified as a cause of autosomal recessive anophthalmia and microphthalmia in 54 individuals to date. Among these families, 50 individuals are from consanguineous families [3, 5, 6, 13–19], one from a non-consanguineous family, [5] and three are sporadic or individual cases [5, 20]. Recently, Liu and coworkers identified compound heterozygous variants in *ALDH1A3* in a proband from a non-consanguineous family with anophthalmia [21]. Among the reported *ALDH1A3*-associated anophthalmia and microphthalmia cases, 30 have been demonstrated in families of Arab origin including families from Egypt [17], Saudi Arabia [14], Lebanan [16], Morocco [6], Israel [15], and the United Arab Emirates [20], 10 in families of Turkish origin [18], and 12 cases have been found in South and East Asian families including families from Pakistan [3, 6], Iran [19], India [3], Sri Lanka [17] and China [21]. Reported consanguinity rates are high (22–55%) in these populations, which has been associated with an increased risk of autosomal recessive diseases due to homozygosity of regional founder mutations [22]. In European populations, where consanguinity rates are generally less than 0.5% [22], anophthalmia and microphthalmia have been reported much less frequently, with only two cases of Spanish and Hispanic origin reported [5, 17]. Our study, together with previously reported studies, thus provides evidence for the notable occurrence of autosomal recessive anophthalmia and microphthalmia in consanguineous families.

Of the 22 previously reported variants, 14 missense, three nonsense, four splice site variants and one small deletion have been documented. In this study, we report a novel

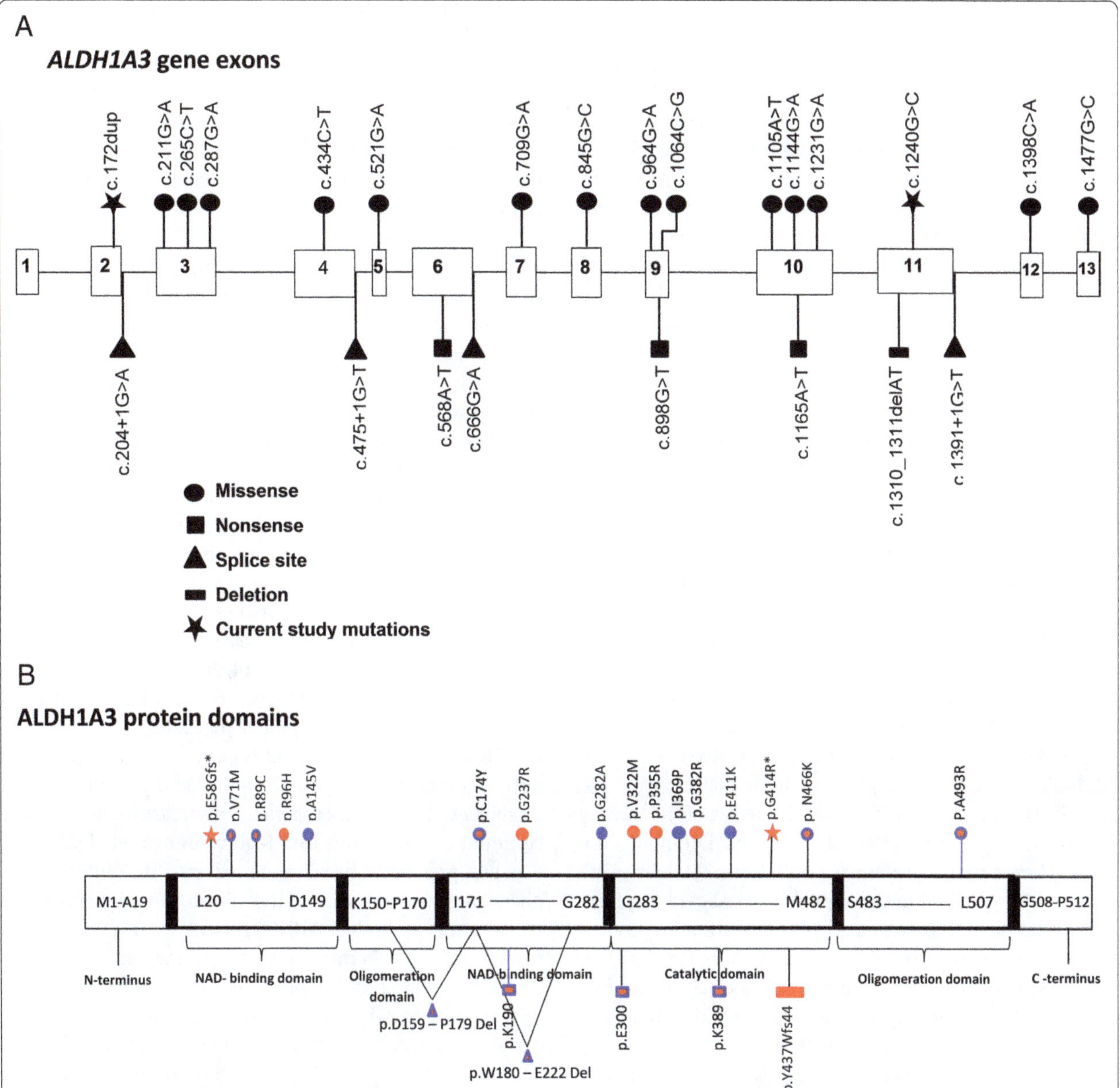

Fig. 2 *ALDH1A3* gene mutations associated with anopthalmia and microphthalmia. **a** Schematic representation of exons of the *ALDH1A3* gene highlighting the positions of all disease causing mutations identified to date. **b** Domains of predicted protein product as described by Moretti and colleagues [11], highlighting the positions of all disease associated variants identified to date. Discrete color pattern of variants shows type of phenotype (red: anophthalmia, blue: micophthalmia and a combination of red and blue: both anophthalmia and microphthlamia

missense mutation (c.1240G > C; p.(Gly414Arg)) in *ALDH1A3* in a consanguineous four generations family of Pakistani origin. This Gly414Arg substitution affects a highly conserved residue across model organisms including humans. This variant, as with the previously documented missense ALDH1A3 variants Val322Met, Ile369Pro, Gly382Arg, Pro355Arg, Glu411Lys and Asn466Lys [3, 14, 17, 18], is presumed to be located in the functionally important catalytic domain that governs substrate specificity. Missense variants in the ALDH1A3 catalytic domain are thought to result in an aberrant tertiary structure with abnormal protein folding, leading to subsequent protein degradation and loss of function, and the novel variant identified in this study is believed to cause disease via a similar mechanism. Two nonsense variants, p.Lys389* and p.Glu300* have also been identified in the catalytic domain of ALDH1A3, resulting in the predicted truncation of the protein product due to mRNA targeted degradation [5, 17]. A single frameshift deletion variant p.Tyr437Trpfs*44 has also been reported in this domain, also predicted to cause loss of function of ALDH1A3 via nonsense-mediated decay [3].

In the oligomerization domain of ALDH1A3, a single missense variant Ala493Pro has been identified, and is expected to hamper the specific activity of the ALDH1A3 tetramer due to the introduction of a helix kink that leads to an incorrect position of the two beta sheets relative to each other within the oligomerization domain at protein level [6]. Fares-Taie et al. [6] found homozygosity for a c.475 + 1G > T splice site mutation in the *ALDH1A3* gene that was predicted to abolish the splice-donor site of intron 4, with an in-frame skipping of exon 5 expected. This would cause a deletion of critical amino acid residues (Asp159-Pro179) in both the oligomerization domain (Asp159-Pro170) and in the NAD-binding domain (Ile171- Pro179) of ALDH1A3 at protein level, presumably affecting both its oligomerization and binding or catalytic abilities. Abouzeid et al. [17] found homozygosity for a c.1391 + 1G > T splice site mutation in the *ALDH1A3* gene that causes alteration of the wild type donor site (http://www.umd.be/HSF3/ or http://krainer01.cshl.edu/cgi-bin/tools/ESE3/esefinder.cgi), (Table 1), and is therefore predicted to affect interaction with core spliceosome proteins resulting in non-functional ALDH1A3 protein production.

Variants in the NAD-binding domain of ALDH1A3 also result in loss of function. The ALDH1A3 variant alleles identified in the NAD-binding domain, important for tetramer stabilization include Val71Met, Arg89Cys, Arg96His, Ala145Val, Cys174Tyr, Gly237Arg and Gly282Ala [6, 14–16, 19–21]. In the present study, a further novel variant (p.Glu58Glyfs*5) was identified in the NAD-binding domain. These variants may impact on tetramer stability, with the newly synthesized unstable proteins predicted to be unstable and therefore subjected to proteasome-dependent degradation in the cells [6, 21]. The Cys174Tyr, Lys190*, Gly237Arg and Gly282Ala variants are located at the foot of the NAD-binding domain (Ile171- Gly282). Variants in this region are important, may directly affect NAD binding by altering the conformation of ALDH1A3 in NAD binding pockets [11], leading to proteasome degradation [5, 21]. A homozygous splice site mutation (c.204 + 1G > A) was found by Abouzeid et al. [17] in the head of NAD binding domain of the ALDH1A3 protein that was predicted to lead to an improperly spliced product by affecting the donor splice site of intron 2. Another homozygous splice site mutation c.666G > A was detected by Semerci et al. [18] in the foot of the NAD-binding domain of the ALDH1A3 protein that was shown to cause an inframe deletion of 43 amino acids (Trp180_Glu222del) at the foot of this domain. These splice site mutations are also likely to affect the tetrameric stability or conformation in NAD binding pockets that are a prerequisite for the normal function of the ALDH1A3 protein.

ALDH1A3-associated anophthalmia and microphthalmia, is frequently reported in association with other ocular and extra ocular anomalies, such as the presence of short eyelids, blepharophimosis and reduced palpebral fissures [5, 13, 17, 21], entropion [5], conjunctival symblepharon [17], conjunctival discoloration [17], large eyebrows and synophrys [17, 18], coloboma [5, 14, 16, 17, 20], hypoplasia of the optic tracts and chiasm [5, 6, 15, 17, 18], hypoplastic extra ocular muscles [15, 18], high arched palate [17], refractive errors including both myopia and hyperopia [14, 16], and esotropia [14]. There is a high variability observed in the phenotypic expression of dysmorphic or extra ocular features associated with anophthalmia and microphthalmia, even in individuals with the same *ALDH1A3* genetic variants [13, 18, 19]. Mild hypoplasia of the vermis (variant of Dandy-Walker malformation), as well as pulmonary stenosis and atrial septal defect, have also been reported in association with *ALDH1A3*-associated anophthalmia and microphthalmia [6, 18]. As these extra ocular findings have only been reported in a single individual, it remains unclear if these features are associated with the *ALDH1A3* mutation, or occur due to a separate genetic disorder. Occasionally, patients with *ALDH1A3*-associated anophthalmia and microphthalmia are also reported to have neurocognitive or behavioral features including intellectual disability, developmental delay and autism [6, 14, 16, 18]. However, this association is controversial due to the wide interfamilial variability in the neurocognitive or behavioral outcomes [14, 16, 18], and the important impact of visual impairment during development [23, 24]. In addition, intellectual disabilities due to other genetic disorders may be more common in populations with high consanguinity [25].

It has previously been suggested that the difference in phenotype between microphthalmia and anophthalmia may be the result of residual ALDH1A3 activity [17]. However, a review of all known disease-causing mutations in *ALDH1A3* (Fig. 2 and Table 1) does not seem to support this hypothesis, with no consistent correlation between a particular phenotype (anophthalmia or microphthalmia) and the nature of variation (missense, nonsense, frameshift or splice variants) or the protein domain affected (NAD--binding domain, catalytic domain or oligomerization domain). This may partly be due to difficulty in distinguishing between anophthalmia from severe microphthalmia in routine clinical practice. True congenital anophthalmia can only be diagnosed radiologically or histologically, and most published cases of clinical anophthalmia probably include cases of severe microphthalmia, where residual ocular tissue may have been present in the orbit despite external appearances of an absent globe [1].

There is a wide phenotypic variation in *ALDH1A3*-associated ocular disease. Individuals with the same *ALDH1A3* variant can display both anophthalmia and microphthalmia in different eyes [5, 17, 20], and affected individuals with the same mutation within the same family have been found to have clinical phenotypes of differing severity [5, 13, 16–

18]. Epidemiological studies have predicted the contribution of both genetic and environmental factors in the pathogenesis of congenital eye defects including anophthalmia and microphthalmia [26], and the wide phenotypic spectrum seen may result from the impact of other factors such as modifying genes or environmental influences affecting the *ALDH1A3*-associated eye disease phenotype. Further studies would be useful to define this interaction and elucidate underlying pathways.

Determining the underlying diagnosis in patients with anophthalmia and microphthalmia is often challenging due to the genetic heterogeneity of the disorder and the wide variation in phenotypic expression. Taken together, these factors makes it extremely difficult to establish an accurate diagnosis based on clinical presentation alone. This problem is particularly significant in developing countries such as Pakistan, where many families reside in highly remote and rural regions with limited access to healthcare and ophthalmic services. There is also limited availability of specific and expensive radiological investigations such as ocular ultrasound or magnetic resonance imaging which are required in cases of clinical anophthalmia to definitively differentiate between true congenital anophthalmia and severe microphthalmia. This has important prognostic implications, as anophthalmia is more frequently associated with a wide range of systemic anomalies including developmental intracranial and hemifacial anomalies, and as such carries a poorer prognosis than microphthalmia [27]. The application of modern genomic technologies in our families enabled an accurate molecular diagnosis of *ALDH1A3*-associated anophthalmia/ microphthalmia to be established and has facilitated informed genetic counselling. Although extraocular features have been reported in association with *ALDH1A3*-associated ocular disease, these are uncommon, and the associations are controversial, providing a relatively good prognosis for affected families when compared to other known causes of anophthalmia.

Conclusions

In summary, our results add to the molecular spectrum of autosomal recessive microphthalmia and anophthalmia in general and of Pakistan in particular. The identification of a novel variants in *ALDH1A3* in the present study consolidates the key role of this gene in autosomal recessive anophthalmia and microphthalmia, contributes to the expanding spectrum of disease-causing *ALDH1A3* gene variants, and emphasizes the key function of *ALDH1A3* in human eye development. Given that *ALDH1A3* gene mutations appear to be the most common cause of anophthalmia and microphthalmia in consanguineous families [3, 6, 15–21], screening for variants in this gene before exome analysis in populations with high rates of consanguinity should be considered.

Acknowledgements
The authors would like to thank the patients and their family members for their participation in this study.

Funding
This research was supported by the Kohat University of Science and Technology, Kohat, Pakistan and RILD Wellcome Wolfson Centre (Level 4), Royal Devon and Exeter NHS Foundation Trust, UK.

Authors' contributions
Clinical data collection, collation, and analysis: SL, ELB, HMR, MY and SS; Genetic testing and data analysis: SL, GVH, ELB, AHC, NM, SK and SS; Manuscript writing and revision: SL, GVH, ELB, AHC, AH and SS; Study supervision and coordination: ELB, AHC, and SS. All authors read and approved the final manuscript.

Competing interests
The authors declare that they have no competing interests.

Author details
[1]Medical Research, RILD Wellcome Wolfson Centre (Level 4), Royal Devon and Exeter NHS Foundation Trust, Exeter, Devon EX2 5DW, UK. [2]Institute of Biomedical and Genetic Engineering (IBGE), Islamabad 44000, Pakistan. [3]Department of Biotechnology and Genetic Engineering, Kohat University of Science and Technology (KUST), Kohat, Khyber Pakhtunkhwa 26000, Pakistan.

References

1. Verma AS, FitzPatrick DR. Anophthalmia and microphthalmia. Orphanet J Rare Dis. 2007;2:47. https://doi.org/10.1186/1750-1172-2-47.
2. Bardakjian TM, Schneider A. The genetics of anophthalmia and microphthalmia. Curr Opin Ophthalmol. 2011;22(5):309–13. https://doi.org/10.1097/ICU.0b013e328349b004.
3. Ullah E, Nadeem Saqib MA, Sajid S, Shah N, Zubair M, Khan MA, et al. Genetic analysis of consanguineous families presenting with congenital ocular defects. Exp Eye Res. 2016;146:163–71. https://doi.org/10.1016/j.exer.2016.03.014.
4. Williamson KA, FitzPatrick DR. The genetic architecture of microphthalmia, anophthalmia and coloboma. Eur J Med Genet. 2014;57(8):369–80. https://doi.org/10.1016/j.ejmg.2014.05.002.
5. Yahyavi M, Abouzeid H, Gawdat G, de Preux AS, Xiao T, Bardakjian T, et al. ALDH1A3 loss of function causes bilateral anophthalmia/ microphthalmia and hypoplasia of the optic nerve and optic chiasm. Hum Mol Genet. 2013; 22(16):3250–8. https://doi.org/10.1093/hmg/ddt179.
6. Fares-Taie L, Gerber S, Chassaing N, Clayton-Smith J, Hanein S, Silva E, et al. ALDH1A3 mutations cause recessive anophthalmia and microphthalmia. Am J Hum Genet. 2013;92(2):265–70. https://doi.org/10.1016/j.ajhg.2012.12.003.
7. Ragge NK, Subak-Sharpe ID, Collin JR. A practical guide to the management of anophthalmia and microphthalmia. Eye (Lond). 2007;21(10):1290–300. https://doi.org/10.1038/sj.eye.6702858.
8. Jimenez NL, Flannick J, Yahyavi M, Li J, Bardakjian T, Tonkin L, et al. Targeted 'next-generation' sequencing in anophthalmia and microphthalmia patients confirms SOX2, OTX2 and FOXE3 mutations. BMC Med Genet. 2011;12:172. https://doi.org/10.1186/1471-2350-12-172.
9. Kumar S, Sandell LL, Trainor PA, Koentgen F, Duester G. Alcohol and aldehyde dehydrogenases: retinoid metabolic effects in mouse knockout models. Biochim Biophys Acta. 2012;1821(1):198–205. https://doi.org/10.1016/j.bbalip.2011.04.004.
10. Xu J, Wang H, Liang T, Cai X, Rao X, Huang Z, Sheng G. Retinoic acid promotes neural conversion of mouse embryonic stem cell in adherent monoculture. Mol Biol Rep. 2012;39(2):789–95. https://doi.org/10.1007/s11033-011-0800-8.
11. Moretti A, Li J, Donini S, Sobol RW, Rizzi M, Garavaglia S. Crystal structure of human aldehyde dehydrogenase 1A3 complexed with NAD+ and retinoic acid. Sci Rep. 2016;6:35710. https://doi.org/10.1038/srep35710.
12. Braun T, Bober E, Singh S, Agarwal DP, Goedde HW. Evidence for a signal peptide at the amino-terminal end of human mitochondrial aldehyde dehydrogenase. FEBS Lett. 1987;215(2):233–6.
13. Plaisancié J, Brémond-Gignac D, Demeer B, Gaston V, Verloes A, Fares-Taie L, et al. Incomplete penetrance of biallelic ALDH1A3 mutations. Eur J Med Genet. 2016;59(4):215–8. https://doi.org/10.1016/j.ejmg.2016.02.004.

14. Aldahmesh MA, Khan AO, Hijazi H, Alkuraya FS. Mutations in ALDH1A3 cause microphthalmia. Clin Genet. 2013;84(2):128–31. https://doi.org/10.1111/cge.12184.
15. Mory A, Ruiz FX, Dagan E, Yakovtseva EA, Kurolap A, Parés X, et al. A missense mutation in ALDH1A3 causes isolated microphthalmia/anophthalmia in nine individuals from an inbred Muslim kindred. Eur J Hum Genet. 2014;22(3):419–22. https://doi.org/10.1038/ejhg.2013.157.
16. Roos L, Fang M, Dali C, Jensen H, Christoffersen N, Wu B, et al. A homozygous mutation in a consanguineous family consolidates the role of ALDH1A3 in autosomal recessive microphthalmia. Clin Genet. 2014;86(3): 276–81. https://doi.org/10.1111/cge.12277.
17. Abouzeid H, Favez T, Schmid A, Agosti C, Youssef M, Marzouk I, et al. Mutations in ALDH1A3 represent a frequent cause of microphthalmia/anophthalmia in consanguineous families. Hum Mutat. 2014;35(8):949–53. https://doi.org/10.1002/humu.22580.
18. Semerci CN, Kalay E, Yıldırım C, Dinçer T, Olmez A, Toraman B, et al. Novel splice-site and missense mutations in the ALDH1A3 gene underlying autosomal recessive anophthalmia/microphthalmia. Br J Ophthalmol. 2014; 98(6):832–40. https://doi.org/10.1136/bjophthalmol-2013-304058.
19. Dehghani M, Dehghan Tezerjani M, Metanat Z, Vahidi Mehrjardi MY. A Novel Missense Mutation in the ALDH13 Gene Causes Anophthalmia in Two Unrelated Iranian Consanguineous Families. Int J Mol Cell Med. 2017; 6(2):131–4. https://doi.org/10.22088/acadpub.BUMS.6.2.7.
20. Alabdullatif MA, Al Dhaibani MA, Khassawneh MY, El-Hattab AW. Chromosomal microarray in a highly consanguineous population: diagnosticyield, utility of regions of homozygosity, and novel mutations. Clin Genet. 2017;91(4):616–22. https://doi.org/10.1111/cge.12872 .
21. Liu Y, Lu Y, Liu S, Liao S. Novel compound heterozygous mutations of ALDH1A3 contribute to anophthalmia in a non-consanguineous Chinese family. Genet Mol Biol. 2017;40(2):430–5. https://doi.org/10.1590/1678-4685-GMB-2016-0120.
22. Bittles AH. A community genetics perspective on consanguineous marriage. Community Genet. 2008;11(6):324–30. https://doi.org/10.1159/000133304.
23. Brambring M, Asbrock D. Validity of false belief tasks in blind children. J Autism Dev Disord. 2010;40:1471–84. https://doi.org/10.1007/s10803-010-1002-2.
24. Brown R, Hobson RP, Lee A, Stevenson J. Are there "autistic-like" features in congenitally blind children? J Child Psychol Psychiatry. 1997;38:693–703.
25. Musante L, Ropers HH. Genetics of recessive cognitive disorders. Trends Genet. 2014;30:32–9. https://doi.org/10.1016/j.tig.2013.09.008.
26. Hornby SJ, Ward SJ, Gilbert CE, Dandona L, Foster A, Jones RB. Environmental risk factors in congenital malformations of the eye. Ann Trop Paediatr. 2002;22:67–77. https://doi.org/10.1179/027249302125000193.
27. Schittkowski MP, Guthoff RF. Systemic and ophthalmological anomalies in congenital anophthalmic or microphthalmia patients. Br J Ophthalmol. 2010;94:487–93. https://doi.org/10.1136/bjo.2009.163436.

Novel mutations of PKD genes in Chinese patients suffering from autosomal dominant polycystic kidney disease and seeking assisted reproduction

Wen-Bin He[1,2†], Wen-Juan Xiao[1†], Yue-Qiu Tan[1,2], Xiao-Meng Zhao[2], Wen Li[1,2], Qian-Jun Zhang[1,2], Chang-Gao Zhong[1,2], Xiu-Rong Li[1,2], Liang Hu[1,2], Guang-Xiu Lu[1,2], Ge Lin[1,2] and Juan Du[1,2*]

Abstract

Background: Autosomal dominant polycystic kidney disease (ADPKD), the commonest inherited kidney disease, is generally caused by heterozygous mutations in *PKD1*, *PKD2*, or *GANAB* (*PKD3*).

Methods: We performed mutational analyses of PKD genes to identify causative mutations. A set of 90 unrelated families with ADPKD were subjected to mutational analyses of PKD genes. Genes were analysed using long-range PCR (LR-PCR), direct PCR sequencing, followed by multiplex ligation-dependent probe amplification (MLPA) or screening of *GANAB* for some patients. Semen quality was assessed for 46 male patients, and the correlation between mutations and male infertility was analysed.

Results: A total of 76 mutations, including 38 novel mutations, were identified in 77 families, comprising 72 mutations in *PKD1* and 4 in *PKD2*, with a positive detection rate of 85.6%. No pathogenic mutations of *GANAB* were detected. Thirty-seven patients had low semen quality and were likely to be infertile. No association was detected between *PKD1* mutation type and semen quality. However, male patients carrying a pathogenic mutation in the Ig-like repeat domain of *PKD1* had a high risk of infertility.

Conclusion: Our study identified a group of novel mutations in PKD genes, which enrich the PKD mutation spectrum and might help clinicians to make precise diagnoses, thereby allowing better family planning and genetic counselling. Men with ADPKD accompanied by infertility should consider intracytoplasmic sperm injection combined with preimplantation genetic diagnosis to achieve paternity and obtain healthy progeny.

Keywords: Autosomal dominant polycystic kidney disease, *PKD1* gene, *PKD2* gene, *GANAB* gene, Novel mutation, Male infertility

Background

Autosomal dominant polycystic kidney disease (ADPKD) is the commonest inherited kidney disease, with an estimated incidence of 1:400 to 1:1000; it accounts for 7–10% of all patients on renal replacement therapy worldwide [1]. It is characterised by the development of renal cysts, hypertension, and extrarenal cysts, and results in end-stage renal disease (ESRD) [2]. In addition, male patients with ADPKD usually show infertility resulting from cystic dilatation of the seminal vesicles [3].

ADPKD is an autosomal dominant inherited disorder resulting from heterozygous mutations in three genes: *PKD1*, *PKD2*, and *GANAB*. Mutations of the first two genes (*PKD1* and *PKD2*) account for 80–85% and 15–20% of resolved cases, respectively [4, 5]. As of January 31, 2018, more than 2000 mutations (2323 in *PKD1* and 278 in *PKD2*) had been described in the Autosomal Dominant Polycystic Kidney Disease Mutation Database

* Correspondence: tandujuan@csu.edu.cn
†Wen-Bin He and Wen-Juan Xiao contributed equally to this work.
[1]Institute of Reproductive and Stem Cell Engineering, School of Basic Medical Science, Central South University, Changsha, Hunan 410078, People's Republic of China
[2]Reproductive and Genetic Hospital of CITIC-Xiangya, Changsha, Hunan 410078, People's Republic of China

(PKDB; http://pkdb.mayo.edu/). Recently, two studies reported the association of the third ADPKD gene *GANAB*, or *PKD3* [6, 7], which accounts for ~ 0.3% of the total cases of ADPKD [7].

In the present study, we performed mutational screening of *PKD1*, *PKD2*, and *GANAB* using long-range PCR (LR-PCR) and direct sequencing, as well as multiplex ligation-dependent probe amplification (MLPA) in 90 unrelated Chinese families with ADPKD. A total of 76 likely pathogenic or pathogenic mutations were identified in 77 families, including 38 novel mutations in PKD genes. These mutation data will contribute to improvement of diagnostics and genetic counselling in a clinical setting. In addition, this study highlights the correlation between men with ADPKD and infertility.

Methods

Study subjects

A total of 90 unrelated families were recruited from the Reproductive and Genetic Hospital of CITIC-Xiangya in China from October 2012 to October 2017, including 72 patients with a positive family history of ADPKD. These patients either sought genetic counselling to avoid delivering a baby with ADPKD due to a positive family history, or sought treatment at our hospital for infertility and were diagnosed with ADPKD based on ultrasound examination before undergoing assisted reproductive technology treatment. All diagnoses were confirmed by ultrasound examination according to previously described criteria: (1) the presence of at least three (unilateral or bilateral) renal cysts in individuals aged 15 to 39 years, or (2) the presence of at least two cysts in each kidney in individuals aged 40 to 59 years, or (3) the presence of four or more cysts in each kidney in individuals aged 60 years and above [8].

All individuals signed a written informed consent form, and blood samples were obtained from all probands and their family members when possible. The study was approved by the Ethics Committee of the Reproductive and Genetic Hospital of CITIC-Xiangya.

Semen analysis and assisted reproductive therapies

Among the 90 unrelated ADPKD probands, 61 were male and 46 provided semen specimens for analysis. Specimens were collected by means of masturbation into a sterile container after 2–7 days of abstinence. All specimens were assessed according to the World Health Organization (WHO) 2010 recommendations [9]. Briefly, within 1 h of ejaculation, the samples were liquefied and analysed for semen volume, sperm concentration, round cells, normal morphology, and sperm motility (defined as WHO motility grades A, B, C, and D, where grade A indicates fast progressive sperm; B, slow progressive sperm; C, nonprogressive sperm; and D, immotile sperm).

All patients providing semen specimens for analysis had a normal 46, XY karyotype, and no Y chromosome abnormalities were detected by microdeletion detection. Other causes of infertility, such as drugs and exposure to toxic substances, were excluded. Physical examination of these male patients showed normal results, including height, weight, hair distribution, mental state, and external genital organs.

Most of individuals who provided semen specimens for analysis have chosen different approaches to conceive offspring, including natural pregnancy, in vitro fertilization (IVF), intracytoplasmic sperm injection (ICSI), and ICSI combined preimplantation genetic diagnosis (PGD).

Mutation analysis of *PKD1*, *PKD2*, and *GANAB*

Genomic DNA (gDNA) was extracted from peripheral blood samples using a QIAamp® DNA blood midi kit (QIAGEN, Hilden, Germany) according to the manufacturer's protocol. All patients were subjected to mutation screening of *PKD1* and *PKD2* using Sanger sequencing, followed by multiplex ligation-dependent probe amplification analysis (MLPA) to detect copy number variation in *PKD1* and *PKD2* in patients lacking definitely pathogenic point mutations in *PKD1* or *PKD2*. Subsequent screening of *GANAB* was carried out in patients for whom no causative genetic aetiology in *PKD1* and *PKD2* had been identified.

For exons 1–34 of *PKD1*, LR-PCR followed by nested PCR was performed with *PKD1*-specific primers, as previously described [10–12], and exons 35–46 of *PKD1* were directly amplified from gDNA by PCR. All exons of *PKD2* and *GANAB*, including the adjacent 30–60 bp intron sequence, were amplified from gDNA by PCR. The primers for amplification of *PKD1* were previously described, with minor modifications [12, 13]; specific primers for *PKD2* and *GANBA* were designed using Primer 3 online (http://primer3.ut.ee) according to reference sequences. The primers and conditions for PCR reactions are provided in Additional file 1: Table S1, Additional file 2: Table S2, Additional file 3: Table S3, Additional file 4: Table S4. If a variant was identified as a putative disease-causative mutation, then mutation site screening of family members was implemented. DNA samples from all patients were screened by bidirectional sequencing on an Applied Biosystems 3130XL genetic analyser (Applied Biosystems, Foster City, CA, USA).

Copy number variation analysis of *PKD1* and *PKD2* was performed by MLPA with a SALSA MLPA probemix P351-C1/P352-D1 *PKD1-PKD2* kit (MRC-Holland, Amsterdam, the Netherlands) according to the manufacturer's instructions [14]. This kit contains probes for 36 of the 46 exons of *PKD1* and 17 probes for *PKD2* exons, covering all PKD2 exons except exon 13 (two probes each for PKD2 exons 1, 2, and 6). The results of MLPA analysis were scanned on an Applied Biosystems 3130XL genetic analyser (Applied Biosystems, Foster City, CA, USA). The raw data were analysed using the Coffalyser MLPA analysis tool (MRC-Holland, Amsterdam, the Netherlands).

Evaluation of the pathogenicity of variations

The PKDB (http://pkdb.mayo.edu), the Human Gene Mutation Database (HGMD; http://www.hgmd.cf.ac.uk/ac/index.php), Exome Aggregation Consortium (EXAC; http://exac.broadinstitute.org), and the gnomAD database (http://gnomad.broadinstitute.org) were searched for previously reported variations. Frameshift variations, typical splicing, nonsense, and in-frame changes of two or more amino acids were defined as definitely pathogenic mutations [2, 15]. A novel mutation was defined as one that had not been described in PKDB or HGMD, or reported in ADPKD patients. The potential pathogenicity of all identified missense variants, indicated by a frequency below 1% in the Asian population of the Exac and gnomAD databases, was evaluated by pedigree analysis and in silico analysis using three different tools: SIFT (http://sift.bii.a-star.edu.sg/), Polyphen-2 (http://genetics.bwh.harvard.edu/pph2), and MutationTaster (http://www.mutationtaster.org/). All variants were classified into five categories: 'pathogenic', 'likely pathogenic', 'uncertain significance', 'likely benign', and 'benign', according to the American College of Medical Genetics and Genomics (ACMG) standards and guidelines for the interpretation of variations [16].

Results

Mutation analysis of *PKD1, PKD2,* and *GANAB*

We performed mutation screening of *PKD1*and *PKD2* for 90 probands using Sanger sequencing and MLPA. The 33 probands for whom no definitely pathogenic mutations were detected in *PKD*1 and *PKD2* were subjected to screening of *GANAB*. A total of 93 variations were identified in this study, comprising 84, 4, and 5 variations in *PKD1*, *PKD2*, and GANAB, respectively (Tables 1 and 2). Among these variations, 51 are novel and have not been described in the ADPKD Mutation Database or HGMD, or been reported in ADPKD patients.

Evaluation of the pathogenicity of variations

We evaluated the potential pathogenicity of all identified missense variants according to the ACMG standards and guidelines for the interpretation of variations. The results are shown in Tables 1 and 2. A total of 84 variations were identified in *PKD1*, including 52 definitely pathogenic variations and 32 missense variants, 20 of which are classified as likely pathogenic mutations. Only four variants were identified in *PKD2*; three of them are definitely pathogenic mutations, and another is classified as likely to be pathogenic. Among the 76 definitely pathogenic or likely pathogenic mutations of *PKD1* and *PKD2*, 38 are novel. We identified five novel variations in *GANAB*. Two variations (p.Arg173Gln, and p.Arg331Cys) have been reported in the gnomAD database 431, and 1979 times, respectively, including 3, and 12 homozygotes, respectively, and are unlikely to be pathogenic. Three other variations (p.Pro123Ala, p.Met360Val, and p.Ile764Met) were identified in the gnomAD database 53,113, and 44 times, respectively, and are not very highly conserved. Two of these (p.Pro123Ala and p.Ile764Met) and a likely pathogenic mutation in PKD1 (p.Leu727Pro) were identified in family 69 with co-occurrence, and segregated with the disease in three affected family members. However, since functional analysis has not been performed, we are unable to determine their pathogenicity thus far, and they are classified as variants of uncertain significance.

Correlation with male infertility

In order to analyze the correlation between ADPKD mutations and male infertility, we analyzed the types of PKD genes mutations and semen quality. In our study, the analysis of semen from 46 male patients revealed that sperm from 37 individuals were abnormal; asthenozoospermia was detected in 18 individuals; 18 other individuals were affected with oligozoospermia or oligoasthenozoospermia; and 1 individual suffered from azoospermia. A total of 28 of the individuals with abnormal sperm were found to harbour definitely pathogenic mutations, and 7 individuals with normal sperm also carried definitely pathogenic mutations (Table 3, Fig. 1). The results showed no correlation between semen quality and types of mutation in PKD genes.

A total of 35 patients who provided semen specimens for analysis have chosen different approaches to conceive. Two patients (one with asthenozoospermia and the other with oligoasthenozoospermia) conceived naturally, and two individuals (one with asthenozoospermia and the other with normal sperm) conceived through ICSI. The 31 other patients chose ICSI combined with PGD; of these patients, genetic diagnosis of embryos has been completed for 22 and the treatment cycle is currently incomplete for 9 patients (Table 4).

Discussion

In the present study, we analysed 90 unrelated patients affected with polycystic kidney disease, including 37 male patients with infertility. Screening of *PKD1, PKD2,* and *GANAB* was performed using a series of molecular genetic analyses. A total of 76 mutations (definitely or likely pathogenic mutations) were identified in 77 of the families, comprising 72 mutations in *PKD1* and 4 in *PKD2*. Pathogenic mutations in *GANAB* have never

Table 1 Defnitely pathogenic mutations in PKD1 and PKD2 identified in this study

cDNA change	Exon/ intron	Amino acid change	Mutation Type	Family No.	Family history	Known/Novel
PKD1						
c.74dupG	1	p.Gly25Glyfs*89	Frameshift	29	Yes	Novel
c.106_107insT	1	p.Pro36Leufs*78	Frameshift	12	Yes	Novel
c.467_487del21	4	p.Ala156_Ala162del	In-frame deletion	49	Yes	Novel
c.856_862delTCTGGCC	5	p.Ser286Serfs*2	Frameshift	30	Yes	Known
c.1198C > T	5	p.Arg400*	Nonsense	17	Yes	Known
c.1297C > T	6	p.Gln433*	Nonsense	48	NA	Known
c.2050A > T	10	p.Arg684*	Nonsense	47	Yes	Novel
c.2659delT	11	p.Trp887Glyfs*11	Frameshift	50	Yes	Known
c.2670 + 1G > A	IVS14	-	Splice	19	Yes	Novel
c.4177C > T	15	p.Gln1393*	Nonsense	51	Yes	Novel
c.4447C > T	15	p.Gln1483*	Nonsense	13	Yes	Known
				14	Yes	
c.4551C > A	15	p.Tyr1517*	Nonsense	39	Yes	Novel
c.4609G > T	15	p.Glu1537*	Nonsense	31	Yes	Known
c.4846G > T	15	p.Glu1616*	Nonsense	37	Yes	Novel
c.4957C > T	15	p.Gln1653*	Nonsense	16	Yes	Known
c.5014_5015delAG	15	p.Arg1672Glyfs*98	Frameshift	53	Yes	Known
c.5120G > A	15	p.Trp1707*	Nonsense	26	Yes	Known
c.5637C > G	15	p.Tyr1879*	Nonsense	20	Yes	Novel
c.6115C > T	15	p.Gln2039*	Nonsense	55	Yes	Known
c.6199C > T	15	p.Gln2067*	Nonsense	34	Yes	Known
c.6804delG	15	p.Trp2268Cysfs*46	Frameshift	63	No	Novel
c.6813_6814delAC	15	p.Arg2272Glyfs*147	Frameshift	7	Yes	Known
c.6945_6946insT	16	p.Gly2316Trpfs*104	Frameshift	1	Yes	Novel
c.7126C > T	17	p.Gln2376*	Nonsense	45	Yes	Known
c.7863 + 1G > C	IVS20	-	Splice	36	Yes	Novel
c.7863 + 2 T > G	IVS20	-	Splice	11	Yes	Novel
c.7915C > T	21	p.Arg2639*	Nonsense	54	Yes	Known
c.7973_7974delTG	21	p.Val2658Glyfs*2	Frameshift	9	Yes	Known
c.8338G > T	23	p.Glu2780*	Nonsense	27	Yes	Known
c.9666_9667delGA	28	p.Glu3222Aspfs*30	Frameshift	32	Yes	Novel
c.10050 + 1G > A	IVS30	-	Splice	44	Yes	Known
c.10220 + 2 T > C	IVS32	-	Splice	3	Yes	Known
c.10397C > G	34	p.Ser3466*	Nonsense	6	Yes	Novel
c.10524_10525delAG	35	p.Glu3509Aspfs*117	Frameshift	2	NA	Novel
c.10710_10715delGGCTGT	36	p.3571_3572del2	In-frame deletion	40	Yes	Known
c.10724G > A	36	p.Try3575*	Nonsense	38	NA	Novel
c.10896_10897delGA	37	p.Ser3633Profs*88	Frameshift	5	No	Novel
c.11240delC	39	p.Pro3747Hisfs*79	Frameshift	33	Yes	Novel
c.11269 + 1G > A	IVS39	-	Splice	10	Yes	Novel
c.11311_11312insGTGCT	40	p.Ser3771Cysfs*57	Frameshift	41	NA	Novel
c.11512C > T	41	p.Gln3838*	Nonsense	15	Yes	Known
c.11538-2A > G	IVS41	-	Splice	18	Yes	Known

Table 1 Defnitely pathogenic mutations in PKD1 and PKD2 identified in this study *(Continued)*

cDNA change	Exon/ intron	Amino acid change	Mutation Type	Family No.	Family history	Known/Novel
c.11617_11637del21	42	p.3873_3879del7	In-frame deletion	4	Yes	Novel
c.11699_11700ins10	42	p.Leu3901Alafs*63	Frameshift	22	Yes	Novel
c.11830_11838dup	43	p.Leu3944_Ala3946dup	In-frame duplication	52	Yes	Novel
c.12101delT	44	p.Val4034Glyfs*5	Frameshift	25	No	Novel
c.12139-2A > T	IVS44	-	Splice	24	Yes	Novel
c.12391G > T	45	p.Glu4131*	Nonsense	43	Yes	Known
c.12570_12571insCTCC	46	p.Ser4190Serfs*21	Frameshift	28	Yes	Novel
c.12682C > T	46	p.Arg4228*	Nonsense	21	Yes	Known
				23	Yes	
c.12712C > T	46	p.Gln4238*	Nonsense	46	Yes	Known
EX31-33del	31–33	-	Large deletion	72	No	Novel
PKD2						
c.973C > T	4	p.Arg325*	Nonsense	8	Yes	Known
c.1094 + 3_1094 + 6delAAGT	IVS4	-	Splice	35	Yes	Known
c.2159dupA	11	p.Asn720Lysfs*5	Frameshift	42	Yes	Known

NA not available; *translation termination codon. Novel mutation defined as one that had not been described in PKDB, HGMD, or reported in ADPKD patients

been identified in Chinese patients. To our knowledge, this is the first report of *GANAB* screening in a cohort of Chinese patients with ADPKD.

PKD1, *PKD2*, and *GANAB* are located in chromosome regions 16p13.3, 4q21–22, and 11q12.3, and they produce the proteins polycystin-1 (PC-1), PC-2, and neutral alpha-glucosidase AB, respectively [17]. A series of molecular genetic analyses were used to screen for mutations of PKD genes. The human genome contains six truncated *PKD1* pseudogenes, which share approximately 97.7% similarity with exons 1–34 of *PKD1* [18]. *PKD1* contains complex reiterated regions, necessitating that LR-PCR be performed prior to sequencing [19]. Screening of *PKD2* was performed by direct Sanger sequencing. Subsequently, MLPA was employed to analyse the copy number variations of *PKD1* and *PKD2* in the genetically unresolved families, followed by screening of *GANAB* using direct Sanger sequencing. This strategy can typically identify almost all variants in PKD genes, as verified by our high mutation detection rate (85.6%,77/90). Recently, targeted next-generation sequencing and whole-exome sequencing have been used to identify mutations involved in ADPKD. Although these methods have high sensitivity, specificity, and accuracy, LR-PCR is still required; furthermore, highly specialised personnel and expensive equipment are required [20]. Thus, the strategy for the identification of mutations in ADPKD used in the present study may be useful in a wide variety of situations.

A total of 2609 variants had been described before January 2018 (2323 in *PKD1*, 278 in *PKD2*, and 8 in *GANAB*). The majority of these variants were missense variants (1225). The others were protein-truncating variants (840), splice site mutations (165), in-frame indels (115), large deletions (24), and variations in the UTR and intervening sequences (228). In our study, a total of 76 mutations (definitely or likely pathogenic variations) were identified in 77 of the families, comprising 41 protein-truncating, 21 missense mutations, and 9 splice site mutations; 4 in-frame indels; and 1 large deletion variants. The positive detection rate was 85.6% (77/90), and 50% (38/76) of all mutations were novel. The proportion of patients with ADPKD with a family history of the disease accounted for 80% (72/90) of all probands, comparable to previously published data [21].

A total of 76 mutations were identified, 72 of which (including 52 definitely pathogenic mutations) were in *PKD1,* accounting for 94.7%. Among all definitely pathogenic mutations of *PKD1*, 39 were truncating mutations, accounting for a large proportion (75%, 39/52), concordant with the results of other recent studies [17]. Furthermore, one large deletion of *PKD1* was identified in our set of patients (1.1%, 1/90), in accordance with previously reported results [22, 23]. A total of 4 mutations were identified in *PKD2,* 3 of which were definitely pathogenic mutations. However, no hot-spots of mutation were identified in *PKD1* or *PKD2,* indicating that for identification of future mutations, all exons of *PKD1* and *PKD2,* including their intron-exon boundaries, should be sequenced.

GANAB has been implicated in the development of autosomal-dominant polycystic kidney and liver disease [7]. In this study, a total of five mutations with a frequency below 1% were identified in the Asian population of the Exac and gnomAD databases; all are missense

Table 2 Evaluation of the pathogenic potential of PKD genes missense variants

cDNA change	Exon	Amino acid change	Co-occurence	SIFT	PolyPhen-2	Mutation Taster	Family No.	Family history	Segregation	Known/Novel	Classification
PKD1											
c.1385G>T	6	p.Arg462Met		NT	PRD	D	77	Yes	Yes	Novel	LP
c.2039A > T	10	p.Tyr680Phe	p.Tyr1879*	NT	POD	P	20	Yes	Yes	Known	LB
c.2180 T>C	11	p.Leu727Pro		NT	PRD	D	69	Yes	Yes	Known	LP
c.2897G>C	12	p.Arg966Pro		NT	PRD	D	73	Yes	Yes	Novel	LP
c.3548C > G	15	p.Ser1183Trp	p.Gln1653*	NT	B	P	16	Yes	Yes	Novel	LB
c.3613G>C	15	p.Asp1205His		NT	POD	P	64	Yes	Yes	Novel	LP
							76	No	NA		
c.3868C > G	15	p.Leu1290Val	p.Gln1653*	T	B	P	16	Yes	Yes	Novel	LB
c.3931G>A	15	p.Ala1311Thr		NT	B	P	80	No	No	Known	LB
c.4273C > T	15	p.Arg1425Cys	p.Gln3838*	NT	B	P	15	Yes	Yes	Novel	LB
c.5600A > G	15	p.Asn1867Ser	p.Arg400*	NT	PRD	D	17	Yes	Yes	Novel	USV
c.5957C>T	15	p.Thr1986Met		NT	PRD	P	87	Yes	NA	Novel	LB
c.6658C>T	15	p.Arg2220Trp		NT	PRD	D	85	Yes	Yes	Known	LP
c.6704C>T	15	p.Ser2235Leu		NT	PRD	D	70	Yes	Yes	Novel	LP
c.6827 T>C	15	p.Leu2276Pro		NT	PRD	D	61	Yes	Yes	Known	LP
c.6878C > T	15	p.Pro2293Leu	p.Pro36Leufs*78	NT	POD	P	12	Yes	NA	Known	LB
c.7099 T>C	17	p.Ser2367Pro		NT	PRD	D	56	Yes	NA	Novel	LP
c.7144A>C	17	p.Ser2382Arg		NT	PRD	D	67	Yes	Yes	Novel	LP
c.7241C > T	18	p.Thr2414Met	c.11269 + 1G > A	NT	PRD	D	10	Yes	Yes	Known	LP
c.7589G>A	19	p.Gly2530Asp		NT	PRD	D	59	No	NA	Known	LP
c.8158A>C	22	p.Thr2720Pro		NT	PRD	D	86	NA	NA	Novel	LP
c.8311G>A	23	p.Glu2771Lys		NT	PRD	D	83	Yes	NA	Known	LP
c.8744A > G	23	p.Asn2915Ser	p.Ser4190Serfs*21	T	B	D	28	Yes	Yes	Novel	USV
c.8750C > T	23	p.Ala2917Val	p.Gln3838*	T	POD	P	15	Yes	Yes	Known	LB
			p.Gln1653*				16	Yes	Yes		
c.10937 T>G	37	p.Val3646Gly		T	PRD	D	68	Yes	Yes	Novel	LP
c.10951G>A	37	p.Gly3651Ser		T	PRD	D	79	Yes	NA	Known	LP
c.11156G>T	38	p.Arg3719Leu		NT	PRD	D	82	Yes	Yes	Novel	LP
c.11248C>G	39	p.Arg3750Gly		NT	PRD	D	74	No	Yes	Known	LP
c.11257C>T	39	p.Arg3753Trp		NT	PRD	D	84	Yes	Yes	Known	LP
c.11351G > T	40	p.Gly3784Val		T	B	P	75	Yes	Yes	Novel	LB
c.11453G>A	41	p.Gly3818Asp		NT	PRD	D	81	Yes	Yes	Known	LP

Table 2 Evaluation of the pathogenic potential of PKD genes missense variants *(Continued)*

cDNA change	Exon	Amino acid change	Co-occurence	SIFT	PolyPhen-2	Mutation Taster	Family No.	Family history	Segregation	Known/Novel	Classification
c.11945A>C	43	p.Gln3982Pro		NT	PRD	P	78	Yes	Yes	Novel	LP
c.12671C>A	46	p.Thr4224Asn		NT	POD	P	66	Yes	NA	Novel	USV
PKD2											
c.965G>A	4	p.Arg322Gln		NT	PRD	D	64	Yes	NA	Known	LP
GANAB											
c.518G>A	5	p.Arg173Gln		T	PRD	D	58	Yes	NA	Novel	B
							86	NA	NA		
c.991C>T	10	p.Arg331Cys		NT	PRD	D	61	Yes	No	Novel	LB
c.1078A>G	11	p.Met360Val		NT	B	D	62	Yes	NA	Novel	USV
c.367C>G	4	p.Pro123Ala		T	POD	D	69	Yes	Yes	Novel	USV
c.2292A>G	19	p.Ile764Met		T	B	D			Yes	Novel	USV

NT Not Tolerated, *T* Tolerated, *PRD* Probably damaging, *B* Benign, *POD* Possibly damaging, *D* Disease causing, *P* Polymorphism, *LB* likely benign variation, *LP* likely pathogenic variation, *USV* uncertain significance variation, *NA* not available, *translation termination codon

Table 3 The semen analysis of 46 male patients

Gene	cDNA change	Exon/ intron	Amino acid change	Predicted location within PKD1 domains	Family No.	Age[a]	Inheriting/age[b]	Semen analysis
PKD1	c.856_862delTCTGGCC	5	p.Ser286Serfs*2	Ig-like repeat domain	30	27	maternal	oligoasthenozoospermia
PKD1	c.1385G>T	6	p.Arg462Met	C-type lectin domain	77	30	paternal/25	asthenozoospermia
PKD1	c.2527 T > C	11	p.Ser843Pro	not defined	45	34	paternal/22	oligoasthenozoospermia
PKD1	c.7126C > T	17	p.Gln2376*	REJ				
PKD1	c.2670 + 1G > A	IVS14	–	Ig-like repeat domain	19	34	maternal	asthenozoospermia
PKD1	c.3613G>C	15	p.Asp1205His	Ig-like repeat domain	64	30	paternal/28	asthenozoospermia
PKD2	c.965G>A	4	p.Arg322Gln	–				
PKD1	c.4447C > T	15	p.Gln1483*	Ig-like repeat domain	13	30	paternal/25	oligoasthenozoospermia
PKD1	c.4551C > A	15	p.Tyr1517*	Ig-like repeat domain	39	31	maternal	asthenozoospermia
PKD1	c.4609G > T	15	p.Glu1537*	Ig-like repeat domain	31	37	paternal/29	asthenozoospermia
PKD1	c.5957C>T	15	p.Thr1986Met	Ig-like repeat domain	87	38	paternal/23	asthenozoospermia
PKD1	c.6115C > T	15	p.Gln2039*	Ig-like repeat domain	55	36	paternal/25	asthenozoospermia
PKD1	c.6199C > T	15	p.Gln2067*	Ig-like repeat domain	34	23	maternal	oligoasthenozoospermia
PKD1	c.6658C>T	15	p.Arg2220Trp	REJ	85	31	paternal/22	oligoasthenozoospermia
PKD1	c.6704C>T	15	p.Ser2235Leu	REJ	70	30	paternal/29	asthenozoospermia
PKD1	c.7241C > T	18	p.Thr2414Met	REJ	10	30	maternal	oligoasthenozoospermia
PKD1	c.11269 + 1G > A	IVS39	–	not defined				
PKD1	c.7863 + 1G > C	IVS20	–	REJ	36	42	maternal	oligoasthenozoospermia
PKD1	c.7863 + 2 T > G	IVS20	–	REJ	11	33	maternal	asthenozoospermia
PKD1	c.7915C > T	21	p.Arg2639*	REJ	54	35	paternal/32	asthenozoospermia
PKD1	c.7973_7974delTG	21	p.Val2658Glyfs*2	REJ	9	33	paternal/28	asthenozoospermia
PKD1	c.8744A > G	23	p.Asn2915Ser	not defined	28	34	maternal	oligoasthenozoospermia
PKD1	c.12570_12571insCTCC	46	p.Ser4190Serfs*21	not defined				
PKD1	c.9666_9667delGA	28	p.Glu3222Aspfs*30	not defined	32	29	paternal/24	oligoasthenozoospermia
PKD1	EX31-33del	31–33	–	not defined	72	35	de novo	oligozoospermia
PKD1	c.10220 + 2 T > C	IVS32	–	not defined	3	44	NA	oligoasthenozoospermia
PKD1	c.12053C > T	44	p.Thr4018Ile	not defined				
PKD1	c.10397C > G	34	p.Ser3466*	not defined	6	27	paternal/22	oligoasthenozoospermia
PKD1	c.10524_10525delAG	35	p.Glu3509Aspfs*117	not defined	2	28	NA	oligoasthenozoospermia
PKD1	c.6804delG	15	p.Trp2268Cysfs*46	REJ	63	35	de novo	azoospermia
PKD1	c.10710_10715delGGCTGT	36	p.3571_3572del2	Putative TM region	40	34	maternal	asthenozoospermia
PKD1	c.10896_10897delGA	37	p.Ser3633Profs*88	not defined	5	37	de novo	oligoasthenozoospermia
PKD1	c.10937 T>G	37	p.Val3646Gly	not defined	68	32	paternal/26	asthenozoospermia

Table 3 The semen analysis of 46 male patients *(Continued)*

Gene	cDNA change	Exon/ intron	Amino acid change	Predicted location within PKD1 domains	Family No.	Age[a]	Inheriting/age[b]	Semen analysis
PKD1	c.10951G>A	37	p.Gly3651Ser	not defined	79	35	maternal	oligoasthenozoospermia
PKD1	c.11240delC	39	p.Pro3747Hisfs*79	not defined	33	33	paternal/25	oligoasthenozoospermia
PKD1	c.11538-2A > G	IVS41	–	not defined	18	36	paternal/30	oligoasthenozoospermia
PKD1	c.11617_11637del21	42	p.3873_3879del7	not defined	4	25	NA	asthenozoospermia
PKD1	c.11699_11700ins10	42	p.Leu3901Alafs*63	Putative TM region	22	29	paternal/22	asthenozoospermia
PKD1	c.11830_11838dup	43	p.Leu3944_Ala3946dup	Putative TM region	52	26	paternal/21	oligoasthenozoospermia
PKD1	c.11945A>C	43	p.Gln3982Pro	Putative TM region	78	33	paternal/28	asthenozoospermia
PKD1	c.12712C > T	46	p.Gln4238*	not defined	46	34	maternal	asthenozoospermia
PKD3	c.518G>A	5	p.Arg173Gln	–	58	37	paternal/27	asthenozoospermia
PKD1	c.1198C > T	5	p.Arg400*	not defined	17	29	maternal	normal
PKD1	c.5600A > G	15	p.Asn1867Ser	Ig-like repeat domain				
PKD1	c.3931G>A	15	p.Ala1311Thr	Ig-like repeat domain	80	27	de novo	normal
PKD1	c.2039A > T	10	p.Tyr680Phe	not defined	20	27	paternal/27	normal
PKD1	c.5637C > G	15	p.Tyr1879*	Ig-like repeat domain				
PKD1	c.4273C > T	15	p.Arg1425Cys	Ig-like repeat domain	15	31	paternal/28	normal
PKD1	c.8750C > T	23	p.Ala2917Val	not defined				
PKD1	c.11512C > T	41	p.Gln3838*	Putative TM region				
PKD1	c.6813_6814delAC	15	p.Arg2272Glyfs*147	REJ	7	32	NA	normal
PKD1	c.7144A>C	17	p.Ser2382Arg	REJ	67	29	maternal	normal
PKD1	c.10050 + 1G > A	IVS30	–	not defined	44	40	paternal/30	normal
PKD1	c.12139-2A > T	IVS44	–	Putative TM region	24	34	maternal	normal
PKD2	c.2159dupA	11	p.Asn720Lysfs*5	–	42	29	maternal	normal

REJ receptor for egg jelly; *NA* not available; [a]the age of the male patients seeking fertility advice from doctors; [b]the age of the patients' fathers fathering their last child; *translation termination codon

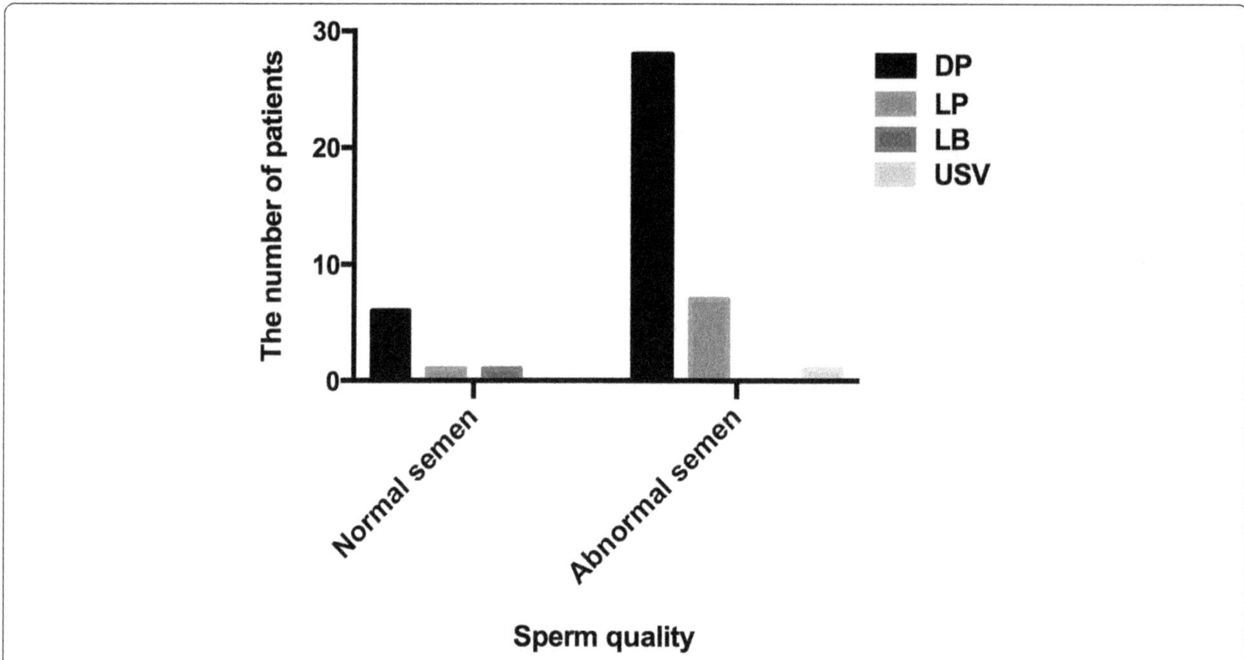

Fig. 1 The semen quality of the male patients who harboured PKD1 mutations. DP, LP, LB and USV are indicated with definitely pathogenic mutations, likely pathogenic variations, likely benign variations and uncertain significance variations, respectively. The results showed that there is no correlation between semen quality and the type of mutation in *PKD1* gene

mutations. Only two mutations (p.Pro123Ala and p.Ile764Met) co-occurred in family 69; these have been described a few times and were found to have segregated with the disease in affected family members, accounting for 1.1%. The patients in this family all suffered from polycystic kidney with liver disease, consistent with earlier findings that the phenotype caused by *GANAB* mutations usually manifests with polycystic liver disease (PLD) [7]. In addition, the patients from family 69 also carried the p.Leu727Pro mutation in *PKD1*, which has been reported in several families and classified as a highly likely pathogenic mutation [17, 24]. As p.Pro123Ala was predicted to be a disease-causing mutation by three tools and p.Ile764-Met was predicted to be benign by PolyPhen-2, the possibility that p.Leu727Pro in *PKD1* and p.Pro123Ala in *GANAB* co-contribute to the development of polycystic kidney with liver disease cannot be excluded. Thus, the fact that no definitely or likely pathogenic mutation was detected in this study suggested that GANAB mutations are rare in Chinese patients with ADPKD.

Earlier studies have reported that *HNF1B* can phenocopy ADPKD [25–27]. In addition, it has been very recently reported that monoallelic mutation in *DNAJB11* can cause atypical ADPKD, which is a phenotypic hybrid of ADPKD and autosomal-dominant tubulointerstitial diseases (ADTKD) [28]. In our study, for the 13 patients with or without a positive family history, the genetic cause remains unknown, but undetected *PKD1*, *PKD2*, or *GANAB* mutations, including deep intronic or synonymous exonic mutations that cause atypical splicing, or large deletions of *GANAB*, could be the underlying reasons. Furthermore, the patients should be reevaluated based on their most recent phenotype, and should be screened for other genes implicated in ADPKD for future analysis, such as *HNF1B* and *DNAJB11*.

ADPKD is a systemic disorder and extrarenal manifestation is not uncommon. Male patients with ADPKD usually suffer from infertility, resulting from abnormal semen, including necrospermia, immotile sperm, asthenozoospermia, and azoospermia [29–31]. PKD1 and PKD2 have been reported to play a pivotal role in the development and maintenance of the male reproductive tract [32, 33]. The potential aetiologies of semen abnormalities in male patients with ADPKD include ejaculatory duct cysts, seminal vesicle cysts, and ultrastructural flagellar defects caused by abnormal polycystins [30]. However, the correlation between the type of PKD gene mutation and semen quality remains unclear. In the present study, 37 individuals were found to have abnormal semen (80%, 37/46). Only some of the male patients with ADPKD carrying definitely pathogenic mutations were infertile, which may indicate that there is no correlation between the type of PKD1 mutation and semen quality. However, 23 of the variations are located in the same four domains of *PKD1*, and more than one third of the mutations (39%,9/23) are located in the Ig-like repeat domain, which is a conserved region of approximately 85 bp surrounding a central sequence consisting of 16 copies [34]. Defects of the Ig-like

Table 4 The assisted reproductive therapies used by the 35 male patients and the clinical outcomes of those therapies

Gene	cDNA change	Amino acid change	Family No.	Semen analysis	Treatment methods
PKD1	c.856_862delTCTGGCC	p.Ser286Serfs*2	30	oligoasthenozoospermia	ICSI+PGD
PKD1	c.1385G>T	p.Arg462Met	77	asthenozoospermia	ICSI+PGD
PKD1	c.2527 T > C	p.Ser843Pro	45	oligoasthenozoospermia	ICSI+PGD
PKD1	c.7126C > T	p.Gln2376*			
PKD1	c.2670 + 1G > A	–	19	asthenozoospermia	ICSI+PGD[a]
PKD1	c.4447C > T	p.Gln1483*	13	oligoasthenozoospermia	ICSI+PGD[a]
PKD1	c.4551C > A	p.Tyr1517*	39	asthenozoospermia	natural pregnant
PKD1	c.4609G > T	p.Glu1537*	31	asthenozoospermia	ICSI+PGD
PKD1	c.6199C > T	p.Gln2067*	34	oligoasthenozoospermia	natural pregnant
PKD1	c.6658C>T	p.Arg2220Trp	85	oligoasthenozoospermia	ICSI+PGD
PKD1	c.6704C>T	p.Ser2235Leu	70	asthenozoospermia	ICSI+PGD
PKD1	c.7863 + 1G > C	–	36	oligoasthenozoospermia	ICSI+PGD
PKD1	c.7863 + 2 T > G	–	11	asthenozoospermia	ICSI+PGD
PKD1	c.10529C > T	p.Thr3510Met			
PKD1	c.7915C > T	p.Arg2639*	54	asthenozoospermia	ICSI+PGD
PKD1	c.7973_7974delTG	p.Val2658Glyfs*2	9	asthenozoospermia	ICSI
PKD1	c.10529C > T	p.Thr3510Met			
PKD1	c.8744A > G	p.Asn2915Ser	28	oligoasthenozoospermia	ICSI+PGD[a]
PKD1	c.12570_12571insCTCC	p.Ser4190Serfs*21			
PKD1	c.9666_9667delGA	p.Glu3222Aspfs*30	32	oligoasthenozoospermia	ICSI+PGD[a]
PKD1	c.10220 + 2 T > C	–	3	oligoasthenozoospermia	ICSI+PGD[a]
PKD1	c.12053C > T	p.Thr4018Ile			
PKD1	c.10524_10525delAG	p.Glu3509Aspfs*117	2	oligoasthenozoospermia	ICSI+PGD
PKD1	c.10896_10897delGA	p.Ser3633Profs*88	5	oligoasthenozoospermia	ICSI+PGD[a]
PKD1	c.10937 T>G	p.Val3646Gly	68	asthenozoospermia	ICSI+PGD
PKD1	c.11240delC	p.Pro3747Hisfs*79	33	oligoasthenozoospermia	ICSI+PGD[a]
PKD1	c.11538-2A > G	–	18	oligoasthenozoospermia	ICSI+PGD
PKD1	c.11699_11700ins10	p.Leu3901Alafs*63	22	asthenozoospermia	ICSI+PGD
PKD1	c.11830_11838dup	p.Leu3944_Ala3946dup	52	oligoasthenozoospermia	ICSI+PGD
PKD1	c.11945A>C	p.Gln3982Pro	78	asthenozoospermia	ICSI+PGD
PKD1	c.12712C > T	p.Gln4238*	46	asthenozoospermia	ICSI+PGD
PKD1	c.1198C > T	p.Arg400*	17	normal	ICSI+PGD
PKD1	c.5600A > G	p.Asn1867Ser			
PKD1	c.3931G>A	p.Ala1311Thr	80	normal	ICSI
PKD1	c.2039A > T	p.Tyr680Phe	20	normal	ICSI+PGD[a]
PKD1	c.5637C > G	p.Tyr1879*			
PKD1	c.4273C > T	p.Arg1425Cys	15	normal	ICSI+PGD[a]
PKD1	c.8750C > T	p.Ala2917Val			
PKD1	c.11512C > T	p.Gln3838*			
PKD1	c.6813_6814delAC	p.Arg2272Glyfs*147	7	normal	ICSI+PGD
PKD1	c.7144A>C	p.Ser2382Arg	67	normal	ICSI+PGD
PKD1	c.10050 + 1G > A	–	44	normal	ICSI+PGD
PKD1	c.12139-2A > T	–	24	normal	ICSI+PGD
PKD2	c.2159dupA	p.Asn720Lysfs*5	42	normal	ICSI+PGD

ICSI intracytoplasmic sperm injection, *ICSI+PGD* ICSI combined preimplantation genetic diagnosis, [a]the treatment cycle is currently incomplete, *translation termination codon repeat domain in PKD1 protein may alter its binding ability, leading to male reproductive tract cysts and infertility [34]. Thus, male patients carrying pathogenic mutations in *PKD1* located in the Ig-like repeat domain may have a high risk of infertility. In addition, 20 and 3 of the mutations identified in the 23 male patients with ADPKD with abnormal semen were paternal and de novo, respectively. However, almost all of these fathers fathered their children when they were younger than the age at which their sons with ADPKD sought fertility advice from their doctors. Furthermore, after the treatment of ICSI, 17 individuals affected with semen abnormalities all achieved paternity or at least obtained embryos. Therefore, we suggest that male patients with ADPKD should achieve paternity as young as possible, and the use of ICSI combined PGD should be considered for patients suffering from low semen quality [30, 31].

In this study, the majority of male patients with ADPKD were found to have abnormal semen (80%), which could due to a selection bias in the study population. Since our hospital specializes in reproductive and genetic disorders, most of the subjects included in the study visited our hospital to seek treatment for infertility. Thus, the proportion of males with abnormal sperm quality is not a true reflection of the proportion of male ADPKD patients with abnormal sperm. Therefore, studies on larger groups of patients with ADPKD recruited from general hospitals are needed to obtain a more accurate estimation of the proportion of ADPKD-affected males with abnormal sperm.

Conclusions

In conclusion, we identified a group of novel mutations in PKD genes, which enriches the PKD mutation spectrum. Male patients with ADPKD are usually affected with infertility, and surgical sperm retrieval combined with assisted reproductive technology may help them to achieve paternity. Our study will provide clinicians with precise diagnoses that have implications for family planning and genetic counselling of affected individuals.

Abbreviations

ACMG: American College of Medical Genetics and Genomics; ADPKD: Autosomal dominant polycystic kidney disease; ESRD: End-stage renal disease; HGMD: Human gene mutation database; ICSI: Intracytoplasmic sperm injection; LR-PCR: Long-range PCR; MLPA: Multiplex ligation-dependent probe amplification; PC-1: Produce the proteins polycystin-1; PC-2: Produce the proteins polycystin-2; PKDB: Autosomal dominant polycystic kidney disease mutation database; PLD: Polycystic liver disease; WHO: World Health Organization

Acknowledgements

We would like to thank the patients and their family members for their support and participation in this research. We would also like to thank the genetic counselling team at the Reproductive and Genetic Hospital of CITIC-Xiangya and the clinicians who referred the patients for the clinical study.

Author' contributions

JD designed the study. WBH, WJX, XMZ, QJZ, and WL performed the mutation analysis of *PKD1*, *PKD2*, and *GANAB*. JD and WBH carried out the evaluation of the pathogenicity of variations. CGZ, XRL, LH, GXL, and GL worked on the clinical study. WBH, WJX and YQT wrote the paper. All authors read and approved the final manuscript.

Funding

This study was supported by grants from the National Natural Science Foundation of China (81771645 and 81471432), Scientific Research Foundation of Reproductive and Genetic Hospital of CITIC-Xiangya (YNXM-201802) and Graduate Research and Innovation Projects of Central South University (Grant 2017zzts372).

Competing interests

The authors declare that they have no competing interests.

References

1. Ong AC, Devuyst O, Knebelmann B, Walz G, Diseases E-EWGIK. Autosomal dominant polycystic kidney disease: the changing face of clinical management. Lancet. 2015;385(9981):1993–2002.
2. Rossetti S, Consugar MB, Chapman AB, Torres VE, Guay-Woodford LM, Grantham JJ, et al. Comprehensive molecular diagnostics in autosomal dominant polycystic kidney disease. J Am Soc Nephrol. 2007;18(7):2143–60.
3. Mieusset R, Fauquet I, Chauveau D, Monteil L, Chassaing N, Daudin M, et al. The spectrum of renal involvement in male patients with infertility related to excretory-system abnormalities: phenotypes, genotypes, and genetic counseling. J Nephrol. 2017;30(2):211–8.
4. European Polycystic Kidney Disease Consortium. The polycystic kidney disease 1 gene encodes a 14 kb transcript and lies within a duplicated region on chromosome 16. The European Polycystic Kidney Disease Consortium. Cell. 1994;77(6):881–94.
5. Kimberling WJ, Kumar S, Gabow PA, Kenyon JB, Connolly CJ, Somlo S. Autosomal dominant polycystic kidney disease: localization of the second gene to chromosome 4q13-q23. Genomics. 1993;18(3):467–72.
6. Iliuta IA, Kalatharan V, Wang K, Cornec-Le Gall E, Conklin J, Pourafkari M, et al. Polycystic kidney disease without an apparent family history. J Am Soc Nephrol. 2017;28(9):2768–76.
7. Porath B, Gainullin VG, Cornec-Le Gall E, Dillinger EK, Heyer CM, Hopp K, et al. Mutations in GANAB, encoding the glucosidase IIalpha subunit, cause autosomal-dominant polycystic kidney and liver disease. Am J Hum Genet. 2016;98(6):1193–207.
8. Pei Y, Obaji J, Dupuis A, Paterson AD, Magistroni R, Dicks E, et al. Unified criteria for ultrasonographic diagnosis of ADPKD. J Am Soc Nephrol. 2009; 20(1):205–12.
9. Cooper TG, Noonan E, von Eckardstein S, Auger J, Baker HW, Behre HM, et al. World Health Organization reference values for human semen characteristics. Hum Reprod Update. 2010;16(3):231–45.
10. Tan YC, Blumenfeld JD, Anghel R, Donahue S, Belenkaya R, Balina M, et al. Novel method for genomic analysis of PKD1 and PKD2 mutations in autosomal dominant polycystic kidney disease. Hum Mutat. 2009;30(2):264–73.
11. Phakdeekitcharoen B, Watnick TJ, Germino GG. Mutation analysis of the entire replicated portion of PKD1 using genomic DNA samples. J Am Soc Nephrol. 2001;12(5):955–63.
12. Zhang S, Mei C, Zhang D, Dai B, Tang B, Sun T, et al. Mutation analysis of autosomal dominant polycystic kidney disease genes in Han Chinese. Nephron Exp Nephrol. 2005;100(2):e63–76.
13. Rossetti S, Chauveau D, Walker D, Saggar-Malik A, Winearls CG, Torres VE, et al. A complete mutation screen of the ADPKD genes by DHPLC. Kidney Int. 2002;61(5):1588–99.
14. Schouten JP, McElgunn CJ, Waaijer R, Zwijnenburg D, Diepvens F, Pals G. Relative quantification of 40 nucleic acid sequences by multiplex ligation-dependent probe amplification. Nucleic Acids Res. 2002;30(12):e57.
15. Liu B, Chen SC, Yang YM, Yan K, Qian YQ, Zhang JY, et al. Identification of novel PKD1 and PKD2 mutations in a Chinese population with autosomal dominant polycystic kidney disease. Sci Rep. 2015;5:17468.
16. Richards S, Aziz N, Bale S, Bick D, Das S, Gastier-Foster J, et al. Standards and guidelines for the interpretation of sequence variants: a joint consensus recommendation of the American College of Medical Genetics and Genomics and the Association for Molecular Pathology. Genet Med. 2015; 17(5):405–24.

17. Cornec-Le Gall E, Audrezet MP, Chen JM, Hourmant M, Morin MP, Perrichot R, et al. Type of PKD1 mutation influences renal outcome in ADPKD. J Am Soc Nephrol. 2013;24(6):1006–13.
18. Symmons O, Varadi A, Aranyi T. How segmental duplications shape our genome: recent evolution of ABCC6 and PKD1 Mendelian disease genes. Mol Biol Evol. 2008;25(12):2601–13.
19. Rossetti S, Strmecki L, Gamble V, Burton S, Sneddon V, Peral B, et al. Mutation analysis of the entire PKD1 gene: genetic and diagnostic implications. Am J Hum Genet. 2001;68(1):46–63.
20. Qi XP, Du ZF, Ma JM, Chen XL, Zhang Q, Fei J, et al. Genetic diagnosis of autosomal dominant polycystic kidney disease by targeted capture and next-generation sequencing: utility and limitations. Gene. 2013;516(1):93–100.
21. Neumann HP, Bacher J, Nabulsi Z, Ortiz Bruchle N, Hoffmann MM, Schaeffner E, et al. Adult patients with sporadic polycystic kidney disease: the importance of screening for mutations in the PKD1 and PKD2 genes. Int Urol Nephrol. 2012;44(6):1753–62.
22. Obeidova L, Elisakova V, Stekrova J, Reiterova J, Merta M, Tesar V, et al. Novel mutations of PKD genes in the Czech population with autosomal dominant polycystic kidney disease. BMC Med Genet. 2014;15:41.
23. Consugar MB, Wong WC, Lundquist PA, Rossetti S, Kubly VJ, Walker DL, et al. Characterization of large rearrangements in autosomal dominant polycystic kidney disease and the PKD1/TSC2 contiguous gene syndrome. Kidney Int. 2008;74(11):1468–79.
24. Rossetti S, Hopp K, Sikkink RA, Sundsbak JL, Lee YK, Kubly V, et al. Identification of gene mutations in autosomal dominant polycystic kidney disease through targeted resequencing. J Am Soc Nephrol. 2012;23(5):915–33.
25. Verhave JC, Bech AP, Wetzels JF, Nijenhuis T. Hepatocyte nuclear factor 1beta-associated kidney disease: more than renal cysts and diabetes. J Am Soc Nephrol. 2016;27(2):345–53.
26. Nishigori H, Yamada S, Kohama T, Tomura H, Sho K, Horikawa Y, et al. Frameshift mutation, A263fsinsGG, in the hepatocyte nuclear factor-1beta gene associated with diabetes and renal dysfunction. Diabetes. 1998;47(8):1354–5.
27. Pace NP, Craus J, Felice A, Vassallo J. Case report: identification of an HNF1B p.Arg527Gln mutation in a Maltese patient with atypical early onset diabetes and diabetic nephropathy. BMC Endocr Disord. 2018;18(1):28.
28. Cornec-Le Gall E, Olson RJ, Besse W, Heyer CM, Gainullin VG, Smith JM, et al. Monoallelic mutations to DNAJB11 cause atypical autosomal-dominant polycystic kidney disease. Am J Hum Genet. 2018;102(5):832–44.
29. Torra R, Sarquella J, Calabia J, Marti J, Ars E, Fernandez-Llama P, et al. Prevalence of cysts in seminal tract and abnormal semen parameters in patients with autosomal dominant polycystic kidney disease. Clin J Am Soc Nephrol. 2008;3(3):790–3.
30. Kim JA, Blumenfeld JD, Prince MR. Seminal vesicles in autosomal dominant polycystic kidney disease. In: Li X, editor. Polycystic kidney disease. Brisbane (AU); 2015.
31. Shefi S, Levron J, Nadu A, Raviv G. Male infertility associated with adult dominant polycystic kidney disease: a case series. Arch Gynecol Obstet. 2009;280(3):457–60.
32. Nie X, Arend LJ. Pkd1 is required for male reproductive tract development. Mech Dev. 2013;130(11–12):567–76.
33. Nie X, Arend LJ. Novel roles of Pkd2 in male reproductive system development. Differentiation. 2014;87(3–4):161–71.
34. Hughes J, Ward CJ, Peral B, Aspinwall R, Clark K, San Millan JL, et al. The polycystic kidney disease 1 (PKD1) gene encodes a novel protein with multiple cell recognition domains. Nat Genet. 1995;10(2):151–60.

Common *FTO* rs9939609 variant and risk of type 2 diabetes in Palestine

Anas Sabarneh[1†], Suheir Ereqat[1,7*†], Stéphane Cauchi[2,3,4,5], Omar AbuShamma[1], Mohammad Abdelhafez[1], Murad Ibrahim[6] and Abdelmajeed Nasereddin[7]

Abstract

Background: Genetic and environmental factors play a crucial role in the development of type 2 diabetes mellitus (T2DM) and obesity. This study aimed to investigate the association of the fat-mass and obesity-associated gene (*FTO*) rs9939609 variant with T2DM and body mass index (BMI) among Palestinian population.

Methods: A total of 399 subjects were recruited, of whom 281 were type 2 diabetic patients and 118 normoglycemic subjects. All of them were unrelated, aged > 40 years and recruited within the period 2016–2017. The A allele of FTO rs9939609 was identified by PCR–RFLP.

Results: Significant association of the minor allele A of *FTO* rs9939609 and T2DM risk was observed with an allelic odd ratio of 1.92 (95% CI [1.09–3.29], $p = 0.02$) adjusted for age and gender, this association partly attenuated when adjusted for BMI with OR of 1.84, (95%CI [1.04–3.05], $p = 0.03$). Stratified data by glycemic status across *FTO* genotypes showed that A allele was marginally associated with increased BMI among diabetic group ($p = 0.057$) but not in control group ($p = 0.7$). Moreover, no significant association was observed between *FTO* genotypes and covariates of age, gender, T2DM complications or any tested metabolic trait in both diabetic and nondiabetic individuals ($p > 0.05$).

Conclusions: The variant rs9939609 of the FTO gene was associated with T2DM in Palestine. This is the first study conducted on this gene in the Palestinian population and provides valuable information for comparison with other ethnic groups. Further analysis with larger sample size is required to elucidate the role of this variant on the predisposition to increased BMI in Palestinians.

Keywords: *FTO*, rs9939609 variant, T2DM, BMI, Palestine

Background

Type 2 diabetes mellitus (T2DM) is the most common type of diabetes as it accounts for more than 90% of all diabetes cases worldwide (World Health Organization) [1]. Polymorphisms within the fat-mass and obesity-associated gene (*FTO*) are of particular interest as they have known effect on obesity which is a major risk factor for T2DM. A genome-wide association study (GWAS) conducted in 2007, confirmed that rs9939609 variant located within the first intron of the *FTO* gene predisposes European populations to diabetes through an effect on body mass index (BMI) [2, 3], while other reports from South Asian population showed that *FTO* gene variants increase the risk of type 2 diabetes independent of BMI [4]. Since then, several studies represent various ethnic populations, confirmed strong associations of the *FTO* rs9939609 with obesity [5, 6]. This association was not replicated in the Chinese Han population and African Americans [7, 8]. It is well-established that dyslipidemia is a risk factor for cardiovascular diseases (CVD) in diabetic patients. However, a study conducted by Doney et al. [9] demonstrated that A allele rs9939609 in the *FTO* gene increases the risk of myocardial infarction in patients with T2DM independent of BMI, glycated hemoglobin, mean arterial pressure and dyslipidemia. Moreover, a significant association of *FTO* variant

* Correspondence: sereqat@staff.alquds.edu
†Anas Sabarneh and Suheir Ereqat contributed equally to this work.
[1]Biochemistry and Molecular Biology Department, Faculty of Medicine, Al-Quds University, Abu Dis-East Jerusalem, Palestine
[7]Al-Quds Nutrition and Health Research Institute – Faculty of Medicine, Al-Quds University-Palestine, Abu Dis-Jerusalem, Palestine
Full list of author information is available at the end of the article

was found in Indian patients with T2DM without dyslipidemia [10].

A sex-specific effect of *FTO* variants on susceptibility to obesity have been shown, a study -in 2016- indicated that the effect of *FTO* variants on T2DM susceptibility in Japanese men but not women is mediated through *FTO* effect on BMI [11]. In 2018, a case control study conducted on obese Iranian women showed that several *FTO* variants including rs9939609 were associated with T2DM and obesity as well [12]. A recent spatial and meta-analysis suggested a region-related associations between *FTO* rs9939609 and T2DM [13]. Thus, the reported results were not consistent in different ethnic population.

In Palestine, the prevalence of DM (for adults aged > 25 years) was 15.3% in 2010, but estimates have placed to be as high as 20.8% by 2020 [14, 15]. Diabetes and its complications are estimated to account for approximately 5.7% of all deaths in Palestine [16]. The prevalence of overweight and obesity is rapidly escalating in the youth and adults, probably due changes in lifestyle, further enhancing the risk of diabetes. In 2016, a cross sectional study among the students at An-Najah National University in Nablus district (North Palestine) showed that the prevalence of overweight and obesity was 26.2%, with significant increase in males (36.4%) compared to females (19.1%) [17]. Genetic association studies of T2DM among Palestinians are scarce. Two studies conducted by Ereqat and colleagues in 2009 [18, 19] investigated the genetic association of Pro12Ala Polymorphism of the PPAR-Gamma 2 gene and rs7903146 variant in the transcription factor 7 like 2 gene (*TCF7L2*) with T2DM. However, no studies have been conducted to determine the genetic association of *FTO* variants with T2DM and/ or obesity. Therefore, our study aimed to examine the association between the *FTO* rs9939609 SNP with the risk of T2DM and its-related phenotypes in Palestinian population.

Methods

Study population

A total of 399 unrelated individuals were recruited from different cities in Palestine. Two-hundred eighty one cases, aged > 40 years, were diagnosed by T2DM according to WHO criteria based on fasting plasma glucose 126 mg/dl and/or currently being treated with medication for diabetes. All participants were recruited within the period of 2016–2017 in collaboration with UNRWA clinics (Hebron and Ramallah, Palestine). The anthropometric measurements were collected from their medical records that included age, sex, family history, drug history, medical history and other related information.

Fasting blood was collected for biochemical tests and DNA studies. All the cases with probable diagnosis of type 1 diabetes were excluded. The control group (n = 118), was selected from individuals who came to the same clinic for health check-up with no past medical history for T2DM and no family history of diabetes in first-degree relations. Age at examination was > 40 years.

Biochemical testing, DNA extraction and genotyping

Five milliliters of blood were obtained after overnight fast, collected in EDTA tubes, centrifuged at room temperature. Plasma glucose, cholesterol, HDL cholesterol, and triglyceride were determined by enzymatic methods as described by manufacturer's instructions (Human, Wiesbaden, Germany). Genomic DNA was extracted from whole blood (300 μl) using genomic DNA purification kit QIAamp according to the manufacturer instructions (Qiagen, Hilden, Germany). DNA samples were stored at 4 °C for further analyses. Genotyping of the *FTO* rs9939609 SNP was done by PCR-based restriction fragment length polymorphism (RFLP) analysis as previously described [20] with the following modifications. The PCR reactions were carried out using 20 ng of purified genomic DNA samples, with 0.4 μM of the forward and reverse primers using PCR-Ready Supreme mix (Syntezza Bioscience, Jerusalem) in a final volume of 25 μl. The genotypes patterns were determined by 2% agarose gel electrophoresis (Agarose; Sigma-Aldrich, Munich, Germany) stained with Ethiduim bromide. A 5% masked, random sample of cases and controls were re-amplified and sent for sequencing to confirm the genotyping method.

Statistical analysis

The genotype frequencies were tested for Hardy–Weinberg equilibrium using a chi-square test through the website http://www.oege.org/software/hwe-mr-calc.html. All statistical analysis was performed using SPSS v23.0 (SPSS, Chicago, IL). Pearson's Chi-square test was used to compare allelic and genotypic frequencies between the diabetic

Table 1 Clinical and biochemical characteristics of case and control groups

Parameters	cases (n=281)	controls (n=118)	*P-value*
M:F ratio	94:187	48:70	
Age at diagnosis (years)	50.39+11.04	NA	
Age at sampling (years)	58.15±12.09	49.62±8.71	0.0001*
BMI	32.9±6.6	29.2±6.2	<0.0001*
SBP (mmHg)	136.21±17.42	122.33±11.44	0.0001*
DBP (mmHg)	80.21±10.83	76.72±9.37	0.0024*
FBS (mg/dl)	163.31±58.72	87.14±7.82	0.0001*
TC (mg/dl)	187.91±47.53	182.15±40.95	0.251
Treatment (OHA,C,I)(n)	204,71,6	NA	

Values are expressed as means ±SD, *P<0.05 is considered to be significant
NA Not applicable. Treatment at time of recruitment *OHA* oral hypoglycemic agent, *C* combination of insulin and hypoglycemic agent, *I* insulin

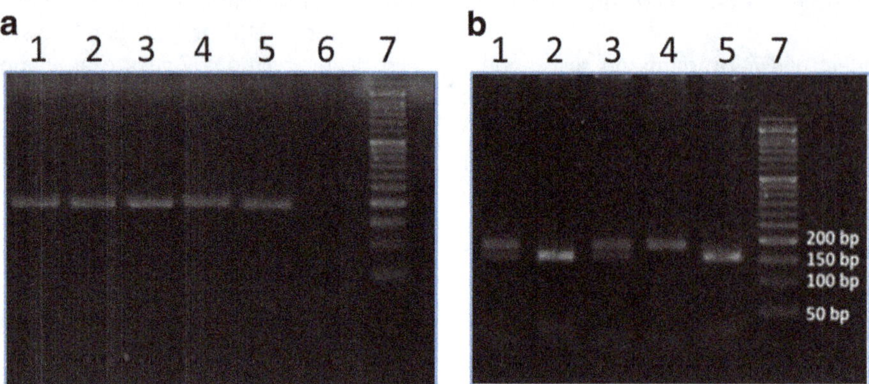

Fig. 1 Agarose gel electrophoresis (2%) of *FTO* gene variant (**a**) PCR products showing 187 bp amplicon (Lanes 1–5), lane 6: Negative control, lane 7: 50 bp ladder. (**b**) Digested PCR product representing different genotypes: Lanes 1, 3: AT genotype; Lanes 2, 5: AA genotype; Lane 4: TT genotype; Lane 7: 50 bp ladder

and nondiabetic groups. ANOVA was used to assess the association between *FTO* genotypes and continuous variables. Logistic regression by R statistics (V 3.4.4) software was used to measure odd ratio (OR) for T2DM adjusted for age, gender and BMI.

Results

Biochemical characteristics of the study participants

The biochemical and anthropometric results of the 281 T2DM patients and 118 nondiabetic subjects are shown in Table 1. As expected, significant differences in biochemical parameters was observed between the two groups ($p < 0.05$). However, the mean total cholesterol was not significant between diabetic and non diabetic groups ($p = 0.25$). Among T2DM group, 64.4% ($n = 181$) were obese (BMI > 30 kg/m2), 30.2% ($n = 85$) were overweight (25–29.9 kg/m2) and 5.3% ($n = 15$) were nonobese (BMI < 30 kg/m2). Of them, 76.6% were treated with oral hypoglycemic agent, 25.3% received a combination of insulin and oral hypoglycemic agents and 2.1% were treated with insulin. Of these patients, 14.6, 12.1, 7.8 and 6% had cardio vascular disease (CVD), nephropathy, diabetic foot and retinopathy, respectively. Noteworthy, 75% of the cases had T2DM first-degree relatives. Among the control group, 44.1% ($n = 52$) were obese, 22.9% ($n = 27$) were overweight and 33.1% ($n = 39$) were not obese.

Analysis of *FTO* variant

FTO genotyping (rs9939609) was performed by PCR followed by RFLP. The presence of product was verified on a 2% agarose gel stained with ethidium bromide, a band of 187 bp was observed as shown in Fig. 1a. The PCR product was digested by *ScaI* restriction enzyme and visualized by 2% agarose gel. A band of 187 bp was observed for the TT genotype, two bands of 154, 33 bp was observed for the AA genotype while three bands of 187, 154, 33 bp were observed for the heterozygous genotype AT as shown in Fig. 1b.

Association of *FTO* variant and T2DM

The genotype and allele frequency of *FTO* gene polymorphism (rs9939609) a;mong the two groups were analyzed and compared as shown in Table 2. Our results revealed that carriers of AA genotype was significantly higher in T2DM subjects compared to non diabetic individuals (36%) vs (16%))($p = 0.003$). The genotyping distribution was in line of Hardy Weinberg equilibrium in all cases and controls ($p = > 0.05$). Logistic regression analysis was performed for AT and AA genotypes with TT as a reference genotype. We found that the AT genotype conferred 2.1 times higher risk for T2DM compared to TT genotypes unadjusted $p < 0.0001$ (Table 3). As our controls were younger than diabetic cases, logistic regression model adjusted for age and gender was used, and showed that allelic odd ratio was 1.92 (95% CI [1.09–3.29], $p = 0.02$). This association remained significant even after adjusting for age, gender and BMI (OR 1.84, 95%CI (1.04–3.05)). The highest risk was observed among AA carriers compared to those with TT genotypes (OR 4.03, 95% CI (2.01–8.06) $p < 0.0001$) as shown in Table 3.

Table 2 Allelic and genotypic frequency of *FTO* variant (rs9939609) among T2DM cases and controls

Genotype	cases(n)	Controls (n)	All Subjects (n)
TT	51	45	96
AT	129	54	183
AA	101	19	120
A allele (%)	58.8	38.9	53

Table 3 Association of *FTO* variant (rs9939609) with T2DM

Genotype	OR(95% CI)	*P*-value	OR(95% CI)	**P*-value
AA vs TT	4.69 (2.49–8.83)	<0.0001	4.03 (2.01–8.06)	<0.0001*
AT vs TT	2.11 (1.26-3.52)	<0.0001	1.84 (1.04-3.05)	0.034*
AA vs (AT+TT)	2.78 (1.72-4.49)	<0.0001	2.71 (1.5-4.9)	0.001*

**P* values were from logistic regression models adjusted for age, gender and BMI, *P*<0.05 was considered significant

Association of *FTO* variant with BMI

The entire data including all the study subjects ($n = 399$) was stratified based on *FTO* genotypes, a significant association was found between *FTO* genotypes and mean BMI, the AA genotypes had the highest BMI (33.29 ± 7.2), unadjusted $p = 0.03$. Because of potential confounding between T2DM and increased BMI as proxy measure of obesity, the data was stratified by glycemic status across *FTO* genotypes. Among diabetic group, a trend of increasing mean BMI was observed among the three genotypes: AA carriers had the highest BMI (34.11 ± 7.1) compared to AT (32.32 ± 6.1) and TT carriers (31.86 ± 6.5) but it was not significant ($p = 0.057$). However, this increasing trend was not found among the control group ($p = 0.7$) as shown in Table 4. Furthermore, no association was found between the *FTO* genotype and gender, age, plasma total cholesterol, as well as systolic and diastolic blood pressure among the two groups. Among diabetic group, no association was found between the *FTO* genotype and cardio vascular disease or diabetes complications ($p > 0.05$).

Discussion

To our knowledge, this study is the first to investigate the association of the *FTO* variant rs9939609 with type 2 diabetes and BMI in Palestine. The significance of common variants in the *FTO* gene for susceptibility to adiposity have been highlighted by large-scale studies among Europeans while conflicting results were reported in Asian populations [21, 22]. Our study showed a significant association of *FTO* variant rs9939609 with T2DM after adjustment by age and gender with an allelic odds ratio of 1.92 (95% CI [1.09–3.29], $p = 0.02$). Moreover, we noted that the association of *FTO* variant rs9939609 with T2DM was partially attenuated by adjusting for BMI with odd ratio of 1.84, 95%CI (1.04–3.05) $p = 0.03$, suggesting that the *FTO* -T2DM association was not completely mediated through *FTO* variant effect on BMI. Similar results were found in Indian, American and Chinese populations [4, 10, 23]. Vasan and colleagues [24] provided evidence that *FTO*-T2DM risk -among Asian Indians- was attenuated but not fully abolished when adjusting to BMI. In contrast, a recent study conducted in Kuwaiti population did not observe an association between the *FTO* rs9939609 with T2DM risk [25]. Two studies in North Indians and Asian Indians demonstrated a strong association of *FTO* rs9939609 with T2DM independent of BMI [4, 26]. However, contradictory results for association of *FTO* variants with T2DM have been reported in different ethnic groups of India [27]. Furthermore, a meta-analysis study conducted in South Asia showed that BMI and central obesity can partly account for the association of A allele of the *FTO* gene and diabetes, whereas this association was much reduced when adjusted for BMI in Europeans indicating ethnic-specific associations [28]. On the other hand, several studies revealed a strong association between different variants within the *FTO* gene and BMI or diabetes supporting that the impact of *FTO* on obesity or diabetes is population-dependent [29–32]. A recent study conducted by Wang and colleagues [33] showed that *FTO* protein expression in T2DM patients was higher than in healthy controls which was positively correlated with T2DM severity, BMI and waist circumference.

Our study revealed that, among all study subjects, the TT carriers had lower BMI compared to AT and AA carriers (unadjusted $p = 0.03$) but when the mean BMI was stratified by glycemic status across *FTO* genotypes, the association with BMI was lost in the control group ($p = 0.7$). In diabetic group, an additive trend of the allele A with increased BMI was observed but was not significant ($p = 0.057$). However, further studies with larger sample size and greater statistical

Table 4 Mean trait values stratified by glycemic status across *FTO* genotypes

	T2DM (*n*=281)				Control (*n*=118)			
	AA	AT	TT	**P*-value	AA	AT	TT	**P*-value
Number	101	129	51		19	54	45	
BMI (kg/m2)	34.11±7.1	32.32±6.1	31.86±6.5	**0.057**	28.89±6.96	29.77±6.1	28.75±5.8	0.688
SBP (mmHg)	133.94±16.9	138.26±16.4	135.47±20.4	0.166	119.3±16.3	124.2±10.7	121.4±9.5	0.222
DBP (mmHg)	78.68±11.9	80.94±10.1	81.35±10.5	0.206	72.8±9.2	76.7±10.2	78.5±8.1	0.087
FBS (mg/dl)	159.11±54.3	163.97±58.9	169.94±65.6	0.553	85.9±6.9	87.7±7.4	86.9±8.8	0.693
TC (mg/dl)	189.16±49.3	188.57±49.2	183.71±39.8	0.783	168.1±40.1	188.5±48.8	180.4±28.2	0.165

**P*<0.05 was considered significant, obtained by ANOVA. Values are expressed as means ±SD. Bold number showed marginally significant association between A allele and increased BMI among diabetic group

power are needed to replicate these findings. In 2016, a study conducted on Egyptian children and adolescents didn't show an association between the polymorphism rs9939609 and BMI. However, that study revealed a significant correlation between LDL and *FTO* rs9939609 supporting the idea that this variant can be a determinant of obesity due to its effect on the lipid profile [34].

The high prevalence of obesity among our diabetic and control group (64 and 44%, respectively) could be attributed to other variants within *FTO* and or other genes which can be modulated by environmental factors and lifestyle. Anyhow, as our diabetic cases were older and had higher BMI than controls, we adjusted for the possible confounding effect of age, sex, and BMI in all the logistic regression analyses while investigating T2DM risk across *FTO* genotypes. Recently, a study conducted by Celis-Morales et al. [35] reported that physical activity attenuates the effect of *FTO* on BMI. Another study conducted on Emirati people showed that the AA carriers who were physically active had a lower mean BMI than those who were physically inactive, while other studies conducted on African Americans and Europeans showed no such interaction [36, 37]. Furthermore, a recent cross sectional study in a multiethnic population suggested that high dietary protein intake may protect against the effects of risk variants in the *FTO* gene on BMI and waist circumference [28]. In this study and due to the lack of data regarding physical activity or diet intake, we were unable to examine the influence of physical activity /diet on the impact of *FTO* variant on BMI. Although *FTO* -T2DM association was found, the lack of association between *FTO* rs9939609 and obesity is most probably due to the small sample size -and thereby decreased statistical power- which was the most important limitation in this study and thus larger sample size is required to verify these results. However, weight, skinfold thicknesses, body fat percentage and waist circumference are reported to be more reliable markers of obesity than BMI [38]. We believe that obesity-related genetic variants also modulate glucose–insulin secretion. Therefore, leaner cases should be recruited while investigating gene–T2DM association among Palestinians.

On the other hand, we did not find any association of *FTO* rs9939609 with the T2DM complications and the prevalence of CVD among the studied population. This is consistent with recent findings showing no association of *FTO* rs9939609 variant with diabetic retinopathy and nephropathy [39]. However, a meta-analysis study reported significant association of the *FTO* rs9939609 variant with CVD risk, which was independent of BMI and other conventional CVD risk factors [40].

Conclusion

The *FTO* rs9939609 variant was significantly associated with T2DM in Palestine. However, further analysis with larger sample size and data on physical activity and diet intake is required to elucidate the role of this variant and other variants of *FTO* gene on the predisposition to increased BMI in Palestinians.

Abbreviations

BMI: Body max index; CVD: Cardiovascular disease; *FTO*: Fat-mass and obesity-associated gene; GWAS: Genome-wide association; OR: Odd ratio; PCR: Polymerase chain reaction; RFLP: Restriction fragment length polymorphism; T2DM: Type 2 diabetes mellitus; *TCF7L2*: Transcription factor 7 like 2; WHO: World Health Organization

Acknowledgments

The authors gratefully acknowledge the UNRWA outpatient clinic members (Hebron and Ramallah, Palestine) who contributed to the patients' recruitment, and all subjects who participated to this study.

Funding

The deanship of scientific research-Al-Quds University provided the financial support.

Authors' contributions

SE and AS performed the experiments and wrote the manuscript; SE and SC analyzed the data; AS, OA and MA collected the samples; AN and MI performed sequencing and analysis; SE, SC and AN designed and supervised the experiments, reviewed and revised the manuscript. All authors read and approved the final manuscript.

Competing interests

The authors declare that they have no competing interests.

Author details

[1]Biochemistry and Molecular Biology Department, Faculty of Medicine, Al-Quds University, Abu Dis-East Jerusalem, Palestine. [2]CNRS, UMR8204, Lille, France. [3]INSERM, U1019, Lille, France. [4]Université de Lille, Lille, France. [5]Institut Pasteur de Lille, Centre d'Infection et d'Immunité de Lille, Lille, France. [6]Microbiology and immunology Department-Faculty of Medicine, Al-Quds University-Palestine, Abu Dis-East Jerusalem, Palestine. [7]Al-Quds Nutrition and Health Research Institute – Faculty of Medicine, Al-Quds University-Palestine, Abu Dis-Jerusalem, Palestine.

References

1. World Health Organization. WHO Media centre. http://www.who.int/mediacentre/factsheets/fs138/en/. Accessed 14 Aug 2018.
2. Frayling TM, Timpson NJ, Weedon MN, Zeggini E, Freathy RM, Lindgren CM, et al. A common variant in the FTO gene is associated with body mass index and predisposes to childhood and adult obesity. Science. 2007;316:889–94.
3. Scuteri A, Sanna S, Chen WM, Uda M, Albai G, Strait J, et al. Genome-wide association scan shows genetic variants in the FTO gene are associated with obesity-related traits. PLoS Genet. 2007;3:e115.
4. Sanghera DK, Ortega L, Han S, Singh J, Ralhan SK, Wander GS, et al. Impact of nine common type 2 diabetes risk polymorphisms in Asian Indian Sikhs: PPARG2 (Pro12Ala), IGF2BP2, TCF7L2 and FTO variants confer a significant risk. BMC Med Genet. 2008;9:59.
5. Cecil JE, Tavendale R, Watt P, Hetherington MM, Palmer CN. An obesity-associated FTO gene variant and increased energy intake in children. N Engl J Med. 2008;359:2558–66.
6. Berentzen T, Kring SI, Holst C, Zimmermann E, Jess T, Hansen T, et al. Lack of association of fatness-related FTO gene variants with energy expenditure or physical activity. J Clin Endocrinol Metab. 2008;93:2904–8.
7. Li H, Wu Y, Loos RJ, Hu FB, Liu Y, Wang J, et al. Variants in the fat mass- and obesity-associated (FTO) gene are not associated with obesity in a Chinese Han population. Diabetes. 2008;57:264–8.
8. Wing MR, Ziegler J, Langefeld CD, Ng MC, Haffner SM, Norris JM, et al. Analysis of FTO gene variants with measures of obesity and glucose homeostasis in the IRAS family study. Hum Genet. 2009;125:615–26.

9. Doney AS, Dannfald J, Kimber CH, Donnelly LA, Pearson E, Morris AD, et al. The FTO gene is associated with an atherogenic lipid profile and myocardial infarction in patients with type 2 diabetes: a genetics of diabetes audit and research study in Tayside Scotland (go-DARTS) study. Circ Cardiovasc Genet. 2009;2:255–9.
10. Raza ST, Abbas S, Siddiqi Z, Mahdi F. Association between ACE (rs4646994), FABP2 (rs1799883), MTHFR (rs1801133), FTO (rs9939609) genes polymorphism and type 2 diabetes with dyslipidemia. Int J Mol Cell Med. 2017;6:121–30.
11. Kamura Y, Iwata M, Maeda S, Shinmura S, Koshimizu Y, Honoki H, et al. FTO gene polymorphism is associated with type 2 diabetes through its effect on increasing the maximum BMI in Japanese men. PLoS One. 2016;11: e0165523.
12. Ghafarian-Alipour F, Ziaee S, Ashoori MR, Zakeri MS, Boroumand MA, Aghamohammadzadeh N, et al. Association between FTO gene polymorphisms and type 2 diabetes mellitus, serum levels of apelin and androgen hormones among Iranian obese women. Gene. 2018;641:361–6.
13. Yang Y, Liu B, Xia W, Yan J, Liu HY, Hu L, et al. FTO genotype and type 2 diabetes mellitus: spatial analysis and meta-analysis of 62 case-control studies from different regions. Genes (Basel). 2017; 8(2):70.
14. Abu-Rmeileh NM, Husseini A, Capewell S, O'Flaherty M. Project M. Preventing type 2 diabetes among Palestinians: comparing five future policy scenarios. BMJ Open. 2013;3:e003558.
15. Abu-Rmeileh NM, Husseini A, O'Flaherty M, Shoaibi A, Capewell S. Forecasting prevalence of type 2 diabetes mellitus in Palestinians to 2030: validation of a predictive model. Lancet. 2012;380:S21.
16. El Sharif N, Samara I, Titi I, Awartani A. Compliance with and knowledge about diabetes guidelines among physicians and nurses in Palestine/ Connaissances et respect des recommandations Sur le diabete chez des medecins et des infirmieres en Palestine. East Mediterr Health J. 2015;21:791.
17. Damiri B, Aghbar A, Alkhdour S, Arafat Y. Characterization and prevalence of metabolic syndrome among overweight and obese young Palestinian students at an-Najah National University. Diabetes Metab Syndr. 2018; 12(3):343–8.
18. Ereqat S, Nasereddin A, Azmi K, Abdeen Z, Amin R. Impact of the Pro12Ala polymorphism of the PPAR-Gamma 2 gene on metabolic and clinical characteristics in the Palestinian type 2 diabetic patients. PPAR Res. 2009; 2009:874126.
19. Ereqat S, Nasereddin A, Cauchi S, Azmi K, Abdeen Z, Amin R. Association of a common variant in TCF7L2 gene with type 2 diabetes mellitus in the Palestinian population. Acta Diabetol. 2010;47(Suppl 1):195–8.
20. Lopez-Bermejo A, Petry CJ, Diaz M, Sebastiani G, de Zegher F, Dunger DB, et al. The association between the FTO gene and fat mass in humans develops by the postnatal age of two weeks. J Clin Endocrinol Metab. 2008; 93:1501–5.
21. Grant SF, Li M, Bradfield JP, Kim CE, Annaiah K, Santa E, et al. Association analysis of the FTO gene with obesity in children of Caucasian and African ancestry reveals a common tagging SNP. PLoS One. 2008;3:e1746.
22. Price RA, Li WD, Zhao H. FTO gene SNPs associated with extreme obesity in cases, controls and extremely discordant sister pairs. BMC Med Genet. 2008;9:4.
23. Bressler J, Kao WH, Pankow JS, Boerwinkle E. Risk of type 2 diabetes and obesity is differentially associated with variation in FTO in whites and African-Americans in the ARIC study. PLoS One. 2010;5:e10521.
24. Vasan SK, Karpe F, Gu HF, Brismar K, Fall CH, Ingelsson E, et al. FTO genetic variants and risk of obesity and type 2 diabetes: a meta-analysis of 28,394 Indians. Obesity (Silver Spring). 2014;22:964–70.
25. Al-Serri A, Al-Bustan SA, Kamkar M, Thomas D, Alsmadi O, Al-Temaimi R, et al.. Association of FTO rs9939609 with obesity in the Kuwaiti population: a public health concern? Med Princ Pract. 2018; 27(2):145–51.
26. Yajnik CS, Janipalli CS, Bhaskar S, Kulkarni SR, Freathy RM, Prakash S, et al. FTO gene variants are strongly associated with type 2 diabetes in south Asian Indians. Diabetologia. 2009;52:247–52.
27. Chauhan G, Tabassum R, Mahajan A, Dwivedi OP, Mahendran Y, Kaur I, et al. Common variants of FTO and the risk of obesity and type 2 diabetes in Indians. J Hum Genet. 2011;56:720–6.
28. Merritt DC, Jamnik J, El-Sohemy A. FTO genotype, dietary protein intake, and body weight in a multiethnic population of young adults: a cross-sectional study. Genes Nutr. 2018;13:4.
29. Saldana-Alvarez Y, Salas-Martinez MG, Garcia-Ortiz H, Luckie-Duque A, Garcia-Cardenas G, Vicenteno-Ayala H, et al. Gender-dependent association of FTO polymorphisms with body mass index in Mexicans. PLoS One. 2016; 11:e0145984.
30. Sentinelli F, Incani M, Coccia F, Capoccia D, Cambuli VM, Romeo S, et al. Association of FTO polymorphisms with early age of obesity in obese Italian subjects. Exp Diabetes Res. 2012;2012:872176.
31. Tan LJ, Zhu H, He H, Wu KH, Li J, Chen XD, et al. Replication of 6 obesity genes in a meta-analysis of genome-wide association studies from diverse ancestries. PLoS One. 2014;9:e96149.
32. Hubacek JA, Dlouha D, Klementova M, Lanska V, Neskudla T, Pelikanova T. The FTO variant is associated with chronic complications of diabetes mellitus in Czech population. Gene. 2018;642:220–4.
33. Wang Q, Wang J, Lin H, Huo X, Zhu Q, Zhang M. Relationship between fat mass and obesity-associated gene expression and type 2 diabetes mellitus severity. Exp Ther Med. 2018;15:2917–21.
34. Abdelmajed SS, Youssef M, Zaki ME, Hassan NA-M, Ismail S. Association analysis of FTO gene polymorphisms and obesity risk among Egyptian children and adolescents. Genes Dis. 2017;4:170–5.
35. Celis-Morales C, Marsaux CF, Livingstone KM, Navas-Carretero S, San-Cristobal R, O'Donovan CB, et al. Physical activity attenuates the effect of the FTO genotype on obesity traits in European adults: the Food4Me study. Obesity (Silver Spring). 2016;24:962–9.
36. Khan SM, El Hajj Chehadeh S, Abdulrahman M, Osman W, Al SH. Establishing a genetic link between FTO and VDR gene polymorphisms and obesity in the Emirati population. BMC Med Genet. 2018;19:11.
37. Liu G, Zhu H, Lagou V, Gutin B, Stallmann-Jorgensen IS, Treiber FA, et al. FTO variant rs9939609 is associated with body mass index and waist circumference, but not with energy intake or physical activity in European- and African-American youth. BMC Med Genet. 2010;11:57.
38. Vasan SK, Fall T, Neville MJ, Antonisamy B, Fall CH, Geethanjali FS, et al. Associations of variants in FTO and near MC4R with obesity traits in south Asian Indians. Obesity (Silver Spring). 2012;20:2268–77.
39. Montesanto A, Bonfigli AR, Crocco P, Garagnani P, De Luca M, Boemi M, et al. Genes associated with type 2 diabetes and vascular complications. Aging (Albany NY). 2018;10:178–96.
40. Liu C, Mou S, Pan C. The FTO gene rs9939609 polymorphism predicts risk of cardiovascular disease: a systematic review and meta-analysis. PLoS One. 2013;8:e71901.

23

Expanding the clinical phenotype of *IARS2*-related mitochondrial disease

Barbara Vona[1,2*], Reza Maroofian[3], Emanuele Bellacchio[4], Maryam Najafi[5], Kyle Thompson[6], Ahmad Alahmad[6], Langping He[6], Najmeh Ahangari[7,8], Abolfazl Rad[5,9], Sima Shahrokhzadeh[8], Paulina Bahena[1], Falk Mittag[10], Frank Traub[10], Jebrail Movaffagh[11], Nafise Amiri[11], Mohammad Doosti[8], Reza Boostani[12], Ebrahim Shirzadeh[13], Thomas Haaf[1], Daria Diodato[14], Miriam Schmidts[5,15], Robert W. Taylor[6] and Ehsan Ghayoor Karimiani[3,7*]

Abstract

Background: *IARS2* encodes a mitochondrial isoleucyl-tRNA synthetase, a highly conserved nuclear-encoded enzyme required for the charging of tRNAs with their cognate amino acid for translation. Recently, pathogenic *IARS2* variants have been identified in a number of patients presenting broad clinical phenotypes with autosomal recessive inheritance. These phenotypes range from Leigh and West syndrome to a new syndrome abbreviated CAGSSS that is characterised by cataracts, growth hormone deficiency, sensory neuropathy, sensorineural hearing loss, and skeletal dysplasia, as well as cataract with no additional anomalies.

Methods: Genomic DNA from Iranian probands from two families with consanguineous parental background and overlapping CAGSSS features were subjected to exome sequencing and bioinformatics analysis.

Results: Exome sequencing and data analysis revealed a novel homozygous missense variant (c.2625C > T, p. Pro909Ser, NM_018060.3) within a 14.3 Mb run of homozygosity in proband 1 and a novel homozygous missense variant (c.2282A > G, p.His761Arg) residing in an ~ 8 Mb region of homozygosity in a proband of the second family. Patient-derived fibroblasts from proband 1 showed normal respiratory chain enzyme activity, as well as unchanged oxidative phosphorylation protein subunits and IARS2 levels. Homology modelling of the known and novel amino acid residue substitutions in IARS2 provided insight into the possible consequence of these variants on function and structure of the protein.

Conclusions: This study further expands the phenotypic spectrum of IARS2 pathogenic variants to include two patients (patients 2 and 3) with cataract and skeletal dysplasia and no other features of CAGSSS to the possible presentation of the defects in *IARS2*. Additionally, this study suggests that adult patients with CAGSSS may manifest central adrenal insufficiency and type II esophageal achalasia and proposes that a variable sensorineural hearing loss onset, proportionate short stature, polyneuropathy, and mild dysmorphic features are possible, as seen in patient 1. Our findings support that even though biallelic *IARS2* pathogenic variants can result in a distinctive, clinically recognisable phenotype in humans, it can also show a wide range of clinical presentation from severe pediatric neurological disorders of Leigh and West syndrome to both non-syndromic cataract and cataract accompanied by skeletal dysplasia.

Keywords: Adrenal insufficiency, CAGSSS, Cataracts, Growth hormone deficiency, *IARS2*, Sensory neuropathy, Sensorineural hearing loss, Skeletal dysplasia, Type II esophageal achalasia

* Correspondence: barbara.vona@uni-wuerzburg.de; eghayoor@gmail.com
[1]Institute of Human Genetics, Julius Maximilians University Würzburg, Würzburg, Germany
[3]Genetics and Molecular Cell Sciences Research Centre, St George's, University of London, Cranmer Terrace, London SW17 0RE, UK
Full list of author information is available at the end of the article

Background

Aminoacyl-tRNA synthetases (ARSs) are evolutionarily conserved enzymes that catalyze amino acid attachment to their cognate tRNA. This catalytic process, termed tRNA charging, is a prerequisite for the translation of genetic sequences into polypeptide chains [1]. Two distinct translation pathways take place in the cytoplasm and in the mitochondria each requiring a separate set of ARSs for the translation of nuclear and mitochondrial genes respectively; in total, there are 37 members of the ARS gene family. Two groups of 17 ARSs are each associated with cytoplasmic or mitochondrial translation, while three so-called bifunctional proteins act in both cellular locations [2, 3]. Based on their cellular localization and function, nomenclature for ARSs follows a systematic scheme that entails the recognised amino acid, followed by ARS for both cytoplasmic and bifunctional enzymes (i.e. IARS for cytoplasmic isoleucyl-tRNA synthetase), and a "2" is added to distinguish mitochondrial ARSs (i.e. IARS2 for mitochondrial isoleucyl-tRNA synthetase) [2, 3]. Although expression of ARSs is ubiquitous and protein synthesis is expected to be systemically impaired, a number of highly diverse clinical phenotypes can emerge from mutations in genes encoding ARSs that affect a wide range of tissues with particularly high metabolic demands [3].

IARS2 is a nuclear-encoded mitochondrial isoleucyl-tRNA synthetase that is imported from the cytosol into the mitochondria where it catalyzes the attachment of an isoleucine residue to a cognate mt-tRNA^{Ile} [4]. Genetic mutations in *IARS2* (OMIM: 612801) on chromosome 1q41 were first described in an extended French-Canadian family with a syndrome abbreviated CAGSSS that is characterised by cataracts, growth hormone deficiency, sensory neuropathy, sensorineural hearing loss, and skeletal dysplasia [5]. A detailed follow-up on two previously published first-cousin probands from a genealogically related French-Canadian family dating back to the nineteenth century was also explored [5, 6]. The three probands in this extended family were homozygous for a pathogenic missense variant (c.2726C > T, p.Pro909Leu) in exon 21 of the 23 exon *IARS2* gene. The proline residue exchange affected a predicted anticodon binding domain. An additional Danish proband presenting CAGSSS features was identified with a homozygous pathogenic variant (c.2620C > A, p.Gly874Arg) also affecting exon 21 [7]. One further proband with compound heterozygous mutations (c.1821G > A, p.Trp607*; c.2122G > A, p.Glu708Lys) was diagnosed with Leigh syndrome and died at the age of 18 months [5]. Furthermore, compound heterozygous variants in *IARS2* (case 6: c.607G > C; p.(Gly203Arg) and c.2575 T > C; p.(Phe859-Leu)); family 10: c.2446C > T; p.(Arg816*) and c.2575 T > C; p.(Phe859Leu)) have been found in two probands from China with sporadic pediatric cataract which characterised by far the mildest clinical presentation of IARS2-related disorders [8]. Moreover, recently identified novel compound missense variants in *IARS2* (c.680 T > C; p.(Phe227Ser) and c.2450G > A; p.(Arg817His)) have been reported in one family with two Japanese siblings showing milder symptoms of CAGSSS and West syndrome concomitant with Leigh syndrome [9]. Thus, these reports assert that mutations in *IARS2* are responsible for a phenotypic spectrum of rare autosomal recessive disorders that require further clinical characterisation.

In this study, we analysed whole exome sequencing data in two unrelated consanguineous Iranian patients presenting with clinical features overlapping with CAGSSS. Exome analysis revealed different novel homozygous variants in *IARS2* in both families. Patient 1 disclosed a homozygous c.2725C > T, p.Pro909Ser variant which interestingly affects the same p.Pro909 amino acid residue that was described in the French-Canadian family. In the exome analysis of patient 2, whose clinical features were limited to only cataract and skeletal dysplasia, we identified a novel homozygous c.2282A > G, p.His761Arg variant in a region of homozygosity spanning 8 Mb. Additionally, we present a detailed and comparative clinical assessment of patients with a phenotypic spectrum of IARS2-related disorders and illustrate the predicted impact of the identified patient mutations on the protein structure. Moreover, cultured fibroblasts of patient 1 were analysed for mitochondrial enzymatic activity and protein extracts were immunoblotted to assess key mitochondrial oxidative phosphorylation (OXPHOS) proteins and steady-state IARS2 levels. Our patients, who have mild forms of CAGSSS, highlight the wide spectrum of clinical severity associated with *IARS2* mutations. Furthermore, as proband 1 displays CAGSSS symptoms concomitant with growth hormone deficiency, central adrenal insufficiency, as well as type II esophageal achalasia, we propose that the phenotypic spectrum of CAGSSS-related disorders resulting from *IARS2* variants could include this constellation of features.

Methods

Informed written consent was obtained from the families prior to their inclusion in the study. This study was performed under the tenets of the Declaration of Helsinki and approved by the Ethics Commission of the University of Würzburg (46/15), as well as the Ethical Commission of Sabzevar University of Medical Sciences (IR.medsab.rec.1395.120). Blood samples were collected from all participants. Genomic DNA was extracted from whole blood using a standard salting out method. DNA samples were quantified using Qubit 2.0 (Life Technologies, Carlsbad, CA, USA).

Next generation sequencing and bioinformatics analysis

Whole exome capture was performed using an Agilent SureSelect Human All Exon V6 Kit according to manufacturer's recommendations and paired-end sequenced on HiSeq 4000 and HiSeq 2500 sequencers.

Exome data were processed for analysis using a GATK-based pipeline [10] that used Burrows-Wheeler alignment [11] to the GRCh37/hg19 human genome assembly. Variant filtering was performed using the following parameters: exonic variants with flanking splice site regions were filtered for quality, and frequency-based data filtering employed MAF ≤ 0.001 as defined by the 1000 Genomes Project [12] and EVS (ESP6500) (http://evs.gs.washington.edu/EVS/) [accessed May, 2017] population data. Artifact-prone gene families (*HLA*s, *MAGE*s, *MUC*s, *NBPF*s, *OR*s and *PRAME*s) were further excluded and the analysis focused on missense, stopgain/stoploss, startgain/startloss, splicing and indel variants. Variant prioritization was aided by the tools FATHMM [13], MutationAssessor [14], MutationTaster [15], PolyPhen-2 [16], and SIFT [17]. Additionally, the EVS, gnomAD [18], GME Variome Project [19], Iranome [20], Ensembl Variant Table [21], ClinVar [22], and HGMD (2017.1) [23] were used for variant analysis. Variants occurring with MAF > 0.01 in the Iranome were also excluded. Splice sites were analysed using the Alamut Visual 2.7 (Interactive Biosoftware, Rouen, France) splicing module. Putative pathogenic variant prioritization followed the following criteria: either three out of five pathogenicity prediction tools score the variant as deleterious or disease causing, or identified variants or adjacent variants affect an amino acid already associated with a genetic disorder entered in databases such as ClinVar or HGMD. In both cases, population frequency database variant entries are in accordance with standards for frequencies of rare disease causing alleles [24]. The remaining variants were filtered for known disease causing genes first and we prioritized homozygous variants due to the autosomal recessive inheritance pattern of disease and family consanguinity.

Variant validation and segregation testing

The *IARS2* (GenBank Reference: NM_018060.3) c.2282A > G and c.2725C > T homozygous variants were subjected to bidirectional Sanger sequencing validation with an ABI 3130xl 16-capillary sequencer (Life Technologies, Carlsbad, CA, USA) for segregation analysis in each respective family. Primer sequences that were designed using Primer3 [25] are available upon request. DNA sequence analysis was performed using Gensearch software (Phenosystems SA, Wallonia, Belgium).

Western blotting

Human fibroblasts were treated as described previously [26]. Proteins of interest were bound by overnight incubation at 4 °C with antibodies against IARS2 (Sigma Prestige cat# HPA024212), COXI (Abcam cat# ab14705, RRID: AB_2084810), SDHA (Abcam cat# ab14715, RRID: AB_301433), Total OXPHOS Human Antibody Cocktail containing antibodies against ATP5A, UQCRC2, SDHB, COXII and NDUFB8 (Abcam cat# ab110411), followed by HRP-conjugated secondary antibodies (Dako Cytomation) and visualised using ECL-prime (GE Healthcare) and BioRad ChemiDoc MP with Image Lab software.

Assessment of mitochondrial respiratory chain enzyme activities

The activities of individual respiratory chain complexes and the mitochondrial matrix marker enzyme, citrate synthase, were assessed as previously described [27].

Homology modelling

Homology modelling of the human mitochondrial isoleucine tRNA ligase (IARS2, NCBI: NP_060530.3) was based on the structure of the isoleucine tRNA ligase from *S. aureus* (PDB 1FFY) as the template. IARS2 was built in the amino acid range 58–1012 (sharing 36% amino acid identity with the bacterial homologue) employing the following procedure. All side chain atoms in the template were removed, amino acids were renamed and renumbered to the corresponding human IARS2 residues according to the pairwise sequence alignment (Additional file 1), and the modified PDB file was parsed to SIDEpro [28] for side chain reconstruction.

The $tRNA^{Ile}$ molecule cocrystallized with isoleucine tRNA ligase from *S. aureus* (PDB 1FFY) and Ile-AMS (an isoleucyl-adenylate analogue) cocrystallized with the isoleucine tRNA ligase from *T. thermophilus* (PDB 1JZQ) were added to the human IARS2 model in same binding poses to this ligase as in the crystal structure complexes. Finally, the side chains of the protein were energy minimised applying the Dreiding force field.

Results

Case presentations

Patient 1 (family 1)

The male proband (Fig. 1a, individual V:3), was born after an uncomplicated pregnancy at 34 weeks gestational age with a 2700 g (25th centile) birth weight and 50 cm (50th centile) length to healthy parents who were first-cousins. At the time of his birth, his father and mother were 29 and 25 years old, respectively. The proband presented with congenital cataracts that required surgery, as well as corneal opacity, bilateral nystagmus, and slight strabismus of the right eye (Table 1, Additional file 2). He was diagnosed with myopia with a

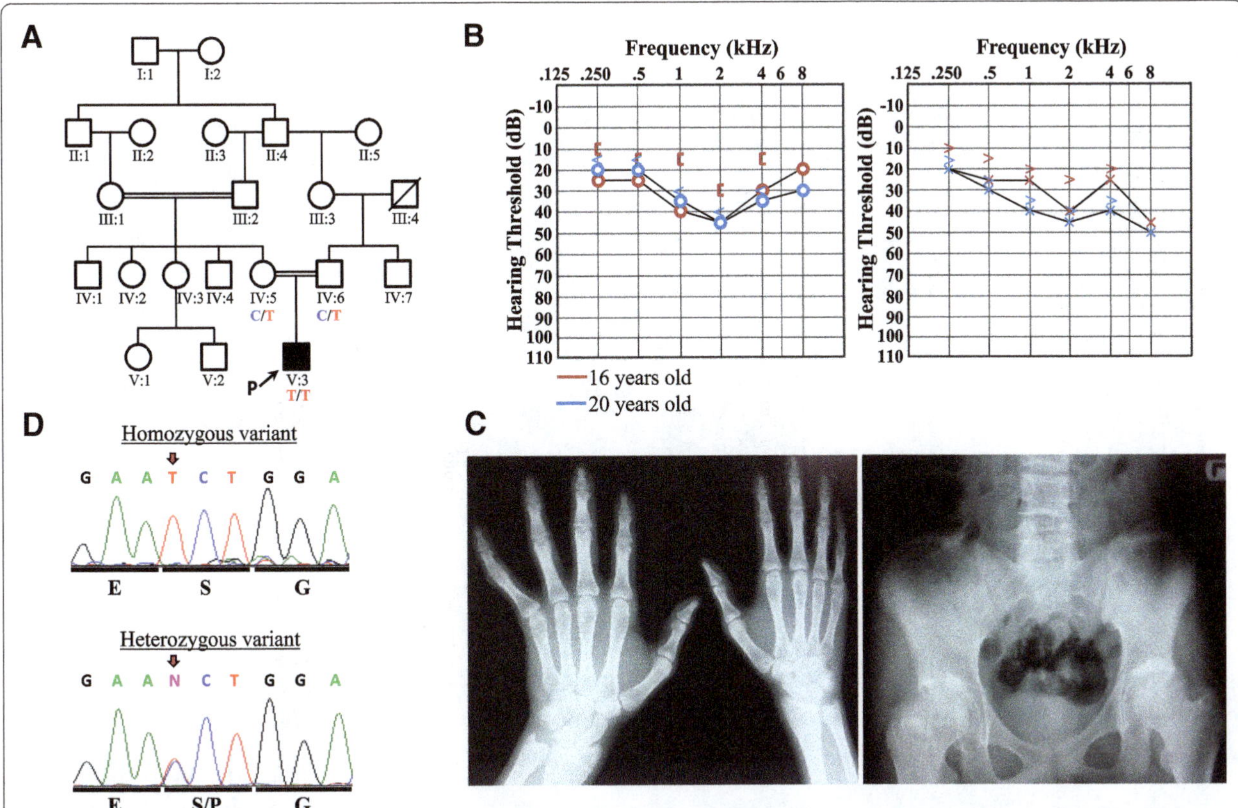

Fig. 1 Pedigree of patient 1, pure-tone audiograms, radiological examinations, and sequence electropherogram. **a** The proband's parents are first-degree cousins. There is no family history of CAGSSS. Genotype results for the c.2725C > T variant are represented under the tested individuals. **b** Pure-tone audiograms from proband 1 at 16 (red) and 20 (blue) years of age reveal stable, sensorineural hearing loss. Right air conduction (circle), unmasked bone conduction (bracket), and masked bone conduction (<) and left air conduction (x) and unmasked bone conduction (>) are shown from left to right, respectively. **c** Radiological images depicting epiphyseal dysplasia of the distal radius and fingers with tapering (left) and right hip with shortened femoral neck due to metaphyseal dysplasia (right). **d** Electropherograms of the homozygous proband (upper panel) and representative heterozygous electrophenogram from a parent (lower panel) showing the nucleotide and amino acid exchange. The variant position is marked with a red arrow

visual acuity of 20/40. At birth, he disclosed spastic features and type II achalasia that was confirmed and treated using endoscopy. Throughout early childhood, he experienced delayed motor development; however, this resolved spontaneously later on. No evidence of cognitive performance limitations has been observed.

The proband is presently 20.6 years old. He shows a proportionate short stature (height of 152 cm (– 3.4 SD), a muscle wasted appearance (weight 30 kg, body mass index of 13 kg/m^2 (– 7.5 SD)) and mild craniofacial dysmorphic features consisting of thick eyebrows, midface retrusion, underdeveloped ala nasi, short philtrum, thin upper lip, vertical crease of the chin, prognatism, and long neck.

A growth hormone deficiency (GHD) was diagnosed, resulting from the combination of severe short stature, delayed bone aged, and very low IGF-1 (– 2 SD) [29]. No growth hormone treatment was available. After repeated measurements, a remarkable decreased serum cortisol level (2.6 μg/dl) and a normal amount of plasmatic adrenocorticotropic hormone (ACTH) in the morning (8 AM) were noted, revealing central adrenal insufficiency. Thyroid-stimulating (TSH), total triiodothyronine (T3), total thyroxine (T4), follicle-stimulating, luteinising, and parathyroid hormones were within reference ranges. An isolated aldosterone measurement showed very high levels at 440 pmol/L (Additional file 2).

Sensorineural hearing loss was diagnosed at 13 years of age (Table 1). Pure-tone audiometry was performed according to best-practice recommendations [30] and revealed a bilateral, stable, mid-to-high frequency moderate hearing loss at ages 16 and 20 years of age (Fig. 1b). Masked bone conduction revealed an air-bone gap at the age of 16 that was later absent. Tympanograms were normal. The patient does not use hearing aids.

Radiological examinations at age 18 years were performed and revealed late manifestations of an underlying spondylo-epi-metaphyseal dysplasia which has been previously described for CAGSSS syndrome. Skeletal

Table 1 Abbreviated clinical summary of patients with pathogenic variants in *IARS2*

	Patient 1 (Present study)	Patient 2 (Present study)	Patient 3 (Present study)	Patient 4 Takezawa et al., 2018 [9]	Patient 5 Takezawa et al., 2018 [9]	Patient 6 Moosa et al., 2017 [7]	Patient 7 (Case 1 in Schwartzentruber et al., 2014 [5]; Jabbour and Harissi-Dagher, 2016 [29]	Patient 8 Case 2 in Schwartzentruber et al., 2014 [5] Patient 1 Liberfarb et al., 1993 [6]	Patient 9 Case 3 in Schwartzentruber et al., 2014 [5] Patient 2 Liberfarb et al., 1993 [6]	Patient 10 Case 4 in Schwartzentruber et al., 2014 [5]
Ethnic descent	Iranian	Iranian	Iranian	Japanese	Japanese	Danish	French-Canadian	French-Canadian	French-Canadian	Scandinavian-Caucasian
Sex	Male	Female	Female	Female	Female	Female	Female	Male	Female	Male
Age at publication	20.6 years	35 years	27 years	8 years	5 years	8 years	33 years	6 years	16.5 years	18 months
Genotype	c.2725C > T p.Pro909Ser	c.2282A > G p.His761Arg	c.2282A > G p.His761Arg	c.680 T > C, p.Phe227Ser; c.2450G > A, p.Arg817His	c.680 T > C, p.Phe227Ser; c.2450G > A, p.Arg817His	c.2620G > A p.Gly874Arg	c.2726C > T p.Pro909Leu	c.2726C > T p.Pro909Leu	c.2726C > T, p.Pro909Leu	c.1821G > A p.Trp607*; c.2122G > A p.Glu708Lys
Ocular evaluation										
Bilateral nystagmus	Yes	Yes	Yes	–	–	Yes	Yes, at 1 month	Yes, at 5 months	Yes, 3 months	–
Cataract	Yes, at birth	Yes, at birth	Yes, at birth	Yes, at birth	–	Yes, at 3 years	Yes, at 17 months; cataract extraction at 22 months	Yes, at 5 months; cataract extraction at 7 months	Yes, 3 months; cataract extracted at 13 months	–
Corneal opacification	Yes	Yes	Yes	–	–	–	Yes, at 5 years, progressive	Yes, at 5 years	Yes, at 16 years 5 months	–
Endocrinology										
Endocrine disturbances	Central adrenal insufficiency, growth hormone deficiency	–	–	–	–	–	Adrenal insufficiency, growth hormone deficiency	–	–	–
Growth hormone replacement therapy	–	–	–	–	–	–	Yes, positive outcome	Yes, positive outcome (cortisol deficiency)	–	–
Hypoglycemic Episodes	–	–	–	–	–	–	Yes	–	Yes	Yes
Auditory evaluation										
Hearing loss	Moderate bilateral sensorineural hearing loss at 13 years of age	–	–	–	–	Bilateral sensorineural hearing loss at 8 years old	Bilateral sensorineural stable hearing loss at 2 years old	Moderate bilateral sensorineural hearing loss at 21 months	–	–
Gastroenterology										
Type II esophageal Achalasia	Yes, from birth	–	–	–	–	–	Yes, 32 years	–	–	–
Musculoskeletal										
Short stature	Yes, proportionate	Yes	Yes	Yes	Yes	Yes, disproportionate	Yes, disproportionate	Yes	Yes	–

Table 1 Abbreviated clinical summary of patients with pathogenic variants in *IARS2* *(Continued)*

	Patient 1 (Present study)	Patient 2 (Present study)	Patient 3 (Present study)	Patient 4 Takezawa et al., 2018 [9]	Patient 5 Takezawa et al., 2018 [9]	Patient 6 Moosa et al., 2017 [7]	Patient 7 (Case 1 in Schwartzentruber et al., 2014 [5]; Jabbour and Harissi-Dagher, 2016 [29]	Patient 8 Case 2 in Schwartzentruber et al., 2014 [5] Patient 1 Liberfarb et al., 1993 [6]	Patient 9 Case 3 in Schwartzentruber et al., 2014 [5] Patient 2 Liberfarb et al., 1993 [6]	Patient 10 Case 4 in Schwartzentruber et al., 2014 [5]
	(−3.4 SD)					(−6 SD),				
Hip dislocation	–	–	–	–	–	Yes, at birth	Yes, at 2 years	Yes, at birth	Yes, at 18 months	–
Spine abnormalities	Yes, mild scoliosis	–	–	Yes	Yes	Yes, abnormal vertebral bodies	Yes, mild scoliosis	Yes, scoliosis	Yes, scoliosis	
Spondylo-epi-meta-physeal dysplasia	Yes	Yes, disproportional shortening of the first metacarpal reduced bone density	Yes, disproportional shortening of the first metacarpal	–	–	Yes	Yes	Yes	Yes	–
Neurological and Developmental Assessment										
Leigh syndrome features	–	–	–	Yes	Yes	–	–	–	–	Yes
West syndrome	–	–	–	Yes	Yes	–	–	–	–	–
Neurodevelopmental Delay	Yes	–	–	Yes	Yes	Yes	Yes, mild	Yes	Yes	Yes
Current normal Intelligence	Yes	Yes	Yes	–	–	Yes	Yes	–	Yes	?
Peripheral neuropathy	Chronic sensorimotor distal axonal polyneuropathy	–	–	–	–	Yes, pain insensitivity in early childhood	Yes, at 9.5 years	Yes, in early childhood	Yes, at 8 months	–

abnormalities in patient 1 included mild scoliosis, bilateral pes planus (with arthrodesis of the right ankle joints performed), wrists showing epiphyseal dyplasia of the distal radius, fingers with tapering and a right hip with a shortened femoral neck due to metaphyseal dyplasia with signs of secondary arthrosis of the hip joint (Fig. 1c).

Electrodiagnostic testing of the left limb at 16 years of age showed abnormal results that were consistent with chronic sensorimotor distal axonal polyneuropathy. It revealed extremely low amplitude or absent sensory nerve action potentials and weakening of the upper and lower limbs with a near-normal motor nerve conduction velocity.

Cranial CT and brain MRI were normal (data not shown).

Patients 2 and 3 (family 2)

Family 2, like family 1, is also of Iranian descent with parents being first cousins (Fig. 2a). Two out of four siblings, both females, were diagnosed with cataract at birth. These females are now 35 years old (patient 2) and 27 years old (patient 3). They were both born after an uneventful pregnancy, had a normal birth weight. At birth, no fundus could be identified in patient 2 during ophthalmological investigations and she showed slight strabismus of the right eye. She received a corneal graft later on, which was rejected when she was 30 years-old. She further presented mild craniofacial dysmorphic features consisting of a flat forehead, protruding upper jaw, mildly thickened eyebrows and deep set eyes. Radiological examination showed a mild deformity of the femoral head, small capital femoral epiphyses and hypoplastic, poorly formed acetabular roofs (Fig. 2b). It may be likely that a waddling gait may later develop. Knees show metaphyseal widening and irregularities while hands show brachydactyly (short fingers) and proximal metacarpal rounding. Hearing tests and growth hormone levels were found to be normal.

Her younger sister, patient 3 presented with a similar phenotype of invisible fundus due to the cataract, light strabismus of the right eye and she also received a corneal graft that was rejected when she was 20 years old. Like her older sister, she had normal hearing tests and normal growth hormone levels. She presented with short stature and a similar mild craniofacial dysmorphology as observed in her sister consisting of flattened forehead, protruding upper jaw and mildly thickened eyebrows, as well as deep set eyes (Table 1, Additional file 2).

Molecular genetic analysis

Patient 1 (family 1)

Whole exome sequencing of patient 1 disclosed 26,052 exonic variants. After applying standard quality filtering (22,603 remaining variants), minor allele frequency (MAF) filtering (≤ 0.001) (1563 remaining variants), known artifact prone gene family filtering (1015 remaining variants) and non-synonymous filters, there were 706 variants remaining of which 648 were heterozygous and 58 homozygous. No putative pathogenic heterozygous variants of interest were found. Of the 58 homozygous variants, a single novel homozygous missense c.2725C > T, p.Pro909Ser variant in the gene *IARS2* (GenBank: NM_018060.3, NP_060530.3) was prioritised as a putative pathogenic variant on the basis that this change affects the same residue that was clinically and functionally proven to be causative in a proband with CAGSSS [5] and the patient had clinical features that fit a CAGSSS diagnosis. Further, this variant was found to reside in a large run of homozygosity spanning nearly 14.3 Mb on chr1q41q42.2 that included 102 additional genes (homozygous interval coordinates: rs10779261 to rs2493145; chr1:216,595,306-230,891,248). No variant in any of the other genes within this interval remained after filtering. In silico analysis of synonymous variants in genes within this interval likewise did not reveal any variants predicted to affect splicing. The homozygous *IARS2* variant was confirmed in patient 1 using Sanger sequencing and both parents were found to be heterozygous (Fig. 1d). A variety of in silico pathogenicity prediction tools were used to assess this missense variant (Table 2): MutationTaster predicted the variant to be disease causing, whereas FATHMM, MutationAssessor, PolyPhen-2 and SIFT ranked the consequence of the exchange as tolerated or benign. This apparently novel variant was not deposited in any of the publicly available population frequency databases such as the Exome Variant Server (EVS), gnomAD, Greater Middle Eastern Variome (GME), Iranome, and Ensembl Variant Table (Table 2).

Patients 2 and 3 (Family 2)

WES was performed on the DNA from patient 2 in the family. On the assumption that the disease follows an autosomal recessive inheritance in the family due to the presence of consanguinity, we prioritised homozygous variants. We further preformed filtering using a minor allele frequency cut off of 0.1% in population databases such as EVS, ExAC, gnomAD, Iranome, and Ensembl given the rare phenotype and excluded non-coding variants except within 10 bp of splice sites as well as synonymous variants. The filtered data narrowed down the variants to a homozygous single nucleotide exchange in exon 18 of *IARS2* currently known monogenic disease-causing genes (c.2282A > G; p.His761Arg) (Fig. 2c) located within an 8 Mb region of homozygosity on chr1q. The variant has not been observed in any public variant database and it is predicted

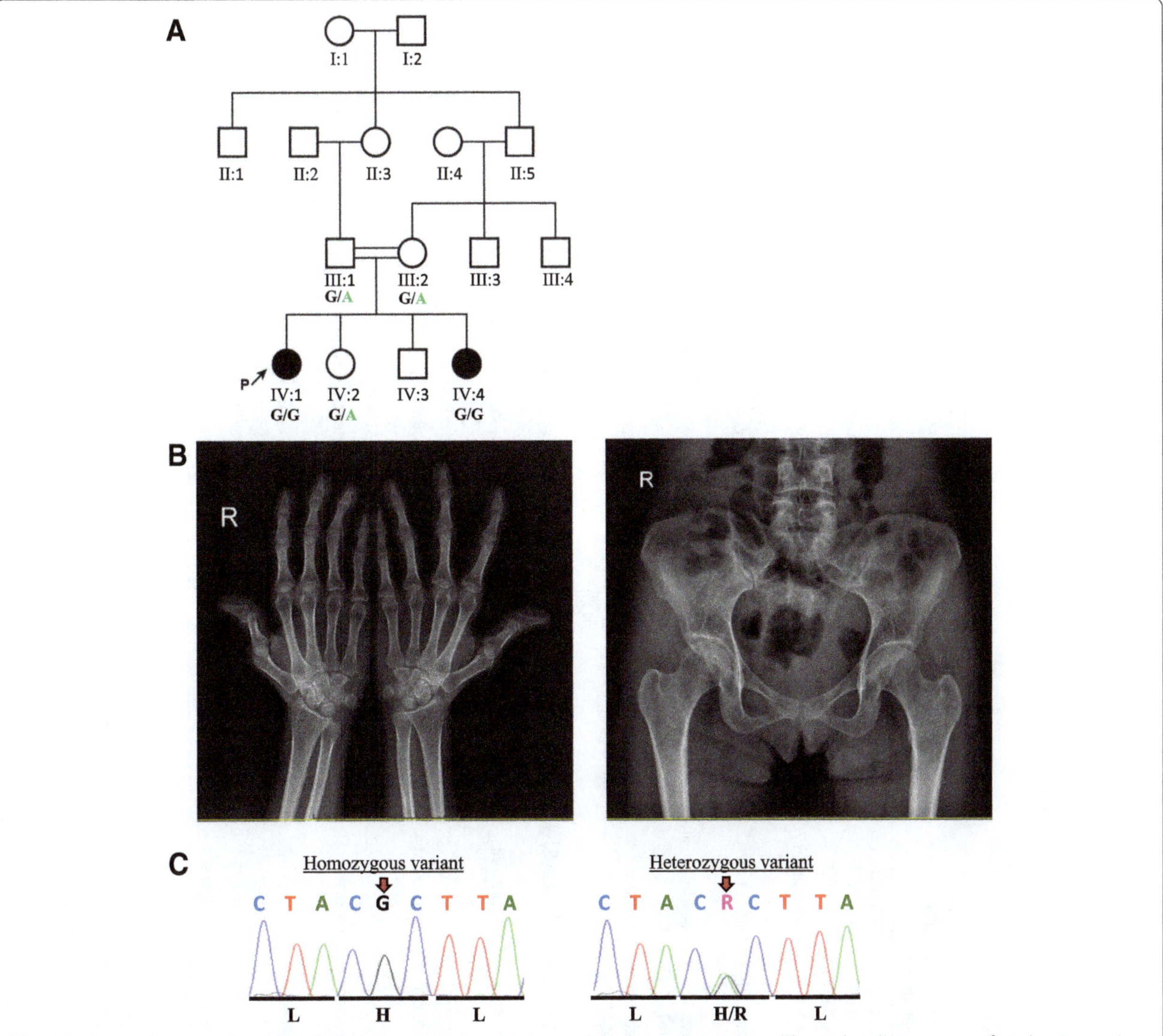

Fig. 2 Pedigree of patients 2 and 3, radiological examinations, and sequence electropherogram. **a** The proband's parents are first-degree cousins. There is no family history of CAGSSS. Genotype results for the c.2282A > G variant are represented under the tested individuals. **b** Radiological images showing that the first metacarpale bone of the right hand (left) projects short and stunted and the plane x-ray the hyperextension of the metacarpophalangeal and the carpophalangeal joints of the thumb is noticeable. The carpal bones show some mild dysplasia and flattening and tapering of the distal phalanges is visible. Some mild dysplasia of the acetabulum is noticeable (right). On both sides a distinct cross over sign is visible. The femoral heads showing some irregular shape with flattened appearance known as pistol grip deformity. The femoral neck seems shortened in comparison to the opposite side. **c** Electropherograms of the homozygous proband (upper panel) and representative heterozygous electropherogram (lower panel) showing the nucleotide and amino acid exchange. The variant position is marked with a red arrow

to affect a highly conserved functionally important isoleucyl-tRNA synthetase domain of the protein. The variant was validated by Sanger sequencing, confirming both patient 2 and 3 having the variant in a homozygous state, whereas parents and the only available healthy sibling were heterozygous. No other pathogenic/highly pathogenic variant in currently known monogenic disease-causing genes was identified from the WES data (Mendeliome filtering).

Both variants identified in Families 1 and 2 have been submitted to the Leiden Open Variation Database v.3.0 (LOVD3) with individual IDs 00163754 and 00181201, respectively (https://databases.lovd.nl/shared/genes/IARS2).

Protein conservation analysis and homology modelling of IARS2 amino acid substitutions

Amino acid conservation analysis and homology modelling of the three previously published and novel IARS2 amino acid substitutions (Glu708Lys, His761Arg, Gly874Glu, Pro909Leu, and Pro909Ser) was performed. For comparative analysis, the Glu708Lys exchange that

Table 2 Pathogenicity and population frequency analysis of *IARS2* variants

IARS2 Alleles	c.2725C > T, p.Pro909Ser (Present study)	c.2726C > T, p.Pro909Leu	c.2620G > A, p.Gly874Arg	c.2282A > G, p.His761Arg (Present study)	c.680 T > C, p.Phe227Ser	c.2450G > A, p.Arg817His	c.2122G > A, p.Glu708Lys	c.1821G > A, p.Trp607*	c.607G > C p.Gly203Arg	c.2446C > T p.(Arg816*)	c.2575 T > C p.(Phe859Leu)
Phenotypes	CAGSSS	CAGSSS	CAGSSS	Cataract,SD	CAGSSS,Leigh, and West syndrome	CAGSSS,Leigh, and West syndrome	Leigh syndrome	Leigh syndrome	Cataract	Cataract	Cataract
FATHMM	Tolerated (2.93)	Tolerated (2.615)	Tolerated (2.77)	Tolerated (2.57)	Tolerated (0.76)	Tolerated (2.38)	Tolerated (0.96)	No entry	Tolerated (−0.77)	No entry	Tolerated (2.62)
MutationAssessor	Low (1.175)	Medium (2.615)	Medium (2.1)	Medium (2.76)	High (4.34)	High (3.89)	Medium (2.955)	No entry	High (4.265)	No entry	Medium (2.63)
MutationTaster	Disease causing (1)	Disease causing (1)	Disease causing (1)	Disease causing (1)	Disease causing (1)	Disease causing (1)	Disease causing (1)	No entry	Disease causing (1)	No entry	Disease causing (1)
PolyPhen-2	Benign (0.426)	Probably damaging (0.983)	Probably damaging (1.00)	Probably damaging (1.00)	Probably damaging (1.00)	Probably damaging (1.00)	Possibly damaging (0.935)	No entry	Probably damaging (1.00)	No entry	Probably damaging (1.00)
SIFT	Tolerated (0.08)	Deleterious (0.03)	Tolerated (0.41)	Tolerated (0.1)	Deleterious (0)	Tolerated (0.06)	Tolerated (0.06)	No entry	Deleterious (0.01)	No entry	Tolerated (0.4)
Ensembl	Not present	Not present	Not present	Not present	Not present	Allele count: 3; 0 homozygous	Allele count: 6; 1 homozygous	Allele count: 1; 0 homozygous	Not present	Allele count: 1; 0 homozygous	Allele count: 2; 0 homozygous
EVS	Not present	Not present	Allele count: 1; 0 homozygous	Not present	Not present	Allele count: 3; 0 homozygous	Allele count: 11; 0 homozygous	Allele count: 1; 0 homozygous	Not present	Not present	Not present
GME	Not present	Not present	Not present	Not present	Not present	Allele count: 4; 0 homozygous	Allele count: 3; 1 homozygous	Not present	Not present	Not present	Not present
gnomAD	Not present	Not present	Allele count: 6; 0 homozygous	Not present	Not present	Allele count: 4; 0 homozygous	Allele count: 369; 6 homozygous	Allele count: 1; 0 homozygous	Not present	Allele count: 3; 0 homozygous	Allele count:39; 0 homozygous
Iranome	Not present	Not present	Not present	Not present	Not present	Not present	Allele count: 1	Not present	Not present	Not present	Not present

GenBank accession IDs: NM_018060.3, NP_060530.3

was reported in compound heterozygosity with a truncating mutation (Trp607*) in the Leigh syndrome proband was included. The Glu708, His761, Gly874, and Pro909 positions are well-conserved to *Danio rerio* (Fig. 3a). IARS2 comprises a tRNA synthetase domain that contains HIGH and KMSKS motifs, an anticodon-binding domain, and an FPG IleRS zinc finger domain (Fig. 3b). The Glu708 residue appears directly involved in the interaction with the tRNA sugar backbone and also in determining IARS2 conformation (Fig. 3c). The Gly874 and Pro909 residues appear to reside in the same anticodon-binding domain.

The His761, Gly874 and Pro909 residues appear to reside in the same anticodon-binding domain. The Gly874Glu substitution affects the N-terminus of an α-helix that interacts with tRNA. Near the latter site of mutation and on another α-helix is where the His761Arg replacement occurs. The Pro909 is part of a loop exposed to the solvent that is not near the active site. It also appears to not be directly involved in tRNA binding (Fig. 3c).

Functional analysis of cultured fibroblasts

We next investigated patient fibroblasts of patient 1 to assess whether we could detect a functional consequence of the p.Pro909Ser variant. We detected no obvious defects in any mitochondrial respiratory chain enzyme activities when related to the activity of the mitochondrial matrix enzyme, citrate synthase (Fig. 4a). In agreement with this, the steady-state levels of OXPHOS subunits were unchanged between patient and control fibroblast samples (Fig. 4b). Moreover, steady-state IARS2 protein levels were also unchanged in the patient samples (Fig. 4b).

Review of clinical presentation of patients with pathogenic variants in *IARS2*

A detailed clinical summary of the seven patients with pathogenic variants in *IARS2* can be found in Additional file 2. A shorter summary presenting the key clinical features observed in the 10 cases known to date can be found in Table 1. The youngest published patient at 8 years of age was from Denmark with a homozygous c.2620G > A, p.Gly874Glu variant [7], whereas the extended French-Canadian family had a segregating c.2726C > T, p.Pro909Leu homozygous variant that involved two previously described patients, patient 1 and patient 2 [6] who were related to an affected individual, case 1 [5]. Also, case 4, with Scandinavian-Caucasian ethnicity had compound heterozygous variants [(c.1821G > A, p.(Trp607*); c.2122G > A, p.(Glu708Lys)] [5]. Of note, case II-1 and II-2 in the Japanese study had segregating compound heterozygous variants [(c.680 T > C; p.[(Phe227Ser)] and c.2450G > A; p. [(Arg817His)] [8]. In the current study, patients in family 1 (patient 1) and family 2 (patient 2 and patient 3) have the c.2725C > T, p.Pro909Ser and c.2282A > G, p.His761Arg homozygous variants, respectively.

Ocular findings

Ocular findings are amongst the most common features associated with *IARS2* loss of function variants in seven out of ten probands affected by bilateral nystagmus and/or cataracts at birth or within the first three years of life (Table 1). Corneal opacifications have likewise been observed in six out of ten patients. Ocular abnormalities generally appear progressive. Particularly excellent follow-up of the ocular findings of patient 7 in Table 1 (case 1 described by Schwartzentruber and colleagues), included the description of a number of failed corneal grafts and severe eye dryness [31]. Furthermore, this patient had a history of congenital neurotropic keratitis, orbital myopathy and ptosis of the right eye (Table S1). Optical coherence tomography also revealed foveal hypoplasia. Unfortunately, the other cases have not been studied in this detailed manner. However, orbital myopathy and slight strabismus of the right eye are also overlapping phenotypes reported in patient 1.

Endocrinology

A main feature of CAGSSS is short stature and growth hormone deficiency that was noted in two of ten patients (Table 1). Not all patients may have been investigated in depth and the Danish proband reported normal growth hormone levels at 4 years of age. However, the authors remarked this may be due to her young age [7]. In Table 1, patient 7 had low growth hormone levels at 15 years of age that worsened to a severe deficiency at 22 years of age [5]. Growth hormone replacement therapy was performed in patient 7 and patient 8 with positive outcomes. The presumed central cortisol deficiency of patient 7 would suggest an adrenal insufficiency is present, although this was not directly described [5]. Patient 1 showed a combination of growth hormone deficiency and central adrenal insufficiency, which could be associated with a hypothalamic-pituitary axis dysfunction. Hypoglycemia, which can be linked to central adrenal insufficiency, was noted in patient 7 and patient 9 [32].

Sensory neuropathy

Half of all patients presented with peripheral neuropathy with a broad age of onset starting as early as 8 months of age (Table 1). A loss of small and medium-sized myelinated fibres, particularly in the hands, was reported in two of these patients. Decreased sensation to pinprick, temperature, and touch in all four extremities was

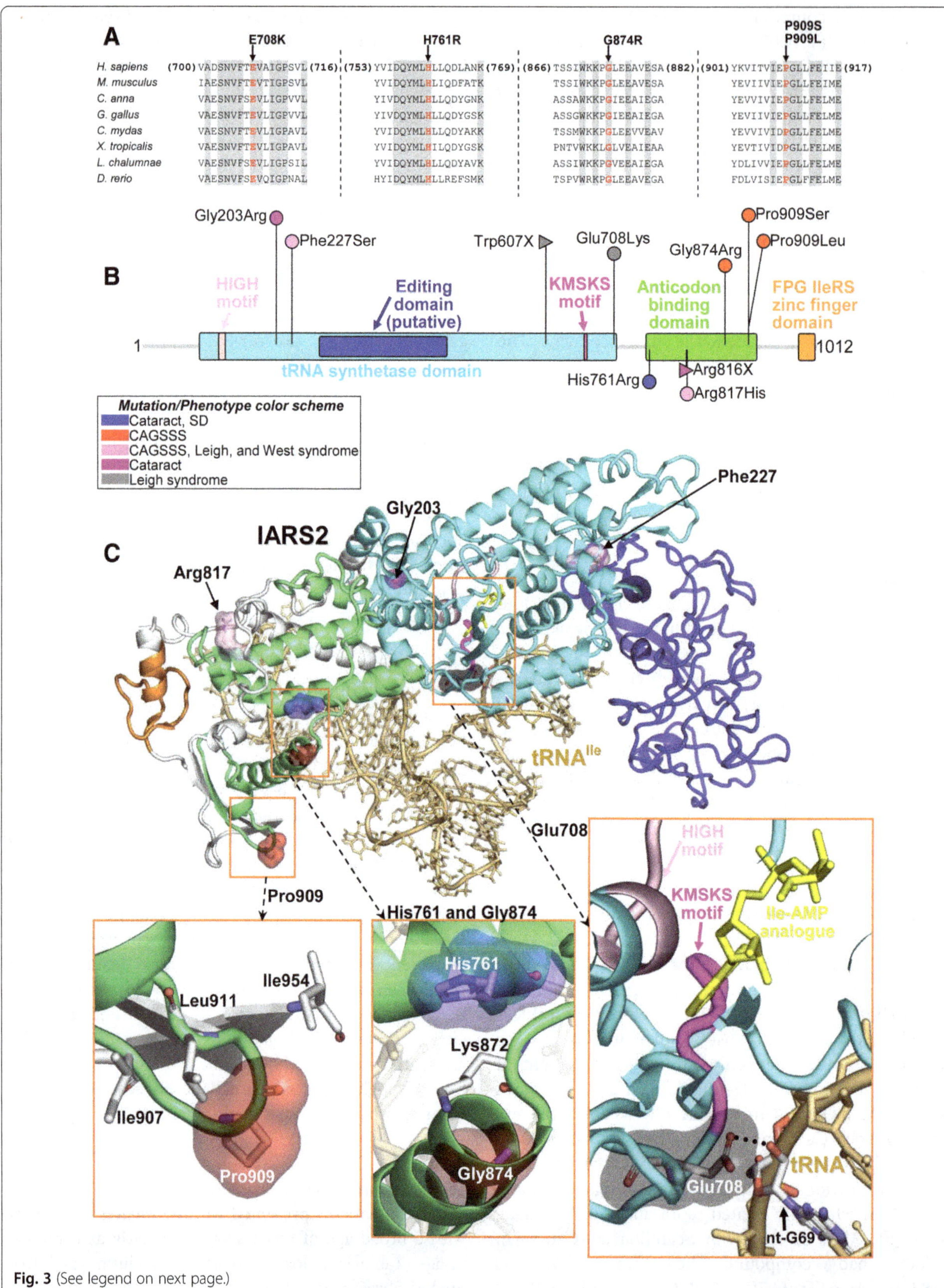

Fig. 3 (See legend on next page.)

(See figure on previous page.)
Fig. 3 IARS2 scheme, sequence alignment and homology model. **a** Sequence alignment among vertebrates (*H. sapiens*, NP_060530.3; *M. musculus*, NM_198653.2; *C. anna*, XM_008492093.1; *G. gallus*, NM_001006397.1; *C. mydas*, XM_007064764.1; *X. tropicalis*, NM_001127043.1; *L. chalumnae*, XM_005998405.2; *D. rerio*, XM_021467083.1) around the sites of the missense mutations discussed in the text (Glu708Lys, His761Arg, Gly874Arg, Pro909Leu, and Pro909Ser). Residues that are invariant in this group of organisms are shown in gray. **b** Schematic view of IARS2 protein indicating mutations (those reported in this study and the published ones) and colored by phenotype. **c** Homology model of IARS2. The protein ribbon has the same colors that are shown in the functional regions of the protein in panel B. The residues affected by the missense mutations are highlighted by surfaces with the same color scheme as in panel B. The bound cognate tRNA ($tRNA^{Ile}$) is shown as ribbon and sticks in light orange, and the Ile-AMP analogue as yellow sticks

reported in patient 7 [5]. Pain insensitivity was noted in early childhood in another patient [7].

Sensorineural hearing loss

Four out of ten patients reported to date were found to exhibit sensorineural hearing loss with a broad age of onset ranging from 18 months to 13 years of age (Table 1). Hearing aids were used in only two of these cases (Additional file 2). Previous publications did not show pure-tone audiograms or in-depth audiological testing results. Patient 8 was described with a 60 to 70 dB low-frequency and 50 dB high-frequency hearing loss at the age of 21 months and brainstem auditory evoked potentials corresponding to a 60 dB bilateral sensorineural hearing loss [6]. The most recent audiogram from patient 1 shows gently sloping mid-to-high-frequency moderate sensorineural hearing loss to 45 to 50 dB (Fig. 1c).

Musculoskeletal alterations

Nine out of ten patients presented with short stature, of which, three exhibited disproportionate short stature and likewise, three cases were diagnosed with spondylo-epi-metaphyseal dysplasia (Table 1). All patients with radiological examinations presented irregular metaphyses and delayed epiphyseal ossification was found in three cases. Seven of ten cases presented with spine abnormalities, of which four presented with scoliosis. Hip dislocation was observed in four cases, joint hypermobility in three cases, and two probands had genu valgum. A muscular wasting appearance was clearly evident in patient 1.

Discussion

CAGSSS is a rare but highly distinctive syndrome with a unique constellation of features, arising from biallelic mutations in *IARS2*. The patients we described here show a considerable phenotypic overlap to previously described patients. However, not all cases fulfill all features of the CAGSSS acronym. We found significant variability regarding onset of symptoms and some individuals show additional symptoms not included in the acronym, suggesting a wider phenotypic spectrum. With only ten molecularly confirmed cases reported to date, genotype-phenotype correlations are difficult to make with certainty, but it seems possible that there is a

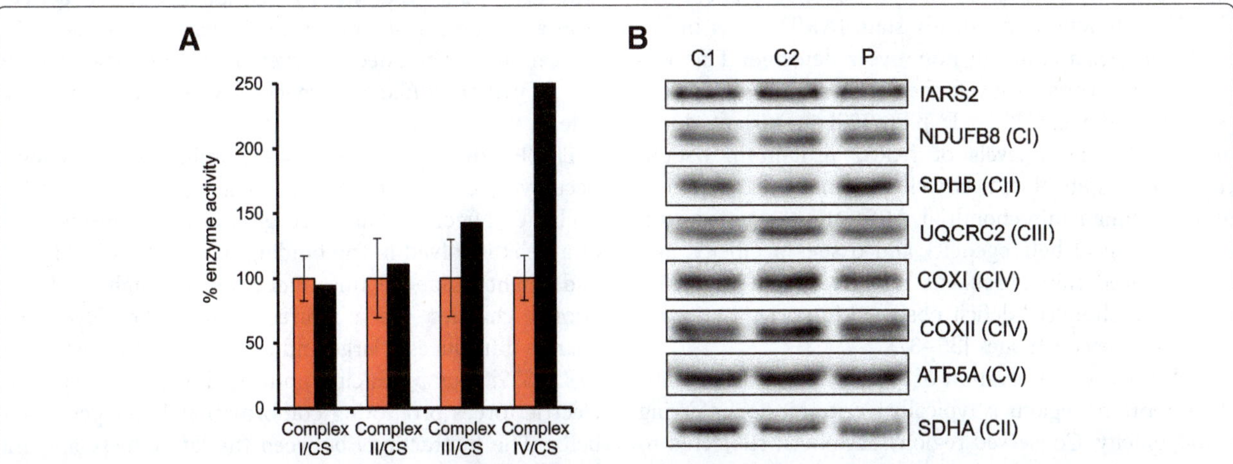

Fig. 4 Biochemical and western blot analyses of patient fibroblasts. **a** Activity of mitochondrial respiratory complexes in control (red) and patient (blue) fibroblast samples. Mean enzyme activities normalised to citrate synthase (CS) of control fibroblasts ($n = 8$) are set to 100% and error bars represent standard deviation. **b** Western blots of protein lysate from patient fibroblasts (P) and two age-matched controls (C1 and C2) immunodecorated with antibodies against IARS2, NDUFB8 (CI), UQCRC2 (CIII), COXI (CIV), COXII (CIV) and ATP5A (CV). SDHA and SDHB (CII) were used as loading controls

predicted milder impact of the p.Pro909Ser variant on IARS2 protein function compared to the other identified alleles (Table 1).

Type II achalasia and adrenal insufficiency were observed in two individuals, patient 1 and patient 7 and interestingly both have a homozygous variant affecting the proline on position 909, p.Pro909Ser in patient 1 and p.Pro909Leu in patient 7 [5]. Due to the low cortisol values in patient 7, we also speculate an adrenal insufficiency that would require further studies. It would be particularly interesting for additional patients with *IARS2* pathogenic variants to be monitored for adrenal insufficiency. The replicated finding of esophageal achalasia suggests an expansion of the CAGSSS phenotypic spectrum. Achalasia, a primary motor disorder of the esophagus, is typically diagnosed in adulthood [33]. Therefore, it is unsurprising that it was not mentioned as a clinical feature in the Danish proband [7]. This may also be an unlikely coincidence that achalasia was also described in a French-Canadian proband [5]. One could speculate that *IARS2* could be one of many genetic factors for this phenotype; however, further reports are required to understand this observation.

In silico analysis suggests the c.2725C > T, p.Pro909Ser variant is likely benign with only one out of five in silico pathogenicity prediction tools ranking this variant as disease causing. Also, two out of five of these tools predicted the novel c.2282A > G, p.His761Arg variant in the current study as disease causing (Table 2). While these tools can be a helpful first insight to the pathogenicity of a variant, no single program provides an error-free prediction result and caution should be used with concluding pathogenicity based exclusively on in silico tools [34]. Based on previous studies, we assessed whether the p.Pro909Ser variant led to any demonstrable effects on OXPHOS function and steady-state IARS2 levels in patient fibroblasts although none were detected. This was somewhat surprising given the earlier report of the patient with the c.2726C > T, p.Pro909Leu variant documented decreased levels of IARS2 protein in patient cells [5]. Despite this, it is well documented that mutation of human mitochondrial ARSs are associated with marked clinical heterogeneity and tissue-specificity, and that cultured skin fibroblasts rarely replicate the functional mitochondrial deficit observed in post-mitotic and clinically-relevant tissues [35–37].

Evolutionary conservation of structurally and functionally important regions is typically a criterion for inferring pathogenicity. Conserved regions have been subjected to negative selection and disease causing variants tend to occur disproportionately in highly conserved amino acids [38]. The homology model of human IARS2 allows the observation that the Glu708Lys variant, a variant associated with Leigh syndrome, affects a glutamic acid directly involved in the binding of mt-tRNA^{Ile} (at the level of nucleotide G69 as inferred from the crystal structure of the complex of tRNA^{Ile} with a bacterial isoleucine tRNA ligase, PDB code 1FFY), and is also very close to the catalytically important KMSKS motif and also nearby the binding site of Ile-AMP (Fig. 3b). The location of Glu708 inside the protein can be reliably assessed from the sequence alignment with the bacterial template (Additional file 1). Thus, it could be expected that the conserved Glu708 might have roles in the correct function of IARS2 and that the Glu708Lys change, which implies a reversal of the electric charge at this site, would somehow influence the enzyme activity. However, the possible clinical importance of the Glu708Lys variant expected from modelling does not appear to be supported by population frequency data, which show a combined eight homozygous (five South Asian individuals, two non-Finnish Europeans, and one Central Asian (GME) individual) and 374 heterozygous carriers from the five population frequency databases used (Table 2) and yielded a combined calculated MAF of 0.00131. In combination with the null Trp607* truncating mutation in the Leigh syndrome patient, [5], we speculate that the Glu708Lys variant alone has moderate severity but may still be functional and provide a viable amount of enzymatic activity but not enough to overcome a null allele. Supported by population frequency data, a homozygous null Trp607* variant is likely to be lethal. We assert that a homozygous Glu708Lys orientation in IARS2 may provide enough enzymatic activity to be viable, and in light of the population frequency data, phenotypically normal. Thus, it remains to be seen whether an association with Leigh syndrome is correct. Phenotypic presentation is also likely absent in the context of variants that mildly disrupt synthetase activity over a certain threshold, since sufficient synthetase activity can be maintained by even low functional activity [39]. Further studies are necessary to understand the role of this variant.

The His761Arg and Gly874Arg amino acid exchanges occur very close to each other (Fig. 3c). The Gly874Arg exchange affects a conserved glycine in the N-terminus of a helix involved in the binding of mt-tRNA^{Ile} (Fig. 3c) and might influence this interaction through conformational changes. As a matter of fact, the Gly874Arg change introduces a large and cationic residue very close to Lys872, thus producing both hindrance and repulsive electric forces promoting conformational changes in the helix. The interactions between the latter helix and the helix bearing His761 might be altered by the replacement of this conserved histidine with an arginine. The Pro909Leu and Pro909Ser variants affect a conserved proline in a solvent exposed loop. Both replacements modify the flexibility of the loop as proline residues provide unique conformational restraints among amino acids. In the case of the Pro909Leu variant, since Pro909 is surrounded by the hydrophobic Ile907, Leu911, and Ile954 residues (Fig. 3c), we foresee that the additional hydrophobic residue introduced by mutation would favour clustering of these hydrophobic residues to minimise their exposure to water. Therefore, the Pro909Leu change is expected to cause more prominent conformational changes compared to the Pro909Ser variant wherein the hydrophilic nature of the loop is preserved by the serine residue. This is consistent with the more severe phenotype associated with the Pro909Leu variant compared to the Pro909Ser variant.

Presently, most of the CAGSSS pathogenic missense variants that have been identified reside in exon 21 (Gly874Arg, Pro909Leu, Pro909Ser) of *IARS2*. It remains unknown whether homozygous variants in this exon tend to be associated with CAGSSS and variants of unknown significance in other affected exons are responsible for Leigh syndrome, a syndrome that is attributed to the death of a patient at 18 months of age that was proposed to be due to compound heterozygous *IARS2* variants (c.1821G > A, p.Trp607* in exon 14 and c.2122G > A, p.Glu708Lys in exon 17) [5]. Japanese siblings who were diagnosed with CAGSSS, Leigh, and West syndrome showed compound heterozygous variants in *IARS2* that affected exons 4 (c.680 T > C, p.Phe227Ser) and 20 (c.2450G > A, p.Arg817His). Patients 2 and 3 presented with ophthalmological and skeletal deficits and had a homozygous variant in exon 18. It can be reasoned that loss-of-function variants result in a more severe phenotype, since tRNA-charging activity would be abolished. This effect is likely independent of the affected exon.

Although no other endocrine disorders have been connected to other patients with mutations in *IARS2*, mitochondrial disease itself represents a high risk for a variety of endocrine diseases. GHD has been related to multiple patients with mitochondrial encephalomyopathy lactic acidosis and stroke-like episodes (MELAS), mtDNA deletions disorders, and nuclear encoded defects [40]. The hypothalamic-pituitary axis dysfunction has been proposed as the underlying pathophysiological mechanism, including chronic ischemia and energy deficiency of the diencephalon, associated with the mitochondrial genetic abnormality of the hypothalamus. This may correlate with our patient, since he shows a co-existing central adrenal insufficiency. Adrenal insufficiency has also been characterised in several patients with other forms of mitochondrial dysfunction, mostly with Kearns-Sayre syndrome, Person syndrome, MELAS, and POLG-related disease [41]. The most accepted pathophysiological mechanism is associated with the high energy demands of endocrine glands; therefore, the impaired mitochondrial ATP production and/ or oxidative stress may greatly reduce the ability to secrete hormone or maintain normal feedback [40].

Whilst this manuscript was in peer review, two additional publications described *IARS2* variants in patients. One of the reports described a Japanese family with two siblings who were diagnosed with Leigh syndrome that was concomitant with some of the features of CAGSSS, as well as West syndrome (Table 1 patients 4 and 5) [9]. Both siblings had novel, compound heterozygous *IARS2* [(c.680 T > C; p.[(Phe227Ser)] and c.2450G > A; p. [(Arg817His)] variants in exons 4 and 20, respectively, and exhibited delayed motor development, as well as infantile spasms and abnormal brain MRI diagnostic imaging leading to a diagnosis of Leigh syndrome. One of the two siblings had cataracts and the other sibling had a neonatal hearing screening result requiring follow-up. Both female children were in their first decade of life at the time of publication.

The second publication which characterised by far the mildest clinical presentation characterized to date described two probands from China with sporadic pediatric cataract [8]. Both probands were identified with compound heterozygous variants in *IARS2* (case 6: c.607G > C; p.(Gly203Arg) in exon 4 and c.2575 T > C; p.(Phe859Leu) in exon 21; family 10: c.2446C > T; p.(Arg816*) in exon 20 and c.2575 T > C; p.(Phe859Leu) in exon 21). Both probands shared the Phe859Leu exchange, which affects the anticodon-binding domain and can be reasoned to exhibit only mild/moderate effects. One of the reasons for this hypothesis is that the amino acid exchange conserves hydrophobicity. Another being that the Gly203Arg that is located in the aminoacyl-tRNA synthetase domain and the Arg816* null allele can reasonably be predicted as causing more severe effects on the protein. If the Phe859Leu exchange were to cause a severe protein change, we would expect a severe or even lethal phenotype in the presence of the null allele. Thus, the allelic protein product with the Phe859Leu exchange should still maintain functionality.

Conclusions

In conclusion, we describe two additional independent families with a total of three affected individuals displaying clinical features overlapping with CAGSSS and novel *IARS2* variants, expanding the clinical and mutational spectrum. Patient 1 also presented with type II esophageal achalasia, as well as growth hormone deficiency and central adrenal insufficiency, which could result from dysfunction of the hypothalamic-pituitary axis. The unusual combination of findings suggest that other endocrine disorders in patients with an *IARS2*-associated mitochondriopathy could likewise be possible and should be excluded. We propose that these additional phenotypes expand the syndromic constellation of symptoms in adults. Early recognition of *IARS2*-related pathophysiology has potentially important implications in clinical management, seeing that undetected adrenal insufficiency could lead to a life threatening crisis.

Abbreviations

ACTH: Adrenocorticotropic hormone; ARS: Aminoacyl-tRNA synthetase; CAGSSS: Cataracts, growth hormone deficiency, sensory neuropathy, sensorineural hearing loss, and skeletal dysplasia; EVS: Exome Variant Server; GHD: Growth hormone deficiency; GME: Greater Middle Eastern Variome project; IARS: Isoleucyl-tRNA synthetase; MAF: Minor allele frequency; MELAS: Mitochondrial encephalomyopathy lactic acidosis and stroke-like episodes; OXPHOS: Oxidative phosphorylation; T3: Total triiodothyronine; T4: Total thyroxine; TSH: Thyroid-stimulating hormone

Acknowledgements

The authors extend their gratitude to the families for their generous participation and to Prof. Mark E. Samuels and Prof. Chari L. Deal at the University of Montreal for helpful discussion.

Funding

RWT is funded by the Wellcome Centre for Mitochondrial Research (203105/Z/16/Z), the MRC Centre for Neuromuscular Diseases (G0601943) and the UK NHS Highly Specialised "Rare Mitochondrial Disorders of Adults and Children" Service. KT and RWT receive funding from The Lily Foundation. AA receives funding for a PhD studentship from the Kuwait Civil Service Commission under the approval of the Kuwait Ministry of Health. MS acknowledges funding from the European Research Council (ERC starting grant TREATCilia, grant agreement number grant No 716344), the "Deutsche Forschungsgemeinschaft" (DFG CRC1140 KIDGEM) and Radboudumc Nijmegen (Hypatia Tenure Track Fellowship). This publication was funded by the University of Würzburg in the funding programme Open Access Publishing.

Authors' contributions

BV, EB, EGK, MS, RM, and RWT designed the study. AR, BV, MD, MN, and RM performed exome data analysis. EB performed protein analysis and homology modelling. AA, KT, and LH performed respiratory chain biochemistry experiments and assessment of protein expression. AR, MD, MN, NA, RM, and SS collected patient samples, extracted gDNA, and performed Sanger sequencing. JM and NA acquired skin biopsy samples for cell culture. ES, FM, NA, PB, RB, and MD collected and analyzed the patient clinical information. MS, RWT, and TH were involved in study supervision. EGK, MS, and RWT provided funding. DD critically revised the manuscript. All authors have participated in manuscript writing and have critically reviewed and approved the final manuscript.

Competing interests

The authors declare that they have no competing interests.

Author details

[1]Institute of Human Genetics, Julius Maximilians University Würzburg, Würzburg, Germany. [2]Department of Otorhinolaryngology, Head and Neck Surgery, Tübingen Hearing Research Centre (THRC), Eberhard Karls University Tübingen, 72076 Tübingen, Germany. [3]Genetics and Molecular Cell Sciences Research Centre, St George's, University of London, Cranmer Terrace, London SW17 0RE, UK. [4]Genetics and Rare Diseases, Research Division, 'Bambino Gesù' Children Hospital, Rome, Italy. [5]Genome Research Division, Human Genetics Department, Radboud University Medical Center and Radboud Institute for Molecular Life Sciences, Geert Grooteplein Zuid 10, 6525KL, Nijmegen, The Netherlands. [6]Wellcome Centre for Mitochondrial Research, Institute of Neuroscience, Newcastle University, Newcastle upon Tyne, UK. [7]Faculty of Medicine, Mashhad University of Medical Sciences, Mashhad, Iran. [8]Next Generation Genetic Clinic, Mashhad, Iran. [9]Cellular and Molecular Research Center, Sabzevar University of Medical Sciences, Sabzevar, Iran. [10]Department of Orthopaedic Surgery, University Hospital of Tübingen, Hoppe-Seyler-Strasse 3, 72076 Tübingen, Germany. [11]Targeted Drug Delivery Research Center, Pharmaceutical Technology Institute, University of Medical Sciences, Mashhad, Iran. [12]Department of Neurology, Faculty of Medicine, Mashhad University of Medical Sciences, Mashhad, Iran. [13]Sabzevar University of Medical Sciences, Sabzevar, Iran. [14]Unit of Neuromuscular and Neurodegenerative Disorders, Laboratory of Molecular Medicine, 'Bambino Gesu' Children's Research Hospital, Rome, Italy. [15]Center for Pediatrics and Adolescent Medicine, University Hospital Freiburg, Faculty of Medicine, Mathildenstrasse 1, 79112 Freiburg, Germany.

References

1. Fujishima K, Kanai A. tRNA gene diversity in the three domains of life. Front Genet. 2014;5:142.
2. Antonellis A, Green ED. The role of aminoacyl-tRNA synthetases in genetic diseases. Annu Rev Genomics Hum Genet. 2008;9:87–107.
3. Meyer-Schuman R, Antonellis A. Emerging mechanisms of aminoacyl-tRNA synthetase mutations in recessive and dominant human disease. Hum Mol Genet. 2017;26(R2):R114–r127.
4. Florentz C, Sohm B, Tryoen-Toth P, Putz J, Sissler M. Human mitochondrial tRNAs in health and disease. Cell Mol Life Sci. 2003;60(7):1356–75.
5. Schwartzentruber J, Buhas D, Majewski J, Sasarman F, Papillon-Cavanagh S, Thiffault I, Sheldon KM, Massicotte C, Patry L, Simon M, et al. Mutation in the nuclear-encoded mitochondrial isoleucyl-tRNA synthetase IARS2 in patients with cataracts, growth hormone deficiency with short stature, partial sensorineural deafness, and peripheral neuropathy or with Leigh syndrome. Hum Mutat. 2014;35(11):1285–9.
6. Liberfarb RM, Jackson AH, Eavey RD, Robb RM. Unique hereditary sensory and autonomic neuropathy with growth hormone deficiency. J Child Neurol. 1993;8(3):271–6.
7. Moosa S, Haagerup A, Gregersen PA, Petersen KK, Altmüller J, Thiele H, Nürnberg P, Cho TJ, Kim OH, Nishimura G, et al. Confirmation of CAGSSS syndrome as a distinct entity in a Danish patient with a novel homozygous mutation in IARS2. Am J Med Genet A. 2017; 173(4):1102–8.
8. Li J, Leng Y, Han S, Yan L, Lu C, Luo Y, Zhang X, Cao LA-Ohoo: Clinical and genetic characteristics of Chinese patients with familial or sporadic pediatric cataract. Orphanet J Rare Dis. 2018;18;13(1):94.
9. Takezawa Y, Fujie H, Kikuchi A, Niihori T, Funayama R, Shirota M, Nakayama K, Aoki Y, Sasaki M, Kure S: Novel IARS2 mutations in Japanese siblings with CAGSSS, Leigh, and West syndrome. doi: https://doi.org/10.1016/j.braindev.2018.06.010. (1872-7131 (Electronic)).
10. McKenna A, Hanna M, Banks E, Sivachenko A, Cibulskis K, Kernytsky A, Garimella K, Altshuler D, Gabriel S, Daly M, et al. The genome analysis toolkit: a MapReduce framework for analyzing next-generation DNA sequencing data. Genome Res. 2010;20(9):1297–303.
11. Li H, Durbin R. Fast and accurate long-read alignment with burrows-wheeler transform. Bioinformatics. 2010;26(5):589–95.
12. Auton A, Brooks LD, Durbin RM, Garrison EP, Kang HM, Korbel JO, Marchini JL, McCarthy S, McVean GA, Abecasis GR. A global reference for human genetic variation. Nature. 2015;526(7571):68–74.
13. Shihab HA, Gough J, Mort M, Cooper DN, Day IN, Gaunt TR. Ranking non-synonymous single nucleotide polymorphisms based on disease concepts. Hum Genomics. 2014;8:11.
14. Reva B, Antipin Y, Sander C. Predicting the functional impact of protein mutations: application to cancer genomics. Nucleic Acids Res. 2011; 39(17):e118.
15. Schwarz JM, Rödelsperger C, Schuelke M, Seelow D. MutationTaster evaluates disease-causing potential of sequence alterations. Nat Methods. 2010;7(8):575–6.
16. Adzhubei IA, Schmidt S, Peshkin L, Ramensky VE, Gerasimova A, Bork P, Kondrashov AS, Sunyaev SR. A method and server for predicting damaging missense mutations. Nat Methods. 2010;7(4):248–9.
17. Ng PC, Henikoff S. Predicting the effects of amino acid substitutions on protein function. Annu Rev Genomics Hum Genet. 2006;7:61–80.
18. Lek M, Karczewski KJ, Minikel EV, Samocha KE, Banks E, Fennell T, O'Donnell-Luria AH, Ware JS, Hill AJ, Cummings BB, et al. Analysis of protein-coding genetic variation in 60,706 humans. Natuere. 2016; 536(7616):285–91.

19. Scott EM, Halees A, Itan Y, Spencer EG, He Y, Azab MA, Gabriel SB, Belkadi A, Boisson B, Abel L, et al. Characterization of greater middle eastern genetic variation for enhanced disease gene discovery. Nat Genet. 2016;48(9):1071–6.
20. Akbari MR, Fattahi Z, Beheshtian M, Mohseni M, Poustchi H, Sellars E, Nezhadi H, Amini A, Arzhangi S, Jalalvand K, et al. Iranome: A human genome variation database of eight major ethnic groups that live in Iran and neighboring countries in the Middle East. Orlando: ASHG Annual Meeting; 2017.
21. Zerbino DR, Achuthan P, Akanni W, Amode MR, Barrell D, Bhai J, Billis K, Cummins C, Gall A, Giron CG, et al. Ensembl 2018. Nucleic Acids Res. 2018; 46(D1):D754–d761.
22. Landrum MJ, Lee JM, Benson M, Brown G, Chao C, Chitipiralla S, Gu B, Hart J, Hoffman D, Hoover J, et al. ClinVar: public archive of interpretations of clinically relevant variants. Nucleic Acids Res. 2016;44(D1):D862–8.
23. Stenson PD, Mort M, Ball EV, Evans K, Hayden M, Heywood S, Hussain M, Phillips AD, Cooper DN. The human gene mutation database: towards a comprehensive repository of inherited mutation data for medical research, genetic diagnosis and next-generation sequencing studies. Hum Genet. 2017;136(6):665–77.
24. Kobayashi YA-O, Yang S, Nykamp K, Garcia J, Lincoln SE, Topper SE: Pathogenic variant burden in the ExAC database: an empirical approach to evaluating population data for clinical variant interpretation. Genome Med. 2017;6;9(1):13.
25. Untergasser A, Cutcutache I, Koressaar T, Ye J, Faircloth BC, Remm M, Rozen SG. Primer3--new capabilities and interfaces. Nucleic Acids Res. 2012;40(15):e115.
26. Thompson K, Majd H, Dallabona C, Reinson K, King MS, Alston CL, He L, Lodi T, Jones SA, Fattal-Valevski A, et al. Recurrent De novo dominant mutations in SLC25A4 cause severe early-onset mitochondrial disease and loss of mitochondrial DNA copy number. Am J Hum Genet. 2016;99(4):860–76.
27. Kirby DM, Thorburn DR, Turnbull DM, Taylor RW. Biochemical assays of respiratory chain complex activity. Methods Cell Biol. 2007;80:93–119.
28. Nagata K, Randall A, Baldi P. SIDEpro: a novel machine learning approach for the fast and accurate prediction of side-chain conformations. Proteins. 2012;80(1):142–53.
29. Xu S, Gu X, Pan H, Zhu H, Gong F, Li Y, Xing Y. Reference ranges for serum IGF-1 and IGFBP-3 levels in Chinese children during childhood and adolescence. Endocr J. 2010;57(3):221–8.
30. Mazzoli M, Van Camp G, Newton V, Giarbini N, Declau F, Parving A. Recommendations for the description of genetic and audiological data for families with nonsyndromic hereditary hearing impairment. Audiol Med. 2003;1:148–50.
31. Jabbour S, Harissi-Dagher M. Recessive mutation in a nuclear-encoded mitochondrial tRNA Synthetase associated with infantile cataract, congenital neurotrophic keratitis, and orbital myopathy. Cornea. 2016;35(6):894–6.
32. Charmandari E, Nicolaides NC, Chrousos GP. Adrenal insufficiency. Lancet. 2014;383(9935):2152–67.
33. Gockel HR, Schumacher J, Gockel I, Lang H, Haaf T, Nöthen MM. Achalasia: will genetic studies provide insights? Hum Genet. 2010;128(4):353–64.
34. Walters-Sen LC, Hashimoto S, Thrush DL, Reshmi S, Gastier-Foster JM, Astbury C, Pyatt RE. Variability in pathogenicity prediction programs: impact on clinical diagnostics. Mol Genet Genomic Med. 2015;3(2):99–110.
35. Sasarman F, Nishimura T, Thiffault I, Shoubridge EA. A novel mutation in YARS2 causes myopathy with lactic acidosis and sideroblastic anemia. Hum Mutat. 2012;33(8):1201–6.
36. Almalki A, Alston CL, Parker A, Simonic I, Mehta SG, He L, Reza M, Oliveira JM, Lightowlers RN, McFarland R, et al. Mutation of the human mitochondrial phenylalanine-tRNA synthetase causes infantile-onset epilepsy and cytochrome c oxidase deficiency. Biochim Biophys Acta. 2014; 1842(1):56–64.
37. Oliveira R, Sommerville EW, Thompson K, Nunes J, Pyle A, Grazina M, Chinnery PF, Diogo L, Garcia P, Taylor RW. Lethal neonatal LTBL associated with Biallelic EARS2 variants: case report and review of the reported Neuroradiological features. JIMD Rep. 2017;33:61–8.
38. Azevedo L, Mort M, Costa AC, Silva RM, Quelhas D, Amorim A, Cooper DN. Improving the in silico assessment of pathogenicity for compensated variants. Eur J Hum Genet. 2016;25(1):2–7.
39. Konovalova S, Tyynismaa H. Mitochondrial aminoacyl-tRNA synthetases in human disease. Mol Genet Metab. 2013;108(4):206–11.
40. Chow J, Rahman J, Achermann JC, Dattani MT, Rahman S. Mitochondrial disease and endocrine dysfunction. Nat Rev Endocrinol. 2017;13(2):92–104.
41. Parikh S, Goldstein A, Karaa A, Koenig MK, Anselm I, Brunel-Guitton C, Christodoulou J, Cohen BH, Dimmock D, Enns GM, et al. Patient care standards for primary mitochondrial disease: a consensus statement from the mitochondrial medicine society. Genet Med. 2017;19(12).

24

The estrogen receptor 1 gene affects bone mineral density and osteoporosis treatment efficiency in Slovak postmenopausal women

Vladimira Mondockova[1], Maria Adamkovicova[1], Martina Lukacova[1], Birgit Grosskopf[2*], Ramona Babosova[3], Drahomir Galbavy[4], Monika Martiniakova[3] and Radoslav Omelka[1]

Abstract

Background: The study investigated the associations of rs9340799:A > G (XbaI) and rs2234693:T > C (PvuII) polymorphisms in the estrogen receptor 1 gene (*ESR1*) with femoral neck (BMD-FN) and lumbar spine bone mineral density (BMD-LS), biochemical markers of bone turnover, calcium and phosphate levels, fracture prevalence, and a response to two types of anti-osteoporotic therapy in postmenopausal women from southern Slovakia.

Methods: We analysed 343 postmenopausal Slovak women (62.40 ± 0.46 years). The influence of rs9340799 (AA vs. AG + GG) and rs2234693 (TT vs. TC + CC) genotypes on BMD and biochemical markers was evaluated by covariance analysis adjusted for age and BMI. Binary logistic regression was used to evaluate the genotype effect on fracture prevalence. Pharmacogenetic part of the study included women who received a regular therapy of HT (17ß estradiol with progesterone; 1 mg/day for both; $N = 76$) or SERMs/raloxifene (60 mg/day; $N = 64$) during 48 months. The genotype-based BMD change was assessed by variance analysis for repeated measurements.

Results: Women with AA genotype of rs9340799 had higher BMD-FN (+ 0.12 ± 0.57 of T-score) and BMD-LS (+ 0.17 ± 0.08 of T-score) in comparison with AG + GG. The rs2234693 polymorphism did not affect any of the monitored parameters. No effect of any *ESR1* polymorphisms was found on fracture prevalence. Both types of anti-osteoporotic therapy had a positive effect on BMD improvement in FN and LS sites. Considering the effect of the *ESR1* gene within the HT, the subjects with rs9340799/AA genotype showed worse response than those with GG genotype (− 0.26 ± 0.10 of BMD-FN T-score; − 0.35 ± 0.10 of BMD-LS T-score) and also with AG genotype (− 0.22 ± 0.08 of BMD-LS T-score). The rs2234693/TT genotype responded poorer in BMD-LS in comparison with TC (− 0.22 ± 0.08 of T-score) and CC (− 0.35 ± 0.09 of T-score). The effect of the *ESR1* gene on raloxifene therapy was reported only in BMD-LS. Subjects with rs9340799/AA genotype had a − 0.30 ± 0.11 of T-score worse response compared to AG genotype. The rs2234693/TT genotype showed − 0.39 ± 0.11 and − 0.46 ± 0.15 lower T-scores in comparison with TC and CC genotypes, respectively.

Conclusions: The rs9340799 polymorphism may contribute to decreased BMD in postmenopausal women from southern Slovakia; however, this is not related to higher fracture prevalence. Concurrently, both polymorphisms affected a response to analysed anti-osteoporotic therapies.

Keywords: Osteoporosis, *ESR1* gene, Polymorphisms, BMD, Fractures, HT, Estradiol, Raloxifene

* Correspondence: birgit.grosskopf@biologie.uni-goettingen.de
[2]Institute of Zoology and Anthropology, Georg-August University, Göttingen, Germany
Full list of author information is available at the end of the article

Background

Osteoporosis is a common disease, characterized by reduced bone mass, defects in the microarchitecture of bone tissue, and an increased risk of fragility fractures [1]. The presence of fractures together with bone mineral density (BMD) measurements forms the basis of diagnostic techniques that guide targeted intervention strategies. The etiology of osteoporosis is multifactorial in which a polygenic background is modulated by the integrated effects of hormonal, environmental and nutritional factors. Although many environmental factors play an important role in BMD variation, genetic influences account for 60–85% of individual variance. So far, genetic studies have revealed candidate genes included in the regulation of BMD and in the osteoporosis progression [2–4]. Estrogen deficiency represents a major mechanism of the rapid bone loss in postmenopausal women. Interactions of estrogens with the receptors in target cells of bone and other tissues regulate growth and bone development, acquisition of peak bone mass, bone metabolism and inhibition of bone loss [5]. Therefore, the gene encoding estrogen receptor 1, one of two mediators of estrogen action, has been considered as an important candidate for the determination of osteoporosis risk [6, 7]. The principal role of the *ESR1* gene in skeletal maintenance has recently been confirmed using mice with targeted deletion of *ESR1* from specific bone cells and their precursors. Lack of the estrogen receptor in osteoblast progenitor and precursor cells affected the periosteum while the absence of the receptor in differentiated osteoblasts, osteocytes, and osteoclasts resulted in reduced cancellous bone mass [8]. Genetic screening of the *ESR1* gene locus has revealed several polymorphic sites. The most widely studied are rs2234693:T > C (PvuII), rs9340799:A > G (XbaI) polymorphisms in intron I, and the (TA)n repeat polymorphism within the promoter region of the gene [6]. Several studies showed a relationship between low number of TA repeats and increased fracture risk or BMD in different populations [9, 10]. Within the rs2234693 and rs9340799 polymorphisms, the results have not always been consistent in different population analyses. However, despite conflicting results, associations of rs2234693 and rs9340799 polymorphisms with BMD have been found in some studies [4, 11–15].

Considering the mechanisms of drug action within specific treatment procedures, such as hormone therapy (HT) or selective estrogen receptor modulators (SERMs) application, the genetic variability in the *ESR1* gene may also have important pharmacogenetic implications. The HT is a treatment commonly used to relieve symptoms and some undesirable consequences of menopause including osteoporosis. Exogenous estrogens also belong to the primary osteoporosis prevention in postmenopausal women, as these agents reduce the risk of vertebral and hip fractures [16]. SERMs are used for prevention and treatment of postmenopausal osteoporosis and breast cancer prevention in high-risk postmenopausal women with osteoporosis [17]. Raloxifene, a member of SERMs, simulates estrogen action on the skeletal system through agonistic binding to estrogen receptors without the negative effects on breast and endometrium [18]. As in the case of association studies, the results of pharmacogenetic ones have not always been consistent. Positive effects of TT genotype on fracture risk [19] and BMD [12, 20, 21] were found in different populations. In addition to HT and SERMs, other currently approved therapies for osteoporosis include bisphosphonates (BPs), applications of vitamin D derivates, parathyroid hormone and teriparatide (a recombinant human parathyroid hormone), calcitonin, strontium ranelate, and anti-RANK ligand monoclonal antibodies [22]. Response to drugs can be affected by many factors, such as sex, age, ethnicity, lifestyle, and concomitant diseases or drug therapy. The individual variation of response to anti-osteoporotic treatments ranges from good to little response or nonresponse (estimated proportion from 5 to 10%), and it may be due to individual genetic factors or environmental influences that could interfere with drug dynamics and kinetics [23]. Common variations in the human genome are today considered as the most important cause of variable drug responses [18].

The aim of this study was to analyse the associations of rs2234693 and rs9340799 polymorphisms in the *ESR1* gene with BMD, biochemical markers of bone turnover, calcium and phosphate levels, fracture prevalence, and a response to two types of anti-osteoporotic therapy in postmenopausal women from southern Slovakia.

Methods

Studied population

Our study included 343 postmenopausal women from southern region of the Slovak Republic aged from 45 to 85 years (62.40 ± 0.46 years) and monitored under the basic diagnostic screening for osteoporosis. Women were selected according to strict inclusion criteria. We excluded women with serious internal, endocrine, chronic and hereditary diseases, patients treated with certain medicaments (glucocorticoids, hormones) and with previous antiosteoporotic treatment, obese women (BMI = 30.0 kg/m^2 and above), women with a significant abuse (alcoholism, nicotinism, caffeinism), individuals with late-onset or premature menopause, and women with serious disturbances in the menstrual cycle. Clinical characteristics and parameters of the study population are shown in Table 1. The proportion of subjects with diagnosed osteoporosis accounted for 60.1% (*N* = 206) of all women.

The studied women came from a Slovak southern region and, from a historical point of view, they could be

Table 1 General characteristics of the studied groups of women

Variable	Total $N = 343$	HT study $N = 76$	Raloxifene study $N = 64$
Age (years)	62.40 ± 0.46	63.22 ± 1.00	65.30 ± 0.98
Body mass index (BMI)	27.60 ± 0.08	27.30 ± 0.18	27.64 ± 0.17
BMD-FN (T-score)	−1.79 ± 0.03	− 2.13 ± 0.04	−2.16 ± 0.06
BMD-FN (g/cm^2)	0.65 ± 0.01	0.60 ± 0.01	0.60 ± 0.01
BMD-LS (T-score)	−2.37 ± 0.04	−2.87 ± 0.04	− 2.95 ± 0.05
BMD-LS (g/cm^2)	0.73 ± 0.01	0.68 ± 0.01	0.67 ± 0.01
Bone isoenzyme of alkaline phosphatase (μkat/l)	0.56 ± 0.04	1.17 ± 0.11	0.68 ± 0.08
Osteocalcin (μg/l)	3.85 ± 0.05	3.92 ± 0.11	4.25 ± 0.13
BetaCrosslaps (ng/l)	709.65 ± 13.57	795.23 ± 24.21	876.86 ± 28.06
Serum calcium (mmol/l)	2.40 ± 0.01	2.39 ± 0.02	2.46 ± 0.03
Serum phosphate (mmol/l)	1.20 ± 0.01	1.19 ± 0.02	1.23 ± 0.03

Data are presented as Mean ± SE (SE – standard error of the mean)
BMD bone mineral density, *HT* hormone therapy (17ß estradiol/progesterone)

considered as descendants of a mixed Hungarian-Slavic population. This territory has been an important Hungarian-Slavic contact zone for more than thousand years [24] and it has homogeneously merged the overlapping populations with a different cultural, linguistic and geographic origin.

Clinical data acquisition

Personal and family history, age and life style habits were examined using a questionnaire (Additional file 1) that was completed by the subjects and reviewed by the qualified physician. BMI was calculated as weight in kilograms divided by height in meters squared. A prevalence (presence or absence) of total, femoral, radial, and spinal fragility fractures (also included compression fractures) in a period of last 5 years was diagnosed by clinical evaluation and using X-rays radiographs. A detailed personal history was considered to avoid counting traumatic fractures. BMD expressed by T-score and g/cm^2 of femoral (BMD-FN) and lumbar spine vertebrae (BMD-LS) was measured at the femoral neck and at the lumbar spine (L2-L4) by dual energy X-ray absorptiometry (HOLOGIC Discovery DXA system). All women were tested with the same densitometer. Biochemical markers of bone remodeling included osteoformation and osteoresorption markers - bone isoenzyme of alkaline phosphatase (ALP; μkat/l), serum osteocalcin (OC; μg/l), serum beta CrossLaps (CTx; ng/l). The ALP was determined by immunoenzymatic assay (Beckman Coulter Access Ostase assay, Beckman Coulter), the OC and CTx were measured by electrochemiluminescence immunoassay with cobas e411 (Roche Diagnostics) within a diagnostic screening. Concentrations of serum calcium (mmol/l) and phosphate (mmol/l) were analysed by photometric assay with cobas c311 (Roche Diagnostics). All measurements were performed by accredited clinical laboratories in Nitra (Slovakia).

Genetic analysis of the *ESR1* gene

Genomic DNA was extracted from EDTA blood samples using the blood isolation kit (SiMax™ Genomic DNA Extraction Kit, China). DNA was amplified by PCR using primers according to Kobayashi et al. [11]. PCR was performed with the following steps: 95 °C for 5 min and then 94 °C for 30 s, 60 °C for 30 s, and 72 °C for 1 min. The PCR consisted of 35 cycles and it was completed by a final extension cycle at 72 °C for 7 min. The PCR product was a 1.3-kb long fragment including a part of intron 1 and exon 2 of the *ESR1* gene. After amplification, the PCR product was digested with XbaI and PvuII restriction endonucleases (Invitrogen) separately at 37 °C overnight and separated by electrophoresis in 2.0% agarose gel containing ethidium bromide. The gels were documented by DNR Bio-Imaging Systems (MiniBIS Pro, Israel). The "G" and "C" alleles indicate the absence of XbaI and PvuII restrictrion site, respectively, the "A" and "T" alleles indicate a presence of these restriction sites (Fig. 1).

Pharmacogenetic study

Data from osteoporotic women, who received regular anti-osteoporotic therapy during 48 months, were analysed (Table 1). BMDs (BMD-FN and BMD-LS) were measured before and after the treatment period. The therapy types included application of hormone therapy (HT) of 17ß estradiol in combination with progesterone (1 mg/day for both; $N = 76$) or SERMs/raloxifene (60 mg/day; $N = 64$). During a treatment, all women received a supplementation of calcium (1000 mg/day) and vitamin D (800 IU/day).

Statistical analysis

The data were summarized as Mean ± SE (Standard Error of the Mean) for quantitative variables and as

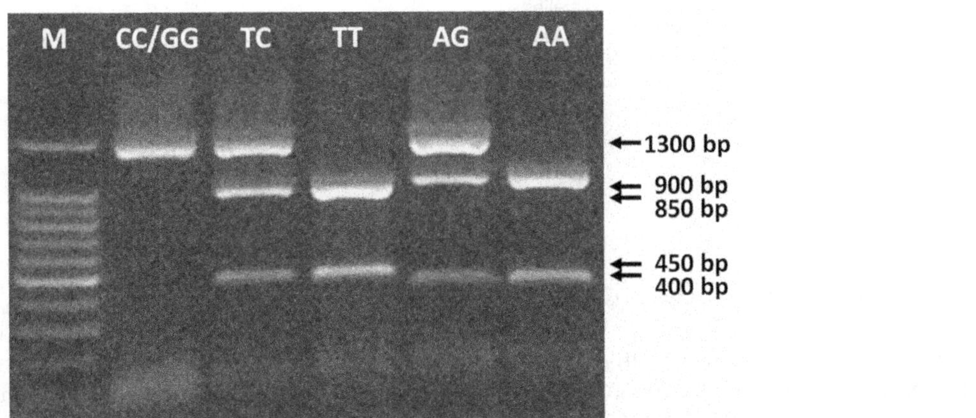

Fig. 1 Representative results of *ESR1* genotypes detection. Lane M – 100 bp ladder; lane CC/GG – amplified *ESR1* gene (1300 bp) and CC or GG genotypes; the other lanes represent combinations of DNA fragments related to the rest *ESR1* genotypes

frequencies for qualitative variables. Genotype distribution was tested for Hardy–Weinberg equilibrium using the chi-square test. The differences of quantitative variables among the genotypes were analysed in quantitative design by covariance analysis (General Linear Model procedure, GLM) after correction of the measurements for age and BMI. A dominant genetic model (TT vs. TC + CC for rs2234693; AA vs. AG + GG for rs9340799) was chosen according to calculations by SNPStats (Institut Català d'Oncologia). Possible interactions (significance interval) were tested using Johnson-Neyman procedure [25]. For evaluation of fracture prevalence Binary Logistic Regression with the genotype, age and BMI as covariates was used. The effect of genotypes on BMD change during a treatment was assessed by variance analysis for repeated measurements using GLM, where the evaluated BMD before and after treatment represented a repeat dependent variable and the individual genotypes were fixed effects. The BMD improvement within a genotype was tested by the same procedure but without between subject factors. Corrections for multiple testing of genotype effects were performed by Bonferroni correction. Statistical analysis was realized using SPSS software version 17.0 (SPSS Inc.; Chicago, IL, USA). The same software package was used to calculate the observed power of the association and pharmacogenetic studies. According to the relatively small sample size, the ideal power analysis parameters for our study were expected at 80% for the observed power with small to medium effect size. The *p*-value less than 0.05 was considered to be statistically significant.

Results

In our studied group we found the highest frequencies of heterozygous genotypes for both polymorphisms (Table 2). The distribution of genotypes agreed with that expected according to the Hardy-Weinberg equilibrium. In addition, rs2234693 and rs9340799 polymorphisms in the *ESR1* gene were in linkage disequilibrium ($\chi^2 = 363.56$; $P < 0.001$). The frequencies of the haplotypes counted 0.52, 0.37, 0.10, and 0.01 for TA, CG, CA, and TG haplotypes, respectively.

Associations of rs9340799 and rs2234693 genotypes with the osteoporosis-related characteristics are presented in Table 3. The results of statistical analysis for rs9340799 polymorphism showed that femoral and spinal BMD were significantly higher in women with the AA genotype in comparison with AG + GG genotypes ($P < 0.05$). No statistically significant difference between the rs9340799 genotypes was observed for other analysed traits (ALP, OC, CTx, Ca, P). Moreover, no association of rs2234693 genotype with BMD, biochemical markers of bone turnover and other serum parameters was found. A haplotype analysis revealed non-significant effects of TA and CG haplotypes on any of the analysed trait.

None of the polymorphisms of the *ESR1* genotypes had an effect on fracture prevalence (Table 4). Femoral fractures were not included in the analysis because of a small number of femoral fracture carriers ($N = 4$).

The findings from the pharmacogenetic analysis showed that both evaluated treatment types had a significant effect on positive BMD change after 48 months of treatment (Table 5; Fig. 2). Within HT, an increase in T-score of 0.347 ± 0.043 and 0.687 ± 0.057 was found for BMD-FN and BMD-LS, respectively. Raloxifene increased the T-score by 0.242 ± 0.070 and 0.463 ± 0.063 in BMD-FN and BMD-LS, respectively. The treatment efficiency of the therapies ranged from + 5.2 to + 11.3% of BMD increase. However, when considering the effects of the *ESR1* gene, significant differences in treatment efficiency also between *ESR1* genotypes were revealed (Tables 6, 7; Fig. 2). Significant changes were found in femoral neck, as well as in lumbar spine BMD. Among HT treated women, the subjects with GG genotype of rs9340799 had significantly

Table 2 Distribution of *ESR1* genotypes and alelles

Polymorphism	Genotype	Number	Genotype frequency (%)	HWE *P* value	Alelle frequency
rs9340799	GG	52	15.2	χ2 = 0.209 *P* = 0.90	G = 0.38 A = 0.62
	AG	157	45.8		
	AA	134	39.0		
rs2234693	CC	73	21.3	χ2 = 0.188 *P* = 0.91	C = 0.47 *T* = 0.53
	CT	175	51.0		
	TT	95	27.7		

HWE Hardy-Weinberg equilibrium (the chi-square test value)

better response to HT than those with AA genotype in both, BMD-FN (P<0.05) and BMD-LS (*P*<0.01). In these cases, the T-scores were different by 0.262 ± 0.103 and 0.345 ± 0.100 at BMD-FN and BMD-LS, respectively. Moreover in BMD-LS, the women with AA genotype responded poorly to the therapy when compared also with AG genotype (− 0.221 ± 0.077 of T-score; *P*<0.05). Within the rs2234693 genotypes, individuals with CC (+ 0.354 ± 0.094 of T-score; *P* ≤ 0.001) and TC (+ 0.215 ± 0.080 of T-score; *P*<0.05) genotypes had better response to HT in BMD-LS in comparison with TT genotype carriers. Despite these differences, all genotypes (except for TT in BMD-FN) showed significant increase in BMD during HT treatment, counting from + 3.4 to + 17.4%.

The effect of the *ESR1* gene on raloxifene therapy was reported only in relation to BMD-LS. Subjects with AA genotype had significantly worse response to raloxifene, counting − 0.299 ± 0.113 of T-score (P<0.05), when compared with AG genotype. Finally, patients with TT genotype showed 0.394 ± 0.110 and 0.461 ± 0.145 lower T-score in BMD-LS (P<0.01) than those with the TC and CC genotypes, respectively. No changes were detected in the femoral neck BMD in relation to the raloxifene therapy.

Table 3 Associations of the rs9340799 and rs2234693 genotypes with osteoporosis-related traits

Parameter	rs9340799:A > G genotypes		Sig. (*P* value)	Sig. Cov.	BMD difference
	AA *N* = 134	AG + GG *N* = 209			
BMD-FN (T-score)	−1.716 ± 0.044	−1.837 ± 0.035	0.035	A	0.120 ± 0.570
BMD-FN (g/cm^2)	0.587 ± 0.07	0.566 ± 0.06	0.035	A	0.020 ± 0.010
BMD-LS (T-score)	−2.262 ± 0.062	−2.432 ± 0.049	0.033	A, B	0.170 ± 0.079
BMD-LS (g/cm^2)	0.741 ± 0.07	0.723 ± 0.05	0.033	A, B	0.018 ± 0.008
ALP	0.493 ± 0.057	0.588 ± 0.046	NS	A, B	
OC	3.833 ± 0.086	3.853 ± 0.069	NS	A	
CTx	691.442 ± 21.246	721.324 ± 16.992	NS	A	
sCa	2.400 ± 0.017	2.399 ± 0.014	NS	A	
sP	1.191 ± 0.015	1.206 ± 0.012	NS	B	
Parameter	rs2234693:T > C genotypes		Sig. (P value)	Sig. Cov.	BMD difference
	TT *N* = 95	TC + CC *N* = 248			
BMD-FN (T-score)	−1.714 ± 0.053	−1.818 ± 0.032	NS	A	
BMD-FN (g/cm^2)	0.585 ± 0.09	0.570 ± 0.05	NS	A	
BMD-LS (T-score)	−2.277 ± 0.073	− 2.400 ± 0.045	NS	A, B	
BMD-LS (g/cm^2)	0.739 ± 0.08	0.726 ± 0.05	NS	A, B	
ALP	0.582 ± 0.068	0.547 ± 0.042	NS	A, B	
OC	3.926 ± 0.102	3.814 ± 0.063	NS	A	
CTx	696.002 ± 25.214	714.878 ± 15.592	NS	A	
sCa	2.394 ± 0.020	2.401 ± 0.013	NS	A	
sP	1.170 ± 0.018	1.208 ± 0.011	NS		

Data are presented as Estimated Marginal Mean ± SE (SE – standard error of the mean); values are adjusted for age and *BMI* BMD-FN – femoral neck BMD (T-score and g/cm^2), *BMD-LS* – lumbal spine BMD (T-score and g/cm^2), *ALP* – bone isoenzyme of alkaline phosphatase (μkat/l), *OC* - osteocalcin (μg/l), *CTx* - BetaCrosslaps (ng/l), *sCa* - serum calcium (mmol/l), *sP* - serum phosphate (mmol/l), *Sig.* – significance of GLM/BMD differences, *NS* – non-significant GLM, *P* values determine significant GLM/BMD differences (*P* < 0.05), *Sig. Cov.* - significance of covariates, *A* – significant (*P* < 0.05) covariate Age, *B* - significant (*P* < 0.05) covariate BMI

Table 4 The effects of the rs9340799 and rs2234693 genotypes on fracture prevalence

Fracture location	Genotypes	Presence of fractures	Absence of fractures	*P* value	OR	95% CI
rs9340799:A > G genotypes						
Spinal	GG	12	40	0.744	0.869	0.373–2.024
	AG	43	114	0.464	0.764	0.437–1.458
	AA	36	98			
Radial	GG	8	44	0.501	0.722	0.279–1.868
	AG	27	130	0.371	0.735	0.375–1.442
	AA	21	113			
Total	GG	13	39	0.913	1.046	0.469–2.330
	AG	48	109	0.632	0.871	0.495–1.533
	AA	42	92			
rs2234693:T > C genotypes						
Spinal	CC	17	56	0.861	0.930	0.414–2.092
	TC	48	127	0.759	0.903	0.472–1.729
	TT	26	69			
Radial	CC	10	63	0.856	0.918	0.363–2.322
	TC	31	144	0.501	0.779	0.377–1.610
	TT	15	80			
Total	CC	18	55	0.858	1.073	0.497–2.315
	TC	56	119	0.583	0.843	0.458–1.552
	TT	29	66			

The total number values count a presence of any fracture in an individual, *OR* - the odds ratio, *CI* - confidence interval, AA and TT genotypes were set as baseline categories in a regression model; femoral fractures were not evaluated

Discussion

At older ages, osteoporosis may be the cause of diminished life quality, decreased functional independence, increased morbidity and, even sometimes, mortality. Genetic research helps to reveal responsible genetic factors, which can expand our possibilities in the treatment of the disease or an identification of individuals at risk.

Our results point to similar genetic variability in rs2234693 and rs9340799 polymorphisms as in other Caucasian populations [9, 19, 26, 27]. Differences in genotype distribution of both polymorphisms can be found between Caucasian and other populations. Data from Asian populations [11, 28–30] showed differential range of allele and genotype frequency. The rs2234693 genotype distribution moves in the range of 14.0–19.3%, 43.6–54.8%, and 29.4–39.1% for CC, TC, and TT genotypes, respectively. The rs9340799 genotype distribution counts 3.5–7.0%, 27.4–35.0%, and 58.6–67.2% for GG, AG, and AA genotype, respectively.

In our study, an association between rs9340799 polymorphism of the *ESR1* gene and BMD was found. The AA genotype individuals had a significantly higher BMD

Table 5 The effect of a treatment type on BMD change

Treatment type	Skeletal site	BMD before treatment	BMD after treatment	BMD difference after treatment	Sig. (*P* value)
HT	FN T-score	−2.132 ± 0.044	−1.784 ± 0.041	0.347 ± 0.043	0.001
	FN BMD	0.603 ± 0.06	0.649 ± 0.05	0.046 ± 0.05 (+ 7.3%)	0.001
	LS T-score	−2.871 ± 0.044	− 2.184 ± 0.048	0.687 ± 0.057	0.001
	LS BMD	0.674 ± 0.005	0.755 ± 0.005	0.081 ± 0.006 (+ 11.3%)	0.001
raloxifene	FN T-score	−2.155 ± 0.059	−1.913 ± 0.078	0.242 ± 0.070	0.002
	FN BMD	0.597 ± 0.008	0.635 ± 0.010	0.038 ± 0.009 (+ 5.2%)	0.002
	LS T-score	−2.947 ± 0.054	−2.484 ± 0.070	0.463 ± 0.063	0.001
	LS BMD	0.670 ± 0.007	0.725 ± 0.008	0.055 ± 0.007 (+ 7.7%)	0.001

BMD of femoral neck (FN) and lumbal spine (LS) is expressed as Estimated Marginal Mean ± SE (SE – standard error of the mean) of T-score (FN and LS T-score) and g/cm^2 (FN and LS BMD); HT – hormone therapy (17ß estradiol/progesterone); Sig. – significance of BMD difference after treatment, P values determine significant differences ($P < 0.05$)

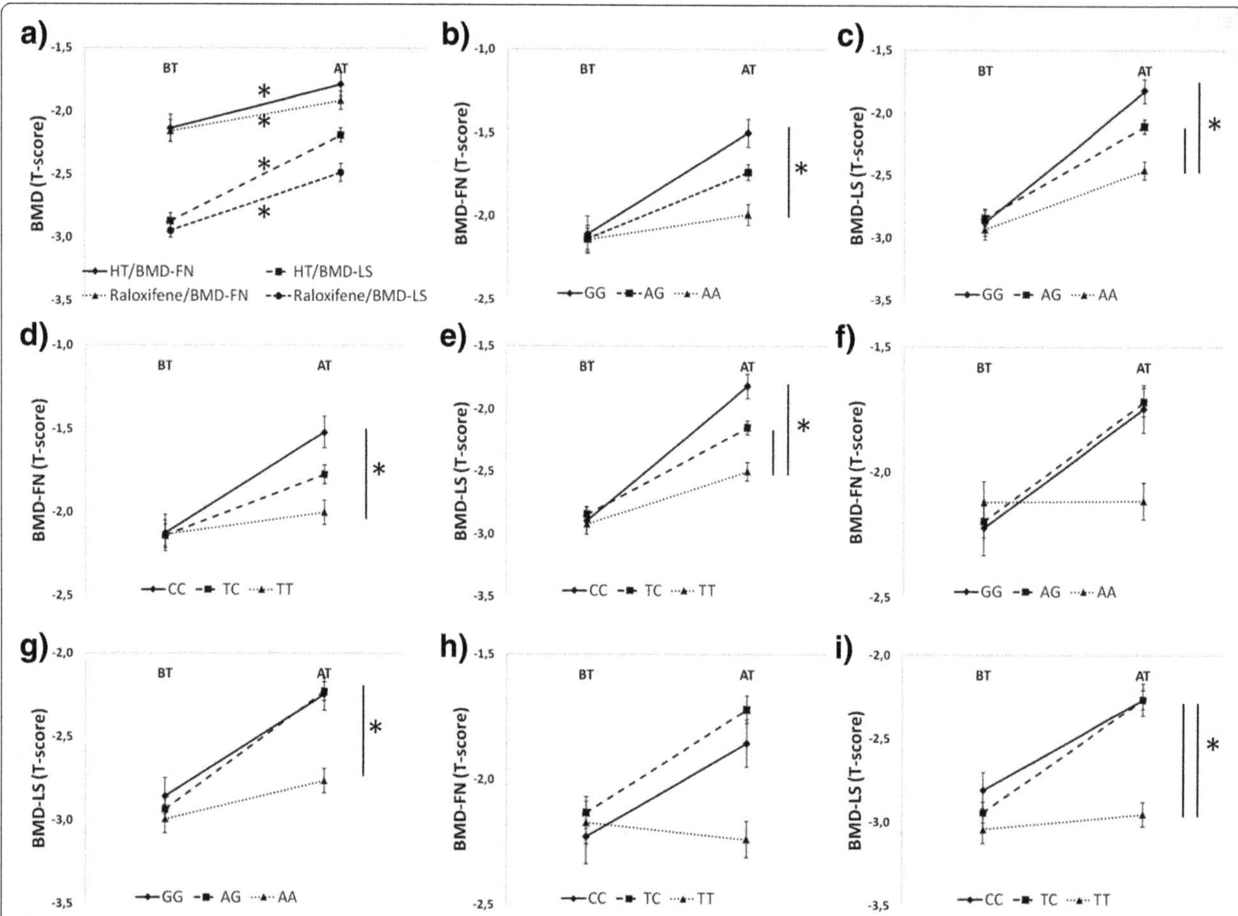

Fig. 2 Effects of the treatment on BMD change. **a** effect of a treatment type on BMD-FN and BMD-LS change; **b-e** effect of HT on BMD-FN and BMD-LS change according to the rs2234693 and rs9340799 genotypes; **f-i** effect of raloxifene treatment on BMD-FN and BMD-LS change according to the rs2234693 and rs9340799 genotypes; BT – before treatment; AT – after treatment; * indicates significant differences ($P < 0.05$)

values compared to AG + GG genotypes. Previous association studies, involving different populations, have produced inconsistent results. In most studies of Caucasian populations, significant associations of rs2234693 and rs9340799 polymorphisms and BMD have not been recorded [31, 32]. Higher BMD-FN was revealed in women from the United States, who were homozygous for C and G alleles of the *ESR1* gene [13]. Van Meurs et al. [10] investigated the impact of rs2234693/rs9340799 haplotypes on BMD in a large population sample of white postmenopausal women, and found a significant association of the TA haplotype with a decreased BMD-LS, whereas the CG haplotype was associated with an increased BMD-LS; no association was found with BMD-FN. In addition, Albagha et al. [26] analysed white women from the United Kingdom, and found that only the CA haplotype was associated with lower values of BMD. Inconsistent results of association studies can be observable also in Asian populations [28–30]. A meta-analysis of 30 studies published by Ioannidis et al. [33] showed a positive effect of GG genotype on BMD and fracture risk, whereas rs2234693 polymorphism was not associated with these traits. In a recent review and meta-analysis of Zhu et al. [34] the authors found significant associations of *ESR1* polymorphisms with BMD in Caucasian women. The GG and AG genotypes were associated with increased FN BMD and FN Z value, respectively. These genotypes also had a higher LS Z value in comparison with AA genotype. CC genotype was associated with a low LS Z value, TC genotype in osteoporotic women was significantly correlated with low FN Z value. The discrepancies between different studies and populations can be explained by ethnic differences or higher variability in studied samples (peri-, pre-, post-menopausal women, multiple pregnancies, different sample size). Interactions between *ESR1* gene and other genetic polymorphisms should also be considered [29, 35].

We did not find any association between *ESR1* genotypes and a presence of fractures. Within a meta-analysis of Tang et al. [36], rs2234693/T allele was strongly identified as a significant risk factor for hip fracture among Caucasian populations, but not in Asian ones. However, in addition to BMD, genetic factors may contribute to

Table 6 BMD changes after hormone therapy in relation to the rs9340799 and rs2234693 genotypes

Genotypes	Skeletal site	BMD before treatment	BMD after treatment	BMD difference after treatment	GLM Sig. (*P* value)	PC Sig. (*P* value)
rs9340799:A > G genotypes						
GG	FN T-score	−2.108 ± 0.106	−1.500 ± 0.082	0.608 ± 0.090	0.001	
	FN BMD	0.605 ± 0.013	0.678 ± 0.010	0.073 ± 0.011 (+ 12.6%)	0.001	
AG	FN T-score	−2.138 ± 0.063	−1.738 ± 0.049	0.400 ± 0.061	0.001	
	FN BMD	0.601 ± 0.008	0.649 ± 0.006	0.048 ± 0.007 (+ 8.4%)	0.001	
AA	FN T-score	−2.141 ± 0.082	−1.991 ± 0.063	0.150 ± 0.066	0.035	
	FN BMD	0.601 ± 0.010	0.619 ± 0.008	0.018 ± 0.008 (+ 3.4%)	0.035	
GG-AG	FN T-score			0.134 ± 0.952	0.042 for FN T-score and FN BMD	NS
	FN BMD			0.016 ± 0.011		NS
GG-AA	FN T-score			0.262 ± 0.103		0.035
	FN BMD			0.031 ± 0.012		0.035
AG-AA	FN T-score			0.128 ± 0.795		NS
	FN BMD			0.015 ± 0.010		NS
GG	LS T-score	−2.877 ± 0.109	−1.823 ± 0.094	1.054 ± 0.053	0.001	
	LS BMD	0.675 ± 0.012	0.788 ± 0.010	0.113 ± 0.006 (+ 16.9%)	0.001	
AG	LS T-score	−2.843 ± 0.064	− 2.105 ± 0.056	0.738 ± 0.073	0.001	
	LS BMD	0.679 ± 0.007	0.758 ± 0.006	0.079 ± 0.008 (+ 11.9%)	0.001	
AA	LS T-score	−2.932 ± 0.083	− 2.459 ± 0.073	0.473 ± 0.125	0.001	
	LS BMD	0.669 ± 0.009	0.720 ± 0.008	0.051 ± 0.013 (+ 8.3%)	0.001	
GG-AG	LS T-score			0.124 ± 0.092	0.002 for FN T-score and FN BMD	NS
	LS BMD			0.013 ± 0.010		NS
GG-AA	LS T-score			0.345 ± 0.100		0.003
	LS BMD			0.037 ± 0.011		0.003
AG-AA	LS T-score			0.221 ± 0.077		0.014
	LS BMD			0.024 ± 0.008		0.014
rs2234693:T > C genotypes						
CC	FN T-score	−2.124 ± 0.093	−1.518 ± 0.072	0.606 ± 0.081	0.001	
	FN BMD	0.603 ± 0.011	0.676 ± 0.09	0.073 ± 0.010 (+ 12.6%)	0.001	
TC	FN T-score	−2.139 ± 0.064	−1.772 ± 0.049	0.367 ± 0.058	0.001	
	FN BMD	0.601 ± 0.008	0.645 ± 0.006	0.044 ± 0.007 (+ 7.7%)	0.001	
TT	FN T-score	−2.132 ± 0.088	−2.000 ± 0.068	0.132 ± 0.077	NS	
	FN BMD	0.602 ± 0.011	0.618 ± 0.008	0.016 ± 0.009 (+ 3.0%)	NS	
CC-TC	FN T-score				NS for FN T-score and FN BMD	
	FN BMD					
CC-TT	FN T-score					
	FN BMD					
TC-TT	FN T-score					
	FN BMD					
CC	LS T-score	−2.894 ± 0.095	−1.818 ± 0.079	1.077 ± 0.067	0.001	
	LS BMD	0.673 ± 0.010	0.789 ± 0.008	0.115 ± 0.007 (+ 17.4%)	0.001	
TC	LS T-score	−2.844 ± 0.065	−2.147 ± 0.054	0.697 ± 0.064	0.001	
	LS BMD	0.679 ± 0.007	0.753 ± 0.006	0.075 ± 0.007 (+ 11.2%)	0.001	
TT	LS T-score	−2.921 ± 0.090	− 2.500 ± 0.075	0.421 ± 0.146	0.010	
	LS BMD	0.670 ± 0.010	0.715 ± 0.008	0.045 ± 0.016 (+ 7.6%)	0.010	

Table 6 BMD changes after hormone therapy in relation to the rs9340799 and rs2234693 genotypes *(Continued)*

Genotypes	Skeletal site	BMD before treatment	BMD after treatment	BMD difference after treatment	GLM Sig. (*P* value)	PC Sig. (*P* value)
CC-TC	LS T-score			0.140 ± 0.083	0.001 for FN T-score and FN BMD	NS
	LS BMD			0.015 ± 0.009		NS
CC-TT	LS T-score			0.354 ± 0.094		0.001
	LS BMD			0.038 ± 0.010		0.001
TC-TT	LS T-score			0.215 ± 0.080		0.026
	LS BMD			0.023 ± 0.009		0.026

BMD of femoral neck (FN) and lumbal spine (LS) is expressed as Estimated Marginal Mean ± *SE* (SE – standard error of the mean) of T-score (FN and LS T-score) and g/cm^2 (FN and LS BMD), *GLM Sig.* – significance of GLM, *PC Sig.* – significance of pairwise comparisons, *NS* – non-significant GLM/BMD differences, *P* values determine significant BMD differences ($P < 0.05$)

fracture risk through mechanisms other than bone mass. These factors can include various skeletal characteristics like bone size and shape, cortical porosity, trabecular microarchitecture, and osteocyte cell function that may not be well captured by BMD measurements alone [37]. Some studies point to the importance of bone micro-damage accumulation in the initiation of bone resorption and remodeling [38]. It would be perspective to include these factors into analyses in relation to fractures. Moreover, BMD changes have a long-term character, while bone turnover markers can directly infer about processes in bone tissue (formation/resorption). In our study, no differences in bone turnover markers between *ESR1* genotypes were observed. In recent years, large genome-wide association studies (GWAS) have brought new insights into the genetics of osteoporosis. Some of the studies replicated previously reported candidate genes (including the *ESR1* gene) in association with BMD and fracture risk [3]. The largest meta-analysis [39] included 17 genome-wide association studies with individuals of European and East Asian ancestry and identified 56 loci (with 24 reported previously) associated with BMD variation and 14 loci associated with risk of fracture. Further studies should be directed towards polymorphisms that have shown significant results in genome-wide association studies to evaluate their effect in specific populations.

Pharmacogenetic research has a potential to allow efficacious treatments, with consequent better chances for the patient health and reduced economic loss [40]. In our study, the effect of rs2234693 and rs9340799 polymorphisms on antiosteoporotic treatment efficiency was revealed. Similar outcomes, where genotypes with C or G alleles were associated with greater sensitivity to HT, have been documented in other studies. Salmen et al. [19] analysed Finnish postmenopausal women during 5-years of HT. They found that women with the TT genotype had a greater fracture risk in comparison with C allele carriers. In study of Giguere et al. [41], women with combined *VDR*-bb/*ESR1*-CC genotype who received HT for more than 5 years, had a 21% greater ultrasound heel stiffness index z score (comparable with BMD scores) than those with the same genotype receiving HT for less than 5 years. The study included post-menopausal women of French-Canadian origin. Rapuri et al. [20] reported significantly higher BMD response to HT treatment in women with the CC genotype compared to TT genotype. Similar findings with a positive effect of the C allele on vertebral BMD were found in the study by Ongphiphadhanakul et al. [21]. Subjects consisted of Thai post-menopausal women and the effect was not found on femoral BMD. Greater increase in lumbar spine BMD was recorded in CC genotypes in postmenopausal Japanese women [12]. No differences in HT efficiency have also been demonstrated in other studies [42, 43].

SERMs have the ability to bind to the estrogen receptor and act as a receptor agonist or antagonist in a tissue-specific manner. Raloxifene (the estrogen receptor agonist in bone) was the first SERM approved for the prevention and treatment of postmenopausal osteoporosis [44]. According to our results, individuals with CC or TC genotypes of rs2234693 and AG genotype of rs9340799 better responded on raloxifene therapy with higher BMD-LS changes in comparison with homozygous TT or AA genotypes. Similarly, postmenopausal osteoporotic women with the CC or AA genotypes on chronic hemodialysis exhibited a better lumbar spine BMD response in a study by Heilberg et al. [45]. Higher increase in total hip BMD was also noticed in postmenopausal women with osteoporosis carrying CC or TC genotypes [46]. Positive efficacy of raloxifene on BMD was also monitored in relation to other genes [47, 48].

Focusing on the percent change in BMD, a very high treatment efficacy in our study is remarkable, reaching up to 11.3 and 7.7% for HT and raloxifene in LS site, respectively. A meta-analysis of Wells et al. [49] showed a BMD-LS gain of 8% using high-dose estrogen (equivalent to 0.9 mg Premarin) during 2 years. The BMD-LS improvement after raloxifene therapy usually reaches around 2.5% after 2 years [50]. Several factors may contribute to the differences between studies. From the

Table 7 BMD changes after raloxifene therapy in relation to the rs9340799 and rs2234693 genotypes

Genotype	Skeletal site	BMD before treatment	BMD after treatment	BMD difference after treatment	GLM Sig. (*P* value)	PC Sig. (*P* value)
GG	FN T-score	−2.222 ± 0.160	−1.744 ± 0.201	0.478 ± 0.105	0.002	
	FN BMD	0.591 ± 0.019	0.649 ± 0.024	0.057 ± 0.013 (+ 10.2%)	0.002	
AG	FN T-score	−2.196 ± 0.100	−1.717 ± 0.126	0.478 ± 0.157	0.006	
	FN BMD	0.595 ± 0.012	0.652 ± 0.015	0.057 ± 0.019 (+ 9.9%)	0.006	
AA	FN T-score	−2.119 ± 0.086	−2.113 ± 0.108	0.006 ± 0.058	NS	
	FN BMD	0.604 ± 0.010	0.604 ± 0.013	0.001 ± 0.007 (+ 0.46%)	NS	
GG-AG	FN T-score				NS for FN T-score and FN BMD	
	FN BMD					
GG-AA	FN T-score					
	FN BMD					
AG-AA	FN T-score					
	FN BMD					
GG	LS T-score	−2.856 ± 0.145	−2.244 ± 0.167	0.611 ± 0.082	0.001	
	LS BMD	0.677 ± 0.016	0.743 ± 0.018	0.065 ± 0.009 (+ 9.7%)	0.001	
AG	LS T-score	−2.935 ± 0.091	−2.226 ± 0.105	0.709 ± 0.087	0.001	
	LS BMD	0.669 ± 0.010	0.745 ± 0.011	0.076 ± 0.009 (+ 11.5%)	0.001	
AA	LS T-score	−2.994 ± 0.078	−2.765 ± 0.090	0.229 ± 0.094	0.021	
	LS BMD	0.663 ± 0.008	0.687 ± 0.010	0.025 ± 0.010 (+ 4.1%)	0.021	
GG-AG	LS T-score			0.030 ± 0.161	0.016 for FN T-score and FN BMD	NS
	LS BMD			0.003 ± 0.017		NS
GG-AA	LS T-score			0.329 ± 0.155		NS
	LS BMD			0.035 ± 0.017		NS
AG-AA	LS T-score			0.299 ± 0.113		0.028
	LS BMD			0.032 ± 0.012		0.028
CC	FN T-score	−2.227 ± 0.145	−1.855 ± 0.177	0.373 ± 0.093	0.002	
	FN BMD	0.591 ± 0.017	0.635 ± 0.021	0.045 ± 0.092 (+ 7.8%)	0.002	
TC	FN T-score	−2.132 ± 0.086	−1.719 ± 0.106	0.413 ± 0.124	0.002	
	FN BMD	0.602 ± 0.010	0.652 ± 0.013	0.050 ± 0.015 (+ 8.6%)	0.002	
TT	FN T-score	−2.171 ± 0.105	−2.238 ± 0.128	0.067 ± 0.060	NS	
	FN BMD	0.597 ± 0.013	0.589 ± 0.015	−0.008 ± 0.007 (−1.0%)	NS	
CC-TC	FN T-score				NS for FN T-score and FN BMD	
	FN BMD					
CC-TT	FN T-score					
	FN BMD					
TC-TT	FN T-score					
	FN BMD					
CC	LS T-score	−2.809 ± 0.130	−2.264 ± 0.140	0.546 ± 0.092	0.001	0.001
	LS BMD	0.682 ± 0.014	0.741 ± 0.015	0.058 ± 0.010 (+ 8.6%)	0.001	0.001
TC	LS T-score	−2.942 ± 0.077	−2.265 ± 0.084	0.677 ± 0.074	0.001	0.001
	LS BMD	0.668 ± 0.008	0.741 ± 0.009	0.073 ± 0.008 (+ 11.0%)	0.001	0.001
TT	LS T-score	−3.043 ± 0.094	−2.952 ± 0.102	0.091 ± 0.114	NS	NS
	LS BMD	0.657 ± 0.010	0.667 ± 0.011	0.010 ± 0.012 (+ 2.0%)	NS	NS

Table 7 BMD changes after raloxifene therapy in relation to the rs9340799 and rs2234693 genotypes *(Continued)*

Genotype	Skeletal site	BMD before treatment	BMD after treatment	BMD difference after treatment	GLM Sig. (*P* value)	PC Sig. (*P* value)
CC-TC	LS T-score			0.067 ± 0.137	0.001 for FN T-score and FN BMD	NS
	LS BMD			0.007 ± 0.015		NS
CC-TT	LS T-score			0.461 ± 0.145		0.007
	LS BMD			0.049 ± 0.016		0.007
TC-TT	LS T-score			0.394 ± 0.110		0.002
	LS BMD			0.042 ± 0.012		0.002

BMD of femoral neck (FN) and lumbal spine (LS) is expressed as Estimated Marginal Mean ± *SE* (SE – standard error of the mean) of T-score (FN and LS T-score) and g/cm^2 (FN and LS BMD); GLM Sig. – significance of GLM, *PC Sig.* – significance of pairwise comparisons, *NS* – non-significant GLM/BMD differences, *P* values determine significant BMD differences ($P < 0.05$)

point of view of our study, we can consider especially limited sample size, differences from other studies in BMD baseline, population composition, or inclusion criteria (e.g. adequacy of calcium/vitamin D intake, previous anti-resorptive treatment). The effect of a therapy was also found to be a dose and time dependent.

Considering limitations of our study, the small sample size seems to be the most important. Despite the ability to calculate optimal sample size, the number of observations is often dependent on the existing economic and human resources or the time available for carrying out the study. The observed power for our study, where the model was significant, ranged from 69 to 73% and from 78 to 94% for association and pharmacogenetic analyses, respectively. Moreover, the revealed effects of the polymorphisms cannot be confirmed on the molecular level. The mechanisms by which the polymorphisms may influence bone mass are still not clear, since these polymorphisms lie in an intronic area of the gene. However, a study of Herrington et al. [51] showed that a functional binding site for the transcription factor B-myb is absent with the T allele, which, in turn, may reduce *ESR1* transcription rates or produce a functionally different ESR1 isoform. It has also been demonstrated that the *ESR1* gene expression can be regulated by epigenetic mechanisms [52]. Moreover, there is still the possibility that both polymorphisms are only linkage markers and the effect itself is caused by another, closely related region of the *ESR1* gene. In any case, all the mechanisms may also be the cause of different impacts of individual polymorphisms on the analysed parameters. Other limitations can involve gene-gene and gene-environment interactions, or epigenetic factors which could influence the pharmacodynamics and pharmacokinetics of individual drug response [18]. Nevertheless, the pharmacogenetic research is promising, especially for osteoporosis, that require long-term treatments and where different therapy types exist to be alternatively chosen.

Conclusion

We found that rs9340799 polymorphism may contribute to decreased BMD in postmenopausal women from southern Slovakia, whereas rs2234693 polymorphism did not affect any of the analyzed parameters. The *ESR1* gene was not significantly related to fracture prevalence. Our study also demonstrated the effect of both *ESR1* gene polymorphisms on the effectiveness of HT (17ß estradiol/progesterone), as well as SERMs/raloxifene therapies with poorer response in patients with rs2234693/TT and rs9340799/AA genotypes. The results can contribute to a more comprehensive insight to the genetics and pharmacogenetics of osteoporosis. The evaluation of effects of previously revealed candidate genes in specific populations may get closer to the practical use of results in predictive genetics and personalized medicine.

Abbreviations

ALP: Bone isoenzyme of alkaline phosphatase; BMD: Bone mineral density; BMD-FN: Femoral neck bone mineral density; BMD-LS: Lumbar spine bone mineral density; BMI: Body mass index; BPs: Bisphosphonates; CI: Confidence interval; CTx: Beta CrossLaps; *ESR1*: Estrogen receptor 1 gene; FN: Femoral neck; GLM: General linear model; GWAS: Genome-wide association studies; HT: Hormone therapy; HWE: Hardy-Weinberg equilibrium; LS: Lumbar spine; NS: Non-significant; OC: Osteocalcin; OR: The odds ratio; PC Sig.: Significance of pairwise comparisons; PCR: Polymerase chain reaction; sCa: serum calcium; SE: Standard error of the mean; SERMs: Selective estrogen receptor modulators; Sig. Cov.: Significance of covariates; Sig.: Significance; sP: serum phosphate; *VDR*: Vitamin D receptor gene

Funding

The study was supported by the projects VEGA 1/0505/18 and KEGA 031UKF-4/2016.

Authors' contributions

The conception and design of the work: RO, VM. Performed the experiments: VM, MA, ML, RB. The acquisition and interpretation of data: RO, VM, DG, BG, MM. Drafting the work or revising it critically for important intellectual content: RO, VM, MA, BG, MM. Final approval of the version to be published: RO, VM, MA, ML, RB, BG, DG, MM. All authors read and approved the final manuscript.

Competing interests

The authors declare that they have no competing interests.

Author details

[1]Department of Botany and Genetics, Constantine the Philosopher University in Nitra, Nitra, Slovak Republic. [2]Institute of Zoology and Anthropology, Georg-August University, Göttingen, Germany. [3]Department of Zoology and Anthropology, Constantine the Philosopher University in Nitra, Nitra, Slovak Republic. [4]Private Orthopedic Ambulance, Nitra, Slovak Republic.

References

1. Ralston SH, Uitterlinden AG. Genetics of osteoporosis. Endocr Rev. 2010; 31(5):629–62.
2. Ralston SH. Genetic determinants of susceptibility to osteoporosis. Curr Opin Pharmacol. 2003;3(3):286–90.
3. Duncan EL, Danoy P, Kemp JP, Leo PJ, McCloskey E, Nicholson GC, Eastell R, Prince RL, Eisman JA, Jones G, Sambrook PN, Reid IR, Dennison EM, Wark J, Richards JB, Uitterlinden AG, Spector TD, Esapa C, Cox RD, Brown SD, Thakker RV, Addison KA, Bradbury LA, Center JR, Cooper C, Cremin C, Estrada K, Felsenberg D, Glüer CC, Hadler J, Henry MJ, Hofman A, Kotowicz MA, Makovey J, Nguyen SC, Nguyen TV, Pasco JA, Pryce K, Reid DM, Rivadeneira F, Roux C, Stefansson K, Styrkarsdottir U, Thorleifsson G, Tichawangana R, Evans DM, Brown MA. Genome-wide association study using extreme truncate selection identifies novel genes affecting bone mineral density and fracture risk. PLoS Genet. 2011;7(4):e1001372. https://doi.org/10.1371/journal.pgen.1001372.
4. Wang C, Zhang Z, Zhang H, He JW, Gu JM, Hu WW, Hu YQ, Li M, Liu YJ, Fu WZ, Yue H, Ke YH, Zhang ZL. Susceptibility genes for osteoporotic fracture in postmenopausal Chinese women. J Bone Miner Res. 2012;27(12):2582–91.
5. Eastell R. Pathogenesis in postmenopausal osteoporosis. In: Murray JF & Associate editors: Primer on the metabolic bone diseases and disorders of mineral metabolism. USA: American society for bone and mineral research; 6th. 2006. p. 259–262.
6. Gennari L, Merlotti D, De Paola V, Calabró A, Becherini L, Martini G, Nuti R. Estrogen receptor gene polymorphisms and the genetics of osteoporosis: a HuGE review. Am J Epidemiol. 2005;161(4):307–20.
7. Gennari L, De Paola V, Merlotti D, Martini G, Nuti R. Steroid hormone receptor gene polymorphisms and osteoporosis: a pharmacogenomic review. Expert Opin Pharmacother. 2007;8(5):537–53.
8. Rooney AM, Van der Meulen MCH. Mouse models to evaluate the role of estrogen receptor α in skeletal maintenance and adaptation. Ann N Y Acad Sci. 2017;1410(1):85–92.
9. Becherini L, Gennari L, Masi L, Mansani R, Massart F, Morreli A, Falchetti AA, Gonelii S, Fiorelli G, Tanini A. Evidence of a linkage disequilibrium between polymorhism in the human estrogene receptor alpha gene and their relationship to bone mass variation in postmenopausal Italian woman. Hum Mol Genet. 2000;9(13):2043–50.
10. Van Maeurs JB, Schui SC, Weel AE. Associations of 5′ estrogen receptor alpha gene polymorphism with bone mineral density, vertebral bone area and fracture risk. Hum Mol Genet. 2003;12(14):1745–54.
11. Kobayashi N, Inoue S, Hosoi T, Ouchi Y, Shiraki M, Orimo H. Association of bone mineral density with polymorphism of the estrogen receptor gene. J Bone Miner Res. 1996;11(3):306–11.
12. Kobayashi N, Fujino T, Shirogane T, Furuta I, Kobamatsu Y, Yaegashi M, Sakuragi N, Fujimoto S. Estrogen receptor alpha polymorphism as a genetic marker for bone loss, vertebral fractures and susceptibility to estrogen. Maturitas. 2002;41(3):193–201.
13. Sowers TD, Jannausch ML, Liang W, Willing M. Estrogen receptor genotypes and their associations with the 10-years changes in bone mineral density and osteocalcin concentrations. J Clin Endocrin Metab. 2004;89(2):733–9.
14. Jeedigunta Y, Reddy PRB, Kolla VK, Munshi A, Anathapur V, Narasimilu G, Akka J. Association of estrogen receptor α gene polymorphisms with BMD and their affect on estradiol levels in pre- and postmenopusal woman in south Indian population from Andhra Pradesh. Clin Chim Acta. 2010;411(7–8):597–600.
15. Kurt O, Yilmaz-Aydogan H, Uyar M, Isbir T, Seyhan MF, Can A. Evaluation of ERα and VDR gene polymorphisms in relation to bone mineral density in Turkish postmenopausal women. Mol Biol Rep. 2012;39(6):6723–30.
16. Chen JS, Sambrook PN. Antiresorptive therapies for osteoporosis: a clinical overview. Nat Rev Endocrinol. 2012;8(2):81–91.
17. Pickar JH, Komm BS. Selective estrogen receptor modulators and the combination therapy conjugated estrogens/bazedoxifene: a review of effects on the breast. Post Reprod Health. 2015;21(3):112–21.
18. Marini F, Brandi ML. Pharmacogenetics of osteoporosis. Best Pract Res Clin Endocrinol Metab. 2014;28(6):783–93.
19. Salmen T, Heikkinen AM, Mahonen A, Kroger H, Komulainen M, Saarikoski S, Honkanen R, Maenpaa PH. Early postmenopausal bone loss is associated with Pvu II estrogen receptor gene polymorphism in Finnish woman: effect of hormone replacement therapy. J Bone Miner Res. 2000;15(2):315–21.
20. Rapuri P, Gallagher J, Knezetic J, Haynatzka V. Estrogen receptor alpha gene polymorphisms are associated with changes in bone remodeling markers and treatment response to estrogen. Maturitas. 2006;53(4):371–9.
21. Ongphiphadhanakul B, Chanprasertyothin S, Payatikul P, Tung SS, Piaseu N, Chailurkit L, Chansirikarn S, Puavilai G, Rajatanavin R. Oestrogen-receptor-alpha gene polymorphism affects response in bone mineral density to oestrogen in post-menopausal women. Clin Endocrinol. 2000;52(5):581–5.
22. Pavone V, Testa G, Giardina SMC, Vescio A, Restivo DA, Sessa G. Pharmacological therapy of osteoporosis: a systematic current review of literature. Front Pharmacol. 2017;8:803.
23. Nguyen TV, Eisman JA. Pharmacogenomics of osteoporosis: opportunities and challenges. J Musculoskelet Neuronal Interact. 2006;6:62–72.
24. Csákyová V, Szécsényi-Nagy A, Csősz A, Nagy M, Fusek G, Langó P, Bauer M, Mende BG, Makovický P, Bauerová M. Maternal genetic composition of a medieval population from a Hungarian-Slavic contact zone in Central Europe. PLoS One. 2016;11(3):e0151206. https://doi.org/10.1371/journal.pone.0151206 eCollection 2016.
25. D'Alonzo KT. The Johnson-Neyman procedure as an alternative to ANCOVA. West J Nurs Res. 2004;26(7):804–12.
26. Albagha OM, McGuigan FE, Reid DM, Ralston SH. Estrogen receptor alpha gene plymorphism and bone mineral density: haplotype analysis in woman from the UnitedKingdom. J Bone Min Res. 2001;16(1):128–34.
27. Bustamante M, Nogués X, Enjuanes A, Elosua R, García-Giralt N, Pérez-Edo L, Cáceres E, Carreras R, Mellibovsky L, Balcells S, Díez-Pérez A, Grinberg D. COL1A1, ESR1, VDR and TGFB1 polymorphisms and haplotypes in relation to BMD in Spanish postmenopausal women. Osteoporos Int. 2007;18(2):235–43.
28. Matsushita H, Kurabayashi T, Tomita M, Tanaka K. Effects of vitamin D and estrogen receptor gene polymorphisms on the changes in lumbar bone mineral density with multiple pregnancies in Japanese women. Hum Reprod. 2004;19(1):59–64.
29. Nam HS, Shin MH, Kweon SS, Park KS, Sohn SJ, Rhee JA, Choi JS, Son MH. Association of estrogen alpha receptor gene polymorphism with bone mineral density in Korean women. J Bone Min Metab. 2005;23(1):84–5.
30. Dai X, Wang C, Dai J, Shi D, Xu Z, Chen D, Teng H, Jiang Q. Association of single nucleotide polymorphisms in estrogen receptor alpha gene with susceptibility to knee osteoarthritis: a case-control study in a Chinese Han population. Biomed Res Int. 2014;2014:151457.
31. Bagger YZ, Jorgensen HL, Heegard AM, Bayer L, Hansen L, Hassager C. No major effect of estrogen receptor gene polymorphisms on bone mineral density of bone loss in postmenopausal Danish women. Bone. 2000;26(2):111–6.
32. Tanriover MD, Tatar GB, Uluturk TD, Erden DD, Tanriover A, Kilicarlslan A, Oz SG, Yurter HE, Sozen T, Guven GS. Evaluation of the effects of vitamin D receptor and estrogen receptor 1 gene polymorphisms on bone mineral density in postmenopausal women. Clin Rheumatol. 2010; 29(11):1285–93.
33. Ioannidis JP, Stavrou I, Trikalinos TA, Zois C, Brandi ML, Gennari L, Albagha O, Ralston SH, Tsatsoulis A. ER-alpha genetics meta-analysis. Association of polymorphisms of the estrogen receptor alpha gene with bone mineral density and fracture risk in women: a meta-analysis. J Bone Miner Res. 2002; 17(11):2048–60.
34. Zhu H, Jiang J, Wang Q, Zong J, Zhang L, Ma T, Xu Y, Zhang L. Associations between ERα/β gene polymorphisms and osteoporosis susceptibility and bone mineral density in postmenopausal women: a systematic review and meta-analysis. BMC Endocr Disord. 2018;18(1):11.
35. Correa-Rodríguez M, Viatte S, Massey J, Schmidt-RioValle J, Rueda-Medina B, Orozco G. Analysis of SNP-SNP interactions and bone quantitative ultrasound parameter in early adulthood. BMC Med Genet. 2017;18(1):107.
36. Tang L, Cheng GL, Xu ZH. Association between estrogen receptor α gene (ESR1) PvuII (C/T) and XbaI (a/G) polymorphisms and hip fracture risk: evidence from a meta-analysis. PLoS One. 2013;8(12):e82806. https://doi.org/10.1371/journal.pone.0082806.
37. Zmuda JM, Cauley JA, Ferrell RE, Nevitt MC, Feingold E, Ensrud K, Stone KL, Hochberg MC, Harris EL, Cummings SR. Familial resemblance in fall-related risk factors in older woman. Calcif Tissue Int. 2000;67:497.

38. Boyde A. The real response of bone to exercise. J Anat. 2003;203(2):173–89.
39. Estrada K, Styrkarsdottir U, Evangelou E, et al. Genome-wide meta-analysis identifies 56 bone mineral density loci and reveals 14 loci associated with risk of fracture. Nat Genet. 2012;44(5):491–501.
40. Massart F, Brandi ML. Genetics of the bone response to bisphosphonate treatments. Clin Cases Miner Bone Metab. 2009;6(1):50–4.
41. Giguère Y, Dodin S, Blanchet C, Morgan K, Rousseau F. The association between heel ultrasound and hormone replacement therapy is modulated by a two-locus vitamin D and estrogen receptor genotype. J Bone Miner Res. 2000;15(6):1076–84.
42. Silvestri S, Thomsen AB, Gozzini A, Bagger Y, Christiansen C, Brandi ML. Estrogen receptor α and β polymorphisms: is there an association with bone mineral density, plasma lipids, and response to postmenopausal hormone therapy. Menopause. 2006;13(3):451–61.
43. Masi L, Ottanelli S, Berni R, Cacudi E, Giusti F, Marcucci G, Cavalli L, Fossi C, Marini F, Ciuffi S, Tanini A, Brandi ML. CYP19 and ESR1 gene polymorphisms response of the bone mineral density in post-menopausal women to hormonal replacement therapy. Clin Cases Miner Bone Metab. 2014;11(1):36–43.
44. Ettinger B, Black DM, Mitlak BH, Knickerbocker RK, Nickelsen T, Genant HK, Christiansen C, Delmas PD, Zanchetta JR, Stakkestad J, Gluer CC, Krueger K, Cohen FJ, Eckert S, Ensrud KE, Avioli LV, Lips P, Cummings SR. Reduction of vertebral fracture risk in postmenopausal women with osteoporosis treated with raloxifene: results from a 3-year randomized clinical trial. Multiple outcomes of raloxifene evaluation (MORE) investigators. JAMA. 1999;282(7):637–45.
45. Heilberg IP, Hernandez E, Alonzo E, Valera R, Ferreira LG, Gomes SA, Bellorin-Font E, Weisinger JR. Estrogen receptor (ER) gene polymorphism may predict the bone mineral density response to raloxifene in postmenopausal women on chronic hemodialysis. Ren Fail. 2005;27(2):155–61.
46. Zhang ZL, He JW, Qin YJ, Huang QR, Liu YJ, Hu YQ, Li M. Association of bone metabolism related genes polymorphisms with the effect of raloxifene hydrochloride on bone mineral density and bone turnover markers in postmenopausal women with osteoporosis. Zhonghua Yi Xue Yi Chuan Xue Za Zhi. 2006;23(2):129–33.
47. Palomba S, Numis FG, Mossetti G, Rendina D, Vuotto P, Russo T, Zullo F, Nappi C, Nunziata V. Raloxifene administration in post-menopausal women with osteoporosis: effect of different BsmI vitamin D receptor genotypes. Hum Reprod. 2003;18(1):192–8.
48. Mencej-Bedrač S, Zupan J, Mlakar SJ, Zavratnik A, Preželj J, Marc J. Raloxifene pharmacodynamics is influenced by genetic variants in the RANKL/RANK/OPG system and in the Wnt signaling pathway. Drug Metabol Drug Interact. 2014; 29(2):111–4.
49. Wells G, Tugwell P, Shea B, Guyatt G, Peterson J, Zytaruk N, Robinson V, Henry D, O'Connell D. Cranney a; osteoporosis methodology group and the osteoporosis research advisory group. Meta-analyses of therapies for postmenopausal osteoporosis. V. Meta-analysis of the efficacy of hormone replacement therapy in treating and preventing osteoporosis in postmenopausal women. Endocr Rev. 2002;23(4):529–39.
50. Delmas PD, Davis SR, Hensen J, Adami S, van Os S, Nijland EA. Effects of tibolone and raloxifene on bone mineral density in osteopenic postmenopausal women. Osteoporos Int. 2008;19(8):1153–60.
51. Herrington DM, Howard TD, Hawkins GA, Reboussin DM, Xu J, Zheng SL, Brosnihan KB, Meyers DA, Bleecker ER. Estrogen receptor polymorphisms and effects of estrogen replacement on HDL cholesterol in women with coronary disease. N Engl J Med. 2002;346(13):967–74.
52. Lau KM, LaSpina M, Long J, Ho SM. Expression of estrogen receptor (ER)-alpha and ER-beta in normal and malignant prostatic epithelial cells: regulation by methylation and involvement in growth regulation. Cancer Res. 2000;60(12):3175–82.

Multimodal imaging in a pedigree of X-linked Retinoschisis with a novel *RS1* variant

Kirk Stephenson[1*†], Adrian Dockery[2†], Niamh Wynne[3], Matthew Carrigan[2], Paul Kenna[3], G. Jane Farrar[2] and David Keegan[1]

Abstract

Background: To describe the clinical phenotype and genetic cause underlying the disease pathology in a pedigree (affected $n = 9$) with X-linked retinoschisis (XLRS1) due to a novel *RS1* mutation and to assess suitability for novel therapies using multimodal imaging.

Methods: The Irish National Registry for Inherited Retinal Degenerations (Target 5000) is a program including clinical history and examination with multimodal retinal imaging, electrophysiology, visual field testing and genetic analysis. Nine affected patients were identified across 3 generations of an XLRS1 pedigree. DNA sequencing was performed for each patient, one carrier female and one unaffected relative. Pedigree mapping revealed a further 4 affected males.

Results: All affected patients had a history of reduced visual acuity and dyschromatopsia; however, the severity of phenotype varied widely between the nine affected subjects. The stage of disease was classified as previously described. Phenotypic severity was not linearly correlated with age. A novel *RS1* (Xp22.2) mutation was detected (NM_000330: c.413C > A) resulting in a p.Thr138Asn substitution. Protein modelling demonstrated a change in higher order protein folding that is likely pathogenic.

Conclusions: This family has a novel gene mutation in *RS1* with clinical evidence of XLRS1. A proportion of the older generation has developed end-stage macular atrophy; however, the severity is variable. Confirmation of genotype in the affected grandsons of this pedigree in principle may enable them to avail of upcoming gene therapies, provided there is anatomical evidence (from multimodal imaging) of potentially reversible early stage disease.

Keywords: X-linked Retinoschisis, Retinoschisin, Inherited retinal dystrophy, Inherited maculopathy

Background

Target 5000 [1, 2] (Fighting Blindness, Ireland), the Irish National Inherited Retinal Degeneration Registry, aims to phenotype and genotype all patients in Ireland with inherited retinal degenerations (IRD). A concurrent goal of the study is to facilitate the implementation of individualised management plans including, where appropriate, novel therapeutic options for those patients with modifiable disease. This paper is focused on the application of this process for a pedigree with X-Linked Retinoschisis (OMIM: 312700, XLRS1) and the clinical and genetic workup of these patients for potential new therapies and future participation in appropriate trials now emerging for this form of IRD.

XLRS1 is a rare IRD (1:15000–30,000 [3]) due to variants in the *RS1* gene encoding the retinoschisin protein (OMIM: 300839, Xp22.1). XLRS1 is a mutationally heterogeneous disorder with over 230 known variants [4–6], the majority of mutations falling in exons 4–6 (the structurally important discoidin domain of the retinoschisin protein [7]). Congenital poor vision in males is due to macular schisis and results in variable outer retinal atrophy with age. As novel gene therapies are in clinical trials [8, 9], to

* Correspondence: kirkstephenson@hotmail.com
†Kirk Stephenson and Adrian Dockery contributed equally to this work.
1The Catherine McAuley Centre, Mater Private Hospital, Nelson Street, Dublin 7, Ireland
Full list of author information is available at the end of the article

optimise options for patients, confirmation of the presence of an *RS1* variant is essential and moreover must be supplemented with various clinical assays to assess the stage of disease and potential suitability for treatment.

With wide variability in phenotype between and within families [10–12], clinical diagnosis can be challenging. Multimodal imaging has been an excellent addition for confirming phenotype and guiding molecular genetic testing. Optical Coherence Tomography (OCT) imaging may detect intraretinal cystic spaces [13], which may appear in multiple retinal planes. Fundus autofluorescence (AF) imaging can detect subtle patterns of change in the retinal pigment epithelium (RPE), which allows staging of severity [14]. Microperimetry can delineate areas of residual function [15]. Thus, multimodal imaging can be used to demonstrate maintenance of anatomy which may determine suitability for novel treatments.

The *RS1* genomic location was first implicated as pathogenic using multipoint linkage analysis of Dutch families affected by XLRS1 [16]. Locus localization was later refined and the *RS1* gene was identified by positional cloning. Mapping and expression analysis led to the discovery of the then novel transcript (XLRS1) [17] encoding the retinoschisin protein.

Retinoschisin, a 224 amino acid protein, is secreted from photoreceptors and bipolar cells in retina and has been shown to be crucial for cell adhesion during retinal development [18]. It has been suggested that retinoschisin may also be involved in mitogen-activated protein kinase signaling and apoptosis in retina [18] and recently has been shown to influence Na/K-ATPase signaling and localization [19]. Employing cryo-electron microscopy, it has been discovered that functional retinoschisin forms a dimer of octamer rings comprising a hexadecamer. Given this intricate structure, a mutation that affects the folded structure of the RS1 protein monomer is likely to inhibit the proper assembly of the 16-subunit oligomer [20, 21] as evidenced by the large number of reported pathogenic mutations [5]. Pathogenic RS1 mutations are typically associated with XLRS1, although some mutations show greater phenotypic variability than others, including greater ranges of onset age and severity of condition [12].

Methods

Clinical phenotyping

A large pedigree with a clinical diagnosis of XLRS1 was invited to participate given informed consent. Nine affected males (7 adults, 2 children), one carrier female and one unaffected male attended the recruiting hospitals as specified above to take part in the IRD registry (Fig. 1).

Phenotyping included an ophthalmic and medical history, pedigree mapping, and dilated ophthalmic examination. Colour photography, autofluorescence (AF, Optos plc, Scotland) and spectral domain optical coherence tomography (SD-OCT, Cirrus HD-OCT, Carl Zeiss Meditec AG, CA, USA) images were acquired. This multimodal imaging was assessed and the macular findings were categorised into their appropriate stages. Stage was assessed by individual eye, not entire patient.

DNA isolation and next generation sequencing

Blood samples were taken from patients after clinical assessment. DNA was isolated from 2 ml of blood and fragmented for targeted sequencing to an average fragment size of 200–250 base pairs. Sequencing libraries were generated and target capture was performed with the Nimblegen SeqCap EZ kit (Roche), incorporating the exonic regions of over 200 genes implicated in IRDs. Capture regions also included intronic regions in the CEP290, ABCA4 and USH2A genes that are known to potentially contain pathogenic mutations [22–24]. The total size of the captured region was approximately 750 kb.

Captured patient DNA was multiplexed into 24-sample pools and sequenced using an Illumina MiSeq. Confirmatory single-read sequencing was also performed to verify the presence of candidate mutations.

Polymerase chain reaction and sanger sequencing

To validate the *RS1* variant identified by NGS, an amplicon for direct Sanger sequencing was designed incorporating the variant. The sequence used for primer design was Human reference transcript NM_000330.3. Forward primer: 5′- GCAGATGATCCACTGTGCTG – 3′. Reverse primer: 5′ - TTTCTTGGGAGGTGGAGATG – 3′. Oligonucleotides were purchased from Sigma-Aldrich (www.sigmaaldrich.com/). The target DNA products were

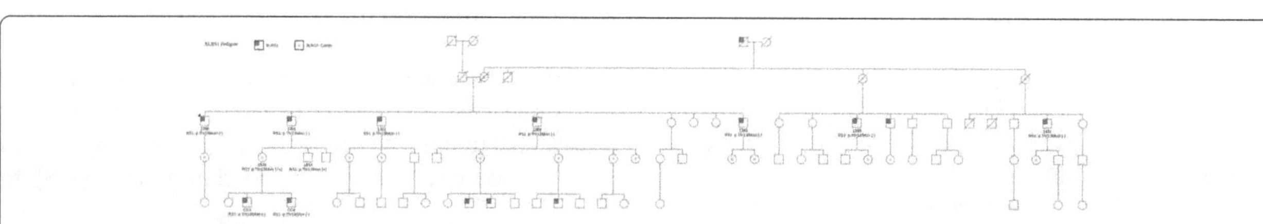

Fig. 1 Pedigree of 5 generations of an XLRS1 pedigree. Individuals marked with a red square were confirmed to be clinically affected. *RS1* genotype has been annotated within the pedigree tree for those investigated

amplified using Q5 High-Fidelity 2x Master Mix (New England Biolabs Inc). The annealing temperature for reactions was 65 °C; all other details were executed as per the supplier's recommendations. PCR products were purified using the GeneJET Gel Extraction Kit (Thermo Fisher Scientific). Sanger sequencing was performed by Eurofins Genomics (www.eurofinsgenomics.eu).

Data analysis

Data obtained from NGS was subsequently demultiplexed and mapped to the human genome (hg38) using BWA version 0.7.15 [25]. Duplicate reads were flagged using Picard version 2.5.0 [26] and downstream analysis and variant calling performed using Freebayes version 1.1.0 [27].

Variants were identified and scored based on methods outlined in Carrigan et al. [1]. Synonymous variants, polymorphisms and mutations with high frequency in any population were filtered out, and the remaining list of rare variants with the potential to affect protein sequence was output for manual inspection. Output scores from the following ensemble variant pathogenicity predictor tools are shown in Table 1. The scale for each score ranges from 0 (likely benign) to 1 (likely pathogenic).

MetaLR

Meta Logistic Regression (LR) [28] incorporates pathogenicity prediction scores and maximum minor allele frequency from nine different tools for more accurate and thorough evaluation of deleterious effect of missense mutations. This allows for the more accurate assessment of variants than any of the singular methods alone.

M-CAP

Mendelian Clinically Applicable Pathogenicity (M-CAP) Score [29] was the first high sensitivity pathogenicity classifier for rare missense variants in the human genome aimed at the clinic. It combines pathogenicity scores from other tools and databases (including SIFT, Polyphen-2 and CADD) with novel features to create a more powerful model.

Revel

REVEL (rare exome variant ensemble learner) [30], is also an ensemble predictor tool and was trained with recently discovered pathogenic and rare benign missense variants, excluding those previously used to train its constituent tools. REVEL also claims to have the best performance for categorising pathogenic from rare benign variants with allele frequencies < 0.5%.

The American College of Medical Genetics and Genomics (ACMG) criteria for classifying pathogenic variants was utilised [31]. The other rare variants detected were for autosomal recessive conditions and showed pathogenic variants in only 1 allele. This was consistent between affected male relatives in this study.

Protein modelling

3D models of single subunit wildtype RS1 (NM_000330.3) and the Thr138Asn mutant were generated using Iterative Threading ASSEmbly Refinement, I-TASSER [32]. Polymer structures of RS1 were obtained from the Protein Data Bank (PDB, ID#3JD6,) [33]. The effect of single point mutations on protein stability was measured using STRUM [34]. Protein alignments were generated using Clustal Omega [35].

Results

Mean patient age of affected adult males ($n = 7$) was 67 +/− 5.38 years. The recruited carrier female (daughter) was 47 years of age. Mean age of the 2 affected grandsons was 13 +/− 1.41 years. Mean visual acuity for adult affected males was LogMAR 0.78 +/− 0.16 for right eyes and 0.74 +/− 0.28 for left eyes. Two eyes were not assessable due to one case of dense cataract (amblyopic eye) and one enucleation (due to complications following previous retinal surgery, presumed post vitreous haemorrhage or detachment). Only one of 14 adult eyes developed either a retinal detachment or haemorrhage previously (indeterminable). Mean visual acuity of affected grandsons was LogMAR 0.6 +/− 0.14 for right eyes and 0.5 for both left eyes.

Macular changes varied in severity, which showed no correlation to patient age. A severity staging was proposed by Tsui and Tsang [14], outlined in Table 2. Of 12 assessable adult eyes, 1 was in Stage 1 (8%, mean age 74y), 6 were in Stage 2 (50%, mean age 65.6 +/− 5.72y) and 5 were in Stage 3 (42%, mean age 68.8 +/− 4.55y). The predominantly advanced stage of disease here is likely due to advanced patient age. Corresponding images from this series are in accordance with this and are shown in Fig. 2. Both affected grandsons had bilateral Stage 1 disease. Electrophysiology data for the 2 affected grandsons is shown in Fig. 3. Confirmation of this *RS1* variant's pathogenicity will

Table 1 A direct comparison of the novel mutation, p.Thr138Asn, and a known pathogenic variant in *RS1*. Both variants were analysed with the same bioinformatic pipeline and have been scored by the same computational tools

Variant	Nucleotide	Protein	DBSNP ID	MetaLR	M-CAP	REVEL	ClinVar Report
Novel	c.413C > A	p.Thr138Asn	None	0.9742	0.8775	0.929	None
Known	c.636G > A	p.Arg209His	rs281865362	0.9446	0.9233	0.796	Pathogenic

Table 2 The clinical staging of Retinoschisis [14]

Stage	Colour	AF	SD-OCT
1	Macular schisis, classically radial (A)	Macular pigments displaced between schitic areas (B)	≥1 intraretinal schisis plane (C)
2	RPE pigment mottling (D)	Hyperautofluorescent ring at macula (E)	Collapse of schisis plane(s) (F)
3	Macular atrophy (G)	Large area of central hypoautofluorescence with surrounding hyperautofluorescent ring (H)	Outer retinal atrophy (I)

be of most benefit for this younger generation with potentially reversible macular changes.

Figure 2 demonstrates the clinical staging of XLRS using multimodal imaging. Patient 1 (74y) demonstrates the features of Stage 1 (mild) disease with BCVA LogMAR 0.6. There are subtle pigmentary changes on colour photography (A), with displacement of macular pigment leading to radial pattern of hyper- vs hypo-autofluorescence (B). The most striking feature is on OCT with intraretinal cystic spaces (C) in the inner plexiform and inner nuclear layers.

Patient 2 (60y) shows Stage 2 (intermediate) disease with BCVA of LogMAR 0.9. Colour photography reveals a hypopigmented ring at the macula, surrounding an area of normal pigmentation (D). Autofluorescence confirms this as hypoautofluorescent with a surrounding ring of hyperautofluorescence and a preserved iso-autofluorescent foveal area (E). OCT reveals the absence/collapse of intraretinal cystic spaces, but lacking complete outer retinal atrophy (F). Incidental vitreo-foveal traction is noted in this case.

Patient 3 (71y) has stage 3 (advanced) disease with BCVA of LogMAR 1.0. The colour photograph demonstrates macular atrophy (G), which appears as hypoautofluorescence with a hyperautofluorescent ring (H). This corresponds to outer retinal atrophy without schitic intraretinal space on OCT (I).

Next generation sequencing detected a novel missense mutation in *RS1* (c.413C > A; p.Thr138Asn [1]) falling within exon 5 of the discoidin domain [7]. This is a variant of unknown significance; however, due to its location adjacent to known pathogenic loci, it was deemed to be

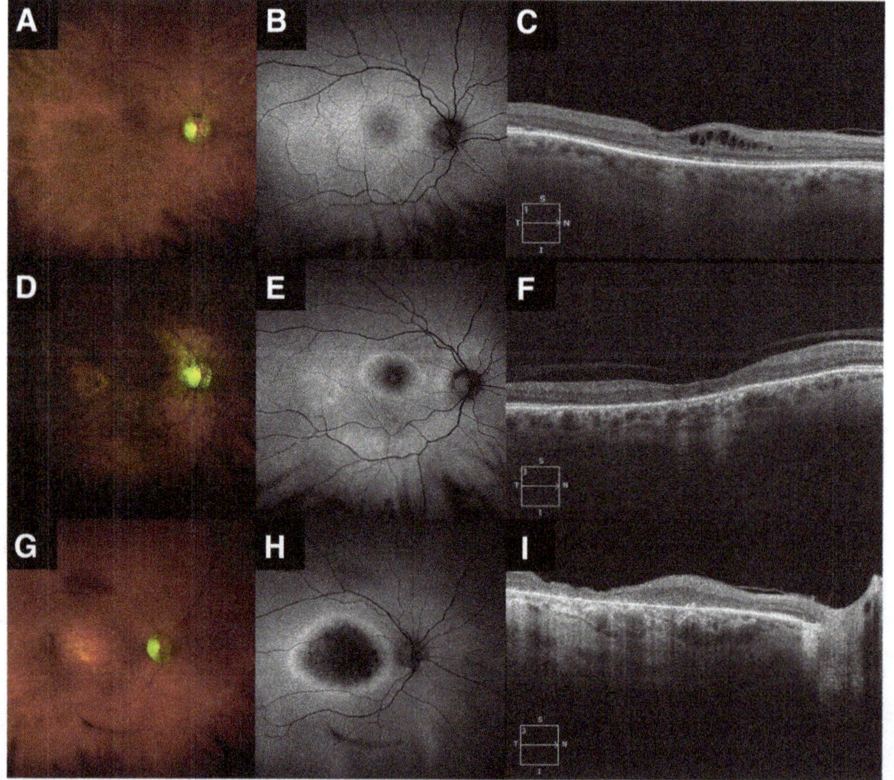

Fig. 2 Phenotypic features of selected cases from this XLRS1 pedigree. Colour photographs (left column), autofluorescence (middle column), and SD-OCT (right column) of the right eyes of 3 patients in Stage 1 (top row), Stage 2 (middle row) and Stage 3 (bottom row). Further description is available in Table 2 and the 'Results' section

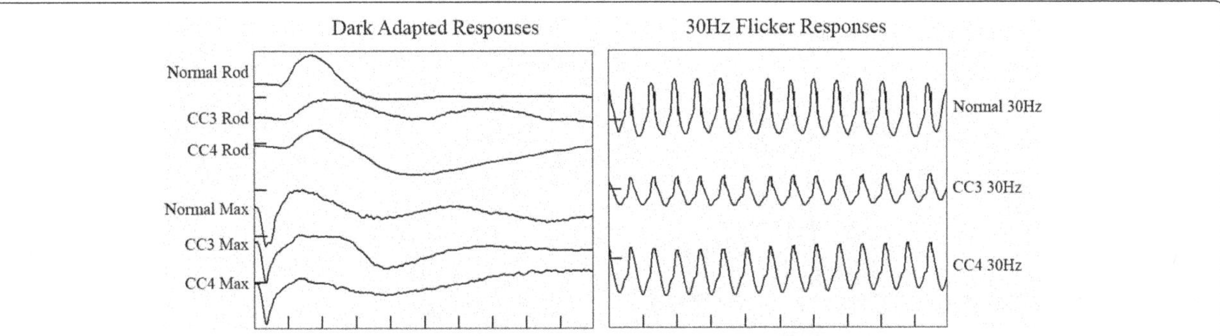

Fig. 3 ISCEV full-field electroretinogram [45] responses from affected grandsons (CC3 and CC4). Horizontal axis: 50 msec per division; Vertical axis: Dark Adapted Responses 500 µV per division; 30 Hz Flicker Responses 250 µV per division. The rod-isolated responses of CC3 and CC4 were slightly, but significantly reduced in amplitudes. The mixed rod and cone responses to the maximal intensity flash stimulus presented to the dark-adapted eye showed a normal a-wave amplitude in each subject, (CC3 445 µV, CC4 441 µV). The b-wave amplitudes were significantly reduced in each patient (CC3 515 µV, CC4 502 µV) and approximated the a-wave amplitudes. Ordinarily, the b-wave amplitude greatly exceeds that of the a-wave. The normal a-wave and selective reduction of the b-wave indicates preserved photo-transduction but impaired post-receptoral retinal function. This has been reported in RS1-associated X-linked retinoschisis [44]

potentially pathogenic and in silico analysis was undertaken.

Mutational analysis

The exonic regions from a panel of 218 IRD genes were sequenced by NGS in the proband from this pedigree. An additional 5 affected males were sequenced with a subsequent panel of the exonic regions of 254 IRD genes. Analysis of this NGS data led to the identification of a mutation in the *RS1* gene within the pedigree. Further analysis of each of the members of the family by PCR amplification of *RS1* and Sanger sequencing demonstrated that each affected male was found to have a hemizygous nonsynonymous mutation in exon 5 of the *RS1* gene (NM_000330.3:c.413C > A, p.Thr138Asn). In addition, the single carrier female analyzed was heterozygous for the same *RS1* mutation while the unaffected male was hemizygous for the reference base at that position (Fig. 4a, b).

The p.Thr138Asn *RS1* mutation involves a polar to polar amino acid substitution. Given that this novel as yet previously unreported mutation is located in the critical discoidin domain of the retinoschisin protein, where many pathogenic mutations have been identified previously, additional in silico analysis was undertaken to explore the potential pathogenicity of this *RS1* mutation on protein structure and conformation. The destabilizing effect of this mutation as predicted in silico is shown below in terms of a prediction of the changes to fold stability (Table 3), where a negative delta delta G (ddG) score is indicative of a destabilizing effect. This change is also represented visually as theoretical structural changes to the retinoschisin monomeric protein structure (Fig. 5a, b). Notable secondary structural changes are identified with arrows in Fig. 5a while Fig. 5b clearly visualizes the position of the specific amino acid substitution. The complexity of the hexadecameric structure of retinoschisin is shown in Fig. 6 for reference.

Table 1 displays the comparative output scores of three highly regarded variant pathogenicity prediction tools for this novel variant and a known pathogenic variant. As seen in the respective columns of the tools, both variants have been deemed likely pathogenic by all three tools. Also, the novel variant described in this study is scored more likely to be pathogenic by two out of three methods listed.

The ACMG guidelines [31] have also been implemented to classify the novel variant. The relevant information has been outlined in Table 4 along with supporting evidence where appropriate [20, 36, 37]. The guidelines state that there is sufficient evidence to classify this variant as pathogenic as there are one strong (PS1) and three moderate (PM1, PM2 and PM5) lines of evidence.

Discussion

A key function of retinoschisin is in retinal adhesion [7]. There is some debate over which retinal plane is affected by the schisis, which has been documented on OCT at the level of the photoreceptor inner segments, the inner nuclear layer and the nerve fibre layer [13, 38]. Decreased retinoschisin protein function may, and likely does, cause multiple planes of schisis.

There is significant variability of the severity of disease phenotype between the two eyes of the same individual, between different members of this XLRS1 pedigree and, as previously documented, between unrelated individuals [10–12]. This variability appears greater with age with some patients progressing through the clinical stages at different rates, possibly due to acquired/environmental factors or other genetic modifiers (see below). Although this variability is noted, there are clinical characteristics that guide the clinician to this diagnosis (e.g. pedigree,

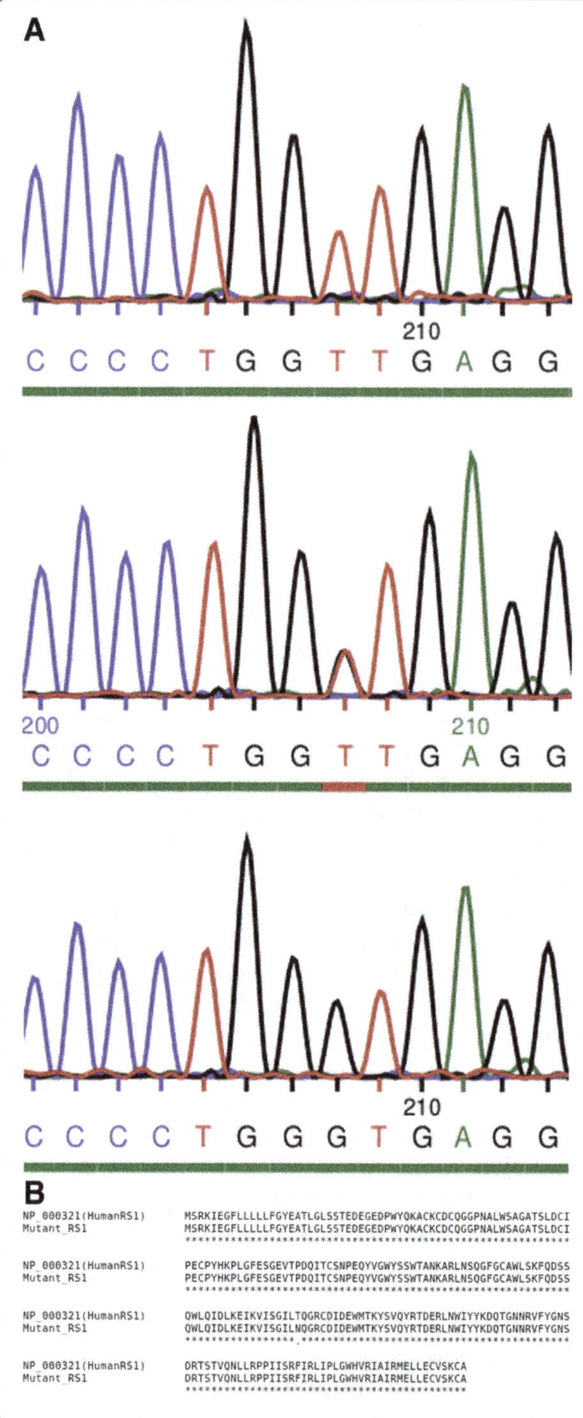

Fig. 4 a Sanger sequencing of *RS1*-exon 5 polymerase chain reaction (PCR) products from members of the pedigree. Top: Sanger sequencing result for affected male (ID#1392) showing a T nucleotide trace at sequencing position 208. Middle: Sanger sequencing result for carrier female (ID#1534) showing a heterozygous result at sequencing position 207, revealing traces from both signals of wild-type G allele and the mutant T allele. Bottom: Sanger sequencing result for unaffected male (ID#1634) showing a G nucleotide trace at sequencing trace position 208. **b** Clustal Omega results for protein alignment of reference RS1 protein sequence against the observed mutant protein sequence. "." denotes the position of the substitution

peripheral retinoschisis, lack of subretinal flecks or vitelliform changes) which are supported by a likely-pathogenic *RS1* variant and lack of other known pathogenic genetic variants. This supports the bimodal presentation of XLRS1. Severe cases of the disease (approximately 30%) are detected in infancy with poor fixation and/or strabismus. Milder cases (approximately 70%) are detected at school entry or in adulthood [39]. The current study highlights that the underlying genetic variant on the *RS1* gene is not predictive of phenotypic severity for this, or indeed any of the other, genetic variant(s) that have been described [12]. Thus, in assessing patients for trial/intervention suitability both a genetic and full phenotypic analysis is required. For example, gene therapy will not be beneficial if there is significant structural change (i.e. stage 3). However, the combination of a stage 1 or 2 case with confirmed genotype would suggest a possible role for genetic manipulation/replacement. As our knowledge of the impact of multiple variants increases we may better predict the molecular effects of each on retinal structure and function thus tailoring our approach to intervention further.

The clinical findings may be subtle in early stage or mild forms of disease. Classically, radial cystic maculopathy at the fovea is seen in 98–100% of cases [40] (Fig 2a-c). Ancillary tests have proven useful, particularly in subtle cases. An electronegative electroretinogram is suggestive of, but not specific, to XLRS1 [41] as this feature may be seen in acquired disease of the inner retina (e.g. central retinal artery occlusion). Microperimetry may assist in detection of subclinical disease [15]. Late stage disease is a diagnostic challenge; however, clinical examination, family history and genotyping as outlined above will aid in determining the diagnosis.

Colour photography, Autofluorescence and Optical Coherence Tomography are non-invasive and accessible

Table 3 Output results of the STRUM program. The change in stability scores between the mutant and wild type RS1 protein is given as delta delta G (ddG)

Position	Wild Type	Mutant Type	ddG
138	T	N	−0.78

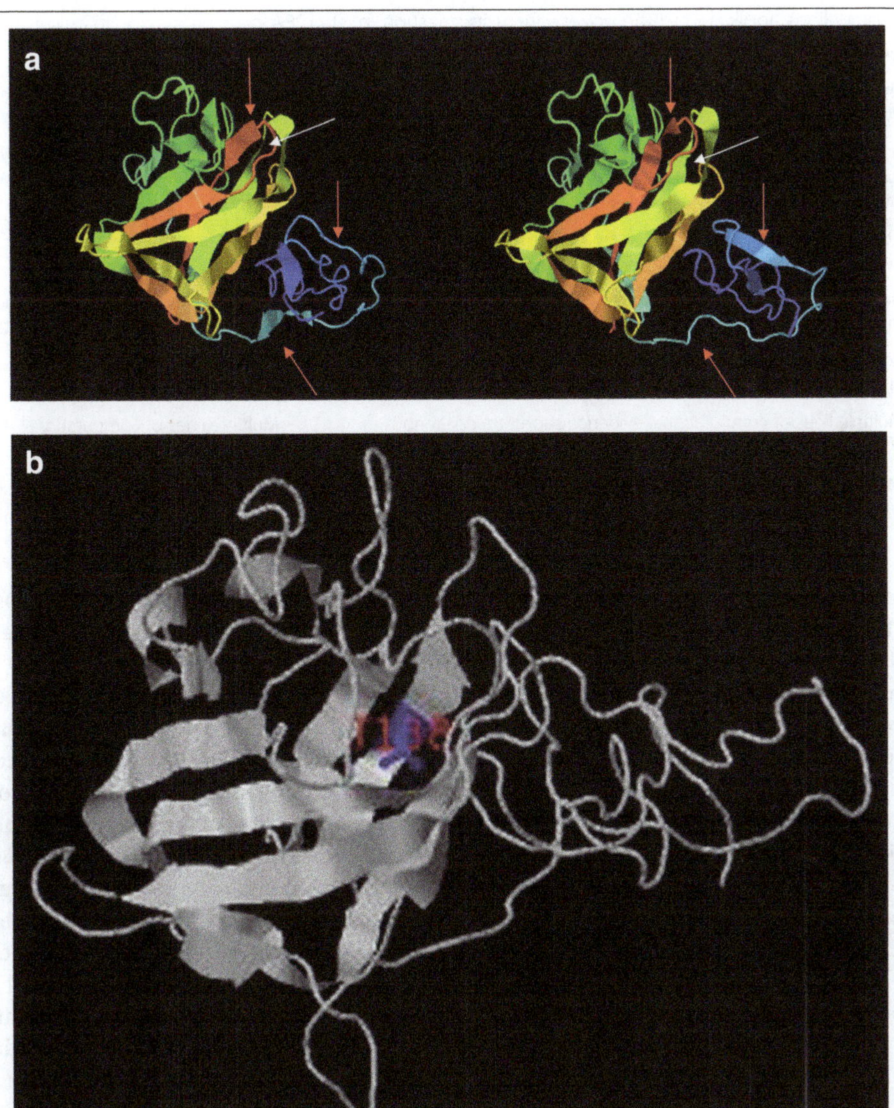

Fig. 5 a Protein models of reference RS1 (left) and mutant T138 N (right) proteins generated by the I-TASSER program. Red arrows denote obvious structural changes to protein structures. A white arrow highlights the position of the amino acid change at codon 138. **b** Protein model of RS1 mutant T138 N generated by STRUM. The affected amino acid residue is displayed in blue and annotated in red

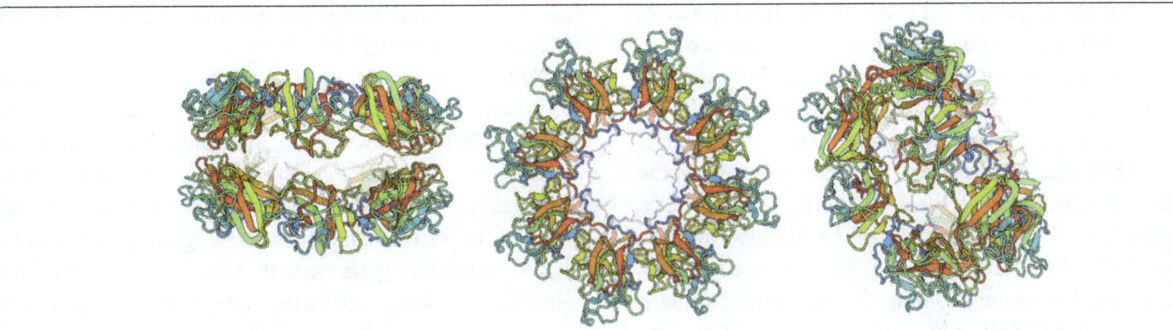

Fig. 6 Different views of the back-to-back octamer rings of wild type RS1 obtained from the Protein Data Bank. (Left) Objective view. (Middle) Plan view. (Right) Perspective view

Table 4 The ACMG guidelines applicable to the novel variant in question, p. Thr128Asn

Category Code	Qualifying Criteria	Relevance to Case
PS4	The prevalence of the variant in affected individuals is significantly increased compared to the prevalence in controls.	This variant is found in a sufficient number of relatives to qualify it as strong evidence of pathogenicity [36].
PM1	Located in a mutational hot spot and/or critical and well-established functional domain (e.g. active site of an enzyme) without benign variation.	Located in well established functional domain as reported by several studies [20, 37].
PM2	Absent from controls (or at extremely low frequency if recessive) in Exome Sequencing Project, 1000 Genomes or ExAC.	Absent from every databased queried.
PM5	Novel missense change at an amino acid residue where a different missense change determined to be pathogenic has been seen before.	Novel mutation at same amino acid as previously reported p.Thr138Ala (HGMD Database).
PP1	Co-segregation with disease in multiple affected family members in a gene definitively known to cause the disease.	Cosegregation in a family in a gene known to cause disease.
PP3	Multiple lines of computational evidence support a deleterious effect on the gene or gene product.	Multiple lines of computational evidence presented here (Table 1).
PP4	Patient's phenotype or family history is highly specific for a disease with a single genetic etiology.	Patient phenotype is highly specific for a disease.

tests useful in determining the clinical stage of XLRS1. This is relevant, for current and upcoming gene therapy trials [8, 9], in selecting those cases most likely to benefit from intervention (i.e. early to intermediate disease [40]). Ancillary tests, such as adaptive optics (AO) imaging and microperimetry, can complement assessment of cone structure/spacing in those who are deemed early/intermediate stage [42, 43].

To our knowledge, this specific mutation is currently unreported in any clinical database available including the Leiden University's Open Variation Database for Retinoschisis (LOVD 3.0 [6]) and represents a novel and likely pathogenic mutation given the clear segregation in this pedigree and the significant predicted effects on protein structure.

Recent studies have outlined the importance of certain key residues in correctly assembling a functional RS1 oligomer. Several key residue positions necessary to ensure proper folding of the retinoschisin protein have been identified [20]. Of note, amino acids at positions 137 and 139 were highlighted in that study as fundamental to forming a beta-sheet required in the interaction between subunits essential in the formation of their functional octamer ring structure. It is possible therefore, that an amino acid substitution at position 138 may provide some steric hindrance, that in turn, would interfere with the relationship between different subunits on the same octamer ring. Such interference could in principle have deleterious consequences for the formation and stability of the oligomeric RS1 complex. This hypothesis is further supported by in silico analysis of the p.Thr138Asn mutation. Computational analysis was utilized to predict protein folding changes in the mutant protein (using I-TASSER); physiochemical properties, position specific conservation and secondary structure prediction scores were used to determine the destabilization effect(s) of the protein substitution at position 138 (using STRUM) where significant changes in the above were predicted for the p.Thr138Asn mutation.

The prediction scores in Table 1 are useful for assessing the confidence with which a variant can be called deleterious or not. However, these are confidence scores and not pathogenicity scores, so although the scores listed would be considered to be quite high, these scores cannot indicate the detrimental effect that this mutation may have relative to a similar amino acid substitution elsewhere in the protein. Increased bioavailability of functional retinoschisin protein would logically correlate to the lasting preservation of the retinal layers; however, to assess this dosage effect, each variant would have to be assessed individually for function and half-life. This is a challenging task for retinoschisin as it has typically proven quite difficult to produce in useful quantities [20]. Currently we rely on in silico predictors of a variant's effect on protein structure. This includes protein modelling (Figs. 4a and b) where possible and delta delta g scores (Table 3), to predict the destabilising effects a mutation may have on a protein. However, when all lines of evidence are considered, this novel *RS1* variant is classified as pathogenic under the guidelines outlined by the ACMG [31] (Table 4).

In XLRS1, age is not an absolute factor, particularly in adulthood, when evaluating severity of disease and the likely benefit from novel gene therapies. The individuals in this XLRS1 pedigree exhibited no clear correlation between patient age and 1) stage of disease, 2) visual acuity, 3) central retinal thickness or 4) age at onset despite a shared novel *RS1* gene variant. Advanced cases prove a diagnostic challenge as many inherited and acquired macular diseases follow a final common pathway of outer retinal atrophy. Each case must be judged on its potential (anatomically within Stage 1 or 2 and genetically possessing a pathogenic *RS1* variant) to respond to novel therapies. Furthermore, the variability in clinical presentations between family members with the same mutation suggests the possible involvement of genetic modifier loci and or environmental effect(s).

While there is variability in phenotype between relatives affected by the same genetic variant, the significance is that the clinician not be discouraged from the diagnosis due to these differences but consider them within the spectrum of the 3 described clinical stages. The diagnostic value of ERG, in particular the characteristic decrease in b-wave activity in combination with suggestive clinical findings are powerful tools for diagnosing younger patients, however the diagnostic value of these tests may be less certain with advanced age [44]. Confirmation of extent of severity (clinical stages) and a pathogenic *RS1* variant open a potential avenue of treatment for those in Stage 1 or 2. This information then guides genetic testing for at risk relatives who could possibility benefit from novel disease-modifying therapies.

There is a possibility that there may be some form of modifier or digenic effect which could account for the observed phenotypic variability. With this in mind, the coding regions of known genes associated with retinal degenerations were subjected to sequence analysis. The presence of multiple pathogenic variants within a single patient is extremely rare but has been previously observed, even in our own IRD cohort. Although, as previously mentioned, this method unfortunately did not detect any likely genetic cause of phenotypic variability between the affected patients in this pedigree.

The retinoschisin protein is widely expressed throughout the layers of the retina in childhood and more specifically in rod and cone photoreceptor cells in adulthood and is seen to act as a cellular adhesive when functioning correctly. However, other proteins are also capable of fulfilling similar adhesive functions, for example adherins and cadherins in adherens junctions or claudins and occuldin in tight junctions. Given that some of these other proteins belong to large protein families, it is a possibility that variation in relative composition of these cellular adhesive protein cocktails may have a more notable contribution to a variable phenotype in the absence of functional retinoschisin.

This variability creates a diagnostic challenge in advanced XLRS1 disease. The clinical clues in conjunction with adjunctive testing, confirmed by robust genetic assessment (i.e. ruling out other causes and confirming a pathogenic *RS1* variant) confirm the diagnosis, thus empowering those affected by bringing them closer to accessing novel gene therapies where appropriate and preparing younger generations for those potential therapeutic options.

Conclusions

Here we describe how multimodal imaging in XLRS1 and confirmation of a pathogenic *RS1* variant help to a) confirm diagnosis, b) monitor progression, c) assess clinical stage and thus suitability for novel therapeutic options even in patients of advanced age. Autofluorescence and OCT are non-invasive, well-tolerated and readily available in most clinical centres. Standardisation of clinical assessment and staging criteria, perhaps in conjunction with a central European reading centre, would allow detection of individuals with modifiable XLRS1 who may be suitable for novel gene therapy clinical trial participation.

Abbreviations

ACMG: American College of Medical Genetics; AF: Autofluorescence; AO: Adaptive Optics; IRD: Inherited Retinal Degeneration; I-TASSER: Iterative Threading ASSEmbly Refinement; LogMAR: Logarithm of the Minimum Angle of Resolution; LOVD: Leiden University's Open Variation Database; MMUH: Mater Misericordiae University Hospital, Dublin, Ireland; MPH: Mater Private Hospital, Dublin, Ireland; OCT: Optical Coherence Tomography; OMIM: Online Mendelian Inheritance in Man; PCR: Polymerase Chain Reaction; PDB: Protein Data Bank; RPE: Retinal Pigment Epithelium; RVEEH: Royal Victoria Eye & Ear Hospital, Dublin, Ireland; XLRS1: X-Linked Retinoschisis

Acknowledgements

Fighting Blindness Ireland; Clinical Research Centre: University College Dublin/Mater Misericordiae University Hospital, Dublin, Ireland; The Research Foundation, The Royal Victoria Eye & Ear Hospital, Dublin, Ireland; School of Genetics, Trinity College Dublin, Ireland; Retinal Eye Centre, Mater Private Hospital, Dublin, Ireland.

Funding

All patients were seen as part of the Target 5000 Irish National Inherited Retinal Degeneration Registry which is funded through the Irish charity Fighting Blindness (charity number: 20013349). There are no specific sources of industry or institutional funding supporting this publication. All publications arising as part of this project are independent endeavours of the publishing authors.

Authors' contributions

KS, NW, PK and DK recruited the patients, performed history and clinical examination, and wrote the clinical portions of the manuscript. AD, MC and GJF performed next generation sequencing on blood samples from the patients, performing protein modelling/pathogenicity analysis and wrote the genetic portions of the manuscript. All authors have read and approved the manuscript.

Competing interests

None of the authors have any competing interests as laid out in BioMed Central's guidance document.

Author details

[1]The Catherine McAuley Centre, Mater Private Hospital, Nelson Street, Dublin 7, Ireland. [2]Department of Genetics, Trinity College Dublin, Dublin, Ireland. [3]The Research Foundation, The Royal Victoria Eye and Ear Hospital, Dublin, Ireland.

References

1. Carrigan M, et al. Panel-based population next-generation sequencing for inherited retinal degenerations. Sci Rep. 2016;6:33248.
2. Dockery A, et al. Target 5000: Target Capture Sequencing for Inherited Retinal Degenerations. Genes (Basel). 2017;8(11). https://doi.org/10.3390/genes8110304.
3. George ND, et al. Infantile presentation of X linked retinoschisis. Br J Ophthalmol. 1995;79(7):653–7.

4. Functional implications of the spectrum of mutations found in 234 cases with X-linked juvenile retinoschisis. The Retinoschisis consortium. Hum Mol Genet. 1998;7(7):1185–92. https://www.ncbi.nlm.nih.gov/pubmed/9618178.
5. Stenson PD, et al. The human gene mutation database: building a comprehensive mutation repository for clinical and molecular genetics, diagnostic testing and personalized genomic medicine. Hum Genet. 2014; 133(1):1–9.
6. Leiden University Medical Center, N. Leiden Open Variation Database 3.0. 2018; Available from: http://www.lovd.nl/3.0/home. Accessed 5 July 2018.
7. Bush M, et al. Cog-wheel Octameric structure of RS1, the Discoidin domain containing retinal protein associated with X-linked Retinoschisis. PLoS One. 2016;11(1):e0147653.
8. ClinicalTrials.gov [Internet]. Bethesda (MD): National Library of Medicine (US). 2015 Apr 15. Identifier NCT02416622, Safety and Efficacy of rAAV-hRS1 in Patients With X-linked. Retinoschisis (XLRS); [6 screens]. Available from: https://clinicaltrials.gov/ct2/show/NCT02416622. Accessed 5 July 2018.
9. ClinicalTrials.gov [Internet]. Bethesda (MD): National Library of Medicine (US). 2014 Dec 14. Identifier NCT02317887, Study of RS1 Ocular Gene Transfer for X-linked Retinoschisis; [8 screens]. Available from: https://clinicaltrials.gov/ct2/show/NCT02317887. Accessed 5 July 2018.
10. Eksandh LC, et al. Phenotypic expression of juvenile X-linked retinoschisis in Swedish families with different mutations in the XLRS1 gene. Arch Ophthalmol. 2000;118(8):1098–104.
11. Molday RS, Kellner U, Weber BH. X-linked juvenile retinoschisis: clinical diagnosis, genetic analysis, and molecular mechanisms. Prog Retin Eye Res. 2012;31(3):195–212.
12. Lai YH, et al. A novel gene mutation in a family with X-linked retinoschisis. J Formos Med Assoc. 2015;114(9):872–80.
13. Gregori NZ, et al. Macular spectral-domain optical coherence tomography in patients with X linked retinoschisis. Br J Ophthalmol. 2009;93(3):373–8.
14. Tsui I, Tsang SH. In: Noemi Lois JVF, editor. Fundus autofluorescence in X-linked Retinoschisis, in Fundus Autofluorescence. Philadelphia: Lippincott Williams & Wilkins; 2009.
15. Nittala MG, et al. Spectral-domain OCT and microperimeter characterization of morphological and functional changes in X-linked retinoschisis. Ophthalmic Surg Lasers Imaging. 2009;40(1):71–4.
16. Bergen AA, et al. Multipoint linkage analysis in X-linked juvenile retinoschisis. Clin Genet. 1993;43(3):113–6.
17. Sauer CG, et al. Positional cloning of the gene associated with X-linked juvenile retinoschisis. Nat Genet. 1997;17(2):164–70.
18. Plossl K, et al. Retinoschisin is linked to retinal Na/K-ATPase signaling and localization. Mol Biol Cell. 2017;28(16):2178–89.
19. Plossl K, Weber BH, Friedrich U. The X-linked juvenile retinoschisis protein retinoschisin is a novel regulator of mitogen-activated protein kinase signalling and apoptosis in the retina. J Cell Mol Med. 2017;21(4):768–80.
20. Tolun G, et al. Paired octamer rings of retinoschisin suggest a junctional model for cell-cell adhesion in the retina. Proc Natl Acad Sci U S A. 2016; 113(19):5287–92.
21. Ramsay EP, et al. Structural analysis of X-linked retinoschisis mutations reveals distinct classes which differentially effect retinoschisin function. Hum Mol Genet. 2016;25(24):5311–20.
22. den Hollander AI, et al. Mutations in the CEP290 (NPHP6) gene are a frequent cause of Leber congenital amaurosis. Am J Hum Genet. 2006;79(3): 556–61.
23. Bauwens M, et al. An augmented ABCA4 screen targeting noncoding regions reveals a deep intronic founder variant in Belgian Stargardt patients. Hum Mutat. 2015;36(1):39–42.
24. Steele-Stallard HB, et al. Screening for duplications, deletions and a common intronic mutation detects 35% of second mutations in patients with USH2A monoallelic mutations on sanger sequencing. Orphanet J Rare Dis. 2013;8:122.
25. Li H, Durbin R. Fast and accurate long-read alignment with burrows-wheeler transform. Bioinformatics. 2010;26(5):589–95.
26. Picard. Available from: http://broadinstitute.github.io/picard/. Accessed 18 Aug 2017.
27. Garrison E, Marth G. Haplotype-based variant detection from short-read sequencing. arXiv:1207.3907 2012; Available from: http://arxiv.org/abs/1207.3907.
28. Dong C, et al. Comparison and integration of deleteriousness prediction methods for nonsynonymous SNVs in whole exome sequencing studies. Hum Mol Genet. 2015;24(8):2125–37.
29. Jagadeesh KA, et al. M-CAP eliminates a majority of variants of uncertain significance in clinical exomes at high sensitivity. Nat Genet. 2016;48(12): 1581–6.
30. Ioannidis NM, et al. REVEL: an ensemble method for predicting the pathogenicity of rare missense variants. Am J Hum Genet. 2016;99(4):877–85.
31. Richards S, et al. Standards and guidelines for the interpretation of sequence variants: a joint consensus recommendation of the American College of Medical Genetics and Genomics and the Association for Molecular Pathology. Genet Med. 2015;17(5):405–24.
32. I-TASSER. Available from: http://zhanglab.ccmb.med.umich.edu/I-TASSER/. Accessed 18 Aug 2017.
33. RCSB Protein Data Bank. Available from: https://www.rcsb.org/. Accessed 18 Aug 2017.
34. Quan L, Lv Q, Zhang Y. STRUM: structure-based prediction of protein stability changes upon single-point mutation. Bioinformatics. 2016;32(19): 2936–46.
35. Sievers F, et al. Fast, scalable generation of high-quality protein multiple sequence alignments using Clustal omega. Mol Syst Biol. 2011;7:539.
36. Jarvik GP, Browning BL. Consideration of Cosegregation in the pathogenicity classification of genomic variants. Am J Hum Genet. 2016; 98(6):1077–81.
37. Plossl K, et al. Pathomechanism of mutated and secreted retinoschisin in X-linked juvenile retinoschisis. Exp Eye Res. 2018;177:23–34.
38. Yanoff M, Kertesz Rahn E, Zimmerman LE. Histopathology of juvenile retinoschisis. Arch Ophthalmol. 1968;79(1):49–53.
39. Deutman AF, Pinckers AJ, Aan de Kerk AL. Dominantly inherited cystoid macular edema. Am J Ophthalmol. 1976;82(4):540–8.
40. Wang T, et al. Intracellular retention of mutant retinoschisin is the pathological mechanism underlying X-linked retinoschisis. Hum Mol Genet. 2002;11(24):3097–105.
41. Sergeev YV, et al. Molecular modeling of retinoschisin with functional analysis of pathogenic mutations from human X-linked retinoschisis. Hum Mol Genet. 2010;19(7):1302–13.
42. Akeo K, et al. Detailed morphological changes of Foveoschisis in patient with X-linked Retinoschisis detected by SD-OCT and adaptive optics fundus camera. Case Rep Ophthalmol Med. 2015;2015:432782.
43. Duncan JL, et al. Abnormal cone structure in foveal schisis cavities in X-linked retinoschisis from mutations in exon 6 of the RS1 gene. Invest Ophthalmol Vis Sci. 2011;52(13):9614–23.
44. Bradshaw K, et al. Mutations of the XLRS1 gene cause abnormalities of photoreceptor as well as inner retinal responses of the ERG. Doc Ophthalmol. 1999;98(2):153–73.
45. McCulloch DL, et al. ISCEV standard for full-field clinical electroretinography (2015 update). Doc Ophthalmol. 2015;130(1):1–12.

First molecular study in Lebanese patients with Cockayne syndrome and report of a novel mutation in *ERCC8* gene

Alain Chebly[1*], Sandra Corbani[1], Joelle Abou Ghoch[1], Cybel Mehawej[1], André Megarbane[2] and Eliane Chouery[1]

Abstract

Background: Cockayne Syndrome (CS) is a rare autosomal recessive disorder characterized by neurological and sensorial impairment, dwarfism, microcephaly and photosensitivity. CS is caused by mutations in *ERCC6 (CSB)* or *ERCC8 (CSA)* genes.

Methods: Three patients with CS were referred to the Medical Genetics Unit of Saint Joseph University. Sanger sequencing of both *ERCC8* and *ERCC6* genes was performed: *ERCC8* was tested in all patients while *ERCC6* in one of them.

Results: Sequencing led to the identification of three homozygous mutations, two in *ERCC8* (p.Y322* and c.843 + 1G > C) and one in *ERCC6* (p.R670W). All mutations were previously reported as pathogenic except for the c.843 + 1G > C splice site mutation in *ERCC8* which is novel.

Conclusions: Molecular diagnosis was established in all patients included in our study. A genotype-phenotype correlation is discussed and a link, between mutations and some specific religious communities in Lebanon, is suggested.

Keywords: Cockayne, CS, *ERCC8*, *ERCC6*, Sanger sequencing, Lebanon

Background

Cockayne syndrome (CS; MIM# 133540, 216400) is a rare autosomal recessive disorder belonging to the family of premature aging syndromes. It was first described by Edward Alfred Cockayne, a British physician, in 1936 in a paper entitled "Dwarfism with retinal atrophy and deafness", followed ten years later by another paper reporting a follow up data on the same patients [1, 2]. The incidence of this syndrome is estimated to be 2.7 per million in Western Europe [3]. CS is a multisystem disorder characterized by growth failure, dwarfism, microcephaly, intellectual disability, senile face and photosensitivity [1, 4]. Other symptoms of the disease include retinopathy and hearing loss that are progressive during life and which severity correlates with the severity of the disease [4, 5]. Cataracts, for instance, found in almost 50% of CS patients, are associated with a poor prognosis when occurring at an early age [4, 6, 7]. CS is clinically divided into three subtypes: the classical form or CS type I, the severe form or CS type II and the mild form or CS type III [4, 8, 9]. The onset of symptoms in type I is in the early childhood, usually after one year of age. Type II, involving more severe symptoms, often exists at birth, while type III appears later in childhood [4, 10].

This rare disease is linked to mutations in one of two excision-repair cross-complementation genes *ERCC6* (*CSB)* and *ERCC8* (*CSA).* These genes encode proteins involved in the transcription-coupled sub-pathway of nucleotide excision repair (TC-NER) of UV-induced DNA damage [11, 12]. CS proteins are also implicated in the control of oxidative stress response and in the maintenance of mitochondrial function [13] . *ERCC6* (10q11.2) encodes CSB, a 1493 aa protein that belongs to the SNF2/SW12 ATPases family [14] while *ERCC8* (5q12.1) encodes CSA, a 396 aa protein, comprising WD (tryptophan-aspartic acid dipeptide) repeats. CSA interacts with CSB and

* Correspondence: alain.chebly@usj.edu.lb
[1]Medical Genetics Unit, Faculty of medicine, Saint Joseph University (USJ), Damascus street, B.P. 17-5208, Mar Mikhaël, Beirut 1104 2020, Lebanon
Full list of author information is available at the end of the article

p44, a subunit of the human RNA polymerase II transcription factor IIH [15, 16].

Among the reported CS cases, 62 to 68% had mutations in *ERCC6* gene [17, 18].

The diagnosis of CS in three Lebanese patients was confirmed, in 1999, by Jabre et al. using the recovery of RNA synthesis (RRS) assay after UVC irradiation in patients' fibroblasts. Impaired RRS is typically found in CS cells. Molecular evaluation of these patients was not performed [19]. Here we report the first molecular study of CS in the Lebanese community.

Methods

Patients

Three patients with CS were referred to the Medical Genetics Unit of Saint Joseph University (USJ). Among them, two patients present a classical form and one a severe form. Approval to conduct this study was obtained from the Ethics Committee of Saint Joseph University (USJ), Beirut, Lebanon.

Patient A

Patient A (Fig. 1a, patient III.4) is the fourth child born to non-consanguineous Christian (Greek Orthodox) parents, from the Akkar region in North Lebanon. Among the five children of this family, three were affected. Only patient III.4 presented to the clinical examination and was included in this study. He was born at term weighting 4 kg (90th Percentile). At 3 months of age, the parents noted a hypotonia. Patient A was first referred to us at the age of 16. His clinical examination showed hypotonia, a short stature (104 cm: < 3rd Percentile), a head circumference of 47 cm (< 3d Percentile) and a typical dysmorphic face associating microcephaly, enophtalmy, and an aquiline nose with a sensorial impairment including hearing loss. He had numerous dental caries and some skin lesions due to photosensitivity. Patient A deceased at 17 years of age.

Patient B

Patient B (Fig. 1b, patient III.2) is the second child born to non-consanguineous Muslim parents, from Saida in South Lebanon. She was a term newborn weighting 3,1 kg (15th

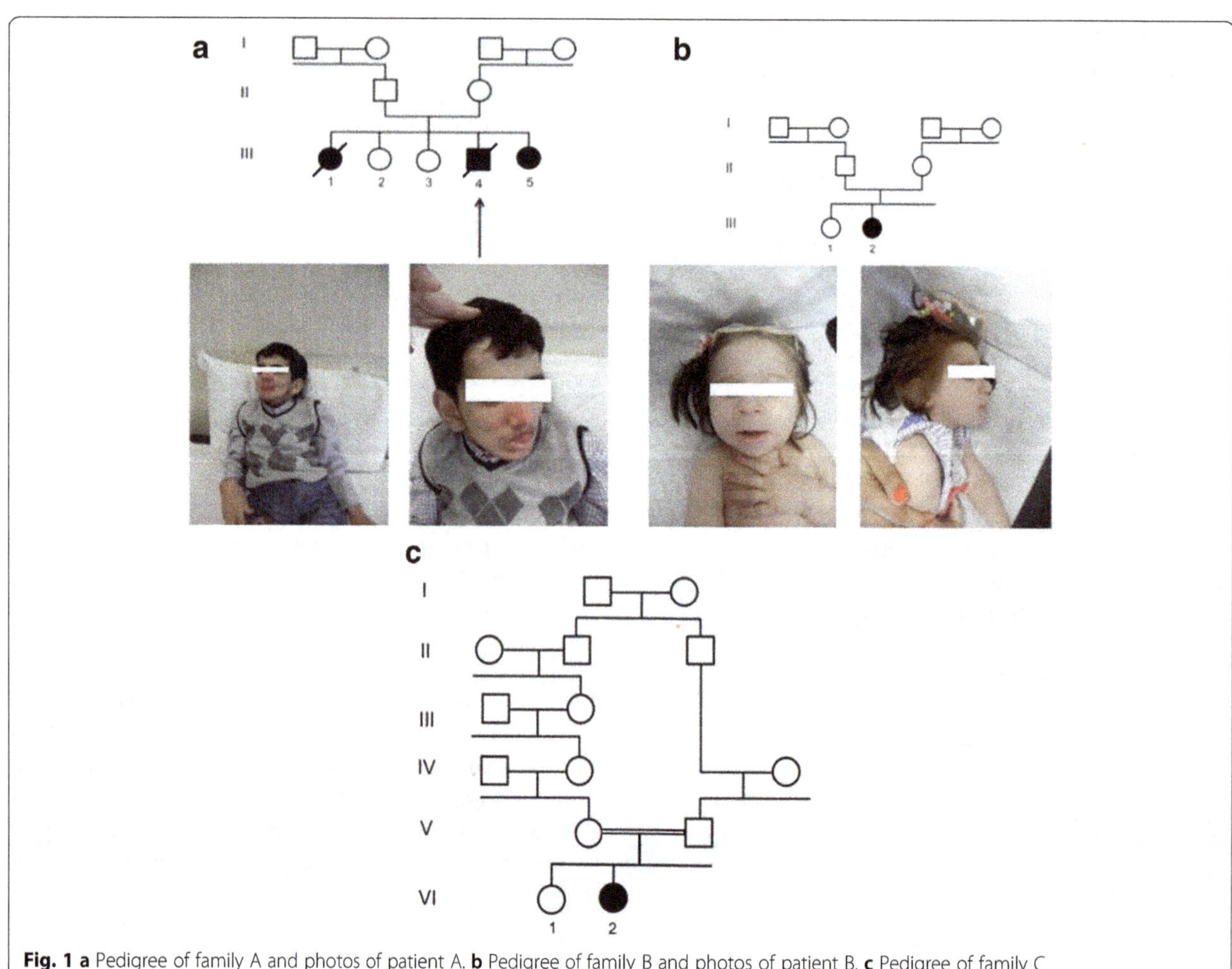

Fig. 1 **a** Pedigree of family A and photos of patient A. **b** Pedigree of family B and photos of patient B. **c** Pedigree of family C

Percentile) with a height of 51 cm (50th Percentile) and a head circumference of 35,5 cm (75th Percentile). Patient B underwent two surgeries for bilateral congenital cataracts, one at the age of 2 months and the other at the age of 4 months. The parents noted the onset of cutaneous photosensitivity and skin lesions at an early age. Patient B presented to us at one year of age, with a height of 67 cm (< 3rd Percentile), a head circumference of 38,5 cm (<3rd Percentile) and a weight of 6.3 kg(< 3rd Percentile). Her clinical examination showed characteristic facial dysmorphisms including microcephaly, aquiline nose, low-set ears, deep-set eyes, dry skin and no teeth.

Patient C

Patient C (Fig. 1c, patient VI.2) is the second child born to consanguineous Druze parents, from Kfarselwan in Mount Lebanon. She was delivered by cesarean section, weighting 2,9 kg (10th Percentile) with a height of 51 cm (50th Percentile) and a head circumference of 34 cm(35th Percentile). The onset of growth failure was first noted at the age of 3 months. Patient C was referred to us at the age of 2 years. Her clinical examination showed a remarkable growth failure in addition to some typical dysmorphic features including microcephaly, exophthalmia and an aquiline nose. At two and a half years old, patient B underwent a surgery for bilateral cataracts. At the age of 3 years, hearing loss started to manifest and led to deafness.

Methods

DNA extraction and sanger sequencing

Peripheral blood samples were obtained from the three patients after obtaining written informed consent from the parents. Genomic DNA was isolated from white blood cells using standard salt-precipitation methods. Genomic sequence of *ERCC8* (NM_000082.3) and *ERCC6* (NM_000124.3) were obtained from UCSC Genomic Browser on Human (hg19).

PCR primers were designed using Primer3 software to amplify each of the 12 exons of *ERCC8* gene and the 21 exons of *ERCC6* gene as well as their flanking intronic sequences (Additional file 1: Table S1). PCR reactions were performed using Taq DNA polymerase (Invitrogen Life Technologies, Carlsbad, CA, USA). PCR fragments were run on 1% agarose gel. The fragments were purified using "SIGMA-ALDRICH™" GenElute PCR clean-up kit and then sequenced using Big Dye_ Terminator v1.1 Cycle sequencing kit (Applied Biosystems, Foster City, CA, USA). Sequence reaction was purified on Sephadex G50 (Amersham Pharmacia Biotech, Foster City, CA, USA) and loaded into an ABI 3500 Sequencer after the addition of Hidi formamide. Electropherograms were analyzed using Sequence Analysis Software version 5.2 (Applied Biosystems) and then aligned with the reference sequences using ChromasPro v1.7.6.1 (Technelysium, Queensland, Australia).

RNA extraction and cDNA sequencing

Peripheral blood samples were obtained from family C (patient C and parents) and RNA was isolated using Chomczynscki and Sacchi method with Trizol (Invitrogen Life Technologies, Carlsbad, CA, USA). Manual method with Phenol Chloroform was performed in order to obtain a better outcome. RT-PCR was used to obtain cDNA from RNA using SuperScript II reverse transcriptase (Invitrogen Life Technologies, Carlsbad, CA, USA) and then cDNA was treated like DNA.

In order to rule out contamination of RNA samples by genomic DNA, PCR of the housekeeping gene β-globin was performed using the following primers: Globin-F (5′-AAG TTG GTG GTG AGG CCC TG-3′) and Globin-R (5′-TTG CCA AAG TGA TGG GCC AG-3′). For each sample, two reactions were performed: the first allowing the amplification of the β-globin transcript (RT+) and the second allowing the exclusion of any contamination by genomic DNA (RT-) (Fig. 4c).

For *ERCC8* RT-PCR, two couples of primers were designed: Couple 1 with primer F in exon 9 and primer R in intron 9 to investigate if intron 9 is included in *ERCC8* mature transcript. Couple 2 with primer F in exon 9 and primer R in exon 10, which should amplify in a normal case. Both couples are shown in Fig. 2, couple 1 in blue and couple 2 in red.

Results

The strategy adopted in this study consisted of initially sequencing exon 10 of the *ERCC8* gene based on the fact that the majority of mutations in CS patients from the Arab community are located in this exon [17]. If no mutations were detected, the rest of the *ERCC8* gene (11 exons) is tested. If *ERCC8* sequencing showed normal results, *ERCC6* is evaluated.

Sequencing led to the detection of a homozygous non-sense mutation in exon 10 of *ERCC8*

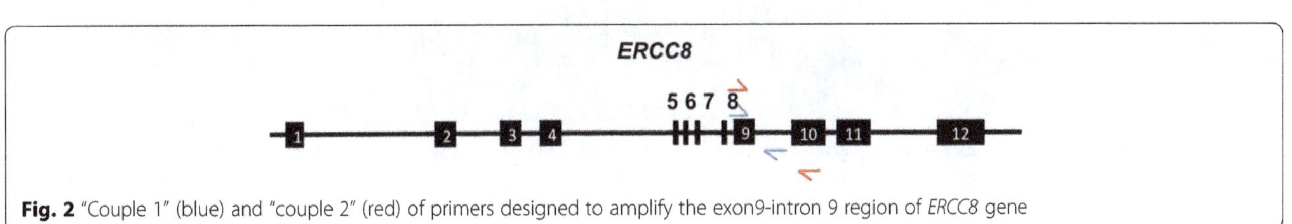

Fig. 2 "Couple 1" (blue) and "couple 2" (red) of primers designed to amplify the exon9-intron 9 region of *ERCC8* gene

(NM_000082.3:c.966C > A; p.Y322*) in patient A (Fig. 3a). Testing of *ERCC8* did not reveal any mutation in patient B, however, a homozygous mutation in exon 10 of the *ERCC6* gene (NM_000124.3:c.2008C > T; p.R670W) was detected in this patient (Fig. 3b). Parents of patient B are heterozygous for the same mutation (Fig. 3b). Genetic evaluation of patient C led to the identification of a novel homozygous variant in *ERCC8* (NM_000082.3:c.843 + 1G > C) altering the donor splice site of intron 9 of the gene (Fig. 3c).

Interpretation of this novel variation using the prediction tool "Human Splicing Finder" revealed that its effect is most probably affecting the splicing. The effect of this splice site mutation was studied on RNA by PCR amplification using a couple of primers (couple 1) that includes a reverse primer specific to intron 9. Contamination with genomic DNA was ruled out using globin as a control (Fig. 4c). Amplification, using couple 1, was observed in patient C, thus suggesting that a part of intron 9 is included in *ERCC8*'s transcript. This result was confirmed by sequencing of the obtained amplicon (Fig. 4a).

The same PCR performed on the parents showed a weak amplification; hypothesizing that they carry one mutated copy of the *ERCC8* gene.

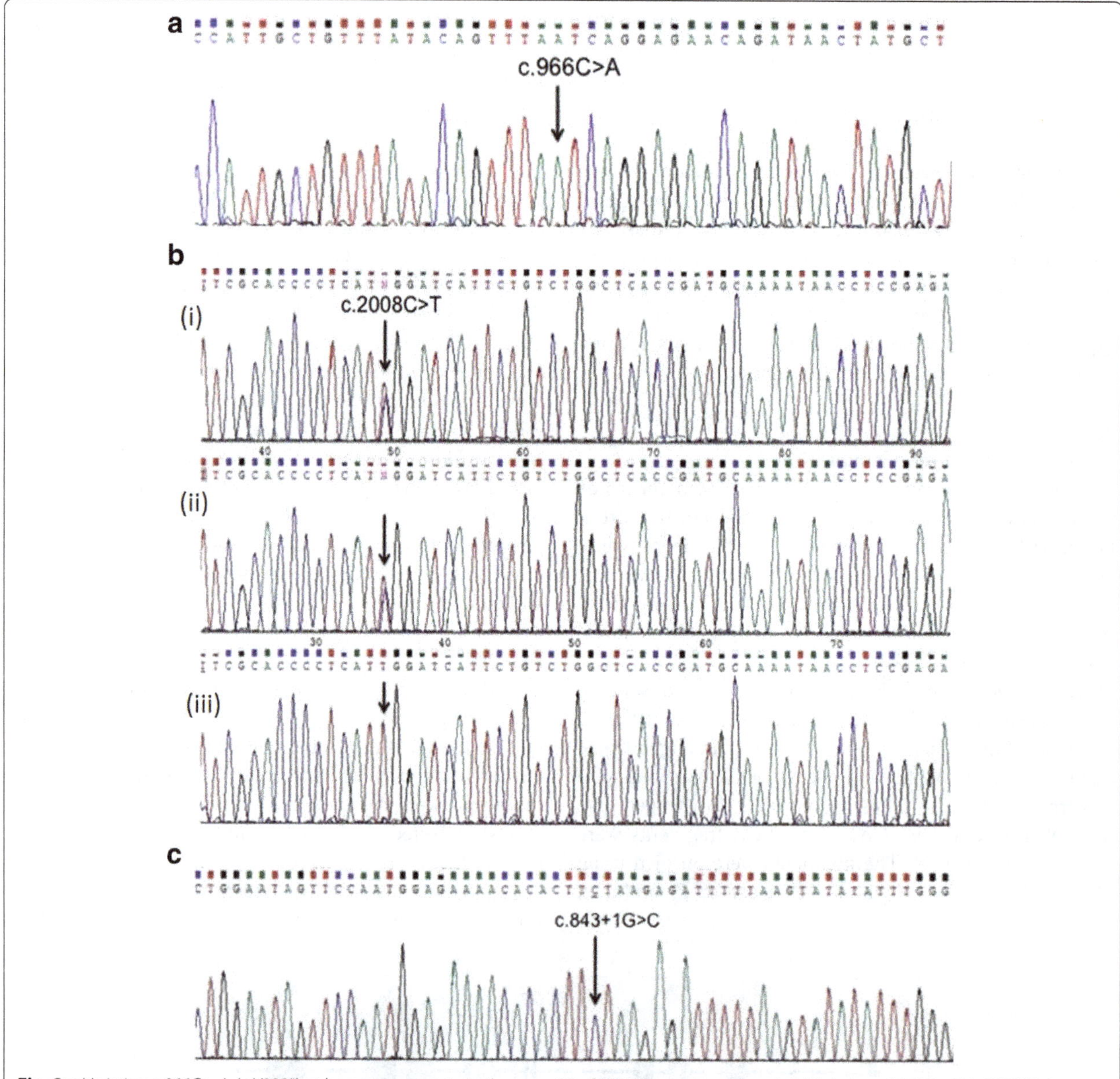

Fig. 3 a Variation c.966C > A (p.Y322*) at homozygous state in the exon 10 of *ERCC8* gene in patient A. **b** Variation c.2008C > T (p.R670W) in *ERCC6* gene in family B: (i)Father, (ii)Mother and (iii)Patient B. **c** The novel variation c.843 + 1G > C in the junction exon9-intron9 of *ERCC8* gene in patient C

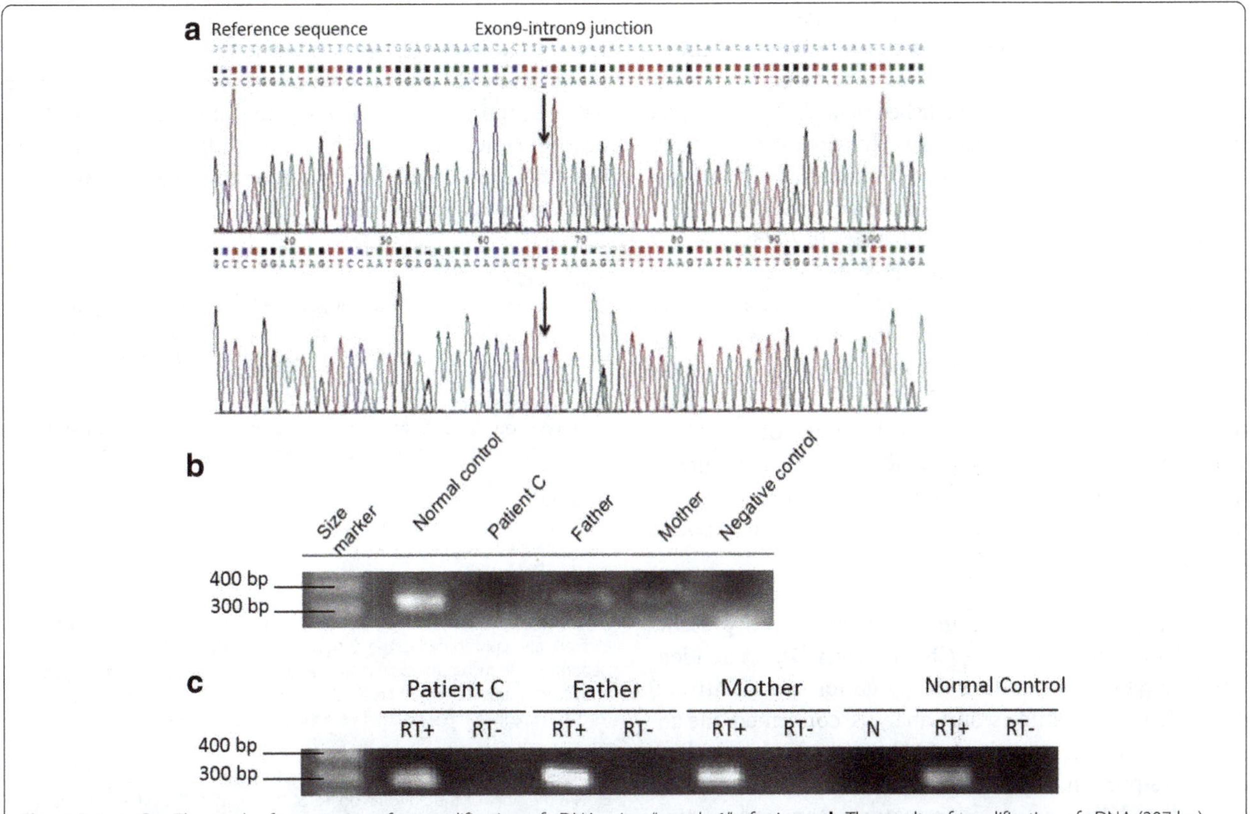

Fig. 4 Patient C: **a** The result of sequencing after amplification of cDNA using "couple 1" of primers. **b** The results of amplification of cDNA (307 bp) using "couple 2" of primers. **c** β-globin PCR: two reactions were performed for each sample RT+ and RT-, and N is the negative control of the PCR

RNA Analysis using primers named "couple 2" showed no amplification for patient C and a normal amplification for a normal control. Absence of amplification is due to the large size of the amplicon including intron 9 in the mRNA (Fig. 4b). The same PCR performed for the parents showed poor amplification (307 bp) in comparison to the normal control (Fig. 4b) thus suggesting that the parents have one normal copy of *ERCC8* gene. Altogether, these data confirm the inclusion of at least a part of intron 9 in the mRNA of *ERCC8* (r.[843 + 1G > C; 843_844ins843 + 1_843 +?]), which is predicted to cause the insertion after the Leucine (281) of three amino acids (Arg, Asp, Phe) and a premature stop codon in CSB, thus mimicking the effect of the p.L281_V282insRDF* mutation.

In conclusion, three different mutations were identified in the Lebanese CS patients included in this study: one in *ERCC6* and two in *ERCC8*.

Discussion

Three Lebanese patients originating from different geographic regions and belonging to different religious communities were included in this study. Of these patients, only one (patient C) is born to consanguineous parents.

All CS patients, including the three patients herein reported, present microcephaly, growth failure, typical face, intellectual disability and photosensitivity. In addition to these symptoms, Patient B has bilateral congenital cataracts and is affected by the severe form of the disease CSII, based on Lowry's classification [8]. Patients A and C, who showed a normal intra uterine growth and symptoms that appeared around the age of 3 months, are affected with the classical form of the disease: CSI.

In order to identify the molecular basis of CS in these patients, *ERCC8* and *ERCC6* genes were analyzed: two different mutations in *ERCC8* (p.Y322* and c.843 + 1G > C) were detected in two patients and one in *ERCC6* (p.R670W) in the third.

The nonsense mutation p.Y322* (c.966C > A) in the *ERCC8* gene was found at a homozygous state in patient A who presents with CS type I, which correlates with a published genotype-phenotype study showing that the majority of patients with *ERCC8* mutations (75% of CSA patients) are classified as CSI [10]. Since consanguinity is not reported in family A and parents of patient A were not analyzed, the occurrence of a large genomic deletion of one *ERCC8* allele cannot be completely ruled out. The identified mutation was previously linked to CS in

Christian Arabs communities and in patients from a Lebanese origin [17]. The detection of the same mutation in patient A who is born to a Christian Lebanese family is in support of the published data. Altogether, these findings might guide the diagnosis strategy for CS patients belonging to the Christian Arabs communities towards the prioritization of the sequencing of exon 10 in *ERCC8*.

The missense mutation p.R670W (c.2008C > T) in *ERCC6* was found at a homozygous state in patient B who is clinically classified as CSII. Patient B thus belongs to the 56% of patients with *ERCC6* mutations (CSB patients) who were shown to present with CSII [10]. The same mutation was found in a CS patient with Caucasian origins who presents with CSI, with an age of onset of a year and a half and without cataracts [17]. The absence of genotype-phenotype correlation, in this case, might be due to the fact that the Caucasian patient is compound heterozygous for this mutation.

The novel mutation c.843 + 1G > C in *ERCC8* was found at a homozygous state in patient C who presents with CSI as the majority of CSA patients [10]. The identified mutation affects the splicing donor site of intron 9 of *ERCC8*. RNA studies and analysis confirmed the inclusion of intron 9 in the mRNA of the patient, which alters the protein sequence. The c.843 + 1G > C variation is predicted to lead to a premature stop codon, thus mimicking a p.V282Lfs*5 mutation. Two different mutations affecting the splicing of exon 9 were already described: the first affecting the donor splice site (c.843 + 2 T > C) and the second (c.843 + 5G > C) predicted to lead to a premature stop codon mimicking a p.A240Gfs*8 mutation [17, 20]. However, in both studies RNA analysis were not performed.

All identified mutations are homozygous, which raises the possibility of the presence of a common ancestor per family, especially that couples of the non-consanguineous families A and B are from the same village and of the same religion. In fact, consanguineous marriages and same-religion marriages are widely practiced in the Middle East region and particularly in Lebanon where the population is divided into different religious groups. Jalkh et al., showed a high prevalence of rare recessive diseases in offspring of related and unrelated couples in Lebanon, which is concordant with the data presented in our study [21].

Conclusions

In conclusion, this is the first molecular study of CS in Lebanon. Here we report mutations in *ERCC8* and *ERCC6*, of which one is a novel splice site variation altering the splicing of *ERCC8*.

The finding of specific mutations in some religious communities suggests the possibility of the existence of a link between the clustering of mutations and the community to which belong a CS patient. Further molecular studies are needed to confirm this hypothesis.

Our study showed a concordance with the trend linking between the severity of CS and the molecular basis of the disease. However, a clear genotype – phenotype correlation has yet to be established in order to pave the way for a rapid molecular diagnosis.

Abbreviations

CS: Cockayne Syndrome; CSA: Cockayne Syndrome A; CSB: Cockayne Syndrome B; *ERCC6*: Excision Repair Cross-Complementation group 6; *ERCC8*: Excision Repair Cross-Complementation group 8; UVC: Ultra Violet C

Acknowledgements

We express our deepest gratitude to the CS patients and their families for their full cooperation throughout this study.

Funding

This work was not supported by any grant.

Authors' contributions

AC wrote the manuscript and prepared the Figs. AM evaluated the patients clinically and contributed to the design of this study. AC, SC and JAG: performed the molecular experiments and analyzed the data. EC wrote the molecular results. EC and CM revised and edited the final version. All authors read and approve the submitted version of the manuscript.

Competing interests

EC is a member of the editorial board of this journal. The other authors declare they have no competing interests.

Author details

[1]Medical Genetics Unit, Faculty of medicine, Saint Joseph University (USJ), Damascus street, B.P. 17-5208, Mar Mikhaël, Beirut 1104 2020, Lebanon. [2]Institut Jérôme Lejeune, Paris, France.

References

1. Cockayne EA. Dwarfism with retinal atrophy and deafness. Arch Dis Child. 1936;11(61):1–8.
2. Cockayne EA. Dwarfism with retinal atrophy and deafness. Arch Dis Child. 1946;21(105):52–4.
3. Kleijer WJ, Laugel V, Berneburg M, Nardo T, Fawcett H, Gratchev A, et al. Incidence of DNA repair deficiency disorders in western Europe: Xeroderma pigmentosum. Cockayne syndrome and trichothiodystrophy DNA Repair. 2008;7(5):744–50.
4. Nance MA, Berry SA. Cockayne syndrome: review of 140 cases. Am J Med Genet. 1992 Jan 1;42(1):68–84.
5. Gandolfi A, Horoupian D, Rapin I, DeTeresa R, Hyams V. Deafness in Cockayne's syndrome: morphological, morphometric, and quantitative study of the auditory pathway. Ann Neurol. 1984;15(2):135–43.
6. Natale V. A comprehensive description of the severity groups in Cockayne syndrome. Am J Med Genet A. 2011;155A(5):1081–95.
7. Wilson BT, Stark Z, Sutton RE, Danda S, Ekbote AV, Elsayed SM, et al. The Cockayne syndrome natural history (CoSyNH) study: clinical findings in 102 individuals and recommendations for care. Genet med off J am Coll. Med Genet. 2016;18(5):483–93.
8. Lowry RB. Early onset of Cockayne syndrome. Am J Med Genet. 1982; 13(2):209–10.
9. Sugita K, Takanashi J, Ishii M, Niimi H. Comparison of MRI white matter changes with neuropsychologic impairment in Cockayne syndrome. Pediatr Neurol. 1992;8(4):295–8.
10. Laugel V. Cockayne syndrome: the expanding clinical and mutational spectrum. Mech Ageing Dev. 2013;134(5–6):161–70.
11. de Boer J, Hoeijmakers JH. Nucleotide excision repair and human syndromes. Carcinogenesis. 2000;21(3):453–60.

12. van Hoffen A, Balajee AS, van Zeeland AA, Mullenders LHF. Nucleotide excision repair and its interplay with transcription. Toxicology. 2003; 193(1–2):79–90.
13. D'Errico M, Pascucci B, Iorio E, Van Houten B, Dogliotti E. The role of CSA and CSB protein in the oxidative stress response. Mech Ageing Dev. 2013; 134(5–6):261–9.
14. Lake RJ, Fan H-YSTRUCTURE. Function and regulation of CSB: a multi-talented gymnast. Mech Ageing Dev. 2013;134(0):202–11.
15. Henning KA, Li L, Iyer N, McDaniel LD, Reagan MS, Legerski R, et al. The Cockayne syndrome group a gene encodes a WD repeat protein that interacts with CSB protein and a subunit of RNA polymerase II TFIIH. Cell. 1995;82(4):555–64.
16. Saijo M. The role of Cockayne syndrome group a (CSA) protein in transcription-coupled nucleotide excision repair. Mech Ageing Dev. 2013; 134(5–6):196–201.
17. Laugel V, Dalloz C, Durand M, Sauvanaud F, Kristensen U, Vincent MC, et al. Mutation update for the CSB/ERCC6 and CSA/ERCC8 genes involved in Cockayne syndrome. Hum Mutat. 2010;31(2):113–26.
18. Calmels N, Botta E, Jia N, Fawcett H, Nardo T, Nakazawa Y, et al. Functional and clinical relevance of novel mutations in a large cohort of patients with Cockayne syndrome. J Med Genet. 2018;55(5):329–43.
19. Jabre P, Mezzina M, Megarbane A. Cockayne syndrome in Lebanon. Description of 3 cases and review of the literature. J Med Liban. 1999;47(2):144–7.
20. Wang X, Huang Y, Yan M, Li J, Ding C, Jin H, et al. Molecular spectrum of excision repair cross-complementation group 8 gene defects in Chinese patients with Cockayne syndrome type A. Sci Rep. 2017;7(1).
21. Jalkh N, Sahbatou M, Chouery E, Megarbane A, Leutenegger A-L, Serre J-L. Genome-wide inbreeding estimation within Lebanese communities using SNP arrays. Eur J Hum Genet. 2015 Oct;23(10):1364–9.

Preliminary study showing no association between G238A (rs361525) tumor necrosis factor-α (TNF-α) gene polymorphism and its serum level, hormonal and biochemical aspects of polycystic ovary syndrome

Fahimeh Kordestani[1], Sahar Mazloomi[1], Yousef Mortazavi[2,3], Saeideh Mazloomzadeh[4], Mojtaba Fathi[3,5*], Haleh Rahmanpour[6] and Abolfazl Nazarian[7]

Abstract

Background: Polycystic ovary syndrome (PCOS) is the main cause of female infertility. Interactions among genetic, biochemical, and immunological factors can affect the pathogenesis of PCOS. As a proinflammatory cytokine, tumor necrosis factor-α (TNF-α) plays an important role in this regard. The present study aimed to evaluate the association of the rs361525 gene single-nucleotide polymorphism (SNP) and TNF-α serum levels with the hormonal and biochemical characteristics of PCOS in Iranian individuals.

Methods: The SNP rs361525 in the *TNF-α* gene was analyzed by polymerase chain reaction–restriction fragment length polymorphism (PCR-RFLP) in a total of 111 PCOS patients and 105 healthy females. Serum levels of TNF-α, lipid and hormone profiles, and biochemical factors were measured using enzyme-linked immunosorbent assay (ELISA) and calorimetric methods, as appropriate.

Results: The TNF-α serum level was higher in women with PCOS compared with the control group ($p < 0.0001$), and it was significantly correlated with the homeostasis model assessment (HOMA) factor ($r = 0.138$, $p < 0.05$). No significant differences were found in the genotype and allelic frequencies between the two groups ($p > 0.05$). Higher levels and significant differences were found for the HOMA factor, luteinizing hormone/follicle-stimulating hormone (LH/FSH), testosterone, and body mass index (BMI) in the PCOS group compared with the control group ($p < 0.0001$). High LH/FSH ratios (odds ratio [OR] = 1.98, 95% confidence interval [CI] = 1.20–3.28, $p < 0.01$), and high HOMA factor (OR = 5.04, 95% CI = 2.82–9.01, $p < 0.001$) were significantly associated with an increased risk of PCOS.

Conclusions: Despite the lack of significant difference between rs361525 polymorphism of the *TNF-α* gene and PCOS, the serum level of TNF-α was increased in PCOS patients and positively correlated with the HOMA factor. Elevation of the LH/FSH ratio and HOMA for insulin resistance (HOMA-IR) increased the risk of PCOS. Therefore, TNF-α could indirectly contribute to PCOS progression.

Keywords: Polycystic ovary syndrome (PCOS), Tumor necrosis factor-alpha (TNF-α), Hormone profile, Polymorphism, Polymerase chain reaction–restriction fragment length polymorphism (PCR-RFLP)

* Correspondence: m_fathi@zums.ac.ir
[3]Zanjan Metabolic Disease Research Center, Valiasr Hospital, Zanjan University of Medical Science, Zanjan, Iran
[5]Department of Biochemistry, School of Medicine, Zanjan University of Medical Sciences, PO Box: 4513956111, Zanjan, Iran
Full list of author information is available at the end of the article

Background

Polycystic ovary syndrome (PCOS) is a major cause of female infertility, affecting 6–10% of women during reproductive age; moreover, it is one of the most prevalent endocrine disorders [1]. This syndrome is associated with increased risks of obesity, type 2 diabetes mellitus, hyperinsulinemia, insulin resistance, cardiovascular disease, and dyslipidemia [1, 2]. Evidence indicates an interaction among genetic, biochemical, environmental, and immunological factors in the pathogenesis of PCOS [2, 3] .Among the immunological factors, a disequilibrium of pro-/anti-inflammatory cytokines has been offered as a key contributor [2].

As a proinflammatory cytokine, tumor necrosis factor-α (TNF-α) is secreted by ovarian macrophages, granulose-luteal cells, and immune cells [4]. In addition to interference in immune and inflammation responses, differentiation, proliferation, and cell death [5], TNF-α has a role in PCOS patients with obesity [6], insulin resistance [7, 8], hyperandrogenism [9], and PCOS patients with hyperandrogenism [10]. In contrast, the production of TNF-α in granulosa cells in PCOS patients decreases aromatase gene expression. This process occurs via the inhibition of adenylyl cyclase and the cyclic adenosine monophosphate (cAMP) signaling pathway, resulting in the reduction of 17-β-estradiol production from the ovary; consequently, elevated ovarian androgen is one of the most common characteristic of PCOS patients [11, 12].

TNF-α induces serine phosphorylation in insulin receptor substrate-1 (IRS-1), resulting in the inhibition of tyrosine kinase activity in the insulin receptor and leading to insulin resistance and hyperinsulinemia [8, 10]. This process is also the cause of a low production of sex hormone–binding globulins in the liver, which increases the free androgen serum level [11]. Accordingly, a direct relationship between the serum levels of TNF-α and androgen in PCOS patients has been identified in some studies [13, 14].

TNF-α is encoded by a gene located on chromosome 6p21.3, and it has a promoter of 1100 bp in length. Nucleotide substitution in this region can affect transcription factors' binding affinity, and subsequently, the level of gene expression. Therefore, different concentrations of serum TNF-α can be produced, leading to many sorts of disorders [3, 15]. Studies in Chinese, Korean, and South Indian populations have revealed a relationship between polymorphisms in the promoter region of the *TNF-α* gene and PCOS [1, 3, 16], hyperandrogenism [9], type 2 diabetes [17], and obesity [18].

In a case-control study of a Korean population, G allele carriers of single-nucleotide polymorphism (SNP) rs361525 in the *TNF-α* gene showed an association with overweight/obesity susceptibility [18]. It has been demonstrated that a G238A *TNF-α* SNP in the promoter region could be associated with diabetes, and the 238A/308G haplotype has been shown to elevate the TNF-α serum level in an Indian population [17]. Overall, based on different studies, it has been shown that *TNF-α* SNPs can elevate the serum levels of TNF-α, and this could be associated with PCOS [13, 19, 20].

In our study, the *TNF-α* G238A SNP (rs361525) was selected based on previous studies showing positive associations between this SNP and serum levels of testosterone and insulin, obesity, and so on which all of them are the properties of PCOS. Therefore, the lack of research regarding the relationship between PCOS and SNP rs361525 in the *TNF-α* gene in the gene databases was the basis for this selection. To the best of our knowledge, this is the first study to investigate the genotyping of rs361525 polymorphism and determination of TNF-α serum levels in Iranian PCOS patients, including an evaluation of the effects of this factor on serum lipid profiles and related endocrine and biochemical factors.

Methods

Study population and sample collection

In the present study, a total of 216 women comprising 111 PCOS patients and 105 controls were recruited from the Endocrinology Clinic of Valiasr Hospital and Gynecology Clinic of Mousavi Hospital, Zanjan, Iran. According to the Rotterdam consensus, PCOS is characterized by two out of three of the following: clinical and/or biochemical signs of hyperandrogenism, polycystic ovaries on sonography, and oligo-/anovulation [21]. Patients with inflammatory diseases, acute or chronic infections, Cushing's syndrome, and androgen-secreting tumors were excluded. The selected participants had not taken any hormonal or anti-inflammatory medicine for 3–6 months before entering the study. All subjects were new cases for PCOS.

This study was approved by ethics committee (No. ZUMS.REC.1394.90) of Zanjan University of Medical Sciences of Iran. Written informed consent was received from all the subjects before blood sampling.

For sample size calculation, we conducted a pilot study including 20 PCOS patients and 20 healthy individuals. After completion of the experiment, 25% of PCOS cases and 10% of healthy control were carrier. Sample size was calculated 100 per group based on $P1 = 0.10$, $P2 = 0.25$, $\alpha = 0.05$, $\beta = 0.20$ using the formula of comparing two proportions.

Blood specimens were collected from subjects in two separate tubes on days 3–5 of their menstrual period, following the World Health Organization (WHO) guidelines. Anticoagulated whole blood samples were taken for DNA extraction and serum for biochemical parameters. Serum samples were kept at − 20 °C until determination of the biochemical parameters. Genomic DNA was extracted from white blood cells using the Bioneer genomic DNA extraction kit (Bioneer, Korea, Cat. No. K-3032). The DNA quality was determined with 260/280 optical density (OD) ratios in all samples, which were stored at − 20 °C until use.

Genotyping

Polymerase chain reaction (PCR)

In this study, polymerase chain reaction–restriction fragment length polymorphism (PCR-RFLP) was used for genotyping of G238A (rs361525) in the promoter region of the *TNF-α* gene. Semi-nested PCR was performed using two pairs of primers with the following sequences: forward, 5′-AGGAAACAGACCACAGACC-3′; reverse, 5′-ATCTGGAGGAAGCGGTAGTGG-3′. These were used in the first PCR reaction. The PCR product size was 264 bp. The primers for the second PCR reaction were 5′-GAAGACCCCCCTCGGAACC-3′ (forward) and 5′ATCTGGAGGAAGCGGTAGTGG-3′ (reverse), with a product size of 151 bp. The restriction site was designed to be situated on the forward primer in the second PCR reaction (Fig. 1).

PCR was performed according to the manufacturer's protocol (Ampliqon, Denmark; PCR Master Mix 2× containing Taq DNA polymerase, buffer, $MgCl_2$, and dNTP). DNA template (200 ng) and 10 μmol/L of each primer were added to the PCR reaction mix (25 μL). Amplification was carried out with a thermal cycler (Flex Cycler^2, Germany) under the following conditions: for the first PCR, an initial denaturation at 95 °C for 5 min, followed by 35 cycles of denaturation at 92 °C for 30 s, annealing at 62 °C for 30 s, and an extension at 72 °C for 45 s. For the second PCR, the initial denaturation took place at 95 °C for 5 min, followed by 40 cycles of denaturation at 92 °C for 30 s, annealing for 63 °C for 30 s, and an extension at 72 °C for 45 s. Finally, both PCRs were followed by a final extension at 72 °C for 5 min. The PCR products were separated using 2.5% agarose (Invitrogen, USA) gel electrophoresis and visualized with an ultraviolet transilluminator after staining with DNA safe stain (EURx, Poland).

Restriction fragment length polymorphism (RFLP)

Products of the first PCR were used as a template for the second PCR, so digestion was performed on the products of the second PCR (151 bp) using 0.5 units of *HpaII* restriction endonuclease (CinnaGen, RD1171), following the manufacturer's recommendations. Briefly, the reaction was incubated at 37 °C for 6 h. Digested fragments were separated on 3% agarose gel by electrophoresis. Fragments of 133 bp and 18 bp were considered to represent the homozygous GG genotype, while segments of 151 bp, 133 bp, and 18 bp represented the heterozygous GA genotype. A single band of a 151-bp fragment was considered a homozygous AA genotype.

Clinical and biochemical parameter measurement

Waist and hip circumferences, body weight, and height were measured in all subjects as anthropometric variables. The body mass index (BMI) and waist–hip ratio (WHR) were calculated as follows:

BMI = body mass/ (height)^2[kg/m^2],

WHR = waist circumference (cm)/hip circumference (cm).

For measurement of the serum levels of follicle-stimulating hormone (FSH; Monobind kit, USA), luteinizing hormone (LH; Monobind kit, USA), testosterone (Monobind kit, USA), estrogen (Monobind kit, USA), insulin (Monobind kit, USA), and TNF-α (eBioscience, Austria), the enzyme-linked immunosorbent assay (ELISA) method was used according to the manufacturer's recommendations. Color intensities at the final step were recorded using an ELISA reader (Stat Fax-2100 microplate reader, Awareness Technology, USA). The biochemical parameters including fasting blood glucose (Pars azmoon, Iran), triglyceride (Pars azmoon, Iran), total cholesterol (Pars azmoon, Iran), low-density lipoprotein (LDL; Pars azmoon, Iran), and high-density lipoprotein (HDL; Pars azmoon, Iran) were measured using a BT3000 autoanalyzer (Biotechnica Instruments, USA). Homeostasis model assessment (HOMA) as an insulin resistance index was computed using the following formula: HOMA = fasting glucose (mg/dl) × fasting insulin (mU/ml)/405.

Statistical analysis

All statistical analyses were performed using SPSS 22.0 (Chicago, IL, USA). Data were tested for normal distribution using the Kolmogorov–Smirnov test. Differences between two variables were measured with an independent sample *t*-test for normal distributions, while the Mann–Whitney test was used for non-normally distributed data. The qualitative or quantitative results were expressed as the frequency or mean ± SD, respectively.

The association between groups and biochemical factors were evaluated using regression logistic binary test by calculating the odds ratios (OR) at a 95% CI. Differences in serum levels of FSH, LH, testosterone, estrogen, insulin, TNF-α, fasting blood glucose, triglyceride, total cholesterol, LDL, and HDL between the groups were tested using the independent student *t*-test or Mann–Whitney test, as appropriate. The correlation between continuous variables was assessed using Pearson's correlation coefficient. A *p*-value less than 0.05 was considered significant.

Differences in the frequency of the alleles and genotypes between the PCOS patients and age-matched healthy subjects were tested using Chi-square tests. The Hardy–Weinberg equilibrium (HWE) was estimated using the Chi-square test.

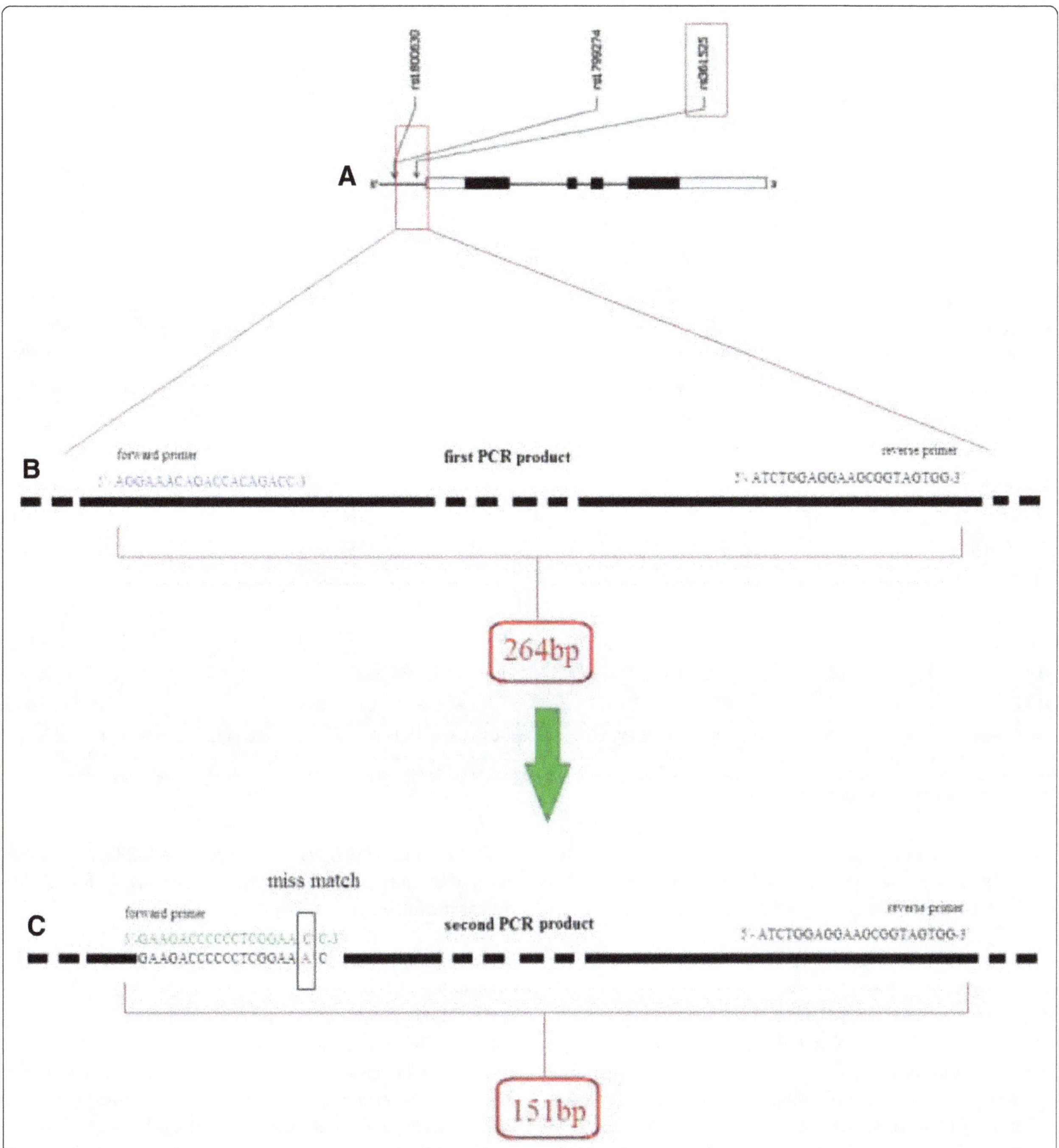

Fig. 1 **a** Gene map of a single-nucleotide polymorphism (SNP) in *TNF-α* gene on chromosome 6. Semi-nested PCR with two pairs of primers. The reverse primer was common for both PCRs. **b** Primers and PCR product size in the first PCR. **c** Primers and PCR product size in the second PCR (semi-nested). (TNF-α: tumor necrosis factor-α)

Results

This study was carried out on 216 subjects, including 111 cases and 105 controls. These groups' demographic characteristics are shown in Table 1. Although the BMI, WHR, total cholesterol, and triglycerides in the PCOS group were significantly higher than they were in the healthy controls ($p < 0.05$), the baseline LDL serum level did not reach statistical significance among the two groups ($p = 0.069$). As indicated in Table 1, LH/FSH ($p < 0.0001$) and testosterone ($p < 0.0001$) were statistically higher in PCOS patients compared with healthy individuals, but estrogen ($p < 0.05$) was statistically higher in the control group. Significant differences were found in the HOMA index between the healthy control and PCOS groups ($p < 0.0001$), and this factor was significantly higher in the obese group

Table 1 Participants' Demographic, Anthropometric, Biochemical, and Hormonal Characteristics

Characteristic	PCOS patients ($n = 111$)	Control ($n = 105$)	p-value
Age (yr)	26.49 ± 6.34	27.46 ± 7.06	0.353
Height (cm)	160.59 ± 5.75	161.31 ± 5.09	0.36
Body weight (kg)	66.74 ± 14.25	62.60 ± 11.70	0.024*
BMI (kg/m^2)	25.88 ± 5.24	24.07 ± 4.5	0.008*
WC (cm)	86.57 ± 12.78	82.14 ± 10.66	0.009*
HC (cm)	102.49 ± 12.53	100.99 ± 10.56	0.37
WHR	0.84 ± 0.1	0.81 ± 0.07	0.007*
SBP (mmHg)	105.90 ± 10.62	106.01 ± 17.38	0.55
TC (mg/dl)	187.89 ± 37.03	178.83 ± 32.79	0.05*
TG (mg/dl)	122.45 ± 24.177	105.25 ± 27.33	< 0.0001*
HDL.c (mg/dl)	41.79 ± 11.61	40.3 ± 9.96	0.377
LDL.c (mg/dl)	119.88 ± 26.86	113.67 ± 23.76	0.069
Insulin (μg/dl)	15.64 ± 5.9	8.99 ± 4.36	< 0.0001*
FBS (mg/dl)	68.83 ± 12.35	71.9 ± 14.41	0.089
HOMA-IR	2.59 ± 1.4	1.18 ± 0.99	< 0.0001*
E2 (pg/ml)	57.08 ± 38.96	73.44 ± 53.68	0.021*
Testosterone (pg/ml)	1.01 ± 0.45	0.89 ± 0.66	< 0.0001*
TNF-α (pg/ml)	2.96 ± 1.37	2.37 ± 0.94	< 0.0001*
FSH (IU/L)	7.42 ± 3.78	8.97 ± 6.62	0.005*
LH (IU/L)	10.25 ± 10.51	6.38 ± 4.44	< 0.0001*
LH/FSH	1.47 ± 1.22	0.86 ± 0.71	< 0.0001*

Data expressed as mean ± standard deviation (SD). *Abbreviations*: *BMI*, body mass index; *WC*, waist circumference; *HC*, hip circumference; *WHR*, waist hip ratio; *SBP*, systolic blood pressure; *TC*, total cholesterol; *TG*, triglyceride; *HDL*, high density lipoprotein; *LDL*, low density lipoprotein; *FBS*, fast blood sugar; *HOMA-IR*, homeostatic model assessment for insulin resistance; *E2*, estradiol; *TNF-α*, tumor necrosis factor-α; *FSH*, follicle-stimulating hormone; *LH*, luteinizing hormone, *indicates that this entity is significant statistically

than the non-obese group ($p < 0.001$). TNF-α serum levels tended to be significantly higher in women with PCOS than controls ($p < 0.0001$).

Genotype frequencies

Using specific primers, 151 bp of PCR products were obtained in semi-nested PCR (Fig. 2). Following digestion of PCR products with *HpaII* restriction enzyme, 151 bp, 133 bp, and 18 bp were obtained (Fig. 3).

The genotype frequencies of G238A SNP (rs361525) in PCOS and healthy controls were calculated by allele counting in the total population. As shown in Table 2, the GG genotype was found in 93.7% of PCOS patients and 91.4% of healthy individuals ($p > 0.05$), and the AG genotype was found in 5.4% of PCOS patients and 5.7% of controls ($p > 0.05$). The AA genotype was found in 0.9% of PCOS patients and 2.9% of controls ($p > 0.05$).

The allelic frequencies were 0.96 and 0.04 for G and A in PCOS patients and 0.94 and 0.06 in controls respectively (not significantly different; Table 2). Thus, the A allele compared with the G allele, and vice versa, was not found to be associated with an increased risk of PCOS. The HWE was tested for the G238A SNP, but no statistically significant differences were found for this assumption ($p < 0.05$).

Correlation analysis

Correlations between TNF-α, HOMA-IR, BMI, and triglycerides were investigated, and the results are shown in Table 3. The TNF-α serum levels were significantly correlated with the HOMA factor ($r = 0.138$, $p < 0.05$). There was a positive correlation between TNF-α serum levels and BMI, or triglyceride, but they were not significant ($p > 0.05$).

The HOMA factor significantly correlated with BMI ($r = 0.444$, $p < 0.001$) and triglyceride ($r = 0.263$, $p < 0.001$). BMI was positively and significantly correlated with triglyceride ($r = 0.395$, $p < 0.001$).

Risk of PCOS and values of hormonal–biochemical factors

The association between the risk of PCOS and biochemical factors was tested with ORs and 95% CIs. The variables that were significantly associated with PCOS were considered in multiple regression analysis. As indicated in Table 4, after adjustment for confounding factors, low estrogen serum levels (OR = 0.97, 95% CI = 0.96–0.99, $p < 0.001$), high

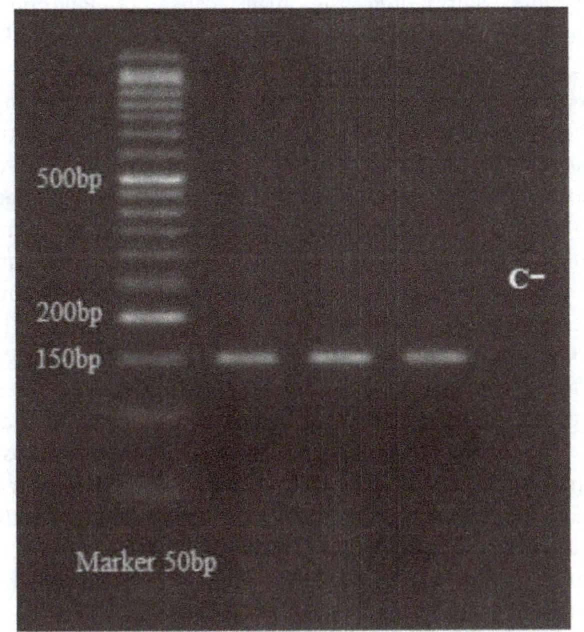

Fig. 2 Nested PCR products gel: The gel photograph represents the amplified fragments of promoter region carrying G238A in TNF-α gene by semi nested PCR. Lane 1: 50 bp ladder size marker; lanes 2, 3, and 4: 151-bp PCR product (semi-nested PCR); Lane 5: no template control

Table 2 Distribution of Genotypes and Allele Frequencies of rs361525 Polymorphism of *TNF-α* Gene in PCOS and Control Groups

TNF-α (– 238; rs361525)	Normal *n* (%)	PCOS *n* (%)	*p*-value
GG genotype	96 (91.4)	104 (93.7)	$P > 0.05$
AG genotype	6 (5.7)	6 (5.4)	$P > 0.05$
AA genotype	3 (2.9)	1 (0.9)	$P > 0.05$

n = Number of individuals; *TNF-α*; tumor necrosis factor-α, *PCOS*; polycystic ovary syndrome

LH/FSH ratios (OR = 1.98, 95% CI =1.20–3.28, $p < 0.01$), and a high HOMA factor (OR = 5.04, 95% CI = 2.82–9.01, $p < 0.001$) were significantly associated with an increased PCOS risk. Less clear trends were observed for testosterone (OR = 1.73, 95% CI = 0.84–3.59, $p < 0.05$), BMI (OR = 0.95, 95% CI = 0.85–1.06, $p < 0.05$), and triglycerides (OR = 1.01, 95% CI = 1.00–1.02, $p < 0.05$) in this test. It seems that hyperinsulinemia and the LH/FSH ratio increase the risk of PCOS by about 5 and 2 times, respectively.

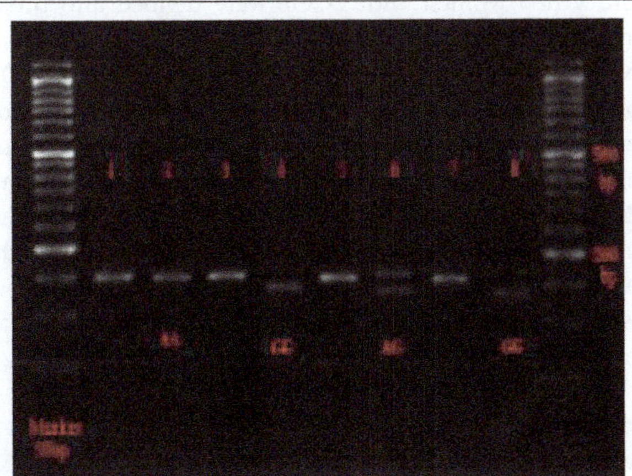

Fig. 3 The gel photograph represents the digestion fragments with *HpaII*. Before *HpaII* digestion: Lanes 1,3, 5 and 7: 151-bp fragments. After *HpaII* digestion: Lane 2: 151-bp band representing the homozygous AA genotype (mutant type); Lanes 4 and 8: 133-bp band representing the homozygous GG genotype (wild type); Lane 6: 151- and 133-bp bands representing AG genotype (heterozygous)

Discussion

As an endocrine-metabolic disorder, PCOS has been demonstrated to be associated with insulin resistance, obesity, and cardiovascular disease [22–24]. Although the etiology of PCOS is not clear, but some types of cytokines, such as TNF-α, have been suggested to be related to PCOS [25].

The relationship between the rs361525 SNP of *TNF-α* polymorphism in the promoter region and PCOS has not been investigated so far, and the associations of this gene polymorphism with some hormonal and biochemical factors are not clear. However, there are a few studies regarding the effects of this *TNF-α* gene polymorphism on obesity and prediabetic individuals. Therefore, this study aimed to evaluate the relationship between the *TNF-α* gene rs361525 polymorphism and PCOS in an Iranian population. Although we found that there were significant differences in TNF-α serum levels between the two studied groups, A allele carriers compared with G allele carriers, and vice versa, were not found to be associated with an increased risk of PCOS. Populations in this study were out of the HWE; this may have been related to the small sample size, regional sample collection, inbreeding, mutation, natural selection, gene drift, gene flow, and so on.

Yu et al. [18] found that SNP rs361525 in the *TNF-α* gene was strongly associated with obesity, and G allele carriers increased the risk of obesity in Korean population. After evaluation of prediabetes and normoglycemic

Table 3 Pearson Correlation Coefficients between TNF-α, HOMA-IR, BMI, and Triglyceride in the Study Subjects

Factors	TNF-α	HOMA-IR	BMI	TG
TNF-α	1	–	–	–
HOMA-IR	0.138*	1	–	–
BMI	0.050	0.444**	1	–
TG	0.113	0.263**	0.395**	1

Abbreviations: *TNF-α*; tumor necrosis factor-α, *HOMA-IR*; homeostasis model assessment for insulin resistance, *BMI*; body mass index, *TG*; triglyceride, *r*; correlation coefficient
*.Correlation is significant at the 0.05 level (*p*-value)
**.Correlation is significant at the 0.01 level (*p*-value)

Table 4 Multiple Logistic Regression Analysis of Participants' Characteristics

Characteristic	OR (Exp)	95% CI	*p*-value
Age (years)	0.95	0.88–1.02	0.17
BMI (kg/m^2)	0.95	0.85–1.06	0.37
E2 (pg/ml)	0.97	0.96–0.99	< 0.001*
Testosterone (pg/ml)	1.73	0.84–3.59	0.13
LH/FSH	1.98	1.20–3.28	0.007*
HOMA factor	5.04	2.82–9.01	< 0.001*
TNF-α (pg/ml)	1.26	0.82–1.93	0.29
Triglycerides (mg/dl)	1.01	1.00–1.02	0.08

Abbreviations: *CI*, confidence interval; *OR*, odds ratio; *BMI*, body mass index; *E2*, estradiol; *HOMA-IR*, homeostasis model assessment for insulin resistance; *TNF-α*, tumor necrosis factor-α, *indicates that this intity is significant statistically

individuals for SNP rs361525 in the *TNF-α* gene, Dutta et al. [17] found that AA/GA genotypes were significantly more common in individuals with prediabetes, and these individuals had higher TNF-α serum levels. Progression to diabetes in these carriers was found, and a lower reversal rate after therapeutic lifestyle interventions was observed. Prediabetes is an aspect of PCOS, so TNF-α serum level results between case and control in our study is in line with this experiment. TNF-α serum levels in our study in PCOS patients compared prediabetes were lower maybe related to different type of diseases, different measurement methods, different ethnic groups.

Recent investigations have shown that rs1799964 polymorphism in the promoter region of the *TNF-α* gene could be associated with PCOS [1, 3, 16]. In contrast, several studies have revealed a lack of direct involvement of rs1800629 polymorphism of the *TNF-α* gene in PCOS patients in South Indian, Turkish, and Australian populations [2, 3, 15]. Korhonen et al. [26] indicated that rs1799724 polymorphism of the *TNF-α* gene did not have an significant association with PCOS, but a 0.17-fold increased risk of PCOS has been demonstrated in T allele carriers of this SNP.

In this study, along with the increase in serum TNF-α values, a significant increase in fasting insulin, LH/FSH ratios, testosterone, cholesterol, triglyceride, and BMI were observed in PCOS patients compared with the controls. Wherever the serum level of TNF-α increased, elevation of the HOMA factor was observed, with a positive correlation. In contrast, an increase of the LH/FSH ratio and HOMA-IR contributed to the progression of PCOS. This result means that TNF-α could indirectly exacerbate PCOS, and it illustrates the importance of serum TNF-α levels, LH/FSH ratios, and HOMA-IR in PCOS diagnosis.

Consistent with our results, Xiong et al. [20] showed that higher serum triglyceride and TNF-α in PCOS patients represented the main cause of low-grade chronic inflammation. Moreover, Pawelczak et al. [19] demonstrated that free testosterone and serum TNF-α were elevated in adolescents with PCOS. It is interesting that the serum TNF-α values were different among various studies. As in our study, fluctuations in the TNF-α serum level in previous research may have been related to variations in hormonal regulation among different subjects, inflammation-mediated synthesis mechanisms, the length of time since PCOS diagnosis, and different hereditary and genetic backgrounds [26].

Consistent with our results, Gao et al. [27] found that TNF-α and the HOMA index were higher in women with PCOS. Accordingly, it has been demonstrated that TNF-α may induce insulin resistance by serine phosphorylation in IRS-1 [9, 11]. Samy et al. [28] reported that such inflammatory markers correlated significantly with the BMI and HOMA index in PCOS patients. It can be postulated that TNF-α and HOMA index may be prognostic and diagnostic factors [27].

There have been reports that the index of insulin sensitivity is inversely correlated with circulating TNF-α, interleukin-6 (IL-6), and C-reactive protein (CRP) levels. Therefore, inflammatory cytokines may induce insulin resistance. Because chronic inflammatory markers enhance insulin resistance and hyperandrogenism, therefore they are involved in the pathogenesis of PCOS [29, 30]. Accordingly, it has been shown that TNF-α facilitates the effects of insulin and insulin-like growth factor 1 (IGF-I) on the ovary, thereby stimulating proliferation and steroid genesis in rat theca cells in vitro [29].

Choi et al. [13] assessed the hormonal and biochemical profiles and TNF-α serum level as an inflammatory cytokine in non-obese PCOS patients in a Korean population. When women with PCOS were divided into those with and without hyperandrogenism, the TNF-α serum level was significantly higher among women with PCOS compared with controls, as well as in the hyperandrogenism group compared with those without hyperandrogenism. In another study, it was shown that serum TNF-α, free and total testosterone, androstenedione, and dehydroepiandrosterone (DHEA) were elevated in PCOS patients compared with the control group [14]. Likewise; testosterone and TNF-α levels were higher in PCOS patients compared with the control group in our study.

Conclusions

Despite a lack of significant difference in the rs361525 polymorphism of the *TNF-α* gene between PCOS and normal individuals, the serum level of TNF-α is increased in PCOS patients and positively correlates with the HOMA factor. In addition, the LH/FSH ratio and HOMA factor increase the risk of PCOS. Therefore, TNF-α could indirectly contribute to PCOS progression.

Abbreviations

BMI: Body mass index; CI: Confidence interval; CRP: C-reactive protein; E2: Estradiol; ELISA: Enzyme-linked immunosorbent assay; FSH: Follicle-stimulating hormone; HOMA-IR: Homeostasis model assessment for insulin resistance; HWE: Hardy–Weinberg equilibrium; IGF-I: Insulin-like growth factor 1; IL-6: Interleukin-6; IRS-1: Insulin receptor substrate-1; LH: luteinizing hormone; OD: Optical density ratios; OR: Odds ratio; PCOS: Polycystic ovary syndrome; PCR-RFLP: Polymerase chain reaction- restriction fragment length polymorphism; SD: Standard deviation; SNP: Single-nucleotide polymorphism; TNF-α: Tumor necrosis factor-α; WHO: World Health Organization; WHR: Waist–hip ratio

Acknowledgements

We are highly grateful to Zanjan University of Medical Sciences for the sincere support offered.

Funding

Grant number is A-12-802-9 which was all provided by Zanjan University of Medical Sciences.

Authors' contributions

MF and YM contributed to the design of the study, and undertook the experiments conduction, analysis of the genotyping for quality control, writing and editing of the manuscript. AN and SMh participated in the coordination and design of the study, performed statistical analysis, and contributed to the editing and writing of the manuscript. FK and SMi assisted in the design and data collection, carried out assays and measurements, and contributed to the editing of the manuscript. HR performed selection of the participants (made the diagnosis) and editing of the manuscript. All authors read and approved the final manuscript.

Competing interests

The author (s) declare that they have no competing interests.

Author details

[1]Department of Biochemistry, School of Medicine, Zanjan University of Medical Sciences, Zanjan, Iran. [2]Department of Medical Biotechnology and Nanotechnology, School of Medicine, Zanjan University of Medical Sciences, Zanjan, Iran. [3]Zanjan Metabolic Disease Research Center, Valiasr Hospital, Zanjan University of Medical Science, Zanjan, Iran. [4]Social Determinants of Health Research Center, Zanjan University of Medical Sciences, Zanjan, Iran. [5]Department of Biochemistry, School of Medicine, Zanjan University of Medical Sciences, PO Box: 4513956111, Zanjan, Iran. [6]Department of Obstetrics and Gynecology, School of Medicine, Zanjan University of Medical Science, Zanjan, Iran. [7]Department of Biochemistry and Nutrition, Faculty of Medicine, Zanjan University of Medical Sciences, Zanjan, Iran.

References

1. Diao X, Han T, Zhang Y, Ma J, Shi Y, Chen Z-J. Family association study between tumour necrosis factor a gene polymorphisms and polycystic ovary syndrome in Han Chinese. Reprod BioMed Online. 2014;29(5):581–7.
2. Vural P, Değirmencioğlu S, Saral NY, Akgül C. Tumor necrosis factor α (– 308), interleukin-6 (– 174) and interleukin-10 (– 1082) gene polymorphisms in polycystic ovary syndrome. Eur J Obstet Gynecol Reprod Biol. 2010;150(1):61–5.
3. Deepika M, Reddy KR, Yashwanth A, Rani VU, Latha KP, Jahan P. TNF-α haplotype association with polycystic ovary syndrome–a south Indian study. J Assist Reprod Genet. 2013;30(11):1493–503.
4. Spaczynski RZ, Arici A, Duleba AJ. Tumor necrosis factor-α stimulates proliferation of rat ovarian theca-interstitial cells. Biol Reprod. 1999;61(4):993–8.
5. MacEwan DJ. TNF receptor subtype signalling: differences and cellular consequences. Cell Signal. 2002;14(6):477–92.
6. Sathyapalan T, Atkin SL. Mediators of inflammation in polycystic ovary syndrome in relation to adiposity. Mediat Inflamm. 2010;2010:758656.
7. Hotamisligil GS, Murray DL, Choy LN, Spiegelman BM. Tumor necrosis factor alpha inhibits signaling from the insulin receptor. Proc Natl Acad Sci. 1994; 91(11):4854–8.
8. Peraldi P, Hotamisligil GS, Buurman WA, White MF, Spiegelman BM. Tumor necrosis factor (TNF)-α inhibits insulin signaling through stimulation of the p55 TNF receptor and activation of sphingomyelinase. J Biol Chem. 1996; 271(22):13018–22.
9. Escobar-Morreale HF, Calvo RM, Sancho J, San Millán JL. TNF-α and hyperandrogenism: a clinical, biochemical, and molecular genetic study. J Clin Endocrinol Metab. 2001;86(8):3761–7.
10. González F. Inflammation in polycystic ovary syndrome: underpinning of insulin resistance and ovarian dysfunction. Steroids. 2012;77(4):300–5.
11. Hara S, Takahashi T, Amita M, Matsuo K, Igarashi H, Kurachi H. Pioglitazone counteracts the tumor necrosis factor-α inhibition of follicle-stimulating hormone-induced follicular development and estradiol production in an in vitro mouse preantral follicle culture system. J ovarian res. 2013;6(1):1.
12. Adashi EY, Resnick CE, Croft CS, Payne DW. Tumor necrosis factor alpha inhibits gonadotropin hormonal action in nontransformed ovarian granulosa cells. A modulatory noncytotoxic property. J Biol Chem. 1989;264(20):11591–7.
13. Choi YS, Yang HI, Cho S, Jung JA, Jeon YE, Kim HY, et al. Serum asymmetric dimethylarginine, apelin, and tumor necrosis factor-α levels in non-obese women with polycystic ovary syndrome. Steroids. 2012;77(13):1352–8.
14. Thathapudi S, Kodati V, Raj AY, Addepally U, Katragadda A, Hasan Q. Role of TNF α in the etiopathogenesis of PCOS: a clinical, biochemical and molecular genetic study. Mol Cytogenet. 2014;7(Suppl 1):P94.
15. Milner C, Craig J, Hussey N, Norman R. No association between the–308 polymorphism in the tumour necrosis factor α (TNFα) promoter region and polycystic ovaries. Mol Hum Reprod. 1999;5(1):5–9.
16. Yun J-H, Choi J-W, Lee K-J, Shin J-S, Baek K-H. The promoter-1031 (T/C) polymorphism in tumor necrosis factor-alpha associated with polycystic ovary syndrome. Reprod Biol Endocrinol. 2011;9(1):1.
17. Dutta D, Choudhuri S, Mondal SA, Maisnam I, Reza AHH, Ghosh S, et al. Tumor necrosis factor alpha– 238G/a (rs 361525) gene polymorphism predicts progression to type-2 diabetes in an eastern Indian population with prediabetes. Diabetes Res Clin Pract. 2013;99(3):e37–41.
18. Yu G-I, Ha E, Park S-H, Park J-H, Jang H-S, Bae J-H, et al. Association of tumor necrosis factor-α (TNF-α) promoter polymorphisms with overweight/obesity in a Korean population. Inflamm Res. 2011;60(12):1099–105.
19. Pawelczak M, Rosenthal J, Milla S, Liu Y-H, Shah B. Evaluation of the pro-inflammatory cytokine tumor necrosis factor-α in adolescents with polycystic ovary syndrome. J Pediatr Adolesc Gynecol. 2014;27(6):356–9.
20. Y-l X, Liang X-y, Yang X, Li Y, L-n W. Low-grade chronic inflammation in the peripheral blood and ovaries of women with polycystic ovarian syndrome. Eur J Obstet Gynecol Reprod Biol. 2011;159(1):148–50.
21. ESHRE TR, Group A-SPCW. Revised 2003 consensus on diagnostic criteria and long-term health risks related to polycystic ovary syndrome. Fertil Steril. 2004;81(1):19–25.
22. Deepika M, Reddy KR, Rani VU, Balakrishna N, Latha KP, Jahan P. Do ACE I/D gene polymorphism serve as a predictive marker for age at onset in PCOS? J Assist Reprod Genet. 2013;30(1):125–30.
23. Elahi MM, Asotra K, Matata BM, Mastana SS. Tumor necrosis factor alpha–308 gene locus promoter polymorphism: an analysis of association with health and disease. Biochimica Biophys Acta. 2009;1792(3):163–72.
24. Saarela T, Hiltunen M, Helisalmi S, Heinonen S, Laakso M. Tumour necrosis factor-α gene haplotype is associated with pre-eclampsia. Mol Hum Reprod. 2005;11(6):437–40.
25. Rojas J, Chávez M, Olivar L, Rojas M, Morillo J, Mejías J, et al. Polycystic ovary syndrome, insulin resistance, and obesity: navigating the pathophysiologic labyrinth. Int j reprod med. 2014;2014:719050.
26. Korhonen S, Romppanen E-L, Hiltunen M, Mannermaa A, Punnonen K, Hippeläinen M, et al. Lack of association between C-850T polymorphism of the gene encoding tumor necrosis factor-α and polycystic ovary syndrome. Gynecol Endocrinol. 2002;16(4):271–4.
27. Gao H, Meng J, Xu M, Zhang S, Ghose B, Liu J, et al. Serum heat shock protein 70 concentration in relation to polycystic ovary syndrome in a non-obese Chinese population. PLoS One. 2013;8(6):e67727.
28. Samy N, Hashim M, Sayed M, Said M. Clinical significance of inflammatory markers in polycystic ovary syndrome: their relationship to insulin resistance and body mass index. Dis Markers. 2009;26(4):163–70.
29. Escobar-Morreale HF, Luque-Ramírez M, San Millán JL. The molecular-genetic basis of functional hyperandrogenism and the polycystic ovary syndrome. Endocr Rev. 2005;26(2):251–82.
30. Dasgupta S, Reddy BM. Present status of understanding on the genetic etiology of polycystic ovary syndrome. J Postgrad Med. 2008;54(2):115.

Targeted gene panel for genetic testing of south Indian children with steroid resistant nephrotic syndrome

Annes Siji[1†], K. N. Karthik[1†], Varsha Chhotusing Pardeshi[1†], P. S. Hari[1] and Anil Vasudevan[1,2*]

Abstract

Background: Steroid resistant nephrotic syndrome (SRNS) is a genetically heterogeneous disease with significant phenotypic variability. More than 53 podocyte-expressed genes are implicated in SRNS which complicates the routine use of genetic screening in the clinic. Next generation sequencing technology (NGS) allows rapid screening of multiple genes in large number of patients in a cost-effective manner.

Methods: We developed a targeted panel of 17 genes to determine relative frequency of mutations in south Indian ethnicity and feasibility of using the assay in a clinical setting. Twenty-five children with SRNS and 3 healthy individuals were screened.

Results: In this study, novel variants including 1 pathogenic variant (2 patients) and 3 likely pathogenic variants (3 patients) were identified. In addition, 2 novel variants of unknown significance (VUS) in 2 patients (8% of total patients) were also identified.

Conclusions: The results show that genetic screening in SRNS using NGS is feasible in a clinical setting. However the panel needs to be screened in a larger cohort of children with SRNS in order to assess the utility of the customised targeted panel in Indian children with SRNS. Determining the prevalence of variants in Indian population and improvising the bioinformatics-based filtering strategy for a more accurate differentiation of pathogenic variants from those that are benign among the VUS will help in improving medical and genetic counselling in SRNS.

Keywords: SRNS, NGS, Targeted re-sequencing, Indian population

Background

Steroid resistant nephrotic syndrome (SRNS) remains one of the most common intractable causes of end-stage renal disease (ESRD) in children with 50–70% of these children developing end-stage renal disease within 5–10 years of diagnosis [1]. The therapeutic options in SRNS are often inefficient, and complicated by significant toxicity adding to the associated morbidities, mortality and cost. There is now compelling evidence that children with pathogenic variations in the genes responsible for maintenance of podocyte structure and function form a distinct subgroup of Nephrotic Syndrome (NS) and these children are generally unresponsive to immunosuppression, but do not have post-transplantation recurrence [2, 3].

More than 53 single gene mutations specific to podocyte or associated with glomerular filtration barrier have been found to be associated with SRNS [4, 5]. Large multi centric studies including population of multiple ethnicities showed genetic mutations in about ~ 30% of SRNS patients with a higher proportion in infants and young children. Most mutations were observed in *NPHS2, WT1* and *NPHS1* genes [4, 6].

However, reports from India including from our center showed that the prevalence of *NPHS2* mutations is much lower in Indian population when compared with Europe and North American population [4% vs. 10.5–28%)] [7–12]. Kumar et al., reported low prevalence of *WT1* mutation in south Indian population, whereas we did not detect any mutation in *WT1* gene in 100 SRNS

* Correspondence: anil.vasudevan@sjri.res.in; anilvasu@hotmail.com
†Annes Siji, K. N. Karthik and Varsha Chhotusing Pardeshi contributed equally to this work.
[1]Division of Molecular Medicine, St. John's Research Institute, Bangalore, India
[2]Department of Pediatric Nephrology, St. John's Medical College Hospital, Bangalore, India

children [13, 14]. These data suggest that a traditional genetic testing using an algorithmic approach based on age of onset of NS to prioritize the genes to be sequenced by Sanger may not be useful [15, 16]. The above data also indicates the need for additional screening of genes implicated in SRNS in order to understand the genetic spectrum of SRNS in Indian population. Given the genetic heterogeneity and phenotypic variability in SRNS, Sanger sequencing is not a feasible approach for routine testing. Next-generation sequencing (NGS) technology is emerging as a cost-effective strategy to screen multiple genes in genetically heterogeneous diseases like SRNS [17].

The aim of our study was to check the feasibility of genetic diagnosis using targeted next-generation sequencing (NGS) approach in Indian children with SRNS. We report the initial results along with the challenges faced in the analysis and interpretation of sequencing data obtained by simultaneously sequencing 17 genes in 25 children with SRNS and 3 healthy individuals.

Methods

Subjects

The Institutional Ethics Committee approved the study and all participants were recruited after informed consent. Twenty five children with idiopathic SRNS (18 males: 7 females) as defined by standard guidelines were included [18]. Socio demographic information, clinical and treatment details were recorded in case record forms. All these children were previously analyzed by Sanger sequencing for all the exons of *NPHS2* and exon 8 and 9 of *WT1* genes [7, 14].We also included three subjects with pathogenic mutations in *NPHS2* reported previously to determine the sensitivity of the targeted-NGS method [7]. Three healthy individuals were included to check sequencing efficiency.

Methods

Blood samples (5 ml) were collected from recruited patients and genomic DNA was extracted from peripheral blood leukocytes by the phenol chloroform method [19]. Quantity of the extracted DNA was estimated using Qubit fluorometric assay (Thermofisher scientific, MA, USA).

Next-generation sequencing

For targeted next-generation sequencing, we selected a panel of 17 genes associated with SRNS based on their prevalence in clinically diagnosed SRNS patients and mutation frequency in the NS cohorts (Table 1) [4, 5, 20]. The genes selected for the panel accounted for 95–100% of the mutations in two large cohorts of SRNS one

Table 1 Genes included in the targeted NS panel to screen genetic variant in Indian SRNS cohort (to be placed after Page 5)

Gene	Accession #	Disease	Inheritance	# exons covered	# exons not covered	# primer pairs
ACTN4[a]	NM_004924	Familial and sporadic SRNS (usually adult)	AD	21	–	25
ADCK4	NM_024876	SRNS	AR	13	1	15
CD2AP	NM_012120	FSGS/SRNS	AD/AR	18	–	20
COQ2	NM_015697	Mitochondrial disease/isolated nephropathy	AR	7	–	9
COQ6	NM_182476	NS + sensorineural deafness; DMS	AR	11	1	13
INF2	NM_022489	Familial and sporadic SRNS, FSGS-associated Charcot-Marie-Tooth neuropathy	AD	22	1	37
LAMB2	NM_002292	Pierson syndrome	AR	32	1	35
LMX1B	NM_002316	Nail patella syndrome; also FSGS without extrarenal involvement	AD	8	2	13
MYO1E	NM_004998	Familial SRNS	AR	28	–	28
NEIL1	NM_024608	childhood SRNS	AR	11	–	12
NPHS1	NM_004646	CNS/SRNS	AR	29	–	32
NPHS2[a]	NM_014625	CNS, SRNS	AR	8	–	10
PDSS2	NM_020381	Leigh syndrome	AR	8	–	9
PLCe1[a]	NM_016341	CNS/SRNS	AR	32	–	42
PTPRO	NM_030667	NS	AR	25	2	28
TRPC6	NM_004621	Familial and sporadic SRNS (mainly adult)	AD	13		18
WT1	NM_024426	Sporadic SRNS (children: may be associated with abnormal genitalia); Denys-Drash and Frasier syndrome	AD	10	–	13

AD autosomal dominant, *AR* autosomal recessive, *DMS* diffuse mesangial sclerosis, *ESRD* end-stage renal disease, *FSGS* focal segmental glomerulosclerosis, *NS* nephrotic syndrome, *SDNS* steroid-dependent nephrotic syndrome, *SRNS* steroid resistant nephrotic syndrome. [a]Genes with a likely or known mutation, or a risk allele, in this cohort

of which included Indian children [6, 21]. A total of 359 primers targeting the exonic regions of the selected 17 genes (307 exons) associated with nephrotic syndrome were designed using Ion Ampliseq Designer (Life Technologies, CA, USA). The amplicon size was designed in a range from 125 to 375 bp. The panel consisted of three primer pools amplicon size ranging from 125 to 375 bp and covering 99.6% exon of the selected genes. The uncovered region was mainly repeat rich region making primer designing difficult. An Ion Torrent adapter-ligated library was prepared using the Ion AmpliSeq Library Kit 2.0 (Life Technologies, CA, USA) by following the manufacturer's protocol. Briefly, 10 ng of DNA was amplified by PCR using the premixed primer pool and Ion AmpliSeq HiFi master mix. After PCR, the amplified targets were treated with FuPa reagent to partially digest primer sequences and phosphorylate the amplicons. For adaptor ligation, amplicons from each sample were combined with a barcode adapter mix that contained Ion P1 adaptor and a unique Ion Xpress Barcode (Life Technologies, CA, USA). The unamplified libraries were purified using AMPure beads (Beckman Coulter, CA, USA) and the purified beads were amplified using Platinum PCR SuperMix High Fidelity and Library Amplification Primer Mix (Life Technologies, CA, USA). The amplified library was purified using AMPure beads. Library quantity and quality was determined using Qubit fluorometric assay and Agilent BioAnalyzer High-Sensitivity DNA kit (Agilent Technologies, CA, USA), respectively.

Template preparation, emulsion PCR, and Ion Sphere Particles (ISP) enrichment were done using the Ion PGM Template OT2 400 kit (Life Technologies, CA, USA) according to the manufacturer's instructions. Next-generation sequencing was carried out on Ion Torrent Personal Genome Machine sequencer (Life Technologies, CA, USA) using the Ion 318 and 314 Chips (Life Technologies, CA, USA) and Ion PGM Hi-Q Sequencing Kit (Life Technologies, CA, USA) according to the manufacturer's instructions.

Variant calling and annotation

The data from the both sequencing runs were analyzed using the Torrent Suite V5 analysis pipeline. Sequence reads were separated according to their barcodes. Human genome sequence (build GRCh37/hg19) was used as a reference sequence. For each individual barcode, the sequence reads were aligned to this reference sequence with a Torrent Mapping Alignment Program optimized to Ion torrent data using the default alignment algorithm and parameters. After alignment, the variants were annotated to determine their clinical significance by using a combination of frequency, structural prediction, or evidence-based data. The DNA variant regions were piled up with Torrent Variant Caller (TVC) plug-in software to identify missense, nonsense, frameshift, obligatory splice variants and short insertion/deletion (indels) across the targeted subset of the reference using germ-line parameters and low stringency settings. The output variant call format (VCF) file was then annotated using Ion Reporter Software v5.0 (Life Technologies, CA, USA) and variants were further investigated. All the variants were filtered based on their coverage (coverage> 30), variant effect (non-synonymous, frameshift, nonsense), location (to detect splice site variants) and allele frequency in public databases (ExAc (http://exac.broadinstitute.org/), and 5000 Exome (http://evs.gs.washington.edu/EVS/) < 1%). The filtered variants were visually examined using Integrative Genomics Viewer (IGV) software (http//www.broadinstitute.org/igv), to further filter out variants with possible strand-bias and variants within homopolymeric region. In silico analysis using Sorting Tolerant From Intolerant (SIFT) and Polymorphism Phenotyping v2 (Polyphen-2) tools was performed to predict the potential deleterious effect of the identified missense variants on protein function [22, 23]. Bioinformatics analysis of the strength of predicted splice site variants was performed with neural networks (NNSPLICE 0.9) [24]. The variants were classified as pathogenic, likely pathogenic, uncertain significance, likely benign, or benign according to the stringent criteria of American College of Medical Genetics and Genomics (ACMG) Standards and Guidelines and Sherloc rules [25, 26]. A scoring system developed by Karbassi et al. was used to determine the pathogenicity of VUS identified in this study [27].

The pathogenic and likely pathogenic variants were validated by Sanger sequencing using variant specific primers in patients as well as in healthy individuals ($n = 30$) (Additional file 1: Table S1).

Results

Demographic and clinical profile

The clinical details of 25 SRNS patients are presented in Table 2 with detailed phenotyping in Additional file 1: Table S2. The median age of onset of NS was 2.5 years-(0.58–16 years) with a median follow up of 2.5 years.. Majority of the patients were non-responsive to non steroidal immunosuppressant, with only 8 children demonstrating partial response to calcineurin inhibitors (Additional file 1: Table S2).

Sequencing results

Two sequencing runs, containing 25 samples (23 patients and 2 healthy individual sample; 318 chip) and 4 samples (2 patients, 1 healthy individual sample and one human standard CEPH DNA sample; 314 chip) were performed.

Table 2 Clinical characteristics of the South Indian nephrotic syndrome cohort

Characteristics		Total (*n* = 25) (%)
Sex	Male	18 (72)
	Female	7 (28)
Age at diagnosis	Median (years)	2.5 years
	Infantile (4–12 months)	3 (12)
	Early childhood (13 months –5 years)	16 (64)
	Late childhood (6–12 years)	4 (16)
	Adolescent (13–18 years)	2 (8)
Family history	Yes	7 (28)
	No	18 (72)
Parental consanguinity	Yes	5 (20)
	No	20 (80)
Steroid resistance	primary steroid resistance	24 (96)
	Secondary steroid resistance	1 (4)
Histopathology subtype	Focal segmental glomerulosclerosis (FSGS)	14 (56)
	Minimal change disease (MCD)	3 (12)
	Mesangial hypercellularity (MHC)	6(24)
	Diffuse mesangial sclerosis (DMS)	1 (4)
	Unknown	1 (4)
Renal outcome	Remission	2 (8)
	Persistent relapse	9 (36)
	Chronic Kidney disease Stage II-IV	4 (16)
	End stage renal disease	5 (20)
	Underwent renal transplant	1 (4)
	Dead	4 (16)

Total 854 M (Q20) and 172 M of Q20 data were obtained per 318 and 314 chips respectively and the coverage was comparable between runs. After filtering out polyclonal, low quality reads, and primer-dimers, the percentage of usable reads were 4.57 M and 0.788 M per 318 and 314 chips respectively (Additional file 1: Table S3). Combining the data derived from two runs, sequencing of the 17 glomerular disease gene panel generated a mean of 0.18 M reads per individual with mean read length of 214 bp. Only 10% of called bases had a quality score of <Q20; About 99% of these reads were mapped to the reference genome (hg19) and 93.9% of mapped reads were on target genes (Additional file 1: Table S4). A mean coverage of 442× was achieved for the genes across all individuals, with 93.1, 63.2 and 17% of the targets having minimum read depth of 20×, 100× and 500× respectively.

Overall, 2916 single-nucleotide variants (SNVs) and indels were identified in the 25 patients and 3 healthy individuals by Torrent Suite software V5, using default germline parameters. These variants were annotated and filtered using the Ion Reporter Software 4.4 with following parameters: inclusion of frameshift, stop loss, missense, nonsense variants and variants located in splice site with a minimum coverage of 20×. After the filtration, a total of 26 variants (23 missense, 2 nonsense and 1 splice site) were identified in 13 genes in 16 subjects (Fig. 1). Among these variants, 1 pathogenic *NPSH2* (R71X), 3 likely pathogenic [*PLCe1* (R752X), *NPHS1* (G968 V) and *NPHS2* (splice site variant, g .179521737C > T)] and 2 VUS (*LMX1B* (V145 M) and *NPHS2* (H141Y) were considered clinically relevant. The remaining 20 variants not considered further for annotation included 15 heterozygous VUS in genes with recessive inheritance, two VUS (P973T and P995L) in *MYO1E* gene in a single patient (SRNS 60) in cis and a likely benign variant (R877Q) in *INF2* gene. A homozygous VUS in *PLCe1* (G222R) gene in SRNS was also excluded from further annotation, as it was observed in a healthy individual. A variant in *ACTN4* gene (R310Q) was excluded from clinically relevant list although it was classified as likely pathogenic based on ACMG criteria. This variant has a very low allele frequency in ExAC database and also has been reported in probands of families with FSGS and individuals with sporadic FSGS [0.0074 (8/1084) controls 0.016 (3/192) sporadic FSGS] [28]. Besides, podocyte transient transfection assay indicates that the mutation inhibited the complex formation between α-actinin-4

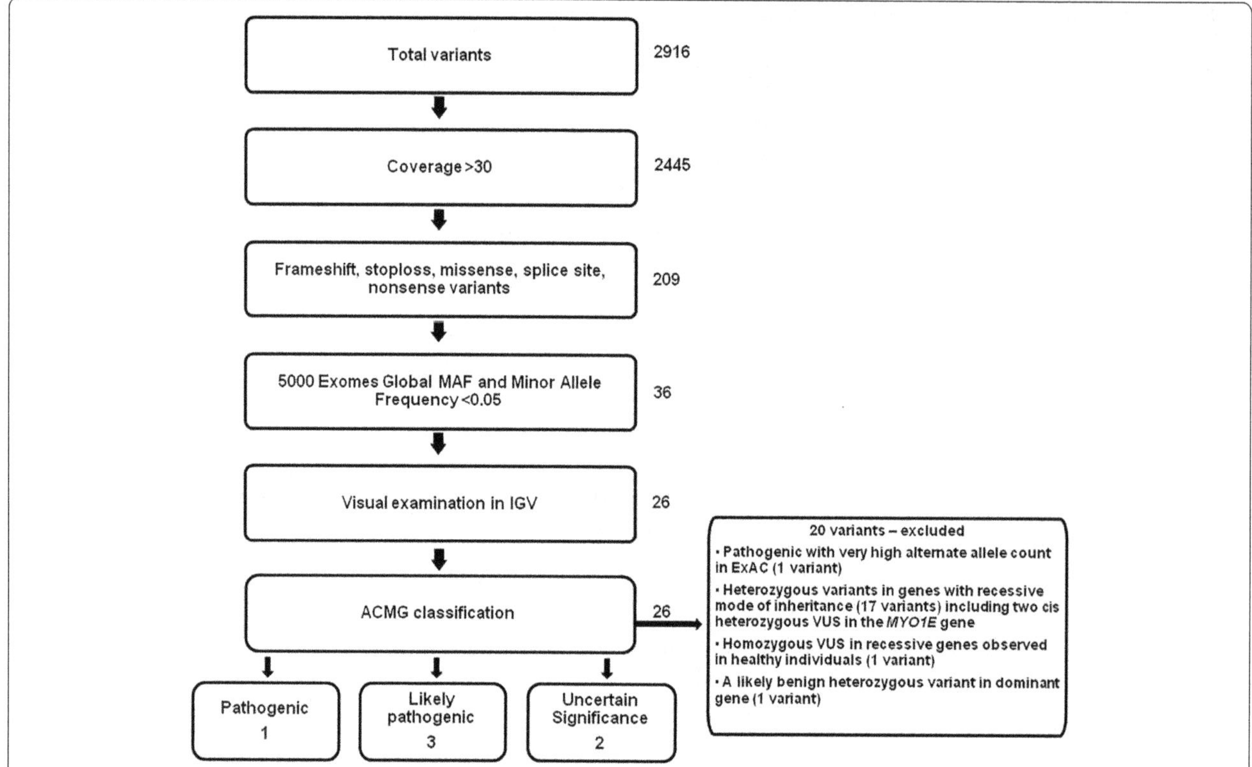

Fig. 1 Flow chart of next generation sequencing variant filtration and annotation. The variants were filtered based on their coverage (minimum coverage of 20×), variant effect, dbSNP, ExAC, 500 exomes and 1000 Genome Project databases status. The filtered variants were visually examined using Integrative Genomics Viewer (IGV) software (http//www.broadinstitute.org/igv), to further filter out variants with possible strand-bias and variants that fall into homopolymeric region. All the filtered variants were annotated as per the ACMG guidelines

and CLP36 causing the podocyte defect although the precise pathways involved were not identified [29]. However, a large number of alternate alleles (n = 1426) have been identified at the same position in general population Although global allele frequency of p.R310Q variant in *ACTN4* was < 1%, total allele count was higher (3138) in gnomAD database (Updated version of ExAC, http://gnomad.broadinstitute.org/variant/19-39207742-G-A). As per the Sherloc rule (EV0161, https://www.ncbi.nlm.nih.gov/pubmed/28492532), variants with allele count > 8, is considered as high allele count and the variant is classified as benign. Therefore although the based on the ACMG criteria p.R310Q variant in ACTN4 was classified as pathogenic, it was considered as benign based on the improved and robust variant classification guidelines of Sherloc.

The pathogenic variant in *NPSH2* (R71X) gene was observed in a pair of sibling (8%). The likely pathogenic variants in *PLCe1* (R752X), *NPHS1* (G968 V) and *NPHS2* (splice site variant, g .179521737C > T) genes were identified in one subject each (4%) (Table 3). All these variants were novel except for the *NPHS2* variant (R71X) [30]. Of the 2 variants, identified by Sangers sequencing previously, one variant (H141Y) was not present in the final filtered variants. A review of the NGS data indicated that the variant was identified by the sequencing but was filtered because of the stringent variant filtration settings (minimum read depth of 30×). A total of 18 reads was obtained for this variant H141Y in *NPHS2*. The pathogenic and likely pathogenic variants were validated using Sanger sequencing in the respective patients and 30 healthy individual samples and no false positives were identified. The pathogenicity score of two variants (*LMX1B*; heterozygous, V145 M, and*NPHS2*; homozygous, H141Y) classified as variants of uncertain significance (VUS) indicated that they could be pathogenic in nature and needed to be explored further for their causality in SRNS (Additional file 1: Table S5).

Genotype –phenotype correlation of disease-causing variants in the cohort

The clinical features and the renal histology were similar between those with pathogenic or likely pathogenic variants. Response to immunosuppressive treatments was not significantly different between those with pathogenic or likely pathogenic variants and those without an abnormal variant. The homozygous nonsense R71X variant in *NPHS2* gene was identified in two siblings (patient SRNS20 and SRNS76). The siblings presented with NS at age of 3.5 and 2.5 years respectively and both showed FSGS on biopsy. Both subjects showed no response to

Table 3 Description of pathogenic and likely pathogenic variants identified in the south Indian steroid resistant nephrotic syndrome cohort

Patient ID	Gene	Zygosity	Nucleotide Change	Amino acid Change	Mutation type	ACMG classification	Prediction							ExAC		
							dbSNP (Build 146)	SIFT	PolyPhen-2	fathmm	Mutation Taster	splicing Predictions-NNSPLICE,ASSP	Alternative allele count	Allele number	No.of h/hemi	Allele frequency
SRNS20, SRNS76	*NPHS2*	Homozygous	c.211C>T	p.R71X	Nonsense	Pathogenic	NA	NA	NA	NA	NA	NA	0	0	0	0
SRNS123	*PLCe1*	Homozygous	c.2254C>T	p.R752X	Nonsense	Likely Pathogenic	NA	NA	NA	NA	NA	NA	1	120380	0	0
SRNS83	*NPHS2*	Homozygous	g.179521737C>T		Splice site	Likely Pathogenic	NA	NA	NA	NA	NA	Y,Y	0	0	0	0
SRNS13	*NPHS1*	Homozygous	c.2903G>T	p.G968V	Missense	Likely Pathogenic	NA	NA	Y (Possibly damaging - 0.887)	Y	Disease causing	NA	0	0	0	0

calcineurin inhibitors. The elder sibling (patient SRNS20) progressed to ESRD by the age of 5 years and died at the age of 6 years with sepsis. The younger sibling currently aged 4.5 years (patient SRNS76) is in CKD stage 3 (Additional file 1: Table S2). Their parents were heterozygous for the point mutation (data not shown). A likely pathogenic homozygous nonsense variant R752X in *PLCe*1 gene was identified in SRNS123 in whom renal biopsy showed DMS (Additional file 1: Table S3). This child presented with symptoms of NS at the age of 1.5 years had renal dysfunction at the time of diagnosis and progressed to ESRD within a year of diagnosis. Similar histopathology has been reported with pathogenic variants in *PLCe1* gene [31]. A splice site likely pathogenic variant was observed in *NPHS2* gene in patient 83 who also had a homozygous VUS in the same gene (H141Y missense, both parents are heterozygous for this particular variant). This child manifested SRNS at the age of 1.2 years, showed FSGS on renal biopsy and progressed to ESRD, 2 years after diagnosis. SRNS 13 was identified to have the homozygous recessive variant (G968 V) in the *NPHS1* gene. The child was diagnosed as SRNS at age of 10 months, with the biopsy report revealing MHC and is in remission at last follow up. Patient 73 in whom a heterozygous variant in *LMX1B* (dominant inheritance) was observed manifested SRNS at the age of 3.5 years with FSGS on biopsy and progressed to ESRD within 7 years of diagnosis. The risk score suggests pathogenicity.

Discussion

Identifying the cause of SRNS is of great importance as it helps in preventing unnecessary exposure to immunosuppressants and their adverse effects, besides establishing a molecular diagnosis and clear prognosis. It also enables targeted treatment as in case of children with pathogenic variants identified in gene encoding enzymes of the co-enzyme Q 10 biosynthesis who are amenable to treatment with coenzyme Q 10 [32].

We report the results of sequencing for molecular diagnosis of SRNS in Indian children by screening 17 genes wherein pathogenic variant in *NPHS2* gene was identified in 8% patients. Siblings carrying this variant along with the patient 83 carrying the *NPHS2* variant H141Y were included as positive samples to check the sensitivity of the present assay. Both these variants were detected (although variant H141Y was initially missed due to low read depth) and no spurious pathogenic mutations were found in any of these samples indicating 85% sensitivity for the assay. Beside these known variants, 3 novel likely pathogenic variants were identified in 3 patients (12%) who were previously sequenced for *NPHS2* and *WT1* genes. These findings demonstrate the utility of NGS in a clinical setting since it allows for rapid and simultaneous screening of multiple SRNS associated genes instead of prioritizing specific genes for genetic testing.

The targeted gene panel was developed based on the results from two largest SRNS cohorts one of which included Indian children with SRNS. The targeted panel included 17 genes which explained the genetic basis in > 95% of children with SRNS in these two cohorts. Previous studies using the targeted multi-gene sequencing to analyze the exon and intron boundaries of genes associated with SRNS in various populations identified mutations in ~ 30% of the patients [4–6, 21, 33–37]. In the present study, disease causing variants were identified in 20% of the cohort which is lesser than that expected probably due to small number of patients included in the cohort.

The most common disease causing variants were identified in the *NPHS2, WT1,* and *NPHS1* genes in the Podonet cohort (1174 patients from 21 countries; included 9 Indian patients = 0.7%), in 1783 unrelated, multinational cohort and in the UK cohort [21]. This in contrast to the Chinese population, wherein the disease causing variants were also identified in *ADCK4* gene (6.67%), in addition to *NPHS1, WT1,* and *NPHS2* genes [37]. In the present study, although the cohort size was small, disease causing variants were identified in *NPHS2* (12%) *NPHS1* (4%) and *PLCe*1 (4%) genes indicating that the genes with variants causing SRNS varies significantly according to ethnic background. While this study and our previous study indicate that *NPHS2* gene is the most common mutated gene in Indian population [7], we also identified *NPHS1* and *PLCe1* genes mutations that would not have been considered in the conventional genetic testing algorithms for SRNS using Sanger sequencing.

All the pathogenic variants were identified in genes associated with recessive Mendelian inheritance, as most of the children (64%) in the cohort developed SRNS at an early age (< 5 years). The age of onset in our study correlated with risk for an as reported in other studies [6, 16]. Surprisingly, we did not find any pathogenic variants in infantile group. This is contrast to the findings from other studies where in ~ 66.3% of SRNS cases (onset between 0 and 1 year) is due to the mutation in one of following four genes: *NPHS1, NPHS2, LAMB2, or WT1* [38]. This indicates that additional SRNS associated genes needs to be screened in this group.

It is well known that SRNS exhibits significant inter and intra familial variability. The use of NGS allows to study the influence of disease causing variants in multiple genes on phenotype variability [33]. In the present cohort, two siblings with identical pathogenic variant (*NPHS2* R71X; SRNS20 and SRNS76) showed different clinical course. The variability in the clinical phenotype of patients carrying the same variant indicate an environmental factor or a possible second-site genetic modification, whereby pathogenic variants in a second gene might modulate the penetrance and/or expressivity of recessive mutations in a primary locus. Although in the siblings we did identify additional variant (R408Q) in *NPHS1*, it was heterozygous and classified as begnin by both ACMG and Karbassi et al. variant scoring system [25, 27]. In patient 83, two variants in the *NPHS2* gene (splice site, g.179521737C > T and missense H141Y) were identified. The splice site variant was classified as likely pathogenic while the H141Y variant was classified as VUS, with the risk score suggesting pathogenic nature. It is difficult to predict which variant is contributing to the disease development in this child. In order determine the role of multiple variants on the phenotypic variability we need to compare patients with different genotype combinations in the various cohorts that have been studied.

The main barrier to determine the pathogenicity of a variant is absence or limited functional testing of variants discovered to identify specific variants that results in dysfunction of the protein product. For example, a novel homozygous variant R752X, in *PLCe1* gene in patient 123 was classified as likely pathogenic instead of pathogenic. Based on the clinical findings and histopathology of patient 123, it is evident that *PLCe1* gene variant can potentially be attributed to the disease development in this patient. However, lack of data which would help with the segregation of alleles in cases and the reference population and absence of functional data, we were unable to classify this variant as pathogenic.

Secondly, guidelines to annotate the heterozygous variants in dominant genes are not very clear. For example the novel *LMX1B* gene variant V145 M with low allele frequency was predicted to be pathogenic in nature as per the Karbassi scoring algorithm but still classified as VUS as per the ACMG criteria. Further functional studies are required to confirm the effect of this variant on protein function and disease phenotype. Since little robust data is available upon which to base an assessment of causality in case of VUS, reporting, genetic and medical counseling can be complex and challenging. There is no consensus on optimal strategies to report such findings and for clinician to communicate them with parents. Counselling parents with an affected child with a VUS is even more challenging in a prenatal setting as quantifying the attributable risk of developing the disease is not possible if the variant is prospectively detected in the unborn fetus. Hence developing appropriate and effective clinical approaches to this challenge including additional training to clinicians in pretest counseling and consenting, interpretation of results and communication of results to the parents is essential. Besides, integrating the data from this study with large publically accessible phenotype and genotype data may help in ascertaining the role of novel variants in disease development and also determine the role of multiple variants on the phenotypic variability.

This study is unique as it is the first Indian study using well phenotyped SRNS cohort and NGS technology for the genetic diagnosis of SRNS. However it had few limitations such as non-random sample selection (majority of the patients were early childhood onset) and selection of small number of patients from a single center. As parental DNA was not available we could not perform segregation studies in the familial cases except in one family.

Conclusions

In conclusion, we demonstrated the feasibility of genetic screening using a targeted gene panel in a clinical setting. However, a larger number of children with SRNS needs to be screened in order to know the genetic profile as well as determine the utility of customizing targeted gene panel to screen Indian children with SRNS. Such screening will help the clinician in better prognostication and rationalizing treatment of SRNS patients. However, there were challenges in the interpretation of variants and uncertainty of some results. Improving bioinformatics-based filtering strategy will help in differentiating pathogenic variants from those that are benign among VUS.

Abbreviations

ACMG: American college of medical genetics; CEPH: Centre d'Etude du polymorphisme; CKD: Chronic kidney disease; DMS: Diffuse mesiangial sclerosis; DNA: Deoxyribo nucleic acid; ESRD: End stage renal disease; FSGS: Focal segmental glomerulosclerosis; IGV: Integrative genomics viewer; ISP: Ion sphere particles; MCD: Minimal change disease; MHC: Mesiangial hypercellularity; NGS: Next generation sequencing; NS: Nephrotic syndrome; SIFT: Sorting tolerant from intolerant; SNV: Single nucleotide variant; SRNS: Steroid resistant nephrotic syndrome; TVC: Torrent variant calling; VCF: Variant call format; VUS: Variants of unknown significance

Acknowledgements

We thank all the patients who participated in the study.

Funding

This work was supported by a grant TATA Educational Trust (Health-CKCC-20141118). We also acknowledge Indian Council of Medical Research (3/ 1/ 2/ 6-RCH; IRIS ID No.2012–26950) for their support.

Authors' contributions

AS was involved in patient recruitment, sample collection and performed the DNA extraction, involved in NGS library preparation and Sequencing. KKN involved in NGS library preparation, sequencing and NGS data analysis. HPS involved in NGS data analysis. VCP involved in NGS sample preparation, QC, sequencing, data analysis and manuscript preparation. AV originated the study, panel gene selection and design, reviewed data analysis and co-wrote the manuscript. All authors read and approved the final manuscript.

Competing interests

The authors declare that they have no competing interest.

References

1. Mekahli D, Liutkus A, Ranchin B, Yu A, Bessenay L, Girardin E, Van Damme-Lombaerts R, Palcoux J-B, Cachat F, Lavocat M-P, Bourdat-Michel G, Nobili F, Cochat P. Long-term outcome of idiopathic steroid-resistant nephrotic syndrome: a multicenter study. Pediatr Nephrol. 2009;24:1525–32.
2. Ding WY, Koziell A, McCarthy HJ, Bierzynska A, Bhagavatula MK, Dudley JA, Inward CD, Coward RJ, Tizard J, Reid C, Antignac C, Boyer O, Saleem MA. Initial steroid sensitivity in children with steroid-resistant nephrotic syndrome predicts post-transplant recurrence. J Am Soc Nephrol. 2014;25:1342–8.
3. Bierzynska A, Saleem MA. Deriving and understanding the risk of post-transplant recurrence of nephrotic syndrome in the light of current molecular and genetic advances. Pediatr Nephrol. 2017;33(11):2027-2035.
4. Bierzynska A, McCarthy HJ, Soderquest K, Sen ES, Colby E, Ding WY, Nabhan MM, Kerecuk L, Hegde S, Hughes D, Marks S, Feather S, Jones C, Webb NJA, Ognjanovic M, Christian M, Gilbert RD, Sinha MD, Lord GM, Simpson M, Koziell AB, Welsh GI, Saleem MA. Genomic and clinical profiling of a national nephrotic syndrome cohort advocates a precision medicine approach to disease management. Kidney Int. 2017;94:884–90.
5. Sen ES, Dean P, Yarram-Smith L, Bierzynska A, Woodward G, Buxton C, Dennis G, Welsh GI, Williams M, Saleem MA. Clinical genetic testing using a custom-designed steroid-resistant nephrotic syndrome gene panel: analysis and recommendations. J Med Genet. 2017;54(12):795–804. https://doi.org/10.1136/jmedgenet-2017-104811.
6. Sadowski CE, Lovric S, Ashraf S, Pabst WL, Gee HY, Kohl S, Engelmann S, Vega-Warner V, Fang H, Halbritter J, Somers MJ, Tan W, Shril S, Fessi I, Lifton RP, Bockenhauer D, El-Desoky S, Kari JA, Zenker M, Kemper MJ, Mueller D, Fathy HM, Soliman NA, Hildebrandt F. A single-gene cause in 29.5% of cases of steroid-resistant nephrotic syndrome. J Am Soc Nephrol. 2015; 26:1279–89.
7. Vasudevan A, Siji A, Raghavendra A, Sridhar TS, Phadke KD. NPHS2 mutations in Indian children with sporadic early steroid resistant nephrotic syndrome. Indian Pediatr. 2012;49(3):231–3.
8. Weber S, Gribouval O, Esquivel EL, Morinière V, Tête M-J, Legendre C, Niaudet P, Antignac C. NPHS2 mutation analysis shows genetic heterogeneityof steroid-resistant nephrotic syndrome and lowpost-transplant recurrence. Kidney Int. 2004;66:571–9.
9. Ruf RG, Lichtenberger A, Karle SM, Haas JP, Anacleto FE, Schultheiss M, Zalewski I, Imm A, Ruf E-M, Mucha B, Bagga A, Neuhaus T, Fuchshuber A, Bakkaloglu A, Hildebrandt F, Arbeitsgemeinschaft Für Pädiatrische Nephrologie Study Group. Patients with mutations in NPHS2 (podocin) do not respond to standard steroid treatment of nephrotic syndrome. J Am Soc Nephrol. 2004;15:722–32.
10. Karle SM, Uetz B, Ronner V, Glaeser L, Hildebrandt F, Fuchshuber A. Novel mutations in NPHS2 detected in both familial and sporadic steroid-resistant nephrotic syndrome. J Am Soc Nephrol. 2002;13:388–93.
11. Caridi G. Broadening the Spectrum of diseases related to Podocin mutations. J Am Soc Nephrol. 2003;14:1278–86.
12. Caridi G, Bertelli R, Carrea A, Di Duca M, Catarsi P, Artero M, Carraro M, Zennaro C, Candiano G, Musante L, Seri M, Ginevri F, Perfumo F, Ghiggeri GM. Prevalence, genetics, and clinical features of patients carrying podocin mutations in steroid-resistant nonfamilial focal segmental glomerulosclerosis. J Am Soc Nephrol. 2001;12:2742–6.
13. Kumar AS, Srilakshmi R, Karthickeyan S, Balakrishnan K, Padmaraj R, Senguttuvan P. Wilms' tumour 1 gene mutations in south Indian children with steroid-resistant nephrotic syndrome. Indian J Med Res. 2016;144:276–80.
14. Siji A, Pardeshi VC, Ravindran S, Vasudevan A, Vasudevan A. Screening of WT1 mutations in exon 8 and 9 in children with steroid resistant nephrotic syndrome from a single Centre and establishment of a rapid screening assay using high-resolution melting analysis in a clinical setting. BMC Med Genet. 2017;18:3.
15. Benoit G, Machuca E, Antignac C. Hereditary nephrotic syndrome: a systematic approach for genetic testing and a review of associated podocyte gene mutations. Pediatr Nephrol. 2010;25:1621–32.
16. Santin S, Bullich G, Tazon-Vega B, Garcia-Maset R, Gimenez I, Silva I, Ruiz P, Ballarin J, Torra R, Ars E, Ikeda M, Honda M, Iijima K. Clinical utility of genetic testing in children and adults with steroid-resistant nephrotic syndrome. Clin J Am Soc Nephrol. 2011;6:1139–48.
17. Drmanac R. The advent of personal genome sequencing. Genet Med. 2011; 13:188–90.
18. Gulati A, Bagga A, Gulati S, Mehta KP, Vijayakumar M. Management of steroid resistant nephrotic syndrome. Indian Pediatr. 2009;46:35–47.
19. Miller SA, Dykes DD, Polesky HF. A simple salting out procedure for extracting DNA from human nucleated cells. Nucleic Acids Res. 1988;16:1215.
20. Brown EJ, Pollak MR, Barua M. Genetic testing for nephrotic syndrome and FSGS in the era of next-generation sequencing. Kidney Int. 2014;85:1030–8.
21. Trautmann A, Bodria M, Ozaltin F, Gheisari A, Melk A, Azocar M, Anarat A, Caliskan S, Emma F, Gellermann J, Oh J, Baskin E, Ksiazek J, Remuzzi G, Erdogan O, Akman S, Dusek J, Davitaia T, Ozkaya O, Papachristou F, Firszt-Adamczyk A, Urasinski T, Testa S, Krmar RT, Hyla-Klekot L, Pasini A, Ozcakar ZB, Sallay P, Cakar N, Galanti M, et al. Spectrum of steroid-resistant and congenital nephrotic syndrome in children: the PodoNet registry cohort. Clin J Am Soc Nephrol. 2015;10:592–600.
22. Ng PC, Henikoff S. SIFT: predicting amino acid changes that affect protein function. Nucleic Acids Res. 2003;31:3812–4.
23. Adzhubei I, Jordan DM, Sunyaev SR. Predicting functional effect of human missense mutations using PolyPhen-2. Current protocols in human genetics. Volume chapter 7. Hoboken, NJ: John Wiley & Sons, Inc.; 2013. 7.20.1–7.20.41
24. REESE MG, EECKMAN FH, KULP D, HAUSSLER D. Improved splice site detection in genie. J Comput Biol. 1997;4:311–23.
25. Richards CS, Bale S, Bellissimo DB, Das S, Grody WW, Hegde MR, Lyon E, Ward BE. ACMG recommendations for standards for interpretation and reporting of sequence variations: revisions 2007. Genet Med. 2008;10:294–300.
26. Nykamp K, Anderson M, Powers M, Garcia J, Herrera B, Ho Y-Y, Kobayashi Y, Patil N, Thusberg J, Westbrook M, Topper S, Topper S. Sherloc: a comprehensive refinement of the ACMG–AMP variant classification criteria. Genet Med. 2017;19:1105–17.
27. Karbassi I, Maston GA, Love A, DiVincenzo C, Braastad CD, Elzinga CD, Bright AR, Previte D, Zhang K, Rowland CM, McCarthy M, Lapierre JL, Dubois F, Medeiros KA, Batish SD, Jones J, Liaquat K, Hoffman CA, Jaremko M, Wang Z, Sun W, Buller-Burckle A, Strom CM, Keiles SB, Higgins JJ. A standardized DNA variant scoring system for pathogenicity assessments in Mendelian disorders. Hum Mutat. 2016;37:127–34.
28. Weins A, Kenlan P, Herbert S, Le TC, Villegas I, Kaplan BS, Appel GB, Pollak MR. Mutational and biological analysis of alpha-actinin-4 in focal segmental glomerulosclerosis. J Am Soc Nephrol. 2005;16:3694–701.
29. Liu Z, Blattner SM, Tu Y, Tisherman R, Wang JH, Rastaldi MP, Kretzler M, Wu C. Alpha-actinin-4 and CLP36 protein deficiencies contribute to podocyte defects in multiple human glomerulopathies. J Biol Chem. 2011;286: 30795–805.
30. Sun H, Zhou W, Wang J, Yin L, Lu Y, Fu Q. A novel mutation in NPHS2 gene identified in a Chinese pedigree with autosomal recessive steroid-resistant nephrotic syndrome. Pathology. 2009;41:661–5.
31. Machuca E, Benoit G, Nevo F, Tete M-J, Gribouval O, Pawtowski A, Brandstrom P, Loirat C, Niaudet P, Gubler M-C, Antignac C. Genotype-phenotype correlations in non-Finnish congenital nephrotic syndrome. J Am Soc Nephrol. 2010;21:1209–17.
32. Heeringa SF, Chernin G, Chaki M, Zhou W, Sloan AJ, Ji Z, Xie LX, Salviati L, Hurd TW, Vega-Warner V, Killen PD, Raphael Y, Ashraf S, Ovunc B, Schoeb DS, McLaughlin HM, Airik R, Vlangos CN, Gbadegesin R, Hinkes B, Saisawat P, Trevisson E, Doimo M, Casarin A, Pertegato V, Giorgi G, Prokisch H, Rötig A, Nürnberg G, Becker C, et al. COQ6 mutations in human patients produce nephrotic syndrome with sensorineural deafness. J Clin Invest. 2011; 121:2013–24.
33. Bullich G, Trujillano D, Santín S, Ossowski S, Mendizábal S, Fraga G, Madrid Á, Ariceta G, Ballarín J, Torra R, Estivill X, Ars E. Targeted next-generation sequencing in steroid-resistant nephrotic syndrome: mutations in multiple glomerular genes may influence disease severity. Eur J Hum Genet. 2014;23: 1192 Publ online 19 Novemb 2014; | doi101038/ejhg2014252.
34. Crawford BD, Gillies CE, Robertson CC, Kretzler M, Otto E, Vega-Wagner V, Sampson MG. Evaluating Mendelian nephrotic syndrome genes for evidence for risk alleles or oligogenicity that explain heritability. Pediatr Nephrol. 2017;32:467–76.
35. McCarthy HJ, Bierzynska A, Wherlock M, Ognjanovic M, Kerecuk L, Hegde S, Feather S, Gilbert RD, Krischock L, Jones C, Sinha MD, Webb NJA, Christian M, Williams MM, Marks S, Koziell A, Welsh GI, Saleem MA. Simultaneous sequencing of 24 genes associated with steroid-resistant nephrotic syndrome. Clin J Am Soc Nephrol. 2013;8:637–48.

36. Weber S, Büscher AK, Hagmann H, Liebau MC, Heberle C, Ludwig M, Rath S, Alberer M, Beissert A, Zenker M, Hoyer PF, Konrad M, Klein H-G, Hoefele J. Dealing with the incidental finding of secondary variants by the example of SRNS patients undergoing targeted next-generation sequencing. Pediatr Nephrol. 2016;31:73–81.
37. Wang F, Zhang Y, Mao J, Yu Z, Yi Z, Yu L, Sun J, Wei X, Ding F, Zhang H, Xiao H, Yao Y, Tan W, Lovric S, Ding J, Hildebrandt F. Spectrum of mutations in Chinese children with steroid-resistant nephrotic syndrome. Pediatr Nephrol. 2017;32:1181–92.
38. Hinkes BG, Mucha B, Vlangos CN, Gbadegesin R, Liu J, Hasselbacher K, Hangan D, Ozaltin F, Zenker M, Hildebrandt F, Arbeitsgemeinschaft für Paediatrische Nephrologie Study Group. Nephrotic syndrome in the first year of life: two thirds of cases are caused by mutations in 4 genes (NPHS1, NPHS2, WT1, and LAMB2). Pediatrics. 2007;119:e907–19.

Permissions

All chapters in this book were first published in MG, by BioMed Central; hereby published with permission under the Creative Commons Attribution License or equivalent. Every chapter published in this book has been scrutinized by our experts. Their significance has been extensively debated. The topics covered herein carry significant findings which will fuel the growth of the discipline. They may even be implemented as practical applications or may be referred to as a beginning point for another development.

The contributors of this book come from diverse backgrounds, making this book a truly international effort. This book will bring forth new frontiers with its revolutionizing research information and detailed analysis of the nascent developments around the world.

We would like to thank all the contributing authors for lending their expertise to make the book truly unique. They have played a crucial role in the development of this book. Without their invaluable contributions this book wouldn't have been possible. They have made vital efforts to compile up to date information on the varied aspects of this subject to make this book a valuable addition to the collection of many professionals and students.

This book was conceptualized with the vision of imparting up-to-date information and advanced data in this field. To ensure the same, a matchless editorial board was set up. Every individual on the board went through rigorous rounds of assessment to prove their worth. After which they invested a large part of their time researching and compiling the most relevant data for our readers.

The editorial board has been involved in producing this book since its inception. They have spent rigorous hours researching and exploring the diverse topics which have resulted in the successful publishing of this book. They have passed on their knowledge of decades through this book. To expedite this challenging task, the publisher supported the team at every step. A small team of assistant editors was also appointed to further simplify the editing procedure and attain best results for the readers.

Apart from the editorial board, the designing team has also invested a significant amount of their time in understanding the subject and creating the most relevant covers. They scrutinized every image to scout for the most suitable representation of the subject and create an appropriate cover for the book.

The publishing team has been an ardent support to the editorial, designing and production team. Their endless efforts to recruit the best for this project, has resulted in the accomplishment of this book. They are a veteran in the field of academics and their pool of knowledge is as vast as their experience in printing. Their expertise and guidance has proved useful at every step. Their uncompromising quality standards have made this book an exceptional effort. Their encouragement from time to time has been an inspiration for everyone.

The publisher and the editorial board hope that this book will prove to be a valuable piece of knowledge for researchers, students, practitioners and scholars across the globe.

List of Contributors

Lingling Li, Genyan Guo, He Chen and Yuxia Zhao
Department of Radiotherapy Oncology, The Fourth Affiliated Hospital of China Medical University, No.4 Chongshan East Road, Huanggu District, Shenyang, Liaoning 110032, People's Republic of China

Haibo Zhang and Ying Yan
Department of Radiation Oncology, The General Hospital of Shenyang Military Command,
No.83 Wenhua Road, Shenhe District, Shenyang, Liaoning 110016, People's Republic of China

Baosen Zhou
Department of Epidemiology, China Medical University, Shenyang, Liaoning, China

Lu Bai
Department of Radiotherapy Oncology, The First Affiliated Hospital of China Medical University, Shenyang, Liaoning, China

José Inácio Salles
Research Division, National Institute of Traumatology and Orthopaedics, Avenida Brasil, 500, Rio de Janeiro, RJ 20940-070, Brazil
Federation International de Volleyball (FIVB) - Coach Commission, Rio de Janeiro, Brazil
Centre for Sports Exercise Medicine, Queen Mary University of London, London, UK

Lucas Rafael Lopes and Jamila Alessandra Perini
Research Division, National Institute of Traumatology and Orthopaedics, Avenida Brasil, 500, Rio de Janeiro, RJ 20940-070, Brazil
Research Laboratory of Pharmaceutical Sciences, West Zone State University, Rio de Janeiro, Brazil
Research Laboratory of Pharmaceutical Sciences, West Zone State University, Rio de Janeiro, Brazil Program of Post-graduation in Public Health and Environment, National School of Public Health, Oswald Cruz Foundation, Rio de Janeiro, Brazil

Maria Eugenia Leite Duarte, Marilena Bezerra Martins and João Antonio Matheus Guimarães
Research Division, National Institute of Traumatology and Orthopaedics, Avenida Brasil, 500, Rio de Janeiro, RJ 20940-070, Brazil

Dylan Morrissey
Centre for Sports Exercise Medicine, Queen Mary University of London, London, UK

Daniel Escorsim Machado
Research Laboratory of Pharmaceutical Sciences, West Zone State University, Rio de Janeiro, Brazil

Isabelle Schrauwen, Imen Chakchouk, Anushree Acharya and Suzanne M. Leal
Center for Statistical Genetics, Department of Molecular and Human Genetics, Baylor College of Medicine, One Baylor Plaza 700D, Houston, TX 77030, USA

Khurram Liaqat
Department of Biotechnology, Faculty of Biological Sciences, Quaid-i-Azam University, Islamabad, Pakistan

Irfanullah, Khadim Shah and Wasim Ahmad
Department of Biochemistry, Faculty of Biological Sciences, Quaid-i-Azam University, Islamabad, Pakistan

Deborah A. Nickerson
Department of Genome Sciences, University of Washington, Seattle, Washington, USA

Michael J. Bamshad
Department of Genome Sciences, University of Washington, Seattle, Washington, USA
Department of Pediatrics, University of Washington, Seattle, Washington, USA

Yu-Liang Jiang
Hebei North University, Zhangjiakou 075061, Hebei Province, China
Department of Gastroenterology, Airforce General Hospital of PLA, Beijing 100142, China

Zi-Ye Zhao
Department of Medical Genetics, Naval Medical University, Shanghai 200433, China
Department of Colorectal Surgery, Changhai Hospital, Shanghai 200433, China

Bai-Rong Li, Jing Li, Xiao-Wei Jin and Shou-Bin Ning
Department of Gastroenterology, Airforce General Hospital of PLA, Beijing 100142, China

Fu Yang and Shu-Han Sun
Department of Medical Genetics, Naval Medical University, Shanghai 200433, China

Hao Wang and En-Da Yu
Department of Colorectal Surgery, Changhai Hospital, Shanghai 200433, China

Lu Zhou, Jiaqi Wang and Tailing Wang
The 3rd Department, Plastic Surgery Hospital of the Chinese Academy of Medical Sciences, Peking Union Medical College, Badachu Road, Shijingshan District, No. 33, Beijing 100041, China

Pavithra Amritkumar
Department of Genetics, Dr. ALM Post Graduate Institute of Basic Medical Sciences, University of Madras, Taramani, Chennai 600113, India
PG and Research Department of Biotechnology, Women's Christian College, Chennai, India

Justin Margret Jeffrey, Jayasankaran Chandru, Paridhy Vanniya S, M. Kalaimathi and C. R. Srikumari Srisailapathy
Department of Genetics, Dr. ALM Post Graduate Institute of Basic Medical Sciences, University of Madras, Taramani, Chennai 600113, India

Rajagopalan Ramakrishnan
Department of ENT, SRM Medical College Hospital and Research Centre, SRM Institute of Science and Technology, Kattankulathur, India

N. P. Karthikeyen
DOAST Hearing Care Center, Anna Nagar, Chennai 600040, India

Zongfu Cao and Xu Ma
Graduate School of Peking Union Medical College, Beijing, China
National Center for Human Genetics, Beijing, China
National Human Genetic Resources Center, National Research Institute for Family Planning, Peking Union Medical College, 12 Da-hui-si, Hai Dian, Beijing 100081, China

Yihua Zhu, Bing Liu and Yi Tong
Department of Ophthalmology, the First Affiliated Hospital of Fujian Medical University, Fuzhou, Fujian, China

Lijuan Liu
Fuzhou Southeast Eye Hospital, Fuzhou, Fujian, China

Shuangqing Wu
Department of Ophthalmology, Hangzhou Red-cross hospital, Zhejiang, Hangzhou, China

Jianfu Zhuang
Xiamen Eye Center of Xiamen University, Xiamen, Fujian, China

Xiaole Chen, Yongqing Xie, Kaimei Nie and Juhua Yang
Biomedical Engineering Center, Fujian Medical University, Fuzhou, Fujian, China

Cailing Lu
Graduate School of Peking Union Medical College, Beijing, China
National Human Genetic Resources Center, National Research Institute for Family Planning, Peking Union Medical College, 12 Da-hui-si, Hai Dian, Beijing 100081, China

Yu Su
Department of Otorhinolaryngology, Head and Neck Surgery, PLA General Hospital, Beijing 100853, People's Republic of China
Department of Otorhinolaryngology, Hainan Branch of PLA General Hospital, Sanya 572000, People's Republic of China

Xue Gao
Department of Otorhinolaryngology, Head and Neck Surgery, PLA General Hospital, Beijing 100853, People's Republic of China
Department of Otolaryngology, The General Hospital of the PLA Rocket Force, 16# Xi Wai Da Jie, Beijing 100088, People's Republic of China

Sha-Sha Huang, Jian-Dong Zhao, Dong-Yang Kang, Xin Zhang and Pu Dai
Department of Otorhinolaryngology, Head and Neck Surgery, PLA General Hospital, Beijing 100853, People's Republic of China

Jing-Ning Mao
Department of Medical Imaging, PLA 307 Hospital, Beijing 100074, People's Republic of China

Bang-Qing Huang
Department of Otorhinolaryngology, Hainan Branch of PLA General Hospital, Sanya 572000, People's Republic of China

Aysha Almas
Department of Public Health Sciences, Karolinska Institutet, 171 77 Stockholm, Sweden
Department of Medicine, Aga Khan University, Karachi, Pakistan

Yvonne Forsell and Jette Möller
Department of Public Health Sciences, Karolinska Institutet, 171 77 Stockholm, Sweden

Vincent Millischer and Catharina Lavebratt
Department of Molecular Medicine and Surgery, Karolinska Institutet, Stockholm, Sweden
Neurogenetics Unit, Center for Molecular Medicine, Karolinska University Hospital, Stockholm, Sweden

Zhiping Tan, Hui Zeng, Jian Wang and Yifeng Yang
Clinical Center for Gene Diagnosis and Therapy, the Second Xiangya Hospital of Central South University, Changsha 410011, China
Department of Cardiovascular Surgery, the Second Xiangya Hospital of Central South University, Changsha 410011, China

Zhaofa Xu, Qi Tian, Xiaoyang Gao, Chuanman Zhou, Yu Zheng and Long Ma
Center for Medical Genetics, School of Life Sciences, Central South University, Changsha 410081, China

Guanghui Ling
Department of Rheumatology, the Second Xiangya Hospital of Cenral South University, Changsha, China

Bing Wang
Department of Spine Surgery, the Second Xiangya Hospital Central South University, Changsha 410011, Hunan, China

Masayuki Sakiyama
Department of Integrative Physiology and Bio-Nano Medicine, National Defense Medical College, 3-2 Namiki, Tokorozawa, Saitama 359-8513, Japan
Department of Dermatology, National Defense Medical College, Tokorozawa, Japan

Hirotaka Matsuo, Yusuke Kawamura, Makoto Kawaguchi, Toshihide Higashino, Akiyoshi Nakayama, Airi Akashi and Nariyoshi Shinomiya
Department of Integrative Physiology and Bio-Nano Medicine, National Defense Medical College, 3-2 Namiki, Tokorozawa, Saitama 359-8513, Japan

Hirofumi Nakaoka
Division of Human Genetics, Department of Integrated Genetics, National Institute of Genetics, Mishima, Japan

Jun Ueyama and Takaaki Kondo
Program in Radiological and Medical Laboratory Sciences, Pathophysiological Laboratory Sciences, Nagoya University Graduate School of Medicine, Nagoya, Japan

Kenji Wakai
Department of Preventive Medicine, Nagoya University Graduate School of Medicine, Nagoya, Japan

Yutaka Sakurai
Department of Preventive Medicine and Public Health, National Defense Medical College, Tokorozawa, Japan

Ken Yamamoto
Department of Medical Chemistry, Kurume University School of Medicine, Kurume, Japan

Hiroshi Ooyama
Ryougoku East Gate Clinic, Tokyo, Japan

Yafei Liu
Division of Biostatistics, School of Public Health, Shandong University, 44 Wenhua Xilu, Jinan 250010, Shandong, China
Shandong Provincial Qianfoshan Hospital, Shandong University, 16766 Jingshi Rd, Jinan 250014, China

Chunxia Wang
Jinan Kingmed Center for Clinical Laboratory Co, Ltd., 554 Zhengfeng Rd, Jinan 250010, Shandong, China

Yafei Chen
Linyi Centre for Adverse Drug Reaction Monitoring, Linyi 276000, Shandong, China

Zhongshang Yuan, Tao Yu, Jianhua Gu, Qinqin Xu, Lijie Ding and Fuzhong Xue
Division of Biostatistics, School of Public Health, Shandong University, 44 Wenhua Xilu, Jinan 250010, Shandong, China

Xiaotong Chi
Department of Imaging and Nuclear Medicine, Taishan Medical University, 619 Changcheng Rd, Tai'an 271016, Shandong, China

Chengqi Zhang, Wenchao Zhang and Fang Tang
Shandong Provincial Qianfoshan Hospital, Shandong University, 16766 Jingshi Rd, Jinan 250014, China

Jenni M. Rimpelä, Kimmo K. Kontula and Timo P. Hiltunen
Department of Medicine, University of Helsinki and Helsinki University Hospital, 00290 Helsinki, Finland

Ilkka H. Pörsti and Antti Tikkakoski
Faculty of Medicine and Life Sciences, University of Tampere and Tampere University Hospital, Tampere, Finland

Antti Jula
National Institute for Health and Welfare (THL), Helsinki, Finland

Terho Lehtimäki
Department of Clinical Chemistry, Fimlab Laboratories and Finnish Cardiovascular Research Center Tampere, Faculty of Medicine and Life Sciences, University of Tampere, Tampere, Finland

Teemu J. Niiranen
National Institute for Health and Welfare (THL), Helsinki, Finland
National Heart, Lung, and Blood Institute's and Boston University's Framingham Heart Study, Framingham, MA, USA

Lasse Oikarinen, Kimmo Porthan and Juha Virolainen
Division of Cardiology, Heart and Lung Center, University of Helsinki and Helsinki University Hospital, Helsinki, Finland

Mahjoubeh Jalali-Sefid-Dashti
South African Medical Research Council Bioinformatics Unit, South African National Bioinformatics Institute, University of the Western Cape, Bellville 7535, South Africa

Melissa Nel
Division of Neurology, Department of Medicine, University of Cape Town, Observatory 7925, South Africa

Jeannine M. Heckmann
E8-74, Neurology, New Groote Schuur Hospital Observatory, Cape Town 7925, South Africa

Junaid Gamieldien
South African National Bioinformatics Institute, University of the Western Cape, Private Bag X17, Bellville 7535, South Africa

Jayesh Sheth, Mehul Mistri and Frenny Sheth
Biochemical and Molecular Genetics, FRIGE's Institute of Human Genetics, FRIGE House, Satellite, Ahmedabad, Gujarat 380 015, India

Lakshmi Mahadevan
Medgenome Labs Pvt Ltd, Bangalore, India

Sanjeev Mehta
Usha Deep Hospital, Ahmedabad, Gujarat, India

Dhaval Solanki
Mantra Child Neurology and Epilepsy Clinic, Bhavnagar, Gujarat, India

Mahesh Kamate
Department of Pediatric Neurology, KLES Prabhakar Kore Hospital, Belgaum, Karnataka, India

Bin Mao, Siyu Chen, Xin Chen, Xiaojia Zhai, Tao Yang, Lulu Li, Zheng Wang, Xiuli Zhao and Xue Zhang
Department of Medical Genetics, Institute of Basic Medical Sciences, Chinese Academy of Medical Sciences and School of Basic Medicine, Peking UnionMedical College, Beijing 100005, China

Xiumei Yu
Department of Obstetrics and Gynecology, the First Affiliated Hospital of Hebei North University, Zhangjiakou 075061, China

Max Drabkin
The Morris Kahn Laboratory of Human Genetics at the National Institute of Biotechnology in the Negev, Ben-Gurion University of the Negev, Beer-Sheva, Israel

Ohad S. Birk
The Morris Kahn Laboratory of Human Genetics at the National Institute of Biotechnology in the Negev, Ben-Gurion University of the Negev, Beer-Sheva, Israel
Genetics Institute, Soroka University Medical Center, Faculty of Health Sciences, Ben-Gurion University of the Negev, Beer-Sheva, Israel

Ruth Birk
Departmentof Nutrition, Faculty of Health Sciences, Ariel University, Ariel, Israel

Cindy George and Andre P Kengne
Non-Communicable Diseases Research Unit, South African Medical Research Council, Parow Valley, PO Box 19070, Cape Town, South Africa

Yandiswa Y Yako
Department of Human Biology, Faculty of Health Sciences, Walter Sisulu University, Mthatha, South Africa

Ikechi G Okpechi
Department of Medicine, Division of Nephrology and Hypertension, University of Cape Town, Cape Town, South Africa
Kidney and Hypertension Research Unit, University of Cape Town, Cape Town, South Africa

Tandi E Matsha
Department of Biomedical Sciences, Faculty of Health and Wellness Science, Cape Peninsula University of Technology, Bellville, Cape Town, South Africa

Francois J. Kaze Folefack
Faculty of Medicine and Biomedical Sciences, University of Yaounde I, Yaounde, Cameroon. 7Medicine Unit, Yaounde University Teaching Hospital, Yaounde, Cameroon

Arati Suvatha and G. K. Chetan
Department of Human Genetics, National Institute of Mental Health and Neuro Sciences, Bangalore, Karnataka 560029, India

M. K. Sibin
Department of Biochemistry, Armed Forces Medical College, Pune 411040, India

Dhananjaya I. Bhat, K. V. L. Narasingarao and Vikas Vazhayil
Department of Neurosurgery, National Institute of Mental Health and Neuro Sciences, Bangalore 560029, India

Siying Lin, Gaurav V. Harlalka, Emma L. Baple and Andrew H. Crosby
Medical Research, RILD Wellcome Wolfson Centre (Level 4), Royal Devon and Exeter NHS Foundation Trust, Exeter, Devon EX2 5DW, UK

Abdul Hameed
Institute of Biomedical and Genetic Engineering (IBGE), Islamabad 44000, Pakistan

Hadia Moattar Reham, Muhammad Yasin, Noor Muhammad, Saadullah Khan and Shamim Saleha
Department of Biotechnology and Genetic Engineering, Kohat University of Science and Technology (KUST), Kohat, Khyber Pakhtunkhwa 26000, Pakistan

Wen-Bin He, Yue-Qiu Tan, Wen Li, Qian-Jun Zhang, Chang-Gao Zhong, Xiu- Rong Li, Liang Hu, Guang-Xiu Lu, Ge Lin and Juan Du
Institute of Reproductive and Stem Cell Engineering, School of Basic Medical Science, Central South University, Changsha, Hunan 410078, People's Republic of China
Reproductive and Genetic Hospital of CITIC-Xiangya, Changsha, Hunan 410078, People's Republic of China

Wen-Juan Xiao
Institute of Reproductive and Stem Cell Engineering, School of Basic Medical Science, Central South University, Changsha, Hunan 410078, People's Republic of China

Xiao-Meng Zhao
Reproductive and Genetic Hospital of CITIC-Xiangya, Changsha, Hunan 410078, People's Republic of China

Anas Sabarneh, Omar AbuShamma and Mohammad Abdelhafez
Biochemistry and Molecular Biology Department, Faculty of Medicine, Al-Quds University, Abu Dis-East Jerusalem, Palestine

Suheir Ereqat
Biochemistry and Molecular Biology Department, Faculty of Medicine, Al-Quds University, Abu Dis-East Jerusalem, Palestine
Al-Quds Nutrition and Health Research Institute - Faculty of Medicine, Al-Quds University-Palestine, Abu Dis-Jerusalem, Palestine

Stéphane Cauchi
CNRS, UMR8204, Lille, France
INSERM, U1019, Lille, France
Université de Lille, Lille, France Institut Pasteur de Lille, Centre d'Infection et d'Immunité de Lille, Lille, France

Murad Ibrahim
Microbiology and immunology Department-Faculty of Medicine, Al-Quds University-Palestine, Abu Dis-East Jerusalem, Palestine

Abdelmajeed Nasereddin
Al-Quds Nutrition and Health Research Institute - Faculty of Medicine, Al-Quds University-Palestine, Abu Dis-Jerusalem, Palestine

Barbara Vona
Institute of Human Genetics, Julius Maximilians University Würzburg, Würzburg, Germany
Department of Otorhinolaryngology, Head and Neck Surgery, Tübingen Hearing Research Centre (THRC), Eberhard Karls University Tübingen, 72076 Tübingen, Germany

Reza Maroofian
Genetics and Molecular Cell Sciences Research Centre, St George's, University of London, Cranmer Terrace, London SW17 0RE, UK

Emanuele Bellacchio
Genetics and Rare Diseases, Research Division, 'Bambino Gesù' Children Hospital, Rome, Italy

Maryam Najafi
Genome Research Division, Human Genetics Department, Radboud University Medical Center and Radboud Institute for Molecular Life Sciences, Geert Grooteplein Zuid 10, 6525KL, Nijmegen, The Netherlands

Kyle Thompson, Ahmad Alahmad, Langping He and Robert W. Taylor
Wellcome Centre for Mitochondrial Research, Institute of Neuroscience, Newcastle University, Newcastle upon Tyne, UK

Najmeh Ahangari
Faculty of Medicine, Mashhad University of Medical Sciences, Mashhad, Iran
Next Generation Genetic Clinic, Mashhad, Iran

Abolfazl Rad
Genome Research Division, Human Genetics Department, Radboud University Medical Center and Radboud Institute for Molecular Life Sciences, Geert Grooteplein Zuid 10, 6525KL, Nijmegen, The Netherlands
Cellular and Molecula Research Center, Sabzevar University of Medical Sciences, Sabzevar, Iran

Sima Shahrokhzadeh and Mohammad Doosti
Next Generation Genetic Clinic, Mashhad, Iran

Paulina Bahena and Thomas Haaf
Institute of Human Genetics, Julius Maximilians University Würzburg, Würzburg, Germany

Falk Mittag and Frank Traub
Department of Orthopaedic Surgery, University Hospital of Tübingen, Hoppe-Seyler-Strasse 3, 72076 Tübingen, Germany

Jebrail Movaffagh and Nafise Amiri
Targeted Drug Delivery Research Center, Pharmaceutical Technology Institute, University of Medical Sciences, Mashhad, Iran

Reza Boostani
Department of Neurology, Faculty of Medicine, Mashhad University of Medical Sciences, Mashhad, Iran

Ebrahim Shirzadeh
Sabzevar University of Medical Sciences, Sabzevar, Iran

Daria Diodato
Unit of Neuromuscular and Neurodegenerative Disorders, Laboratory of Molecular Medicine, 'Bambino Gesu' Children's Research Hospital, Rome, Italy

Miriam Schmidts
Genome Research Division, Human Genetics Department, Radboud University Medical Center and Radboud Institute for Molecular Life Sciences, Geert Grooteplein Zuid 10, 6525KL, Nijmegen, The Netherlands
Center for Pediatrics and Adolescent Medicine, University Hospital Freiburg, Faculty of Medicine, Mathildenstrasse 1, 79112 Freiburg, Germany

Ehsan Ghayoor Karimiani
Genetics and Molecular Cell Sciences Research Centre, St George's, University of London, Cranmer Terrace, London SW17 0RE, UK
Faculty of Medicine, Mashhad University of Medical Sciences, Mashhad, Iran

Vladimira Mondockova, Maria Adamkovicova, Martina Lukacova and Radoslav Omelka
Department of Botany and Genetics, Constantine the Philosopher University in Nitra, Nitra, Slovak Republic

Birgit Grosskopf
Institute of Zoology and Anthropology, Georg-August University, Göttingen, Germany

Ramona Babosova and Monika Martiniakova
Department of Zoology and Anthropology, Constantine the Philosopher University in Nitra, Nitra, Slovak Republic

Drahomir Galbavy
Private Orthopedic Ambulance, Nitra, Slovak Republic

Kirk Stephenson and David Keegan
The Catherine McAuley Centre, Mater Private Hospital, Nelson Street, Dublin 7, Ireland

Adrian Dockery, Matthew Carrigan and G. Jane Farrar
Department of Genetics, Trinity College Dublin, Dublin, Ireland

Niamh Wynne and Paul Kenna
The Research Foundation, The Royal Victoria Eye and Ear Hospital, Dublin, Ireland

Alain Chebly, Sandra Corbani, Joelle Abou Ghoch, Cybel Mehawej and Eliane Chouery
Medical Genetics Unit, Faculty of medicine, Saint Joseph University (USJ), Damascus street, Mar Mikhaël, Beirut 1104 2020, Lebanon

André Megarbane
Institut Jérôme Lejeune, Paris, France

Fahimeh Kordestani and Sahar Mazloomi
Department of Biochemistry, School of Medicine, Zanjan University of Medical Sciences, Zanjan, Iran

Yousef Mortazavi
Department of Medical Biotechnology and Nanotechnology, School of Medicine, Zanjan University of Medical Sciences, Zanjan, Iran
Zanjan Metabolic Disease Research Center, Valiasr Hospital, Zanjan University of Medical Science, Zanjan, Iran

Saeideh Mazloomzadeh
Social Determinants of Health Research Center, Zanjan University of Medical Sciences, Zanjan, Iran

Mojtaba Fathi
Zanjan Metabolic Disease Research Center, Valiasr Hospital, Zanjan University of Medical Science, Zanjan, Iran
Department of Biochemistry, School of Medicine, Zanjan University of Medical Sciences, Zanjan, Iran

Haleh Rahmanpour
Department of Obstetrics and Gynecology, School of Medicine, Zanjan University of Medical Science, Zanjan, Iran

Abolfazl Nazarian
Department of Biochemistry and Nutrition, Faculty of Medicine, Zanjan University of Medical Sciences, Zanjan, Iran

Annes Siji, K. N. Karthik, Varsha Chhotusing Pardeshi and P. S. Hari
Division of Molecular Medicine, St. John's Research Institute, Bangalore, India

Anil Vasudevan
Division of Molecular Medicine, St. John's Research Institute, Bangalore, India
Department of Pediatric Nephrology, St. John's Medical College Hospital, Bangalore, India

Index

A

Aldh1a3 Gene, 169-171, 173-176

Aneurysmal Subarachnoid Haemorrhage, 161

Ankdd1b, 88-95

Ankylosing Spondylitis, 88-89, 91, 94-95

Ankyrin Repeat, 88, 93, 95

Autosomal Dominant Polycystic Kidney Disease, 177, 188-189

Autosomal Recessive Anophthalmia and Microphthalmia, 169, 172

B

Basilar Top Aneurysm, 161, 164, 167

Bcl11b, 109, 113, 115, 117, 119

Blepharophimosis, 33-34, 38, 174

Blood Pressure Dipping, 109, 113, 115-118

Body Mass Index, 83-85, 97, 103, 105-106, 113, 118, 143, 145, 156, 159, 190, 195, 214, 222, 242, 244, 246-249

Bone Mineral Density, 212, 214, 222-224

Breast Carcinoma Amplified Sequence 3, 96-97, 100

C

Cardiovascular Disease, 81-87, 102-103, 107-108, 119, 194-195, 247

Chronic Kidney Disease, 147, 151, 156, 159-160, 253, 257

Circadian Gene, 109, 112, 114, 116

Computed Tomography, 71, 74-75, 79

Comt Val158met, 81-87

Congenital Cataract, 63-64, 69-70

D

Dfnb1, 39-40, 54-55, 58-62

Dfnx2, 71-75, 78-79

Digenic Inheritance, 17-22

Dysferlinopathy, 120, 124-125

Dyslipidemia, 102-103, 105, 190, 195, 243

E

End-stage Renal Disease, 147, 151, 156, 159-160, 177, 250-251

Epicanthus Inversus Syndrome, 33, 38

Erap2, 109, 115, 119

Ercc8 Gene, 235, 237-239

Esr1 Gene, 212-218, 220, 222, 224

Exome Sequencing, 17, 19-22, 59, 66, 88-95, 120-121, 123-125, 138, 140-142, 169-170, 181, 196-197, 202, 232, 234

F

Factor Xiii Polymorphism, 161, 163, 165, 167

Fc Receptor-like 3, 7, 15-16

Foxl2, 33-38

Fto Rs9939609, 190-191, 193-195

G

Gene Mutation, 33, 38, 45, 70-71, 80, 121, 125-126, 131, 136, 138, 141, 145, 186, 188, 211, 225, 234

Gjb2 Mutations, 17, 39, 43, 47, 49, 51, 54-56, 58, 61-62

Gjb6 Mutations, 39, 43, 49-51, 53, 55-58, 61

Gout, 96-97, 99-101

Growth Hormone Deficiency, 196-197, 199, 209-210

H

H19, 1-6

Heterozygous Mutations, 18, 176-177, 197

Hexa Gene, 126, 128-130

Hla-b*27, 88-89, 91-95

Homozygous, 1, 17-20, 40, 43, 45-46, 49-51, 53, 55-58, 70, 84, 93, 99, 120-123, 126, 128-129, 140-145, 158, 163, 174, 176, 202-205, 218, 235, 244, 247, 253-257

Hsf4, 63-70

Hyperglycemia, 102-103, 105

Hypertension, 85-86, 102-103, 105, 108-111, 117-119, 147, 150-151, 153, 156, 159-160, 162-164, 177

I

Iars2, 196-198, 200-205, 207-210

Internal Acoustic Meatus, 71, 75, 79

Intracytoplasmic Sperm Injection, 177-178, 187

Ischemic Heart Disease, 81

K

Kcnq1, 96-100, 102-108

L

Lebanon, 235-237, 240-241

Left Ventricular Hypertrophy, 109, 111, 117-118

Lung Cancer, 1-2, 4-6

M
Mc4r, 140-145, 195
Melanin Pigmentation, 23, 26, 31
Metabolic Syndrome, 102, 104, 106-109, 111, 118, 195
Myalgia, 120-121, 123
Myocardial Infarction, 81-82, 85, 87, 168

N
Nephropathy, 150-151, 160, 189, 192, 194, 251
Next-generation Sequencing, 79, 89, 131-133, 135, 137-139, 211, 233, 251-252, 258-259

O
Osteoporosis, 212-213, 215-217, 220, 222-224

P
Pcdh15, 17-20, 22
Peutz-jeghers Syndrome, 23, 31-32
Pkd Gene, 186
Polycystic Ovary Syndrome, 242-243, 247, 249
Polymerase Chain Reaction, 14, 31, 61, 74, 124, 145, 151, 157, 159, 170, 194, 222, 226, 230, 242, 244, 249
Polymerase Chain Reaction-restriction Fragment Length Polymorphism, 242
Pou3f4, 71-75, 77-80
Ptosis, 33-35, 38, 205

R
Raloxifene Therapy, 212, 216, 220-222
Regulatory Factor X3, 96-97, 100
Retinoschisin, 225-226, 229, 232-234

S
Sanger Sequencing, 19, 21, 29, 63, 90, 93, 120, 123, 129, 131-133, 136-137, 141-142, 169, 178-179, 181, 198, 202-203, 210, 226-227, 229-230, 234-235, 237, 254, 256
Sensorineural Hearing Loss, 45, 47, 61, 80, 196-197, 199-200, 207, 210
Serum Uric Acid, 96-97, 100-101
Single Nucleotide Polymorphisms, 1, 5, 14, 18, 78, 96, 100, 107, 147, 168, 210, 223
Skeletal Dysplasia, 196-197, 210
Steroid Resistant Nephrotic Syndrome, 250-251, 255, 257-258
Stk11 Gene, 23-25, 29, 31-32

T
Tay-sachs Disease, 126-127, 130
Tendinopathy, 7-16
Type 2 Diabetes Mellitus, 108, 160, 190, 194-195, 243
Type Ii Esophageal Achalasia, 196-197

U
Ushlg, 17-20

X
X-linked Deafness, 71-72, 78-80
X-linked Retinoschisis, 225, 229, 234

www.ingramcontent.com/pod-product-compliance
Lightning Source LLC
Chambersburg PA
CBHW061313190326
41458CB00011B/3792

* 9 7 8 1 6 3 2 4 1 6 5 3 7 *